Reactions, Rearrangements and Reagents

Somorendra Nath Sanyal, PhD

Bharati Bhawan
PUBLISHERS & DISTRIBUTORS

Published by

BHARATI BHAWAN (Publishers & Distributors)

www.bharatibhawan.in email: editorial@bbpd.in

4271/3 Ansari Road, Daryaganj, NEW DELHI 110 002, Phone: 23286557
A-61 B/2 Sector 63, NOIDA 201 307, Phone: 4757400
Thakurbari Road, PATNA 800 003, Phone: 2670325
10 Raja Subodh Mallick Square, KOLKATA 700 013, Phone: 22250651
No. 98 Sirsi Circle, Mysore Road, BENGALURU 560 018, Phone: 26740560

First edition 1997
Fourth edition 2003
Revised print 2006
2023 print

Reactions, Rearrangements and Reagents
Printed at B B Printers, Patna-800 009

Preface

The first edition of this book was designed as a concise collection of important organic named reactions, rearrangements and reagents, along with their mechanisms and synthetic applications. The response to the book was quite satisfactory and I received numerous suggestions from teachers all over India. A common suggestion was to increase the scope of the original book by adding a chapter on the mechanisms of organic reactions. This has been done in this edition. Apart from this a few reactions and rearrangements have been added in the second chapter.

I am thankful to my colleagues for making valuable suggestions. I hope that this edition will come up to their as well as the students' expectations.

Somorendra Nath Sanyal

Contents

❑

Chapter 1

Mechanism of Organic Reactions

Introduction

Organic reactions involve the breaking and making of covalent bonds. Chemists are not only interested in what happens in a chemical reaction but also in how it happens. With the accumulated knowledge chemists can design newer molecules.

The breaking and making of covalent bonds usually occur in several discrete steps before transformation into products. The detailed sequential description of all the steps of the transformations into product(s) is called the mechanism of a reaction.

The mechanism of a reaction is satisfactorily established if intermediates involved in all the steps can be isolated but which is unfortunately seldom possible. There are a number of guiding principles which help us to predict the different steps of the reaction. By judiciously considering these guiding principles and the stereochemical aspects, the different steps of the reaction can not only be explained but also the products under different conditions can be predicted.

Complete information regarding all the steps is seldom obtained. However, a good deal of data can be gathered from the following: (a) study of the kinetics of the reaction, (b) isolation of the intermediates if isolable, (c) study of the reaction in the presence of other similar substrates, (d) study of the isotopically labelled atoms in the reactants, (e) trapping of free radicals, (f) crossover experiments, (g) stereochemical aspects, etc.

Study of reaction is an important part of theoretical organic chemistry. The knowledge enables us to predict the products from nearly similar substrates and what is more important is to discern a pattern in apparently diverse reactions. The conditions of the reactions may be altered to afford better yield of one or the other product(s) and sometimes a completely different product. The revolutionary advances in organic chemistry, like the wildfire in the wood, have been possible through the knowledge of the pattern of organic reactions. They have thus provided chemists invaluable guidance in synthesizing a large variety of essential organic compounds such as drugs, vitamins, hormones, natural products, cosmetic aids, synthetic fibres, insecticides, fuels, explosives, etc.

As we are interested in carbon compounds, we shall first study as to how the carbon atoms form bonds with each other and with other atoms.

TYPES OF CHEMICAL BONDS

Organic compounds differ from inorganic compounds in the types of bond formation in the two classes of compounds. A brief study of the electronic theory of bond formation will be helpful.

Modern physics states that atoms consist of central positively charged nucleus surrounded by a number of electrons. These electrons arrange themselves in different shells. The shells have different energies and different maximum capacities for electrons—two in the first shell (K shell), eight in the second shell (L shell), eight or eighteen in the third shell (M shell), etc.

It is known that elements with completely filled shell are inert (stable), e.g., He (2 electrons in K shell), Ne (8 electrons in L shell), Ar (18 electrons in M shell). He, Ne, Ar, etc., are, therefore, called inert (noble) gases.

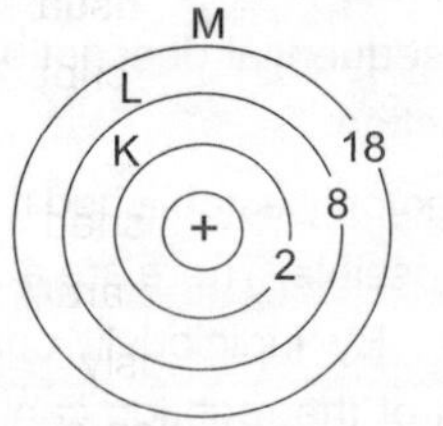

W Kossel and G N Lewis in 1916 suggested that all elements try to achieve the inert gas configurations by changing the number of electrons in their outermost shells. This tendency results in the union of elements or bonds.

Electrovalent or ionic bond

Two elements can achieve stable configuration (i.e., inert gas configuration) by transfer of electrons from one element to the other. This results in the formation of oppositely charged atoms (ions) which are bound together by electrostatic attraction. This type of bond is called electrovalent or ionic bond.

Thus,

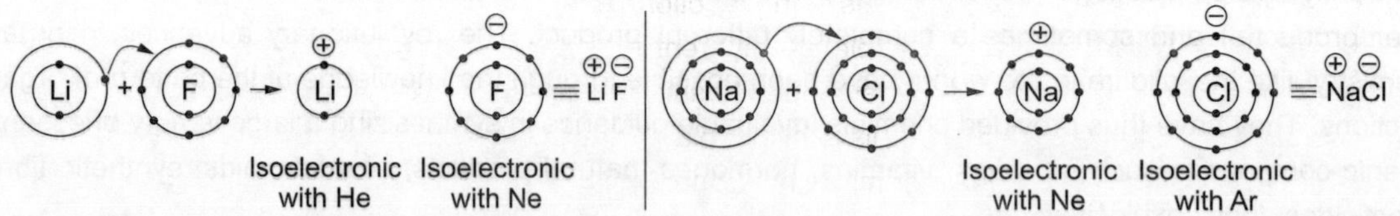

The elements in the beginning of a row in the periodic table can easily acquire their nearest inert gas configuration by losing electrons and those at the end of a row by gaining electrons. The former elements are called electropositive and the latter elements are called electronegative. Thus, ionic bonds are formed between electropositive and electronegative elements.

Covalent bond

Since it is increasingly difficult to extract a number of electrons from an element due to increasing development of positive charge on it, in general the charge on a simple cation is limited to +3 even when the inert gas configuration is not attained. The reverse is similarly true.

Hence, the elements in the middle of a row can neither gain nor lose electrons to achieve inert gas configurations. Also, the transfer of electrons between two electronegative or between two electropositive elements cannot confer inert gas configurations to both the elements.

In such cases, both the elements can acquire the desired inert gas configurations by mutually sharing pairs of electrons—each element contributing an electron to the shared pair. The shared electron pair then belongs to both the elements. The shared electron pair binds the two nuclei, and the bond so formed is called a covalent bond.

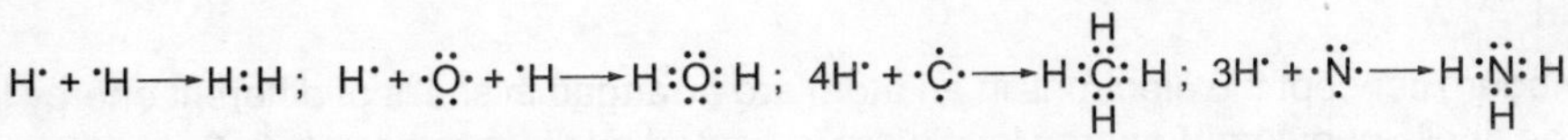

The covalency of an element is the number of covalent bonds it can form. Thus, the covalencies of hydrogen, oxygen, nitrogen and carbon are 1, 2, 3 and 4 respectively. To satisfy the covalency requirement, elements often have to form multiple bonds (double or triple) by sharing more than one pair of electrons. Thus,

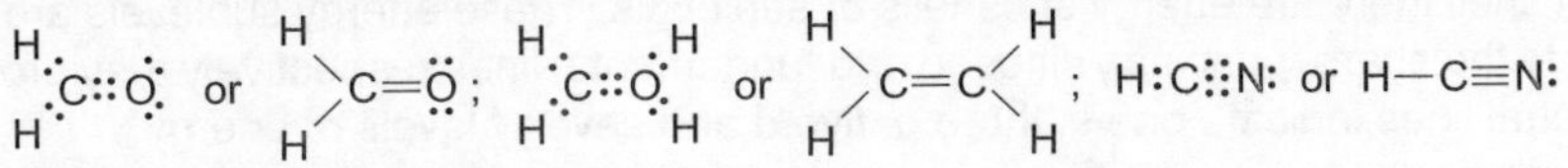

When pair(s) of electrons remains unbonded, as in oxygen and nitrogen in the above compounds, the pair(s) is called lone pair or non-bonding electrons.

The covalent compounds, unlike ionic compounds, are uncharged. However, when the bond is between two dissimilar elements, the shared pair shifts slightly towards the more electronegative of the two elements. The covalent bond, in such case, is slightly polar which is indicated by $+\delta$ and $-\delta$ signs.

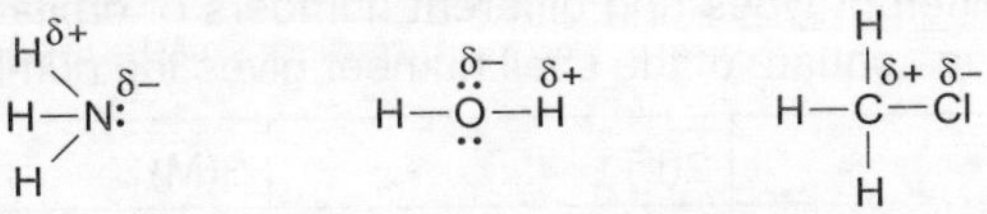

The N—H, O—H and C—Cl bonds are called polar covalent bonds.

Coordinate covalent bond, dipolar bond or semipolar bond

When one element has two electrons short in its outermost shell and the other has a complete outer shell with one or more spare pairs of electrons (lone pair) then the lone pair may be shared by both the elements. Such a bond is called coordinate, dative or polar bond. Thus,

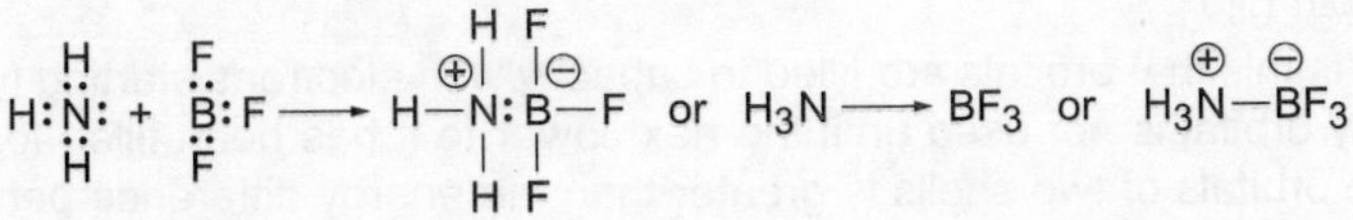

This type of bond is also called a semipolar bond, since a species with completely vacant shell (e.g., a proton) may complete its shell by gaining a share on the pair of electrons of the donor element, which is then positively charged.

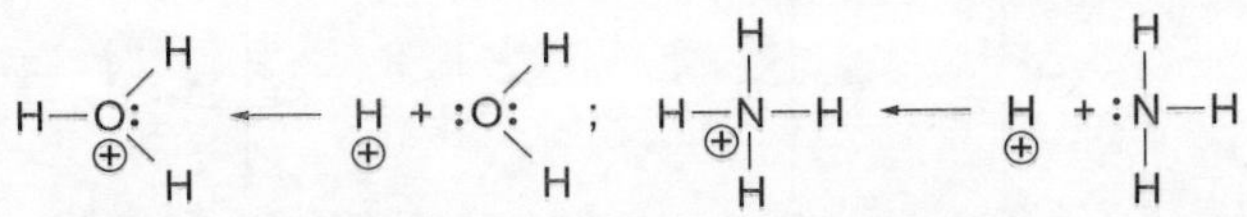

This is essentially a covalent bond, only the resulting species is charged. It is different from ionic bond as also from covalent bond since electrons are neither completely transferred nor mutually shared.

ORBITAL THEORY

The operation of electrostatic force is understandable in ionic bonds but the concept fails to account for the force of attraction between elements bonded by covalent bonds. Thus, the description given in the preceding section does not account for the strength of the covalent bonds and also the shapes of the molecules formed by covalent bonds. To understand this, it is necessary to study the molecular orbital (MO) description of the covalent bonds.

Atomic orbital

According to modern concept the electrons in an atom are arranged in shells of different energy levels around the nucleus. The shells of different energy levels are indicated by the numbers 1, 2, 3, ..., or by the letters K, L, M, ..., starting from the nucleus. The energy of the shells increases in the order: $1 \rightarrow 2 \rightarrow 3 \rightarrow \dots$. Each shell can accommodate a definite number of electrons which is twice the square of the shell number, e.g., the first shell has $2 \times 1^2 = 2$, second shell has $2 \times 2^2 = 8$, third shell has $2 \times 3^2 = 18$ electrons, etc.

Within each shell there are energy subshells or sublevels. These energy sublevels are designated s, p, d and f according to the sharp, principal, diffused and fundamental lines respectively they produce in an X-ray spectra. The spectral lines indicate one s, three p, five d and seven f levels of energy.

Electrons of different energy levels are present in discrete volumes of different shapes, sizes and orientations in the sublevels around the nucleus. The discrete volume in space around the nucleus, where the probability of finding the electron of a particular energy level is greatest, is called an atomic orbital. The concept of orbital emerged from Heisenberg uncertainty principle and wave nature of electrons—an electron does not move in an orbit around the nucleus, it is in a diffused state. Thus, orbitals can be visualised as diffused charge clouds of different shapes, size and orientations within the subshells around the nucleus.

Different shells contain different types and different numbers of orbitals. The shell number gives the number of types of orbitals and the square of the shell number gives the number of orbitals.

Shell no.:	1(K)	2(L)	3(M)	4(N)
Types of orbitals	s	s, p	s, p, d	s, p, d, f
No. of orbitals	$1^2 = 1$	$2^2 = 1 + 3$	$3^2 = 1 + 3 + 5$	$4^2 = 1 + 3 + 5 + 7$

Orbitals of different shells are differentiated by prefixing the shell number: the s orbital of first shell is denoted as 1s orbital, the s and p orbitals of the second shell as 2s and 2p orbitals and so on. The energy of the orbitals increases in the order: $1s \rightarrow 2s \rightarrow 2p \dots$.

According to Pauli exclusion principle, any one orbital can accommodate up to a maximum of two electrons with paired spin ($\uparrow\downarrow$)*.

The general rule is this that orbitals are filled to capacity with electrons starting from the lowest-energy orbital. A higher-energy orbital is not used until the next lower to it has been filled to capacity. The energy difference between the orbitals of two shells is greater than the energy difference between the two types of

* A spinning electron creates a small magnetic field, i.e., it behaves as a tiny magnet. Two oppositely spinning electrons are like two small magnets with their opposite poles in the same direction. This causes attraction between them.

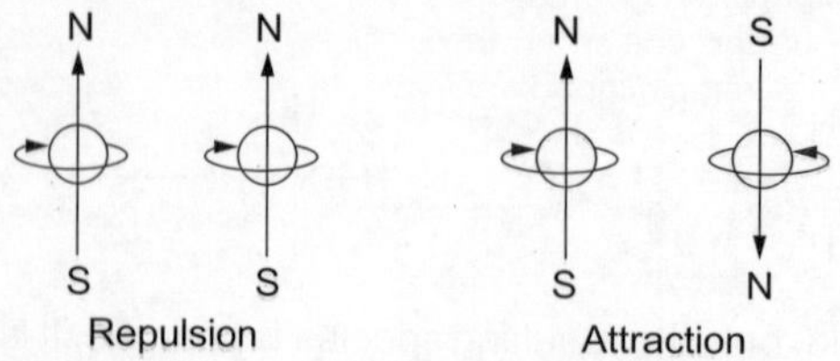

It should, however, be remembered that the spin of an electron is some kind of property and is not actually spin.

orbitals in the same shell. Thus, the energy difference between 1s and 2s orbitals is more than that between 2s and 2p orbitals. The relative energy levels, the maximum capacities of electrons with paired spin of a few shells are given in Table below.

Shell energy	Orbital capacities	No. of electrons
3	↑↓ (3s) ↑↓ ↑↓ ↑↓ (3p) ↑↓ ↑↓ ↑↓ ↑↓ ↑↓ (3d)	18
2	↑↓ (2s) ↑↓ ↑↓ ↑↓ (2p)	8
1	↑↓ (1s)	2

Table

In orbitals of equivalent energies (degenerate), the most stable arrangement is the one where all the unpaired electrons have parallel spin (Hund rule)*.

Thus, the electronic configurations of some elements are:

	1s	2s	2p		
Carbon	↑↓	↑↓	↑	↑	
Nitrogen	↑↓	↑↓	↑	↑	↑
Oxygen	↑↓	↑↓	↑↓	↑	↑

Shape of atomic orbitals

As we are mainly concerned with the first-row elements of the periodic table, we will restrict our discussion to only s and p orbitals without going into the details of how their shapes and orientations bave been determined by quantum mechanics. The s orbitals (1s, 2s, 3s, etc.) are spherically symmetrical about the nucleus. Obviously, the 2s orbital is bigger than the 1s orbital. It surrounds the nucleus from a distance. Between the 1s and 2s orbitals there is a zone called nodal zone where the probability of finding the electrons is zero.

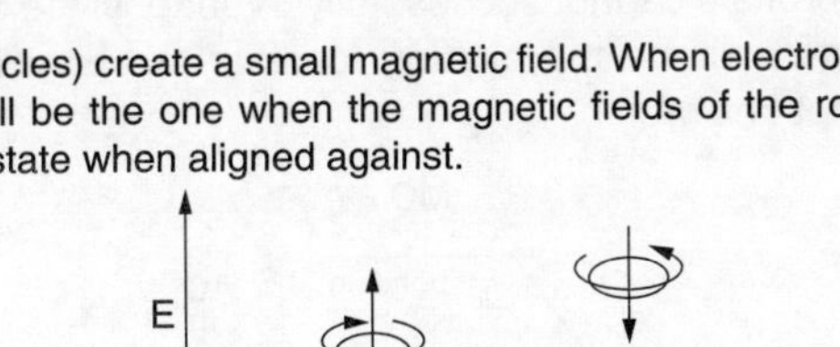

* Rotating electrons (charged particles) create a small magnetic field. When electrons are placed in an external magnetic field, the lowest-energy state will be the one when the magnetic fields of the rotating electrons are aligned with the applied field and higher-energy state when aligned against.

The p orbitals (2p, 3p, 4p, etc.) are dumb-bell-shaped. There are three p orbitals each of the same shape and energy, which are directed at 90° to each other with the point of intersection at the nucleus of the atom.

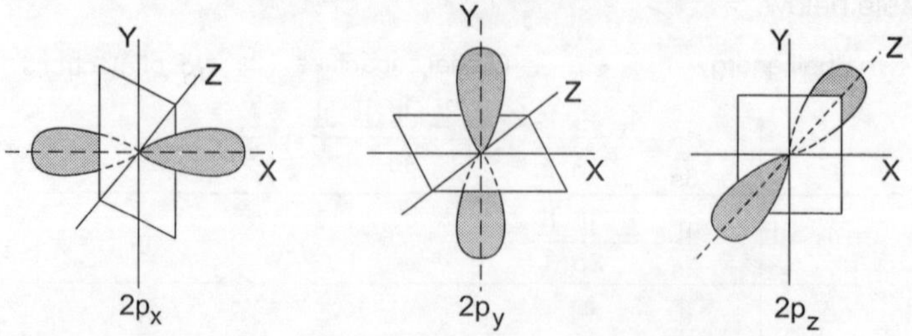

Hence, they are designated $2p_x$, $2p_y$ and $2p_z$ to indicate their directions along the cartesian coordinates. The probability of finding the electrons of $2p_x$ orbital along the yz plane passing through the nucleus is zero. This plane is called the nodal plane. For electrons of $2p_y$ and $2p_z$, the nodal planes are xz and xy respectively. It is for this reason that the three 2p orbitals do not mix up ordinarily. The 2p orbital extends slightly beyond the radius of 2s orbital. The shape of d orbital (five) is double dumb-bell and the shape of f orbital (seven) is rosette.

Overlap of orbitals

When parts of atomic orbitals (AOs) of two atoms occupy the same space on being brought closer, it is called overlap of orbitals. The overlap of two AOs results in the formation of two new orbitals called molecular orbitals (MOs). These MOs are common electron clouds encompassing the nuclei of both the atoms and contain two electrons. Mathematically it has been shown that the addition of two AOs generates a bonding MO and subtraction of one AO from the other generates an antibonding orbital. This method of overlap of AOs is called a linear combination of atomic orbitals (LCAO). [The argument for the generation of the two MOs by LCAO method is this: each AO can accommodate up to a maximum of two electrons so the combination of two AOs should be able to accommodate four electrons for which two MOs should exist.] In the bonding MO both electrons reside mostly between the two nuclei in the ground state and hence aid to the binding of the two nuclei. The bonding MO has lower energy than the two AOs. In the antibonding MO the electrons are at a greater distance from either of the nuclei than in the individual AOs. Hence, the antibonding orbital does not aid to the binding of the two nuclei and is of higher energy than the AOs.

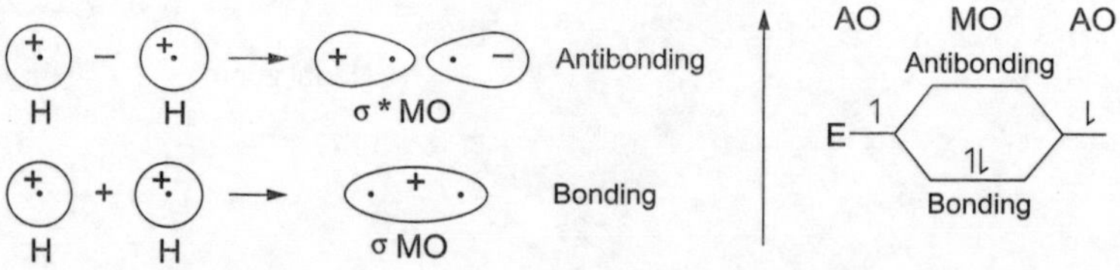

It is for this reason that two filled orbitals cannot successfully overlap, since a pair each will be in bonding and antibonding orbitals. The net result will be the binding force of the bonding MO will be cancelled by the antibonding MO. Hence, He_2 is not known.

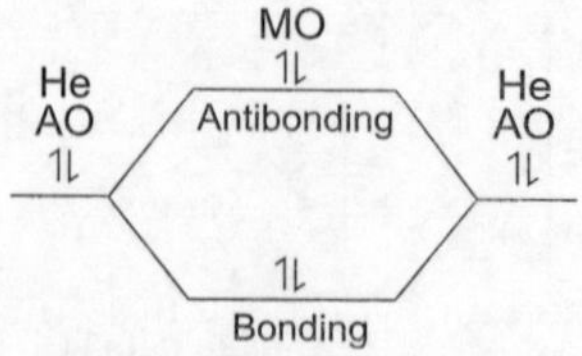

The antibonding orbitals will be ignored as they are not occupied by the electrons in the ground state.

Sigma orbital: Sigma bond When two hydrogen atoms approach close enough, their 1s orbitals, each containing one electron, overlap with the formation of a common molecular orbital.

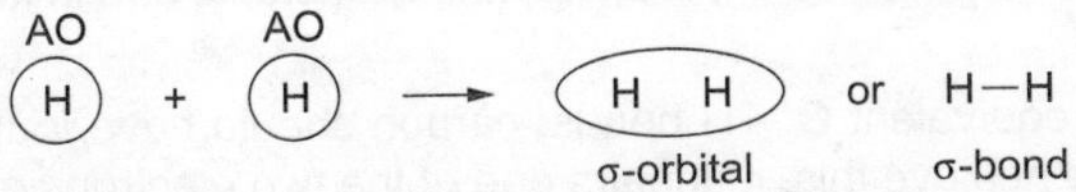

As the MO has a shape nearly similar to s orbital, it is called a σ orbital from the Greek letter σ corresponding to the letter s. The electron cloud is more dense along the internuclear axis and hence binds the two positively charged nuclei firmly. Hence, a σ bond is a very strong bond.

Sigma-bond orbitals can also be formed by the linear overlaps of s and p orbitals, p and p orbitals, between hybridized orbitals and between s and hybridized orbitals. The latter two types will be taken up later.

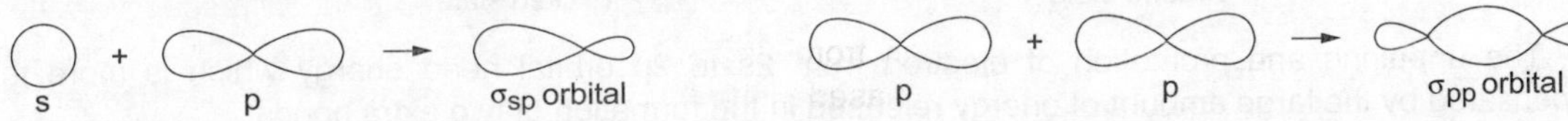

Pi orbital: Pi bond The MO formed by the sideways overlap of two p orbitals perpendicular to the internuclear axis is called a π orbital and the bond called π bond from the Greek letter π corresponding to the letter p. The shape of π orbital is different from that of σ orbital. There are two regions of electron cloud, above and below the line joining the two nuclei. Since the π electrons are not in the internuclear axis, the binding effect is partial. Therefore, the π bond is not as strong as the σ bond; they are loosely held.

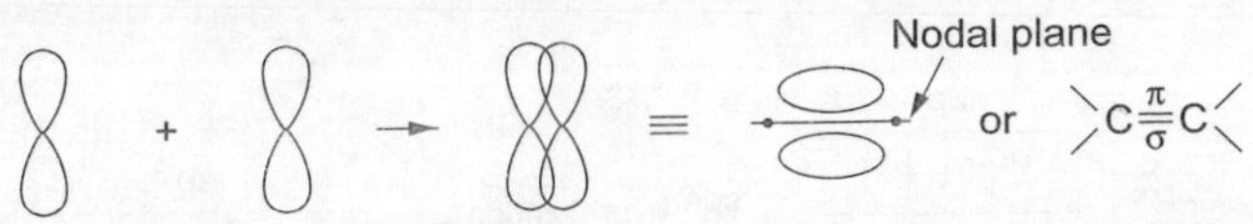

Hybrid orbital Formation of covalent bonds by the overlap of orbitals is accompanied by the release of energy. Greater the overlap, greater is the energy release and greater is the stability. In the formation of molecules, greatest stability is endeavoured. For this, elements try to mobilise all their valence electrons by mixing the atomic orbitals of the outermost shell and producing new type of orbitals called hybrid orbitals. This is in fact a redistribution of energy.

The hybrid orbitals have different shapes from the orbitals from which they have been hybridized. Thus, the hybrid orbital formed on mixing s and p orbitals has the shape of a p orbital but with one lobe smaller than the other.

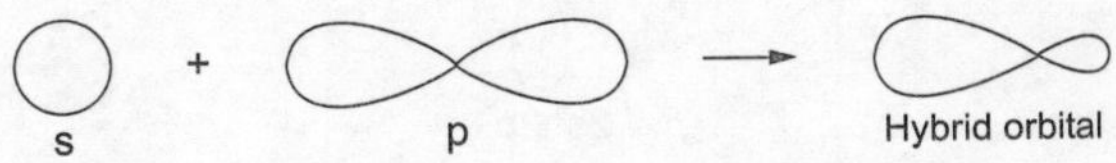

From its shape it is evident that it is more directional and can overlap better with other orbitals than either s or p orbitals, producing stable bonds.

FORMATION OF COMPOUNDS OF CARBONS

Formation of CH_4 (carbon–carbon single bond) Let us consider the formation of a methane molecule. Experimental facts about methane are:

(i) It has four equivalent C – H bonds.
(ii) The H – C – H bond angle is 109°28′.
(iii) It is a tetragonal molecule, i.e., the four hydrogens are at the four apexes of a regular tetrahedron with carbon at the centre.

(iv) The bond energy of a C – H bond is high (102 kcal/mol).

The electronic configuration of an isolated carbon in the ground state is $1s^2 2s^2 2p^2$ in which two unpaired electrons are available for bond formation, i.e., carbon should be divalent. Although divalent carbon compounds such as : CCl_2 or : CH_2 are known, they are highly unstable and in majority of compounds, carbon exhibits tetravalency.

Hybridization To have four equivalent C – H bonds, carbon should have four equivalent orbitals with one unpaired electron in each. To achieve this, it unpairs one of the two electrons of 2s orbital and promotes it to the vacant 2p orbital.

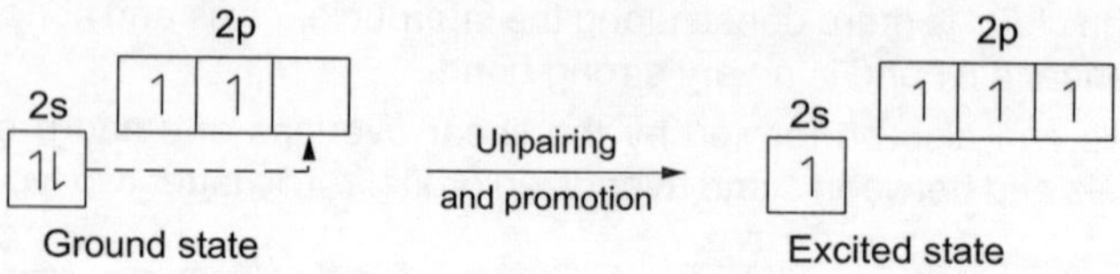

The unpairing and promotion of electron from 2s to 2p orbital need energy which is more than compensated by the large amount of energy released in the formation of two extra bonds.

Now, the four orbitals have one electron each and so can form four C – H bonds. However, these four C – H bonds will not be equivalent since the three 2p orbitals have higher energy than the 2s orbital. Also the 2s and 2p orbitals have different overlapping capacities. Therefore, in order to have four equivalent orbitals, the four orbitals (one 2s and three 2p) are mixed up, i.e., hybridized to produce four new equivalent orbitals called hybrid orbitals. These four hybrid orbitals are called sp^3 orbitals as three p and one s orbitals have been mixed.

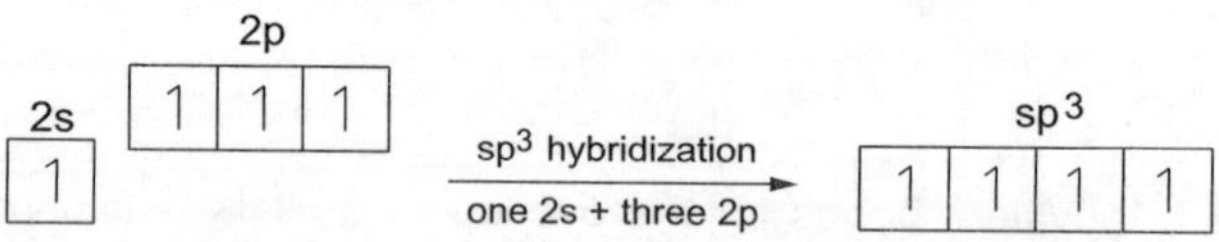

To avoid maximum repulsion between the electrons, the four hybrid orbitals take up a tetrahedral direction. The angle between the axes of any two sp^3 orbitals is 109°28′ when mathematically calculated. Orbital picture of the process is given below.

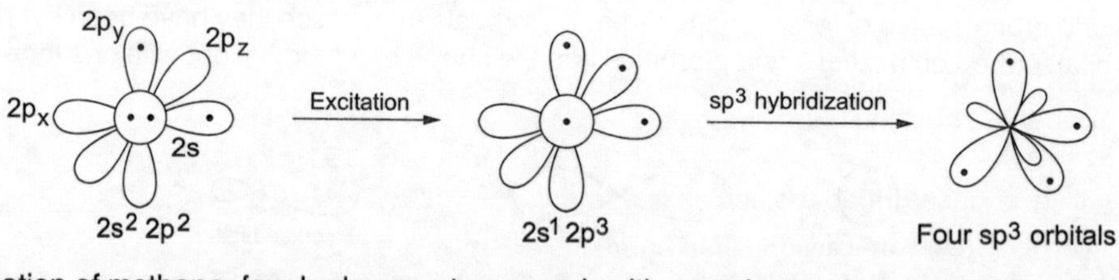

For the formation of methane, four hydrogen atoms, each with one electron in 1s orbital, overlap with each of the four sp^3 orbitals axially. Each bonding MO is a σ orbital, i.e., four C – H σ bonds are formed.

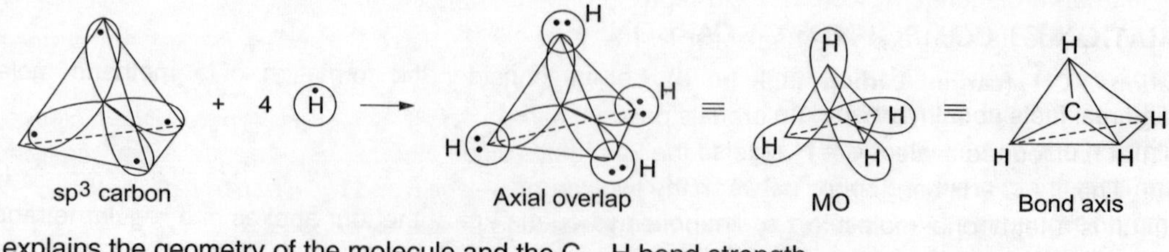

This explains the geometry of the molecule and the C – H bond strength.

Formation of ethylene (carbon–carbon double bond) In ethylene, each carbon is bonded to two hydrogen atoms and one carbon atom with σ bonds. For this, each carbon hybridizes the 2s orbital with two 2p orbitals to produce three sp^2 orbitals to form three strong σ bonds. To attain the state of lowest energy, the three sp^2 orbitals are directed at 120° to each other in a plane. The geometry of sp^2 carbon is, therefore, triangular planar. The remaining unhybridized 2p orbital is perpendicular to the plane.

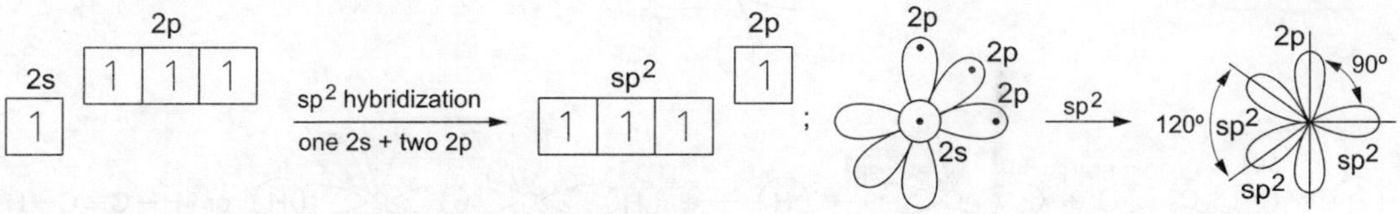

In the formation of ethylene molecule, one of the sp^2 orbitals on each carbon overlap axially to form a strong C – C σ bond. The remaining two sp^2 orbitals on each carbon overlap with the 1s orbitals of four hydrogen atoms to form four C – H σ bonds.

The remaining unhybridized 2p orbitals on each carbon are vertical to the plane containing the carbon and hydrogen atoms. These 2p orbitals are parallel and overlap laterally to form π bond. The bonding π MO is situated above and below the plane containing the atoms of the molecule.

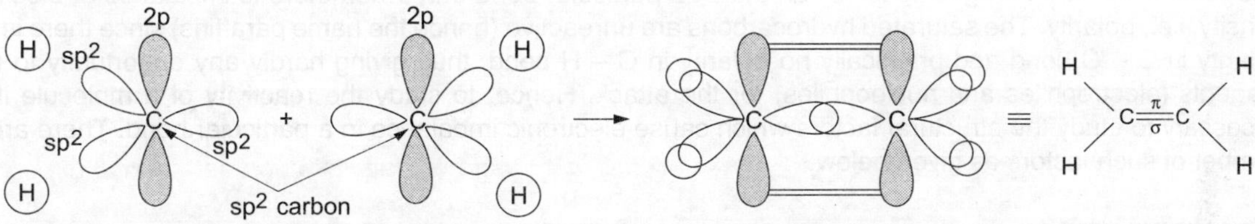

The binding effect of the π bond is reflected in the bond distances, e.g., the C = C distance is 1.33 Å and C – C distance is 1.54 Å. The lateral overlap in π bond is less effective in binding the carbon atoms than the axial overlap in σ bond. Thus, the bond energy of C – C is 83 kcal/mol and that of C = C is 143 kcal/mol and not double of 83 kcal/mol.

The reactivity of unsaturated molecules is due to the more exposed and loosely held π electrons.

Formation of acetylene (carbon–carbon triple bond) In acetylene each carbon is bonded to the other carbon and one hydrogen atom. For this each carbon hybridizes 2s orbital with one 2p orbital to produce two sp^1 hybrid orbitals (Atoms usually mobilize as many hybrid orbitals as it has to form strong σ bonds). The two sp^1 orbitals take up a diagonal position to avoid repulsion, i.e., the angle between the two sp^1 orbitals is 180°. These two sp^1 orbitals on each carbon form two σ bonds—one between the two carbons and one with hydrogen.

The residual two unhybridized 2p orbitals on each carbon are at right angles to each other. Hence, the 2p orbitals on one carbon which are parallel to the 2p orbitals of the other carbon, overlap laterally to form two π bonds. Thus, there are three bonds between the two carbons—one σ and two π bonds. The π-electron cloud is symmetric around the C – C σ bond and exposed to reacting species.

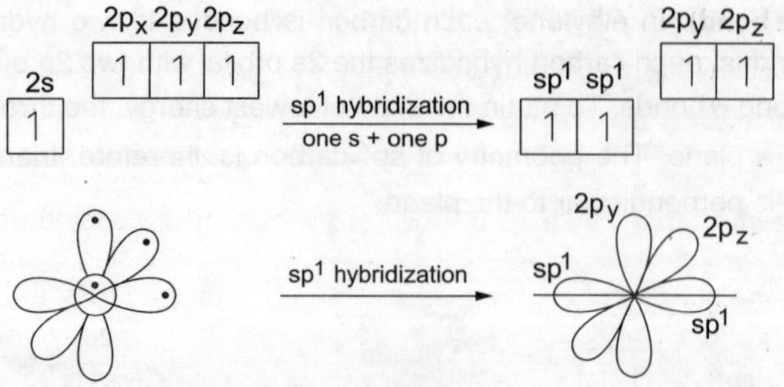

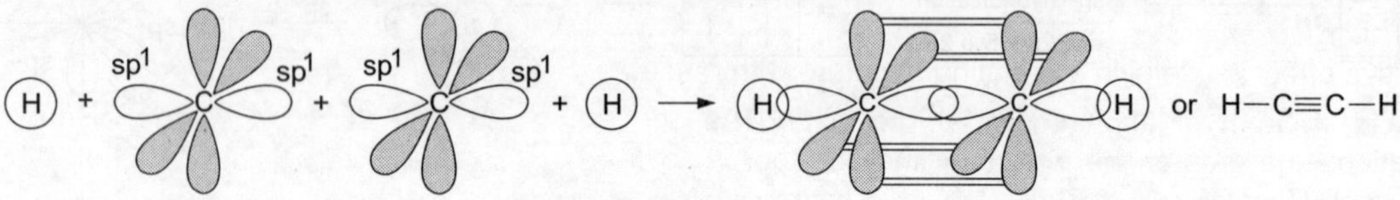

Bond formation

The molecule is linear. The C ≡ C bond distance is 1.20 Å and the bond energy is 194 kcal/mol.

FACTORS INFLUENCING REACTIVITY

Reagents which are charged species can attack a particular bond only when there is imbalance of electron density, i.e., polarity. The saturated hydrocarbons are unreactive (hence the name paraffins) since there is no polarity in C – C bond and practically no polarity in C – H bond, thus giving hardly any opportunity to the reagents (electrophiles and nucleophiles) for the attack. Hence, to study the reactivity of a molecule it is necessary to study the structural factors which cause electronic imbalance in a particular bond. There are a number of such factors as given below.

INDUCTIVE EFFECT

The electron cloud in a σ bond between two unlike atoms is not uniform. It is more dense towards the more electronegative of the two atoms, i.e., the electron pair forming the σ bond is slightly displaced towards X. This permanent state of polarization is called the inductive effect.

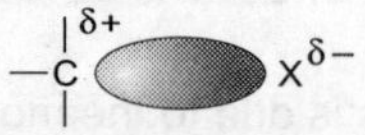

The atom X thus acquires a slight negative charge (δ^-) and the carbon atom a slight positive charge (δ^+), i.e., the bond is polarised. If the electronegative atom is joined to a chain of carbon atoms, the positive charge on the carbon atom is relayed to the other carbon atoms.

$$\overset{\delta+}{C_4} \rightarrow \overset{\delta+}{C_3} \rightarrow \overset{\delta+}{C_2} \rightarrow \overset{\delta+}{C_1} \rightarrow X$$

Since C_1 is slightly positively charged it exerts a pull on the electrons forming covalent bond between C_1 and C_2 but less strongly than X on C_1. The effect thus rapidly dies out. Hence, the effect is not significant beyond the second C-atom. This electron displacement relayed through σ bonds, albeit through a short distance, is known as inductive effect. The effect is permanent but feeble (since it involves shift of strongly held σ-bond electrons) and other stronger factors may overshadow this effect.

Inductive effect may be due to atoms or groups. Relative inductive effects have been measured with reference to hydrogen. The order of electron-withdrawing effect is:

$$NO_2 > F > COOH > Cl > Br > I > OH > OR > C_6H_5 > H > Me_3C- > Me_2CH- > MeCH_2- > CH_3$$

$\longleftarrow$ Electron-withdrawing (– I effect) $\qquad$ $\longleftarrow$ Electron-releasing (+ I effect)

The alkyl groups are less electron-withdrawing than hydrogen and are, therefore, considered as electron-releasing. Electron-withdrawing character is indicated by – I effect and electron-releasing character by + I effect. The effect is additive—the greater the number of electron-withdrawing groups the stronger is the effect.

Applications

Inductive effect is useful in correlating structure with reactivity.

(a) Acid strength of aliphatic carboxylic acids The strength of an acid depends on the extent of its ionization—the greater the ionization the stronger is the acid. The strength of an acid is denoted by the numerical value of pK_a (p$K_a = -\log_{10} K_a$, where K_a is the acidity constant). Smaller the numerical value stronger is the acid.

In acetic acid, the electron-releasing inductive effect of methyl group hinders the breaking of O – H bond; consequently reduces the ionization. This effect is absent in formic acid.

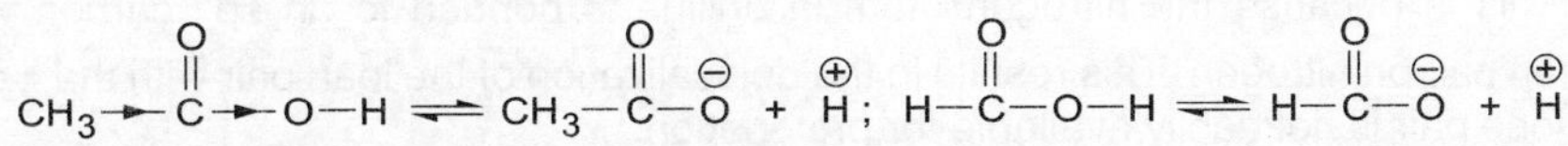

Greater ionization in formic acid over acetic acid makes formic acid (pK_a = 3.77) stronger than acetic acid (pK_a = 4.76). Monochloroacetic acid (pK_a = 2.86) is stronger than formic acid since – I effect of chlorine promotes ionization. As this effect is additive, trichloroacetic acid (pK_a = 0.66) is a still stronger acid.

When an unsaturated carbon is conjugated with the carboxyl group, the acid strength is increased. This is because with the increasing s contribution to the hybrid orbitals, the electrons are progressively drawn closer to the nucleus of the carbon resulting in the increase in – I effect. Since the s contributions in sp, sp^2 and sp^3 orbitals are respectively 50%, 33.3% and 25%, the order of – I effect of hybrid orbitals is $sp > sp^2 > sp^3$. This is reflected in the pK_a values of the following acids.

CH_3-CH_2-COOH	$CH_2=CH-COOH$	$HC\equiv C-COOH$
Propanoic acid (4.88)	Propenoic acid (4.25)	Propynoic acid (1.84)

(b) Aromatic carboxylic acids The α carbon of benzoic acid is sp^2-hybridized. Hence benzoic acid (pK_a = 4.20) is a stronger acid than its saturated analogue, cyclohexane carboxylic acid (pK_a = 4.87). Electron-withdrawing groups substituted at *o*- and *p*-positions enhance the acid strength.

(c) Dioic acids Since carboxyl group is itself an electron-withdrawing group, the dioic acids are in general stronger than their monocarboxyl analogues, e.g.,

$H-COOH$ (3.77) $\quad$ $HOOC-COOH$ (1.23) $\quad$ CH_3-COOH (4.76) $\quad$ $HOOC-CH_2-COOH$ (2.83)

The electron-withdrawing effect of one carboxyl group over the other falls off sharply on separating the two carboxyl groups by at least two saturated carbons.

(d) Aliphatic bases The strength of nitrogenous bases depends on the ease of availability of the unshared electron pair on the nitrogen atom to the proton. Due to the increasing +I effect in amines, the order of base strength should be $NH_3 < MeNH_2 < Me_2NH < Me_3N$. However, the p$K_a$ values are 9.25 (NH_3), 10.64 ($MeNH_2$), 10.77 (Me_2NH) and 9.80 (Me_3N). The pK_a value for the base B: is a measure of the acid strength of its conjugate acid $B^{\oplus}$: H. Stronger the acid $B^{\oplus}H$, weaker is the base B:. In other words, smaller the numerical value of pK_a for the acid, $B^{\oplus}H$, the weaker is the base B:. From the pK_a values it is seen that 2° amine (10.77) is a stronger base than 3° amine (9.80). This is because the base strength of an amine in water depends not only on the ease of availability of lone pair but also on the extent of solvation of the protonated amine by hydrogen bonding. The protonated 3° amine has one and protonated 2° amine has two hydrogens on the nitrogen for hydrogen bonding.

Hence, 2° amine is a stronger base than 3° amine. Solvation is an important factor for the determination of the base strength. This is supported by the fact that the order of base strength of amines is 3° > 2° > 1° in chlorobenzene in which hydrogen bonding is absent.

(e) **Aromatic bases** Aniline is a weaker base (pK_a = 4.62) than its saturated analogue, cyclohexylamine (pK_a = 10.68). This is because the nitrogen atom in aniline is bonded to an sp^2 carbon which pulls the unshared electron pair on nitrogen. This results in the delocalization of the loan pair with the π electrons of the ring. Thus, the lone pair is not easily available for protonation.

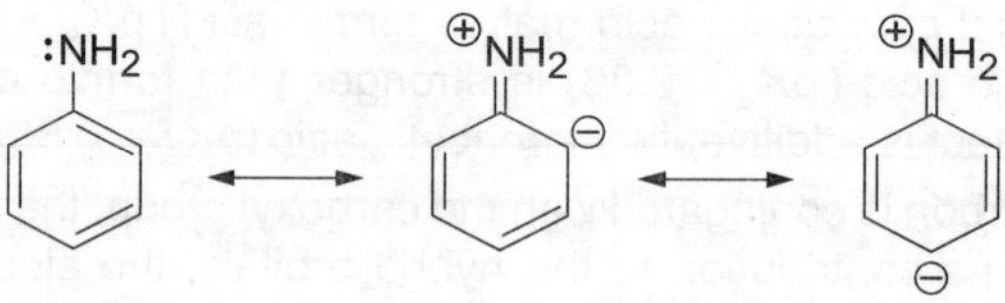

Hence, aniline is a weaker base than ammonia or cyclohexylamine. Electron-withdrawing substituents at *o*- and *p*-positions have marked base-weakening effect. Substituents that have unshared electrons, e.g., $-\ddot{O}H$ or $-\ddot{O}R$ exert electron-donating mesomeric effect from *o*- and *p*-positions increasing the base strength.

Electromeric effect

On the close approach of a reagent, the electronic system of an unsaturated molecule is deformed. When the reagent is removed without allowing the reaction to take place, the electronic system reverts to the original ground state of the molecule. This kind of polarizability of multiple bonds is known as electromeric effect.

Electromeric effect causes complete transfer of the loose π electrons from one carbon to the other. Consequently, one end is positively charged and the other negatively charged which aid the reagent to attack. The shift of the electrons is shown by a curved arrow (⌒) indicating the direction of the electron shift.

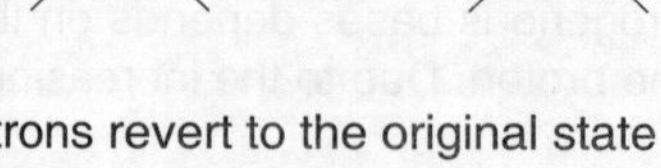

The effect is temporary since the electrons revert to the original state on removing the reagent.

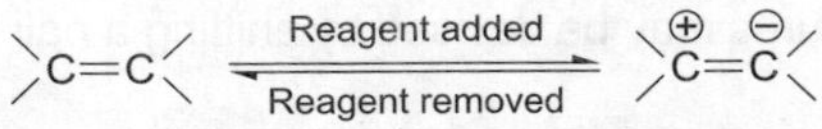

When the multiple bond is between two dissimilar elements the shift of electrons takes place towards the more electronegative of the two. Inductive effect may also determine the direction of the shift of electrons, e.g.,

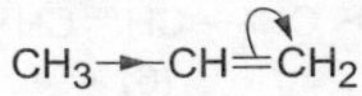

Electromeric effect differs from the inductive effect as given below.

Inductive effect	*Electromeric effect*
1. It is a permanent polarization.	1. It is a temporary polarization.
2. Operates through σ bonds.	2. Operates through π bonds.
3. Weak effect since the σ-bond electrons are strongly held.	3. Strong effect since the loose π electrons shift completely.
4. Charge developed on the carbon joined to the substituent (electron repelling or attracting) is small and is shown as δ^- or δ^+.	4. Complete transfer of electrons causes full charge on the carbons, which is shown by $\oplus$ and $\ominus$ signs.

RESONANCE

Many organic compounds are known which are not adequately represented by single valence bond structrues. All the properties of such a compound are not explained by a single structure. Thus, the valence bond structure of benzene (1) indicates three each carbon–carbon single and double bonds

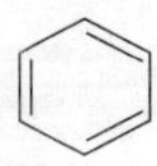

(1)

Measurement of bond distance in benzene, however, shows that all the carbon–carbon bond distances are the same and it is 1.4 Å, i.e., between a single (1.54 Å), and a double bond (1.34 Å). Further, benzene on hydrogenation gives out heat which is less than the heat calculated from its structure (1).

For such compounds it is necessary that other structures be devised to explain all their properties. This is the basis of the concept of resonance. Thus, when two or more good Lewis structures can be devised for a compound, resonance is invoked.

The different structures of a compound devised by different methods of pairing electrons in a fixed atomic skeleton are called resonance or canonical structures. The actual structure of the compound is then a combination of these structures and hence the compound is called a resonance hybrid. A hybrid is more stable than any one of the contributing structures. The contributing resonance structures are shown by double-headed arrows ($\leftrightarrow$) indicating that the real structure involves both ways of pairing electrons.

Each resonance structure represents only partially to the real state of the compound and all of them in combination represent the compound completely. Final structural description of the molecule is then what is obtained on superimposing all the resonance structrues on one another. The actual molecule therefore does not vibrate or oscillate from one structure to another but has one and only one structure which is an average of all the structures. The different resonance structures do not exist, they are drawn by different schemes of pairing electrons to consider the extent of delocalization and hence to assess the stability of the hybrid.

Thus, in 1, 3-butadiene, $\overset{4}{C}H_2 = \overset{3}{C}H - \overset{2}{C}H = \overset{1}{C}H_2$, the $C_1 - C_2$ and $C_3 - C_4$ bonds are found to be longer than a carbon–carbon double bond and $C_2 - C_3$ bond is slightly shorter than a carbon–carbon single bond.

To explain this, several other structures may be devised by shifting a pair of π electrons:

$$\underset{(2)}{CH_2{=}CH{-}CH{=}CH_2} \longleftrightarrow \underset{(3)}{\overset{\ominus}{C}H_2{-}\overset{\oplus}{C}H{-}CH{=}CH_2} \longleftrightarrow \underset{(4)}{CH_2{=}CH{-}\overset{\oplus}{C}H{-}\overset{\ominus}{C}H_2}$$

$$\longleftrightarrow \underset{(5)}{\overset{\ominus}{C}H_2{-}CH{=}CH{-}\overset{\oplus}{C}H_2} \longleftrightarrow \underset{(6)}{\overset{\oplus}{C}H_2{-}CH{=}CH{-}\overset{\ominus}{C}H_2}$$

The structures (3) and (4) show partial single-bond character of $C_1 - C_2$ and $C_3 - C_4$ bonds and structures (5) and (6) show partial double-bond character of $C_2 - C_3$ bond. This explains the observed anomalies in the bond distances in the hybrid.

Thus, in the hybrid structure (i.e., real structure) of the compound, lateral overlaps of all the four p atomic orbitals have taken place, i.e., the electrons are delocalized.

$$\underset{\text{Hybrid}}{\overline{\underline{CH_2{-}CH{-}CH{-}CH_2}}}$$

As a result, two bonding and two antibonding MOs are formed. The hybrid representation shows that each pair of electrons binds four carbon nuclei instead of two. This gives a net stability to the hybrid over any one of the contributing resonance structures.

Experimental confirmation about the stability of the hybrid is afforded from the qualitative measurements of the heat of combustion or hydrogenation.

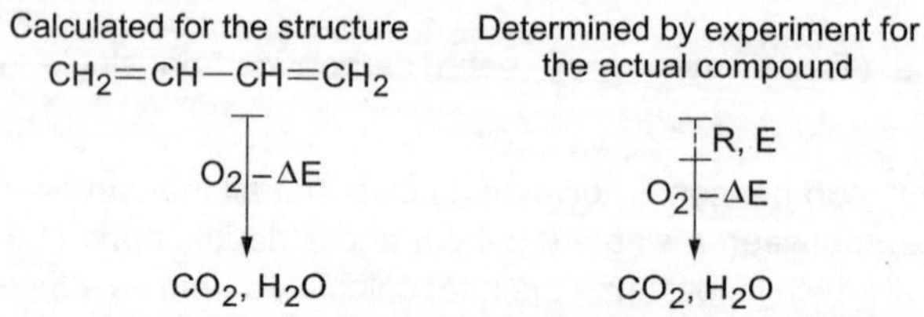

Heat of combustion

It is seen that the actual compound gives out lesser energy than that calculated for the structure $CH_2 = CH - CH = CH_2$. Hence, the actual compound is at a lower-energy state, i.e., more stable.

The difference in the experimental and calculated energies is the amount of energy by which the compound is stable. This difference in the energies is known as the resonance or delocalization energy (RE). It is about 4 kcal/mol for 1, 3-butadiene and 36 kcal/mol for benzene which is also a resonance hybrid.

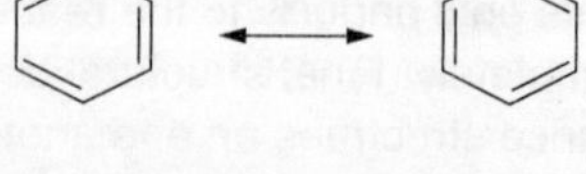

The resonance or stabilization energy of benzene has been calculated from the heat of hydrogenation as given below.

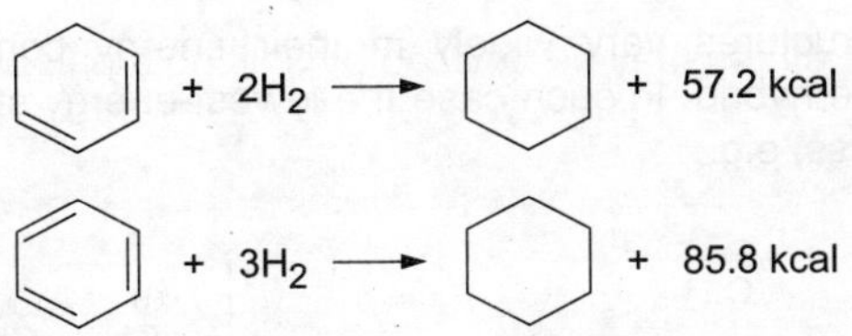

Since benzene has three double bonds, the heat evolved should have been $3 \times 28.6 = 85.8$ kcal/mol but experimentally it is found to be 49.8 kcal/mol, i.e., benzene evolves $85.8 - 49.8 = 36$ kcal/mol less energy than anticipated for the hypothetical cyclohexatriene.

Therefore, the resonance energy of benzene is 36 kcal/mol which is due to the delocalization of the π electrons in a cyclic molecular orbital.

Resonance stability increases with increased number of resonance structures, for larger number of nuclei are brought closer by the binding effect of the loose electrons.

All the resonance structures, however, do not contribute significantly to resonance. Whether a structure will contribute significantly to resonance or not has to be considered from the following rules of resonance.

Rules of resonance

1. All the resonance forms must conform to Lewis structure, e.g., carbon cannot be pentavalent in any of the resonance forms.
2. The positions of the nuclei in all resonance structures must be the same.
3. All the resonance structures must have the same number of paired electrons, e.g., $\dot{C}H_2 - CH = CH - \dot{C}H_2$ is not considered a resonance structure of butadiene (2).
4. Resonance structures with greater number of covalent bonds are more stable than those with lesser numbers. Thus, the nonpolar structure of butadiene (2) is more stable than any of the other resonance structures.
5. Resonance structrues with similar charges on adjacent atoms are insignificant due to electrostatic repulsion and consequent instability, e.g., the resonance form $\overset{\oplus}{C}H_2 - \overset{\ominus}{C}H - \overset{\ominus}{C}H - \overset{\oplus}{C}H_2$ does not contribute to the stability of the hybrid.
6. Structures with positive charge on multiply bonded electronegative element are unimportant since the electronegative element will not adapt to such distribution of electrons. Hence the canonical form, $> \overset{\ominus}{C} - \overset{\oplus}{O}$, of carbonyl group is insignificant.
7. Resonance stabilization is greatest when there are at least two equivalent structures, e.g.,

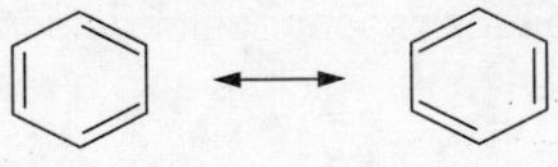 ; $\overset{\oplus}{C}H_2{-}CH{=}CH_2 \longleftrightarrow CH_2{=}CH{-}\overset{\oplus}{C}H_2$

8. Charge-separation structures are less important than those in which the charge is delocalized. This is due to electrostatic attraction between unlike charges.

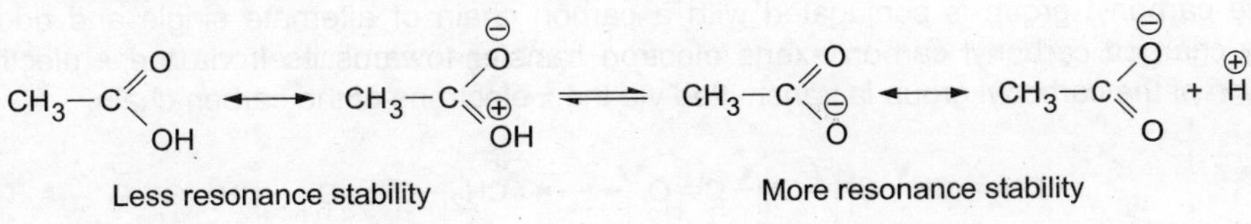

Less resonance stability | More resonance stability

Hence, acetic acid favours ionization.

9. Dissimilar canonical structures vary widely in their energy contents, those of higher energy contribute too little to the hybrid. In such case the lowest-energy structure resembles the hybrid in energy, i.e., the RS is less, e.g.,

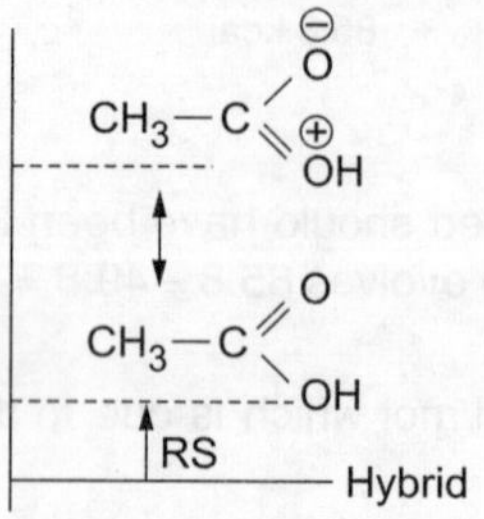

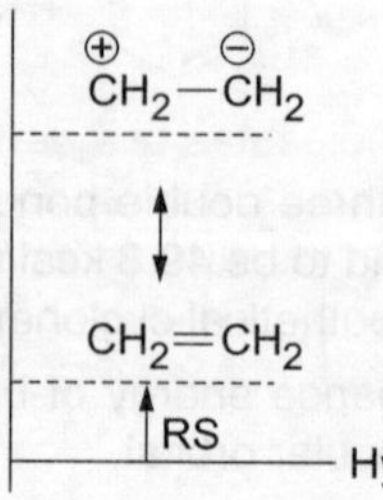

Hence, acetic acid and ethylene are well represented by their conventional structures.

In contrast, similar canonical structures have nearly equal energies and contribute more to the hybrid, so that the RS is more, e.g.,

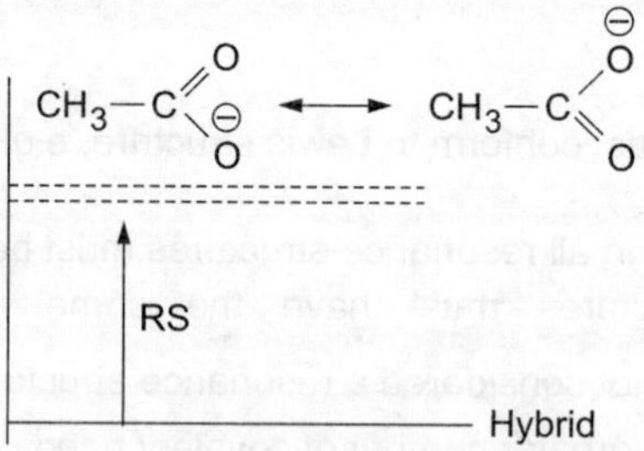

Thus, acetate ion is more stable than acetic acid which therefore ionizes to behave as acid. Similarly, phenol is acidic since phenoxide ion is more stable than phenol (see +M effect).

10. All the atoms in a molecule taking part in resonance should be coplanar. This is necessary for effective overlap of the p orbitals and the delocalization of the electrons. Hence, distortion of planarity will impede resonance with all that is consequent upon.

MESOMERIC EFFECT

The permanent polarization of a group conjugated with a π bond or a set of alternate π bonds is transmitted through the π electrons of the system resulting in a different distribution of electrons in the unsaturated chain. This kind of electron redistribution in unsaturated compounds conjugated with electron-releasing or electron-withdrawing groups or atoms is called mesomeric effect.

We know that carbonyl group is a resonance hybrid.

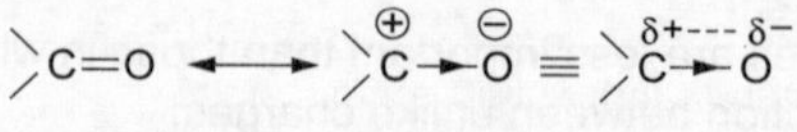

When the carbonyl group is conjugated with a carbon chain of alternate single and double bonds, the positively charged carbonyl carbon exerts electron transfer towards itself via the π electrons. Thus, the polarization of the carbonyl group is transmitted via the π electrons of the carbon chain.

Similarly, the lone pair on the nitrogen atom repels the π electrons of the conjugated chain of the amino compound.

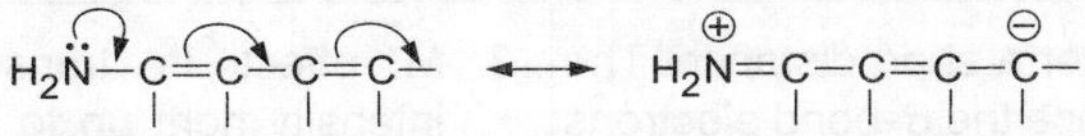

The π electrons of molecules are delocalized due to the mesomeric effect resulting in a number of resonance structures which give stability to the ions. Therefore, this kind of electron transfer is also called resonance effect or conjugative effect besides mesomeric effect.

This is a permanent effect in the ground state of the molecule which is indicated by the dipole moment. The electron-attracting mesomeric effect is indicated by –M effect and the electron-repelling mesomeric effect is indicated by +M effect.

+M effect possessing groups are: $-\ddot{O}H$, $-\ddot{O}R$, $-\ddot{N}H_2$, $-\ddot{N}HR$, $-\ddot{N}R_2$, $-\ddot{S}R$, $-\ddot{X}:$, etc.

–M effect possessing groups are: $-CHO$, $=CO$, $-CN$, $-NO_2$, $-SO_3H$, etc.

The low reactivity of halogens bonded to unsaturated carbon is due to the +M effect of the halogen. The C – Br bond in vinyl bromide has a partial double-bond character due to the +M effect of bromine with consequent low reactivity of bromine.

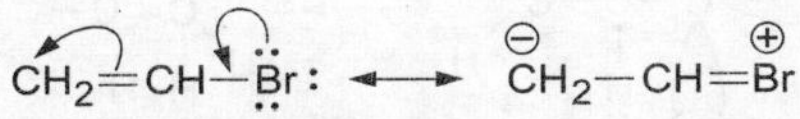

The acidity of phenol is due to the +M effect of OH group. The mesomeric transfer of the lone pair on the oxygen atom of phenol to the π electrons of the benzene ring results in several resonance structures with a positive charge on the oxygen atom. This aids the hydrogen atom of OH group to leave as proton.

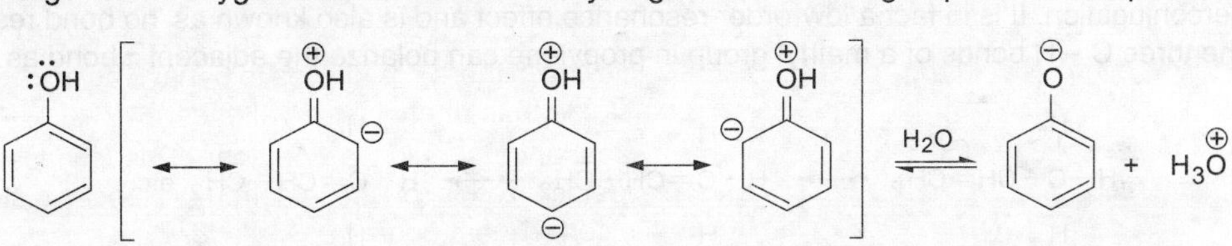

The ionization is specially aided due to the formation of the relatively more stable phenoxide ion.

The charge delocalization in phenoxide ion affords greater stability over phenol in which charge separation occurs in the canonical forms.

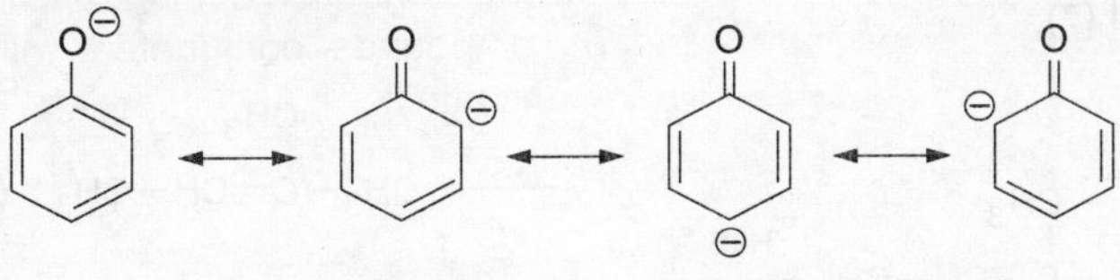

Hence, phenol prefers to ionize, i.e., it is acidic.

The essential differences, between inductive effect and mesomeric effect are:

Inductive effect (I effect)	*Mesomeric effect* (M effect)
1. I effect can operate in saturated and unsaturated compounds.	1. M effect can operate in unsaturated and conjugated compounds.

2. I effect involves electrons of σ bonds.	2. M effect involves electrons of π bonds and lone pairs.
3. I effect is transmitted over a short distance. The effect dies out rapidly since the σ-bond electrons are tightly held.	3. M effect is transmitted with undiminished intensity right up to the end of the unsaturated chain since the effect involves loose π electrons.

HYPERCONJUGATION

The inductive effect of alkyl groups is found to be in the order $Me_3C->Me_2CH->MeCH_2->CH_3-$ when attached to a saturated carbon. When, however, they are attached to an unsaturated carbon (e.g., C = C or aromatic ring) the order is reversed. In this case, electron-releasing effect operates by a different method than in inductive effect.

The electron-releasing effect is explained by assuming that the σ orbital of the α C – H bond overlaps with the adjacent π orbital. The displacement of the electron pair of the α C – H bond causes a partial positive charge on the hydrogen atom without the actual proton release.

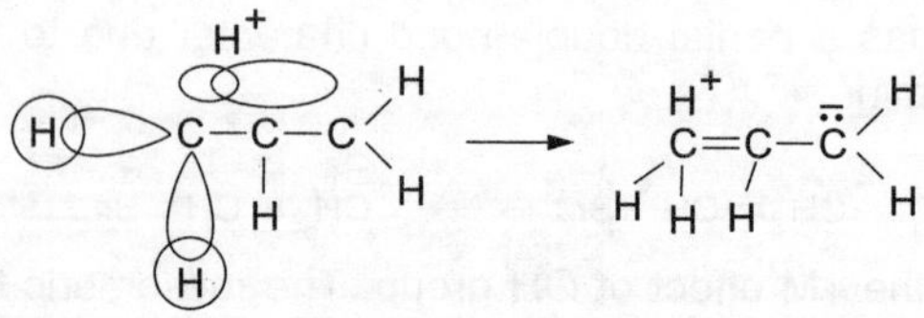

This ability of the σ-bond electrons of an α C – H bond to undergo conjugation with the adjacent π electrons is called hyperconjugation. It is in fact a low-order resonance effect and is also known as 'no bond resonance'. Thus, all the three C – H bonds of a methyl group in propylene can polarize the adjacent π bond as shown:

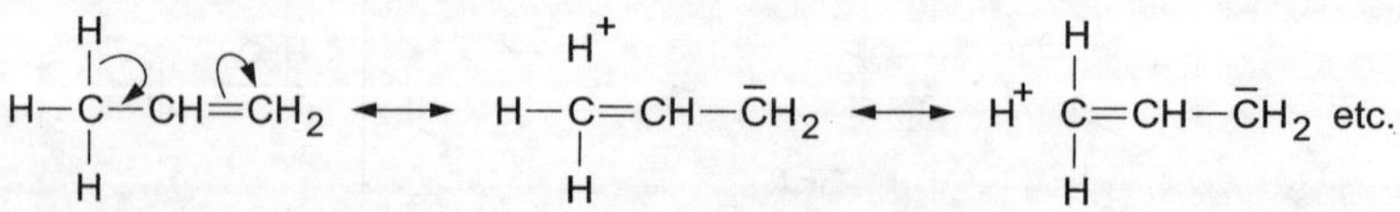

Hence, the site of electrophilic attack is the terminal CH_2 group. As the effect is additive, it is at a maximum with CH_3 group. Hence, the order of this effect is $CH_3 > RCH_2 > R_2CH$.

Hyperconjugation satisfactorily explains the preferential formation of the alkene (8) over (9) on dehydration of the alcohol (7).

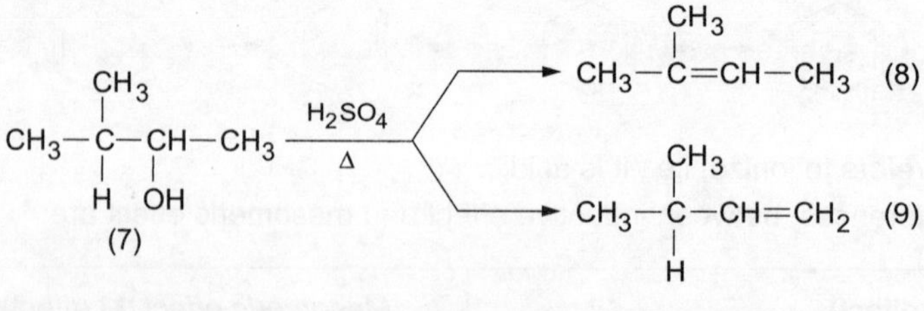

Nine α-hydrogens, by hyperconjugative effect, stabilize the olefin (8) over (9) where there is only one α-hydrogen atom for hyperconjugation.

The ortho- and para-directing effect of methyl group is similarly attributed to electron release by hyperconjugation.

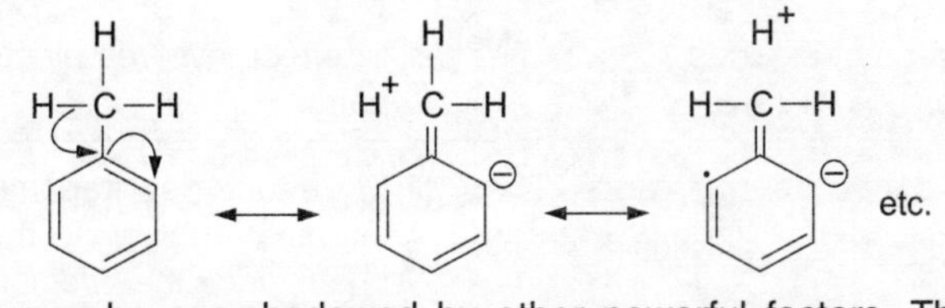

The effect is feeble and may be overshadowed by other powerful factors. Thus, in the dehydration of 3-hydroxy-4-methylpentanal (10)

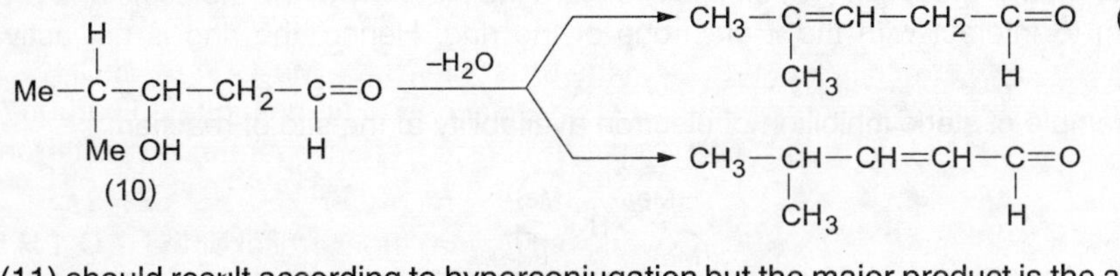

(10) (11) (12)

the aldehyde (11) should result according to hyperconjugation but the major product is the aldehyde (12). This is due to conjugation of the double bond with the carbonyl group in (12) which gives resonance stability, a stronger stabilizing factor.

STERIC EFFECT

The structural feature which influences the chemical reactions due to bulky substituents in the molecule is called steric effect. When the bulky groups hinder the reaction, it is called steric hindrance which may be due to (a) the sheer bulk of the substituents causing the approach of the reagent more difficult or may be due to (b) electronic factor, i.e., promoting or inhibiting electron availability at a particular site. Thus—

(i) Bulky alkyl groups in ketones restrict the space around the carbonyl group to undergo addition reactions. Such hindrance is not observed in aldehydes since one of the groups is hydrogen which occupies small space. Hence aldehydes are more reactive than ketones (inductive effect also plays its part). Cyclohexanone is, however, as much reactive as methyl ketone to addition reactions, since the two groups effecting the ring closure are held back, providing more space for the attack.

(ii) Carboxylic acids with highly substituted α-carbon are esterified with difficulty due to steric hindrance.

(iii) The two substituents at the ortho positions in 2,6-dimethylbenzoic acid block the approach of alcohol towards the carbonyl group so that no esterification occurs under normal conditions.

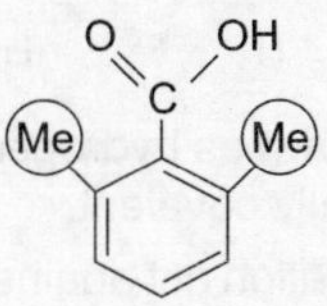

When the carboxyl group is shifted away from the two ortho substituents as in 2, 6-dimethylphenylacetic acid, esterification occurs readily.

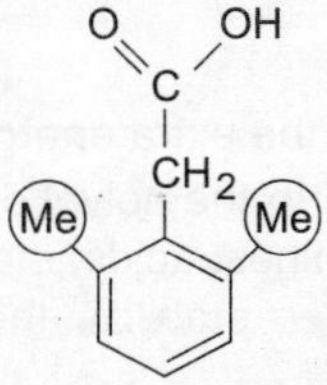

(iv) Tertiary butyl benzene produces exclusively the para isomer since the bulky substituent ($-CMe_3$) sterically blocks attack at the ortho positions.

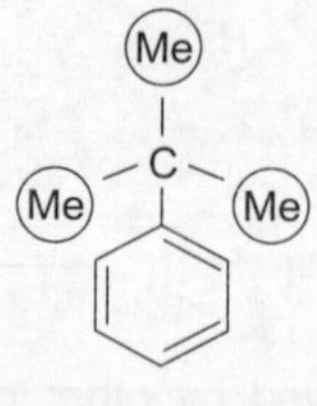

(v) *N, N*-Dimethylaniline undergoes ready azo-coupling but its 2,6-dimethyl derivative (13) does not. Crowding of the four methyl groups in (13) sterically disturb the planarity of the molecule and prevent the lone pair on the N atom to interact with the π electrons of the ring. Hence, the ring is not activated towards azo-coupling.

This is an example of steric inhibition of electron availability at the site of reaction.

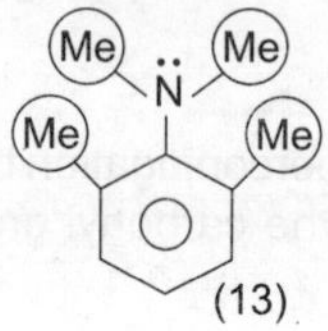

(13)

HYDROGEN BONDING

The covalent bond between a highly electronegative element such as N, O, F, etc., and hydrogen is polar in which the hydrogen forms the positive end of the dipole.

$$\overset{\delta-}{Q} \leftarrow \overset{\delta+}{H} \quad \text{where} \quad Q = N, O, F, \text{etc.}$$

The specificity of hydrogen attached to an electronegative element is due to the development of proton character in hydrogen where there is no core electrons (deshielded nucleus). It can therefore strongly attract a nucleophile (anion or a molecule having an unshared pair of electrons).

An intermolecular attraction between the positively charged hydrogen and the electronegative element of another molecule results in the association of molecules. Thus, water or alcohol is associated as shown below:

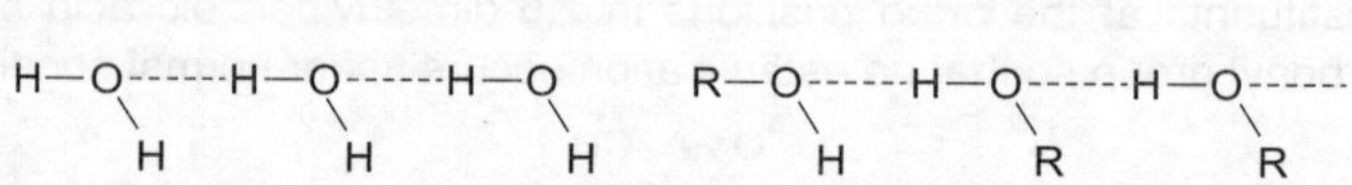

This type of bond (shown by dotted lines) is known as hydrogen bond or proton bond to distinguish it from the covalent bond. The bond may be ionic or partially covalent.

Since the disruptive forces of thermal agitation act against the attractive force (association) between the molecules, three molecules are associated in water, on an average. The strength of a hydrogen bond is about 5 kcal/bond which though small is not insignificant. Hydrogen bonding may be intermolecular or intramolecular.

(a) Intermolecular hydrogen bonding causes:

(i) rise in the b.p. or m.p. which is due to the extra energy required to break the hydrogen bond.

(ii) increase in the solubility which is due to the solvation of the solute molecules in polar solvents by hydrogen bonding. Thus, alcohols, amines, acids, etc., are water soluble.

(b) Intramolecular hydrogen bonding causes:

(i) decrease in the solubility in polar solvents due to restricted hydrogen bonding with polar solvents; thus, the enolate form of ethylacetoacetate is less soluble in water and more soluble in cyclohexane (like dissolves like) since intramolecular hydrogen bonding prevents solvation in water.

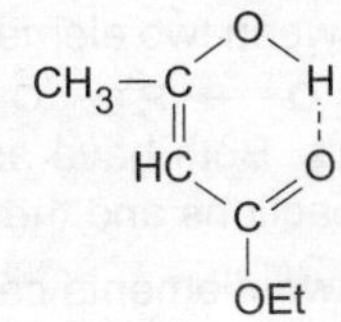

(ii) decrease in the b.p. or m.p.—intramolecular hydrogen bonding prevents association and so less energy is required for b.p or m.p. Thus, *o*-hydroxybenzoic acid has lower m.p. than its isomers.

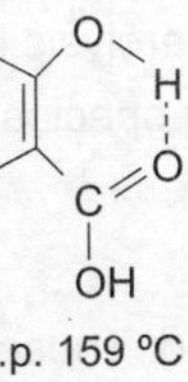

m-isomer m.p. 201 ºC

p-isomer m.p. 214 ºC

m.p. 159 ºC

(iii) increase in acid strength by stabilization of the acidic ion by intramolecular hydrogen bonding, thus, *o*-hydroxybenzoic acid is a stronger acid than its isomers.

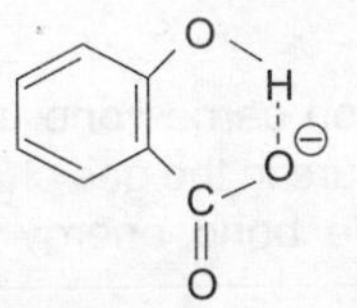

Hydrogen bonding causes shift in the IR spectra. The position of O – H stretching spectra is shifted to longer wavelengths since lower energy is required to stretch the O – H bond which is to some extent already stretched by hydrogen bonding.

Thus, the O – H stretching absorption for alcohol in the vapour phase is 3700 cm^{-1} and for dilute alcohol (i.e., hydrogen-bonded) it is 3300 cm^{-1}.

THE BREAKING AND MAKING OF BONDS

In an organic reaction the molecules undergoing change are called reactants and the new molecules formed are called products.

$$\underset{\text{Reactants}}{CH_4 + Cl_2} \xrightarrow{h\nu} \underset{\text{Products}}{CH_3Cl + HCl}$$

In this reaction a C – H bond and a Cl – Cl bond in the reactants have broken, and a new C – Cl bond and a H – Cl bond are formed in the product. Therefore, an organic reaction is a process of breaking and making of bonds. A reaction is successful if the bonds formed in the products are stronger than the bonds broken in the reactants. There are two possible ways by which a covalent bond can break. When the bond breaks symmetrically, it is called homolytic cleavage or homolysis and when dissymmetrically, it is called heterolytic cleavage or heterolysis.

(a) Homolytic cleavage The covalent bond between two elements can break in such a way that each element retains an electron of the bonding pair, e.g., $P:Q \longrightarrow P^{\bullet} + {}^{\bullet}Q$

The resulting fragments are called free radicals. Both have an unpaired electron (odd electron). Reactions involving free radicals are called free radical reactions and the mechanism is called free radical mechanism.

(b) Heterolytic cleavage The bonds between two elements can break in another way in which one element retains the bonding pair and the other loses, e.g., $P:Q \longrightarrow \overset{\oplus}{P} + :\overset{\ominus}{Q}$. As one element has lost and the other has gained an electron, positively and negatively charged ions (i.e., ion pair) are formed. This process of breaking of bonds is called heterolysis. Since ions are formed, reactions involving heterolytic cleavage are called ionic reactions. Most organic reactions are ionic. Heterolysis occurs more readily in polar solvents.

These radicals or ions may recombine or attack other species to form covalent bonds.

REACTION INTERMEDIATES

In the process of bond breaking, radicals or ions are formed. These are called reaction intermediates. They are of extremely short life but they play a very important role in the reaction. Since we are dealing with the organic compounds, our attention will be focused on the 'carbon fragments' (radicals or ions) of the substrate.

(i) Carbon radical

Carbon radicals are those in which the carbon carries one unpaired electron. They are usually formed on homolytic cleavage of bonds at high temperature in the gas phase, in non-polar solvents, by ultraviolet light or by the addition of other radicals. When the bond energy is low, the carbon radicals may be formed spontaneously or at low temperature, e.g.,

$$Ph_3C:CPh_3 \xrightleftharpoons{\text{solution}} 2Ph_3\dot{C}$$

$$Et_4Pb \xrightarrow{140\ ^\circ C} 4Et^{\bullet} + Pb$$

Carbon radicals are neutral but are extremely reactive due to unpaired electron. Hence a fast chain reaction occurs on homolytic fission.

Some common reactions are:

(a) Propagation of chain reaction—Abstract an atom from a molecule to produce another free radical for the propagation of the reaction.

$$\dot{C}l + CH_4 \longrightarrow \dot{C}H_3 + HCl;\ \dot{C}H_3 + Cl:Cl \longrightarrow CH_3Cl + \dot{C}l$$

(b) Polymerization—Add to multiple bond resulting in polymerization. Vinyl polymerization occurs in this method.

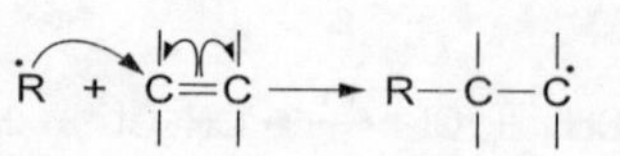

(c) Termination of reaction—They may react with each other to stop the reaction.

$$\dot{C}H_3 + \dot{C}H_3 \longrightarrow CH_3{-}CH_3$$

Geometric shape The carbon carrying the odd electron is supposed to be sp^3- or sp^2-hybridized.

Stability of the carbon radical The stability of the carbon radical increases with the increase in the number of alkyl groups attached to the carbon carrying the odd electron by hyperconjugation.

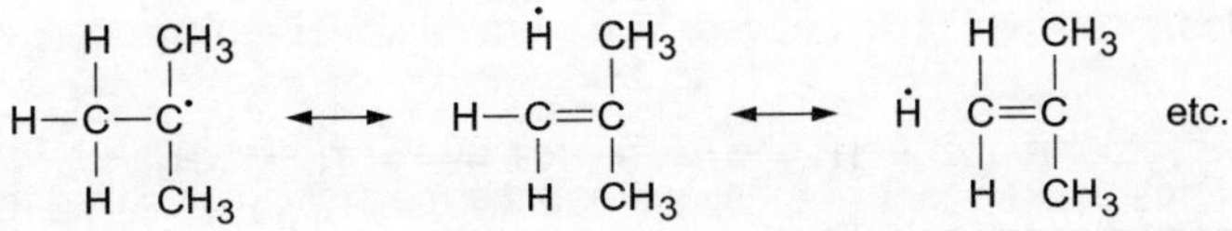

Hence, the stability order of carbon radicals is 3° > 2° > 1° > $\dot{C}H_3$. Carbon radicals in suitable unsaturated systems are more stable than alkyl radicals due to delocalization of the unpaired electron.

$$\dot{C}H_2-CH=CH_2 \longleftrightarrow CH_2=CH-\dot{C}H_2$$

Allylfree radical

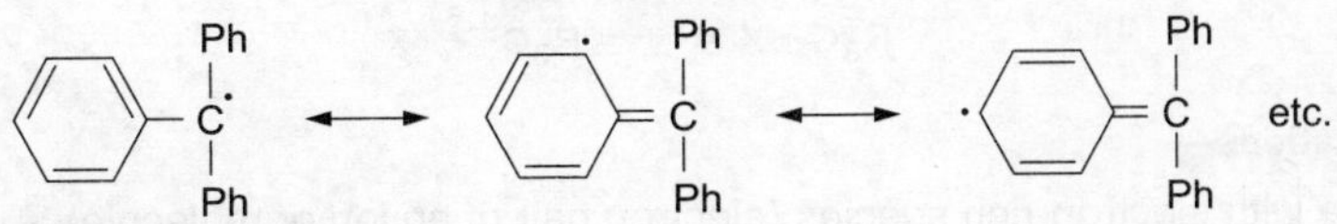

Triphenylmenthyl radical

Hence, allyl and triphenylmethyl radicals are more stable than tertiary carbon radicals.

(ii) Carbocation*

An ion in which the carbon carries a positive charge is called carbocation. They are formed by heterolysis, e.g.,

(a) By the addition of acids to—

(i) Unsaturated compounds.

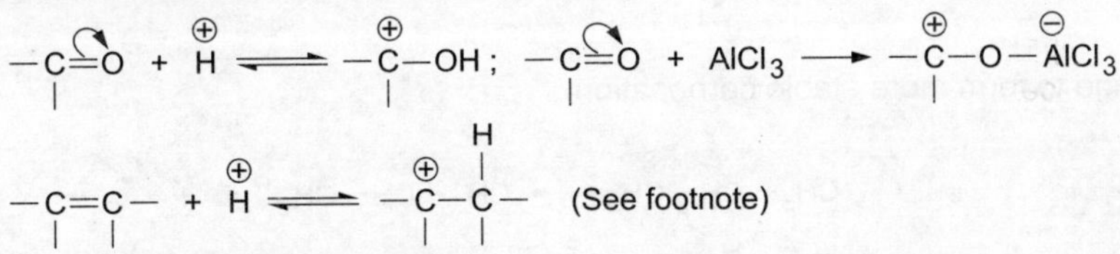

(ii) Compounds containing oxygen atoms.

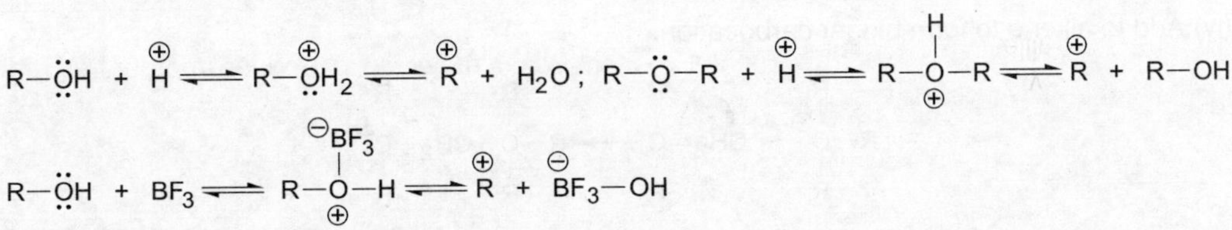

---

* A carbocation is called primary (1°), secondary (2°) or tertiary (3°) when the carbon bearing the positive charge is attached to one, two or three alkyl (i.e., carbon) groups respectively. If the charge on the carbon is negative, it is called 1°, 2° or 3° carbanion in similar way.

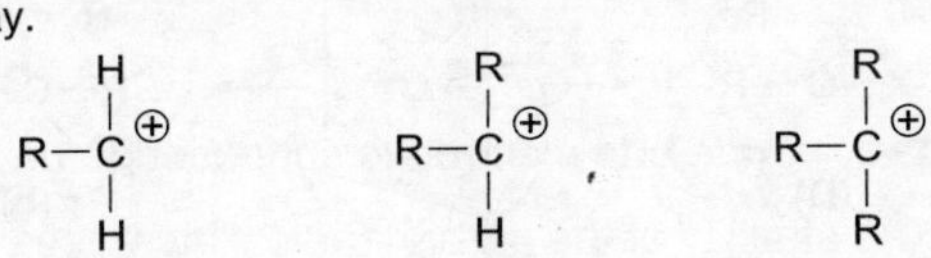

(1°) (2°) (3°)

(iii) Organic halides.

$$R{-}X + \overset{\oplus}{H} \rightleftharpoons R{-}\overset{\oplus}{X}H \rightleftharpoons \overset{\oplus}{R} + XH$$

(b) By the decomposition of diazonium salts.

$$\left[R{-}\overset{\oplus}{N}{\equiv}N{:}\right]\overset{\ominus}{Cl} \longrightarrow \overset{\oplus}{R} + N_2 + \overset{\ominus}{Cl}$$

(c) By ionization.

$$R_3C{-}X \rightleftharpoons R_3\overset{\oplus}{C} + \overset{\ominus}{X}$$

Reactions of carbocations—

(i) Recombine with electron-rich species (electron pair of an ion or molecule).

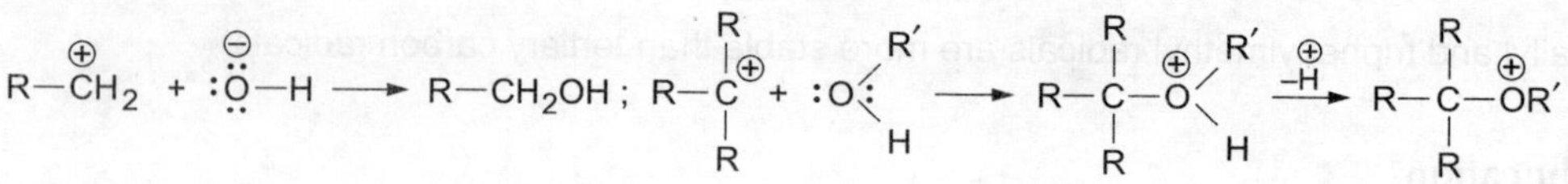

(ii) Eliminate a proton to form olefin.

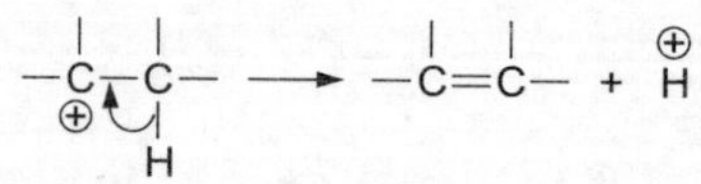

(iii) Rearrange to form more stable carbocation.

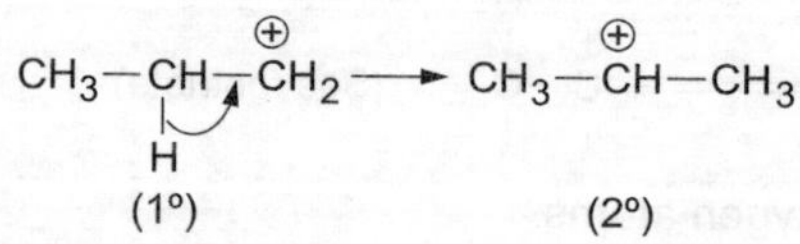

(iv) Add to alkene to form bigger carbocation.

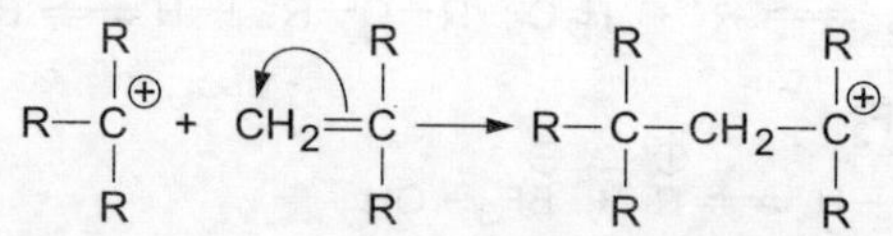

Geometric shape The carbocation takes up the more stable sp^2 configuration with the vacant 2p orbital at right angles to the plane of the sp^2 orbitals.

Stereochemical effect The vacant 2p orbital can be attacked from either side of the plane of the ion by an electron-rich species. This may result in the formation of both the optical isomers in suitable substrates.

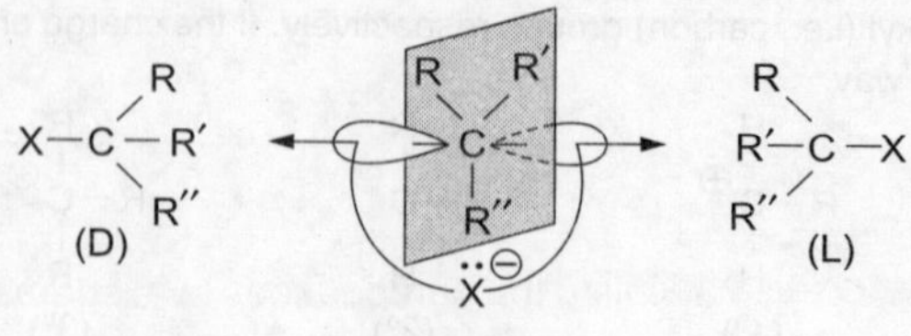

(iii) Carbanion

An ion in which the carbon bears the negative charge is called a carbon anion or carbanion. They are formed by heterolysis when a group departs from a molecule without the bonding pair of electrons.

Carbanions may be formed by the following methods:

(a) When a group or atom departs from a carbon atom without its bonding pair.

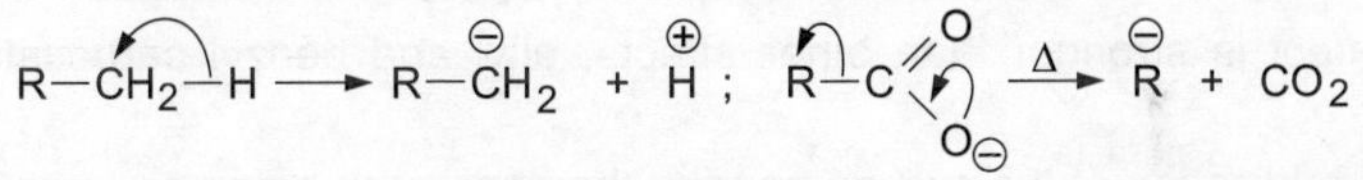

(b) When a negative ion attacks on a multiple bond.

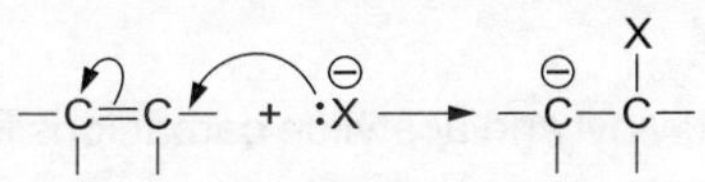

Reactions of carbanions They undergo two types of reactions—displacement and addition.

(i) Displacement reaction.

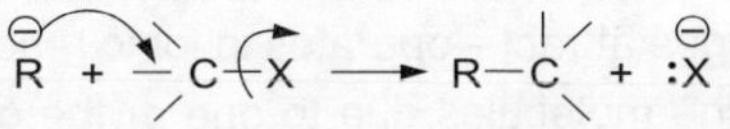 where R = $\overset{\ominus}{C}H(COOR)_2$, $CH_3CO\overset{\ominus}{C}HCOOR$, etc.

(ii) Addition reactions—Add to carbonyl groups and to suitably activated carbon–carbon double bonds.

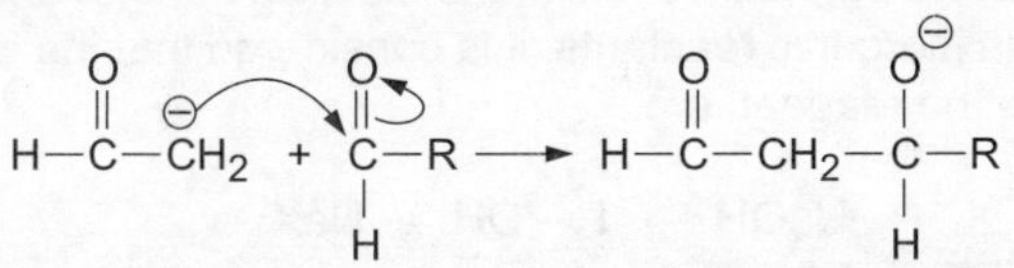

$$PhCH{=}CHCOOEt + \overset{\ominus}{C}H(COOR)_2 \xrightarrow{BH} Ph{-}\underset{\displaystyle CH(COOR)_2}{CH}{-}CH_2COOEt$$

Geometric shape Since in the formation of a carbanion, only an atom or a group departs without the bonding pair of electrons, the unbonded electron pair continues to remain in the same orbital as in the molecule, i.e., the hybridization of the carbanionic carbon is unaltered.

Stabilities of carbanions and carbocations The ionic intermediates are considered as carrying their charges on a carbon atom. However, the ions to some extent are stabilized by delocalization of the charge on other carbon atoms or other elements.

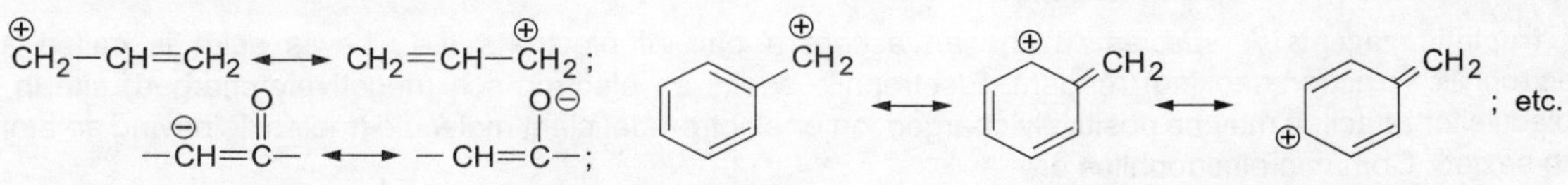

Inductive effect and hyperconjugation also stabilize the carbocations by dispersal of the charge. These effects are additive, hence the stability order of carbocations is 3° > 2° > 1° > $\overset{\oplus}{C}H_3$.

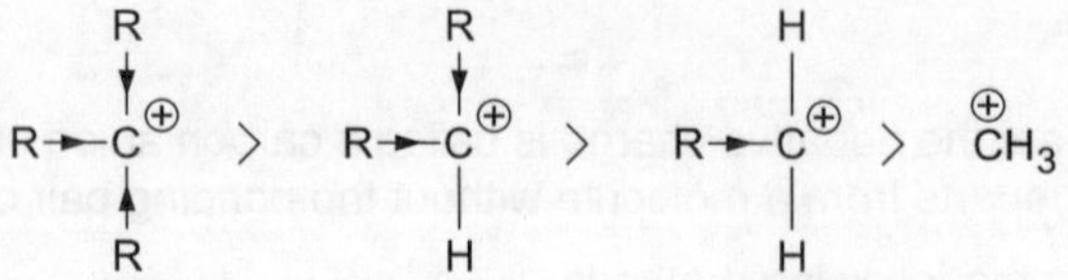

(3°) (2°) (1°)

The order is reversed in case of carbanions due to repulsion between like charges.

As resonance effect is stronger than other effects, allyl and benzyl carbocations are more stable than 3° carbocations.

Change in the hybridization of the carbon bearing the charge on going $sp \rightarrow sp^2 \rightarrow sp^3$ progressively decreases the stability of carbanions. This is due to the greater s character (50%) in sp orbital and least (25%) in sp^3 orbital, i.e., the electrons of sp orbital are more firmly held by the positive nucleus than those of sp^3 orbital with consequent stability.

Hence, the stability order of alkyl, vinyl and acetylide carbanions is $RC \equiv \overset{\ominus}{C} > RCH = \overset{\ominus}{C}H > R\overset{\ominus}{C}H_2$. There are other transient intermediates such as carbenes, R_2C:, chlorocarbenes, $:CCl_2$, nitrenes $R\ddot{N}$ and arynes.

REAGENTS

Majority of organic reactions are ionic and we will be interested in the reagents for ionic reactions. The classical rule of physics—like charges repel and unlike charges attract—operates in ionic reactions.

The electronic imbalance (i.e., dipolarity) created in the molecules due to one or the other structural features or by the approach of the two reactants results in the attraction of oppositely charged species in an ionic reaction. In an ionic reaction, therefore, one reactant donates and the other accepts an electron pair. The reactant which has greater energy takes the aggressive role in the electron transfer and is called the reagent. In a reaction between an organic and an inorganic reactants, it is considered that the organic molecule is the substrate and the inorganic molecule is the reagent, e.g.,

$$\underset{\text{substrate}}{R-X} + \underset{\text{reagent}}{NaOH} \rightarrow R-OH + NaX$$

In a reaction between two organic molecules, it is difficult to specify the reagent and the substrate. Ordinarily, however, the one with full blown charge is more reactive and may be considered as the reagent. Thus, $C_2H_5\overset{\ominus}{O}$ is the reagent in the reaction given below.

$$\underset{\text{substrate}}{R-X} + \underset{\text{reagent}}{C_2H_5\overset{\ominus}{O}\overset{\oplus}{Na}} \rightarrow C_2H_5OR + NaX$$

Broadly, the reagents are of two types. The one which attacks the positive site in the molecule is called the nucleophile or nucleophilic reagent and the one which attacks the negative site in the molecule is called the electrophile or electrophilic reagents.

Electrophilic reagents A species which can accept a pair of electrons (i.e., Lewis acid) is called an electrophilic (electron-seeking) reagent. Electrophile seeks an electron-rich (negatively charged) site in a molecule for attack. It may be positively charged ion or electron-deficient molecule (molecule having an atom with sextet). Common electrophiles are:

(a) Positively charged ions— $\overset{\oplus}{H}$, $H_3\overset{\oplus}{O}$, $\overset{\oplus}{X}$, $\overset{\oplus}{N}O_2$, $\overset{\oplus}{N}O$, $\overset{\oplus}{S}O_3H$, $C_6H_5\overset{\oplus}{N}_2$, $R_3\overset{\oplus}{C}$, etc.

(b) Electron-deficient molecules— BF_3, AlX_3, SO_3, CO_2, ICl, $SnCl_2$, $FeCl_3$, etc.

Nucleophilic reagents A species which can donate an unshared electron pair (Lewis base) is called a nucleophilic (nucleus-seeking) reagent or nucleophile. Nucleophile seeks an electron-deficient site for the attack. It may be a negatively charged ion or a molecule having an unshared electron pair. Some common nucleophiles are:

(a) Negatively charged ion— $\overset{\ominus}{H}$, $H\overset{\ominus}{O}$, $\overset{\ominus}{C}N$, $R\overset{\ominus}{O}$, $R\overset{\ominus}{S}$, $RC\equiv\overset{\ominus}{C}$, $RCO\overset{\ominus}{O}$, $\overset{\ominus}{N}H_2$, $\overset{\ominus}{C}H(COOR)_2$, etc.

(b) Electron-rich molecules— $H_2\ddot{O}$, $R-\ddot{O}-H$, $R-\ddot{N}H_2$, $\ddot{N}H_3$, $R_3\ddot{N}$, RMgBr, RLi, etc.

ENERGETICS OF REACTIONS

An organic reaction is a process of bond breaking and bond making. Since a bond is associated with energy, a chemical reaction essentially involves the energy change of the system. Every system seeks to attain the state of minimum energy. A chemical reaction attains equilibrium when the energy change in the system is complete. If the products have much lower energy than the reactants, a large amount of products will be formed before the equilibrium is attained. In other words, the energy difference between the reactants and products (usually denoted by ΔH) and the position of equilibrium are directly related.

The energies of molecules are dependent on structural features. If some structural feature stabilizes one molecule over the other, however small, the equilibrium will shift towards the more stable molecule.

RATE OF REACTION AND TRANSITION STATE

Wood, paper, etc., when burnt in air are converted into CO_2, H_2O, etc., i.e., the organic molecules (cellulose) react with oxygen and pass to more stable states (CO_2, H_2O, etc.). Although the energy difference between the reactants and products is fairly large, yet it is rarely observed that wood or paper spontaneously burns in the presence of oxygen.

In most chemical reactions increase in temperature results in increase in the reaction rate. Frequency of collision increases with the molecular motion which in turn increases with temperature. Arrhenius postulated that even though there is a net gain of energy in a reaction, yet some extra amount of energy has to be supplied to bring about the reaction. This indicates that without the supply of extra energy, the collision between the reactants is not sufficient to result in the products. The extra amount of energy which must be supplied by collision for a reaction to occur is known as the energy of activation (E_{act}). E_{act} is essential for most reactions. It forms the energy barrier between the reactants and the products. It is this energy barrier which protects us from being burnt out in air.

Reasons for requirement of the extra amount of energy (E_{act}) for reactions:

(i) The energy gained in the process of bond making (in the intermediates and products) is not fully available for bond breaking in the reactants.

(ii) Reactant particles do not move with the same speed. Those moving slowly bounce apart on collision without any effect. Those moving fast can bring home the effect (reaction) on collision.

(iii) The reacting particles having enough energy may not react on collision if they are not properly oriented.

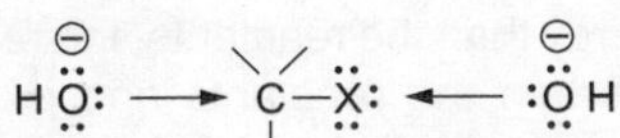

Effective collision — Non-effective collision

Moreover, if the E_{act}, which increases the amplitude of the fundamental vibrations of the particles, results in stretching the wrong bond, it will not assist the reaction. Thus, in the reaction

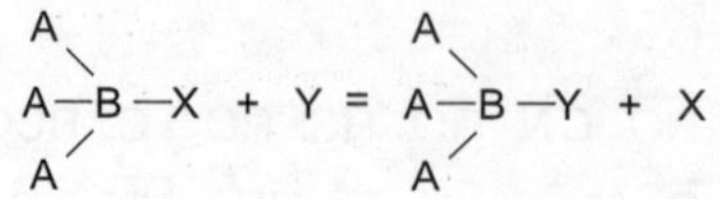

only the stretching of B – X bond will aid the reaction. Hence, a probability factor is involved. We can, therefore, define E_{act} as the minimum amount of energy which must be supplied to surmount the collision and the probability factors. For similar types of reactions the collision and the probability factors are nearly the same. Hence the rate is largely dependent on E_{act}. Lower the E_{act}, faster is the reaction and higher the E_{act}, slower is the reaction.

Transition state

A chemical reaction is a continuous process. The reactants continuously change their geometry under the stress and strain of the reaction conditions and pass through an optimum state when the effective collision has been achieved. This state in the course of reactions is called the transition state, so called because the reactants change from one form to another after this state. The transition state, i.e., the activated complex, is not a real molecule, for partial bonds are formed at the site of reaction. It can be visualized as a complex molecule with a temporary arrangement of atoms with transient existence and which readily passes into a more stable arrangement as products. Transition state is the most important state in a chemical reaction. Transition state and E_{act} are interrelated.

The minimum energy necessary to fulfil all the conditions for the formation of the transition state is the E_{act} of the reaction. Thus, the energy of the transition state is the energy of activation. Higher the energy of the transition state, higher is the energy barrier and slower is the rate of reaction. In a multistage reaction, several transition states are formed but the one with the highest energy controls the rate of the reaction. More stable is the transition state, lower is its energy and more readily it is formed.

Energy diagram The energy changes of a chemical reaction are depicted by energy diagram which shows the progress of the reaction along a path of lowest energy to products. The diagram shows the energy changes against the progress of the reaction. Attention is focused on the starting state, the transition state and the final state.

In the beginning the collision between the reacting particles causes their KE to be used up in increasing their PE until the transition state is formed. As the transition state collapses to form the product, the PE drops and is converted to KE which is given out as heat. The graph starts at the left showing the energies of the reactants, gradually rises to a maximum, as it proceeds along the reaction coordinate, to show the energy of the transition state. The graph then drops to indicate the final energies of the products. The highest point of the graph corresponds to the energy of the transition state.

When the products have lower energy than the reactants, the reaction is called *exothermic* since energy is liberated. The energy difference between the reactants and products is indicated by $-\Delta H$. When the products have higher energy than the reactants, the reaction proceeds by absorption of heat and is called *endothermic.* The energy difference is indicated by $+\Delta H$. For such reaction, a high-energy reagent is used since it is the energy difference of the system which shifts the equilibrium to one direction.

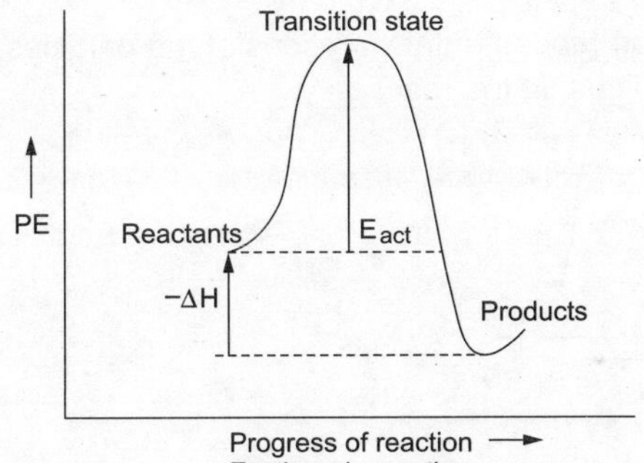

Exothermic reaction

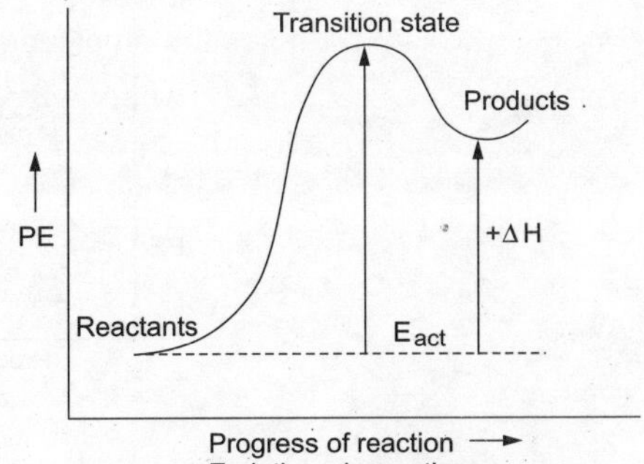

Endothermic reaction

In exothermic reaction the E_{act} may be lower or higher than ΔH. In contrast, it cannot be less than ΔH in endothermic reaction. The endothermic reactions are slower (i.e., difficult) than exothermic reactions. From the diagram it is clear that a reaction cannot be faster than the rate of formation of the transition state. Therefore, the rate-determining step is the energy height of transition state, i.e., E_{act}.

In fact all reactions are in equilibrium. The condition for equilibrium reaction is the energy difference between the reactants and products. When the reaction is very rapid, the E_{act} can be ignored since it is so low that it is available from the thermal changes at room temperature. In such case only ΔH is important since it determines the shift of the equilibrium. The reaction is then equilibrium-controlled. The equilibrium constant K and ΔH are related.

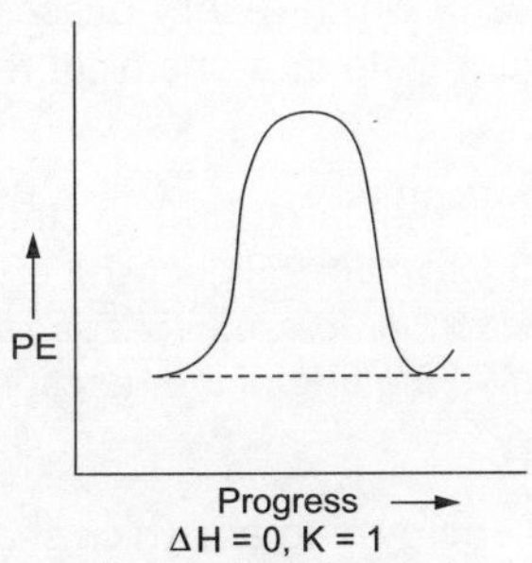

$\Delta H = 0, K = 1$
Reactants and products equally present

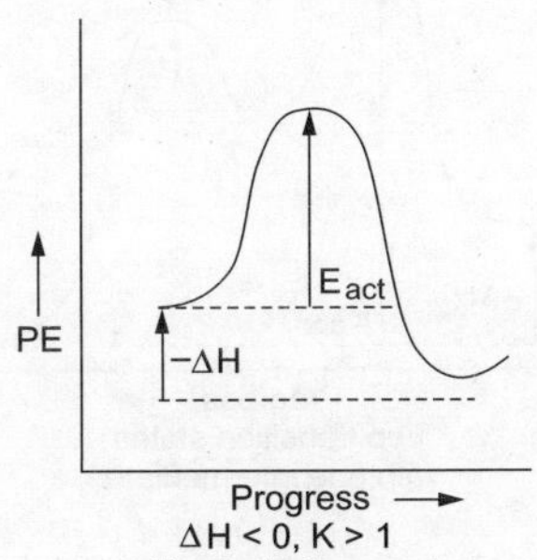

$\Delta H < 0, K > 1$
Products favoured

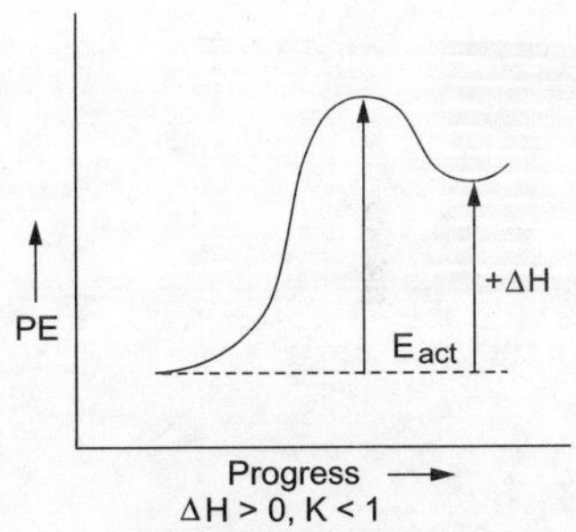

$\Delta H > 0, K < 1$
Reactants favoured

The E_{act} is important for slow reactions.

When several products are formed in a reaction, the one formed at the early stage may not be the most stable product. On prolonging the reaction, the products are brought under equilibrium when the most stable product predominates. The initially formed product in the first step is called kinetically controlled product and the final predominating product is called the equilibrium-controlled product.

A multistage reaction may pass through a number of transition states. In a two-step reaction the minimum of the curve between the two transition states is the energy valley of an intermediate. If the valley is very low, the intermediate is stable enough to be isolated. If the energy height of the adjacent transition state is less than 20 kcal/mol, the intermediate is not isolable at room temperature.

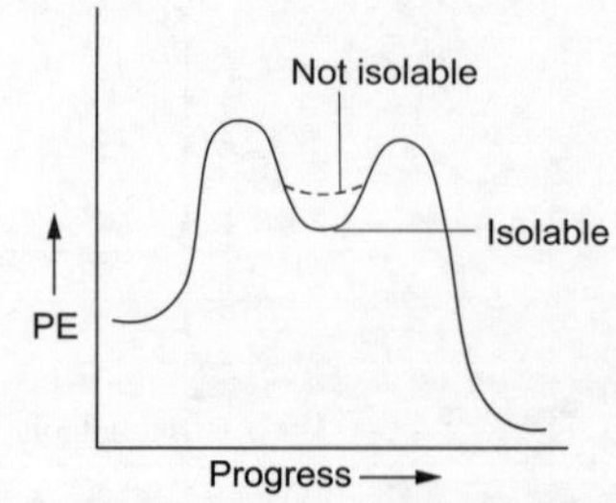

If the E_{act} is low, the transition state is formed early and its geometry will be very nearly that of the substrate. If the transition state is formed late (i.e., the E_{act} is high), its geometry will be nearly that of the product. Any factor that assists in the stabilization of the transition state will lower its energy, i.e., lower the E_{act} and the reaction rate will be fast.

A catalyst is a substance which provides a reaction path of lower energy than the one in its absence. It increases the reaction rate by lowering the energy of the transition state.

Energy diagrams of some common reactions are given below.

Energy diagram of the reaction which proceeds—

(i) In two steps, the first step being slowest, e.g., electrophilic addition, base-catalysed nucleophilic addition, nucleophilic substitution (S_N1), electrophilic aromatic substitution, etc.

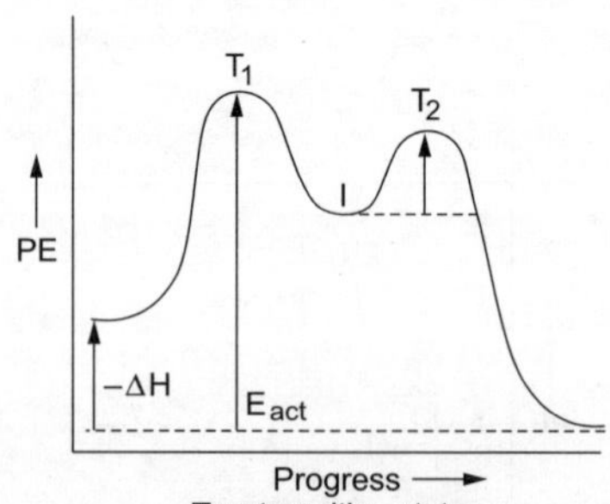

Two transition states with one intermediate

(ii) In two steps, the second step being slowest, e.g., acid-catalysed nucleophilic addition.

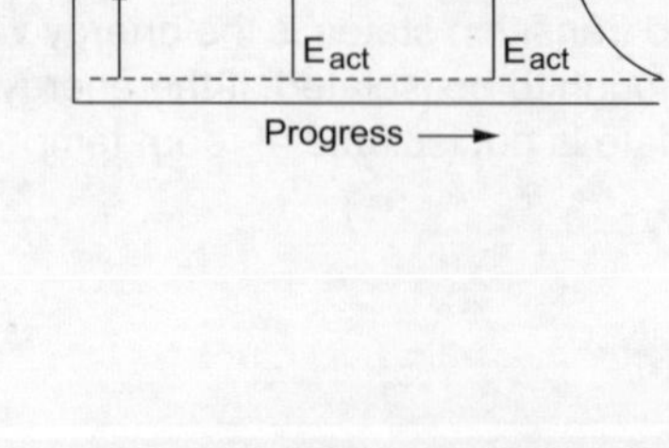

(iii) In one step, e.g., S_N2 reaction.

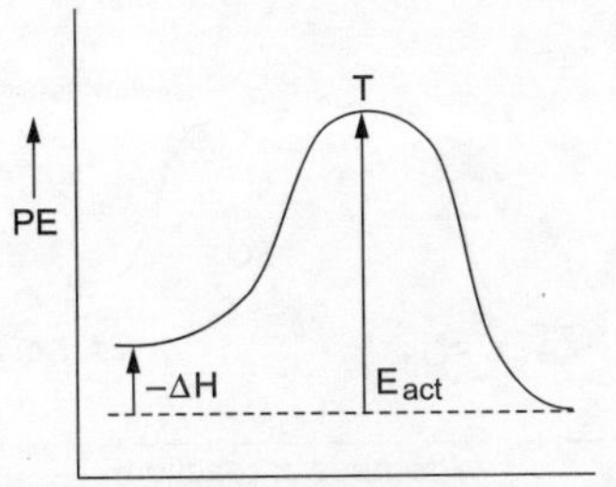

One transition state with no intermediate

Energy diagram of S_N1 vs S_N2—The order of hydrolysis of alkyl halides by S_N1 path is 3° > 2° > 1° and by S_N2 path is 1° > 2° > 3°. Hence, S_N1 vs S_N2 energy diagrams for 1° and 3° halides are:

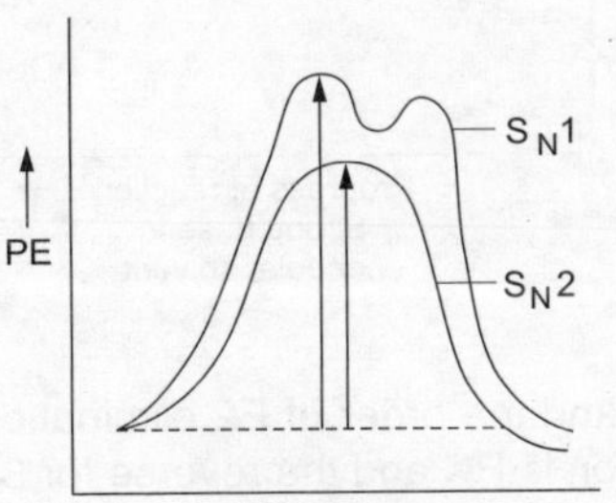

Lower-energy path S_N2 for 1° halides

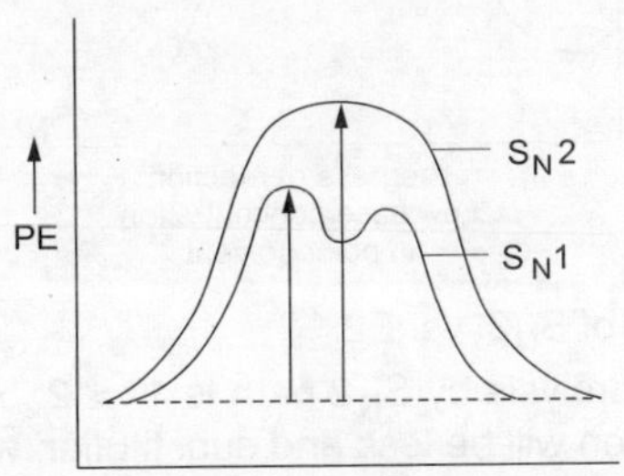

Lower-energy path S_N1 for 3° halides

Energy diagram of electrophilic substitution in benzene with (a) activating substituent and (b) deactivating substituent:

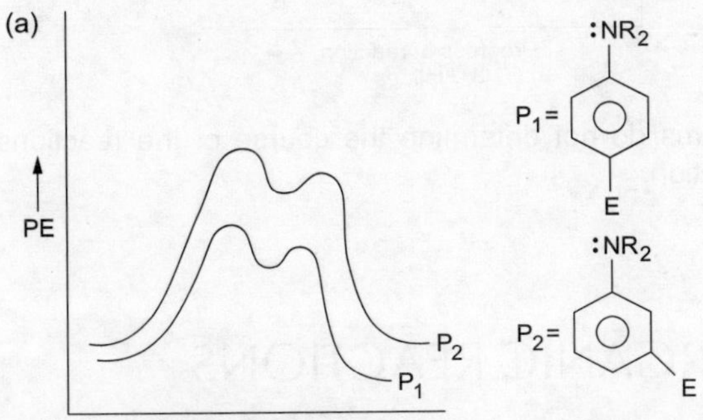

Lower-energy path for *p*-substitution (also for *o*-position)

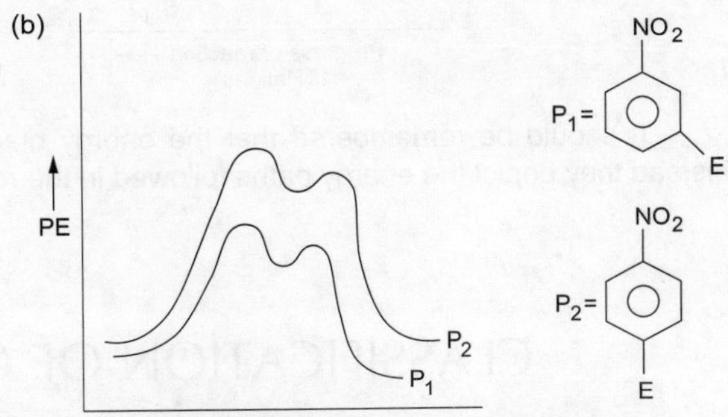

Lower-energy path for *m*-substitution

Energy diagram of sulphonation Sulphonation, unlike other electrophilic aromatic substitution is reversible. Hence, the carbocation formed on attack of SO_3 can lose SO_3 to revert to benzene. Therefore, the energy barrier heights on either side of the carbocation are nearly the same.

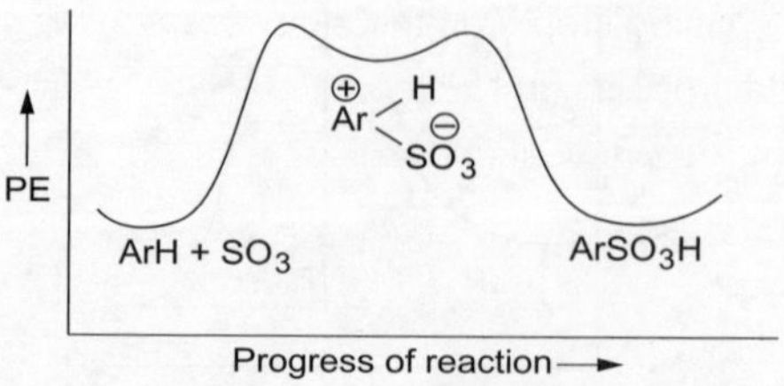

Energy diagram of S_N1 vs E1 for 3° halides—The reactivity order of RX is 3° > 2° > 1° for S_N1 and E1. Hence, the rate depends upon the base concentration and polarity of the solvent.

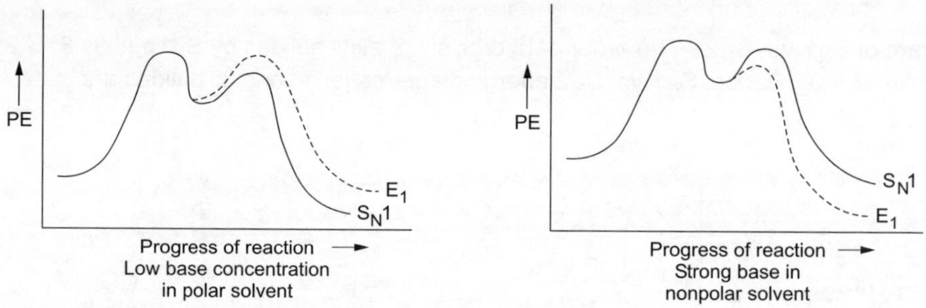

Energy diagram of S_N2 vs E2.

The order of hydrolysis by S_N2 path is 1° > 2° > 3° halides and the order of E2 elimination is 3° > 2° > 1°. Hence, elimination will be less and substitution will be more for 1° RX and the reverse for 3° RX.

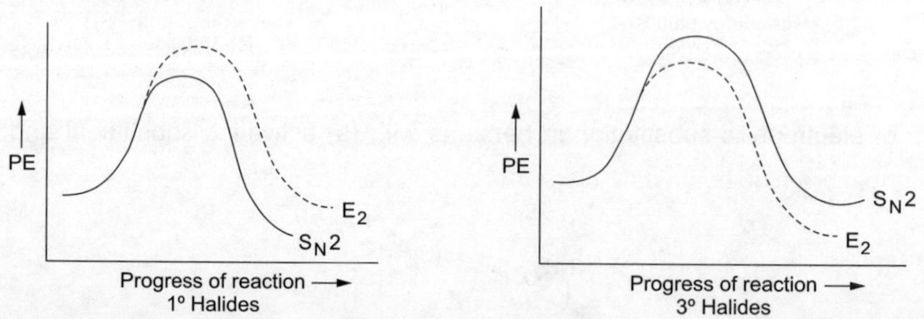

It should be remembered that the energy diagrams do not determine the course of the reactions, instead they depict the energy paths followed in the reaction.

CLASSIFICATION OF ORGANIC REACTIONS

Organic reactions have been broadly classified into two types on the basis of bond cleavage, e.g.,

(i) free radical reactions (homolytic cleavage) and

(ii) ionic reactions (heterolytic cleavage).

A second type of yet another broad classification is on the basis of the products of the reactions, e.g., (a) addition reaction, (b) substitution reaction, (c) elimination reaction and (d) rearrangement.

The above two classifications do not specify the reaction type. A more satisfactory classification has been made by subclassification of the latter three types of reactions (a), (b) and (c) on the basis of the reagents involved in the rate-determining step, i.e., the slowest step. Thus,

1. Addition reactions—(i) Electrophilic (ii) Nucleophilic
2. Substitution reactions—(i) Free radical (ii) Nucleophilic—S_N1, S_N2 and S_Ni (iii) Electrophilic
3. Elimination reactions—E1 and E2
4. Rearrangements

1. ADDITION REACTIONS

A reaction in which the substrate and the reagent add up to form a product is called addition reaction. The reaction occurs at the site of unsaturation in a molecule. Thus, compounds having multiple bonds such as

$$>C=C<, \quad -C\equiv C-, \quad >C=O, \quad -C\equiv N, \text{ etc.}$$

undergo addition reactions.

The reactivity of these compounds is due to the more exposed and easily available π electrons to the electron-seeking (electrophilic) reagent.

(i) Electrophilic addition reaction

This is a characteristic reaction of unsaturated hydrocarbons, e.g.,

$$\underset{\text{Ethylene}}{CH_2{=}CH_2} + Br_2 \xrightarrow{CCl_4} \underset{\text{Ethylene bromide}}{CH_2Br{-}CH_2Br}$$

Both the reactants add to form a single product.

Mechanism The mechanism of the reaction is based on the following observations.

(i) When ethylene is brominated in aqueous solution in the presence of sodium chloride, the product in addition to ethylene dibromide contains 1-chloro-2-bromoethane.

$$CH_2{=}CH_2 \xrightarrow{Br_2 + \overset{\ominus}{Cl}} CH_2Br{-}CH_2Br + BrCH_2{-}CH_2Cl$$

This indicates that a carbocation formed in the first step is attacked by both $\overset{\ominus}{Br}$ (from Br_2) and $\overset{\ominus}{Cl}$ (present in solution) in the second step.

(ii) On bromination *trans*-2-butene gives *meso*-dibromide and *cis*-2-butene gives racemic (DL) modification. This indicates addition of bromine atoms to the π bond from opposite sides of the plane of the ethylene molecule i.e., trans-addition results.

On the basis of the above observations, the following mechanism is suggested: On the approach of the two reactants the Br – Br bond is polarized by the π electrons to form a π complex which breaks down to form a cyclic bromonium ion and the other bromine atom leaves with the bonding pair of electrons in the first step. In the second step the bromide ion attacks either of the carbons (originally double-bonded) from the opposite side to complete the addition. This results in trans-addition.

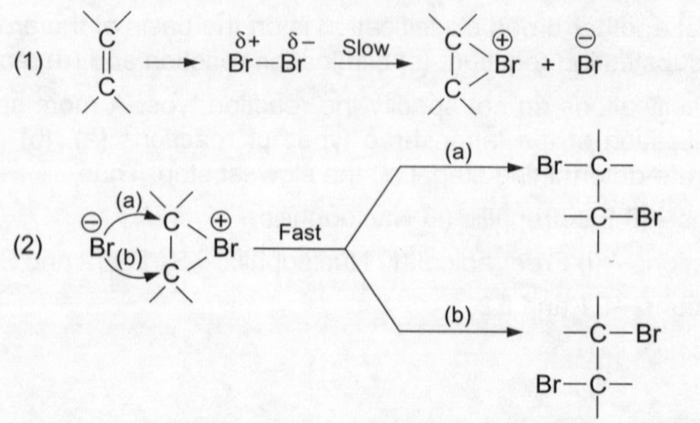

On the basis of the formation of bromonium ion, the formation of *meso*-dibromide from *trans*-2-butene and racemic dibromide from *cis*-2-butene on bromination can now be explained.

Trans

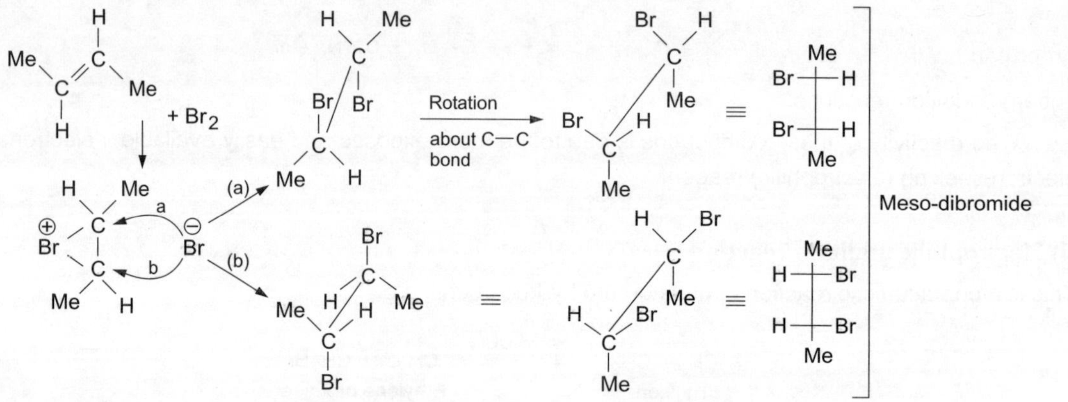

Cis

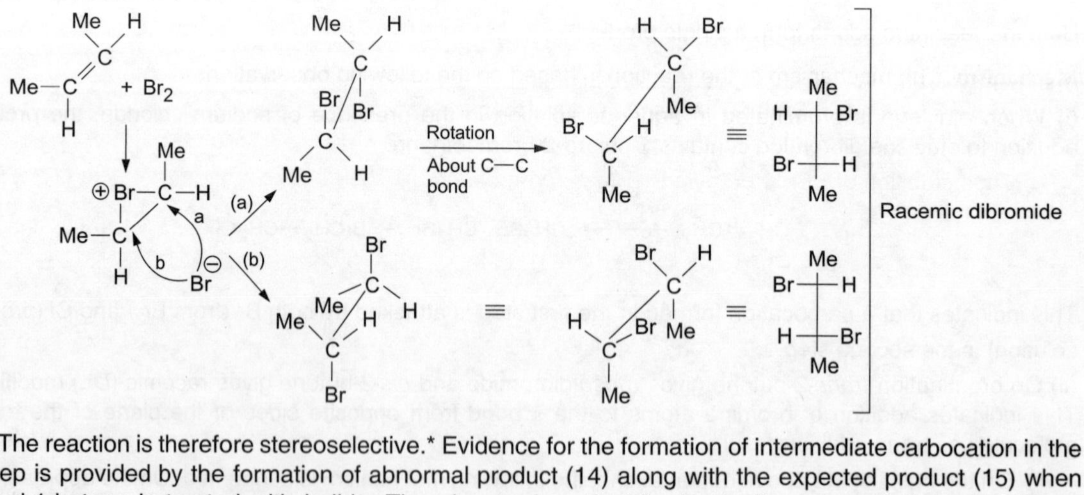

The reaction is therefore stereoselective.* Evidence for the formation of intermediate carbocation in the first step is provided by the formation of abnormal product (14) along with the expected product (15) when 3-methyl-1-butene is treated with halide. The abnormal product is due to the inherent characteristics of rearrangement of carbocations for stability.

* Any reaction in which only one of a set of stereoisomers is formed predominantly or exclusively is called stereoselective.

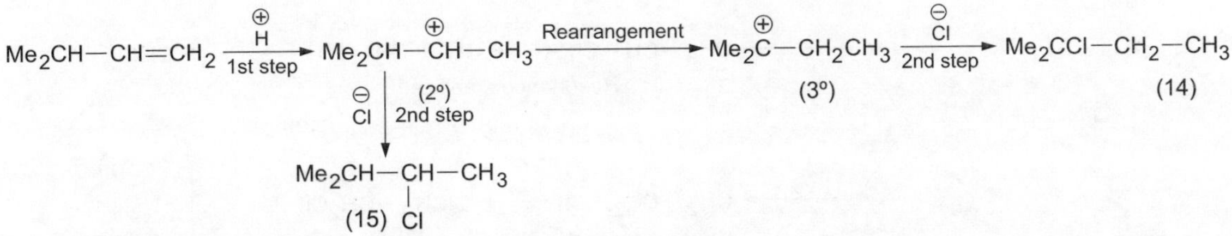

Hence, the bromonium ion may be considered as a resonance hybrid of the following canonical forms, i.e., an alternative canonical form of the carbocation.

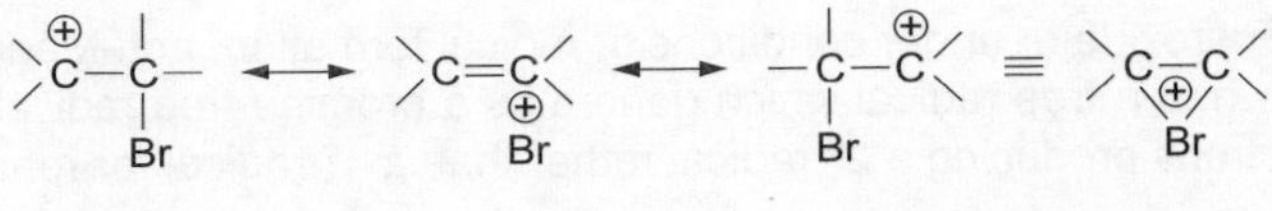

The first step of the reaction is slow due to polarisation of bonds, formation of π complex and bromonium ion or carbocation. In contrast, the second step is fast due to attraction between oppositely charged ions. Since the slowest step is initiated by electrophile and the overall reaction is addition, the reaction has been classed as 'electrophilic addition'.

Effect of substituents It is seen that a bromonium ion or a carbocation is formed in the rate-determining step. It is logical to assume that electron-donating substituents will not only increase the electron density for facile electrophilic attack but also aid to stabilize the carbocation. Thus, the activation energy for the formation of the carbocation is lowered so that the reaction becomes fast. The relative rates of addition of some substituted alkenes are:

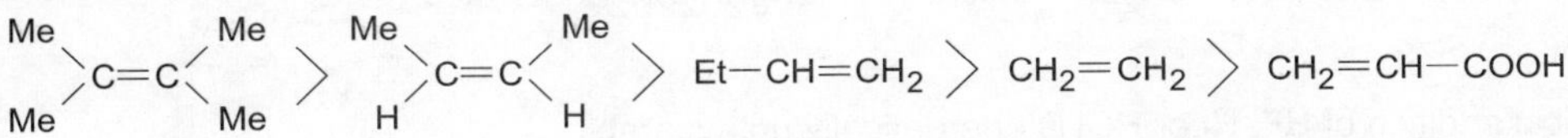

Obviously, electron-withdrawing groups will have reverse effect.

Markovnikov rule In case of addition of unsymmetrical reagents (e.g., HX) to unsymmetrical alkenes, the negative moiety (i.e., nucleophile) of the addendum (reagent) attacks the more highly substituted carbon. This is known as Markovnikov rule.

Thus, addition of HBr to propylene gives 2-bromopropane (16) and not 1-bromopropane (17).

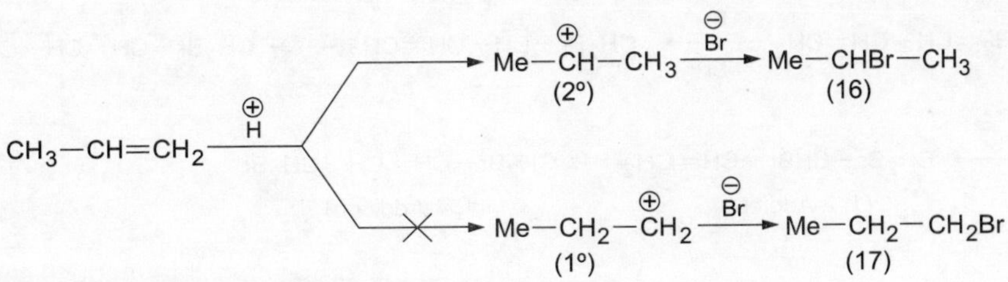

Markovnikov rule is explained on the basis of the stability of the first formed carbocation. Since 2° carbocation is more stable and hence formed more easily than 1° carbocation, the product is (16). Thus, when more than one carbocation formation is possible, the most stable of the carbocations will determine the orientation of the overall addition. This is seen in the addition of HCl to vinyl chloride when ethylidene chloride (18) and not ethylene chloride (19) is obtained.

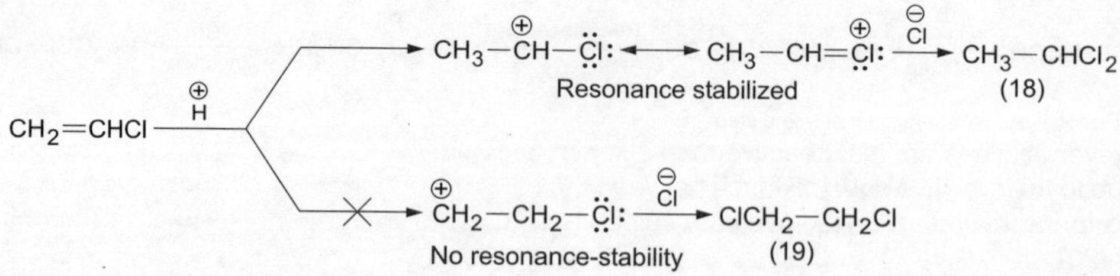

The rate of addition is, however, slower (about 30 times) than with ethane due to the electron-withdrawing effect of chlorine.

In the presence of peroxide or under conditions of radical formation, anti-Markovnikov addition results. The peroxide breaks down to a free radical which generates a bromine-free radical from HBr. The bromine radical attacks the π electrons producing a 2° radical rather than a 1° radical for reasons of stability.

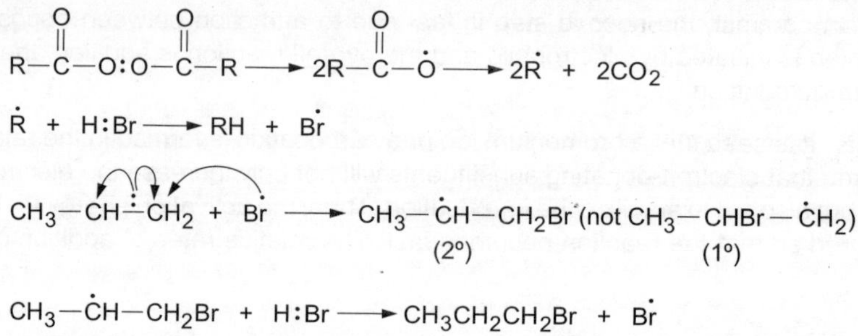

Free radical addition of HF, HI or HCl is energetically unfavourable.

Addition to conjugated dienes Conjugated dienes, e.g., 1, 3-butadiene, undergo electrophilic addition in a similar stepwise process. However, more than one addition product is formed.

This is due to the preferential formation of a resonance-stabilized allylic carbocation in the first step in which the positive charge resides on both C_2 and C_4 either of which can be attacked by the nucleophile in the second step to result in 1, 2, and 1, 4-addition products.

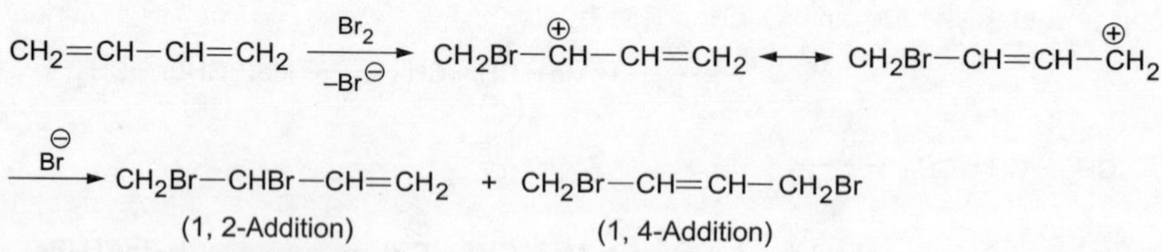

The 1, 2-product predominating at lower temperature and 1,4-product predominating at higher temperature. This may be due to stabilization of 1, 4-product by hyperconjugation.

Addition to alkynes Electrophilic addition to alkynes resembles those of alkenes. For example, one molecule of bromine adds first to acetylene in two steps to give *trans* 1, 2-dibromoethylene and then another molecule of bromine adds to give 1, 1, 2, 2-tetrabromoethane.

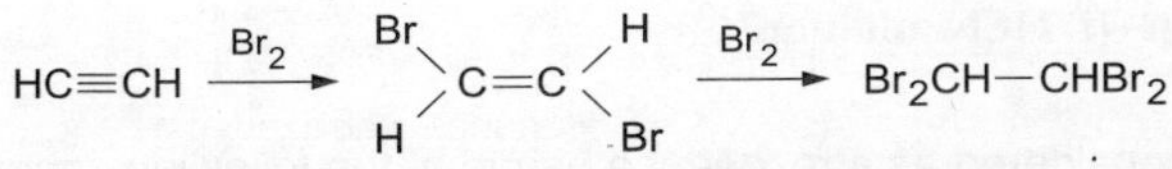

However, alkynes are less reactive than alkenes because the π electrons are more tightly held by the carbons due to their relative short distance between the carbons (1.20 Å for C ≡ C and 1.34 Å for C = C). This is reflected in the hydration of alkynes with sulphuric acid in which the aid of a catalyst (mercuric salt) is necessary (20).

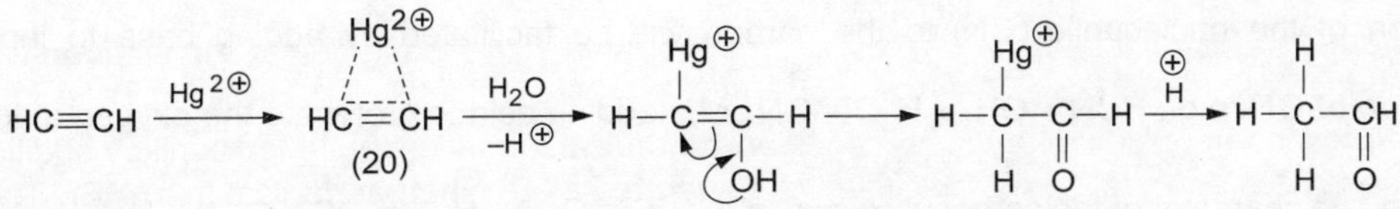

Aromatic compounds (e.g., benzene) have π electrons which are tightly held by several nuclei. Aromatic compounds are, therefore, much less reactive and undergo a few addition reactions. It is more so because addition reaction is energetically unprofitable due to loss of resonance energy.

(ii) Nucleophilic addition reaction

We have seen that electron-releasing groups conjugated to carbon–carbon multiple bonds promote electrophilic addition. In the same way, conjugation of electron-withdrawing groups activate the carbon–carbon multiple bonds towards nucleophilic addition.

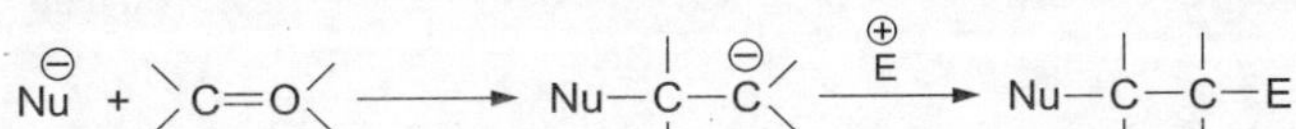

The substituents reduce the π-electron density, thereby aid the attack of the nucleophile and stabilize the carbanion formed on attack by delocalization of the negative charge (cf. Michael reaction). Some common electron-withdrawing groups are:

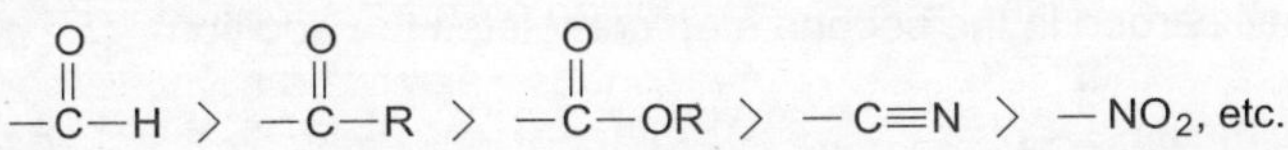

Polar functional groups, e.g., > C = O, – C ≡ N, > C = N, > C = S, etc., also undergo nucleophilic addition. The hetero atoms, like the electron-withdrawing substituents, reduce the π-electron density on the carbonyl carbon and stabilize the anion, formed on attack of the nucleophile, by accommodating the –ve charge.

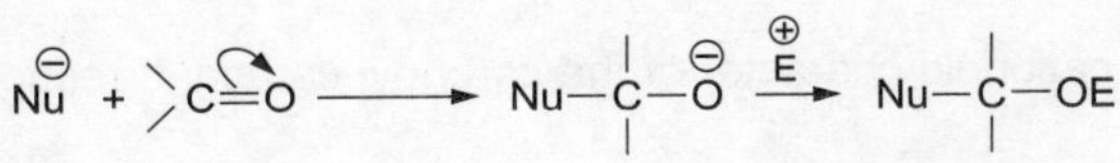

However, the addition product will be stable enough to be isolated provided the carbonyl group is not attached to a good leaving group such as OH, OR, Cl, NH_2, etc. Carboxylic acids and their derivatives, therefore, undergo substitution rather than addition on attack of nucleophiles.

Nucleophilic addition to carbonyl group is, therefore, a characteristic reaction of aldehydes and ketones since $\overset{\ominus}{H}$, $\overset{\ominus}{R}$ and $\overset{\ominus}{Ar}$ are not good leaving groups. Considering the steric and electronic factors (inductive effect) of the group attached to the carbonyl carbon, the reactivity of the carbonyl groups decreases in the order: $H_2C = O > RCHO > R_2CO > ArCHO > Ar_2CO$.

(a) Addition to carbonyl group—(i) HCN addition

Mechanism

The carbonyl group may be considered as a resonance hybrid of the following canonical structures:

$$-\overset{|}{C}=O \longleftrightarrow -\overset{\oplus}{\underset{|}{C}}-\overset{\ominus}{O}$$

The addition of the nucleophile ($\overset{\ominus}{C}N$) to the carbon will be facilitated by adding base to increase the concentration of $\overset{\ominus}{C}N$, e.g., $HCN + \overset{\ominus}{O}H \rightarrow H_2O + \overset{\ominus}{C}N$ or by adding acid to protonate the oxygen atom so as to increase the +ve character of the carbonyl carbon, e.g., $>C=O + \overset{\oplus}{H} \longrightarrow >\overset{\oplus}{C}-O-H$. Hence, the reaction is catalysed by both, acids and bases. However, base-catalysed nucleophilic addition reactions are common.

Base-catalysed—The base removes the weakly acidic protons from the reagent to generate the nucleophile which adds to the carbonyl carbon in the first step. In the second step a fast addition of protons to the negatively charged oxygen completes the addition.

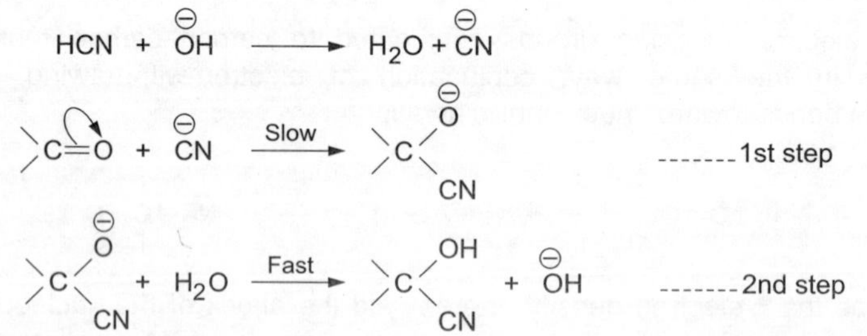

Acid-catalysed—The acid protonates the negatively charged oxygen atom in the first step. The slow attack of the reagent to the carbonyl carbon in the second step completes the addition.

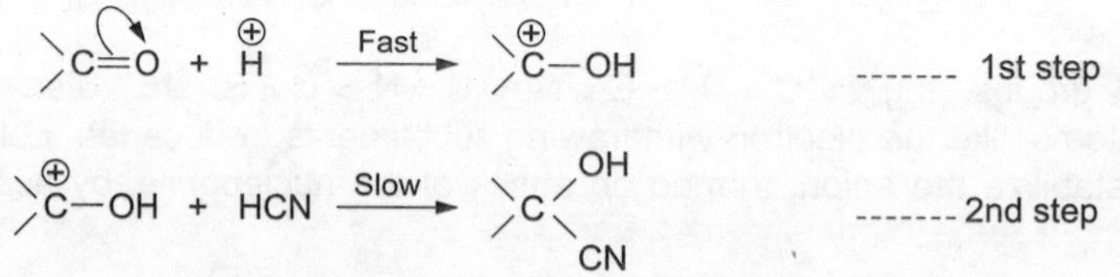

Although acids increase the cationoid character of the carbonyl carbon, it reduces the concentration of the nucleophile, e.g.,

$$\overset{\ominus}{C}N + \overset{\oplus}{H} \longrightarrow HCN\,; \quad R\ddot{N}H_2 + \overset{\oplus}{H} \longrightarrow R\overset{\oplus}{N}H_3$$

Hence, highly acidic medium retards the reaction. Weak acids which can form hydrogen bond are used. In practice the carbonyl compound is mixed with sodium cyanide and acid is added to generate HCN. The acid should be insufficient to consume all the sodium cyanide so that the medium remains alkaline.

In both acid- and base-catalysed additions, the nucleophile is added in the slowest step and hence the reaction is called nucleophilic addition.

Addition product of carbonyl compound with HCl is not isolable. The equilibrium lies far to the left since chlorine is a good leaving group.

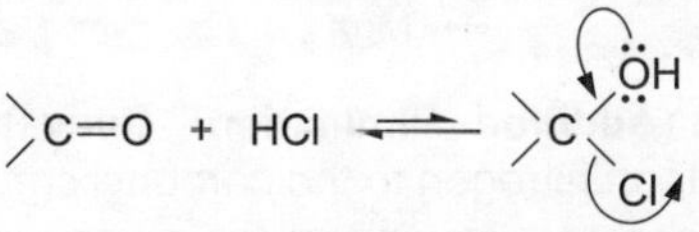

A number of carbonyl addition reactions follow the same mechanistic pattern of cyanohydrine formation. A few of these are mentioned.

(ii) Alcohol addition The addition of alcohol to carbonyl group to form hemiacetal is catalysed by both base and acid but the formation of acetal from hemiacetal is catalysed by acids only.

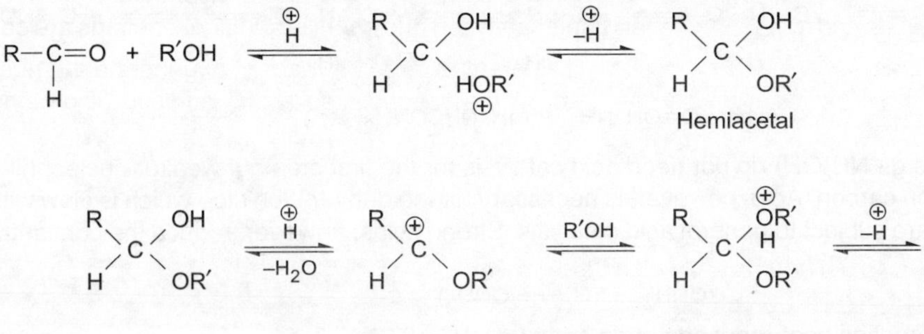

(iii) Bisulphite addition Aldehydes, methyl ketones or cyclic ketones add with sodium bisulphite in aqueous medium to form crystalline adducts. The effective nucleophile is $SO_3^{2\ominus}$ which is a strong nucleophile, and so no catalyst is required for the addition.

$$NaHSO_3 \rightleftharpoons \overset{\oplus}{Na} + \overset{\oplus}{H} + SO_3^{2\ominus}$$

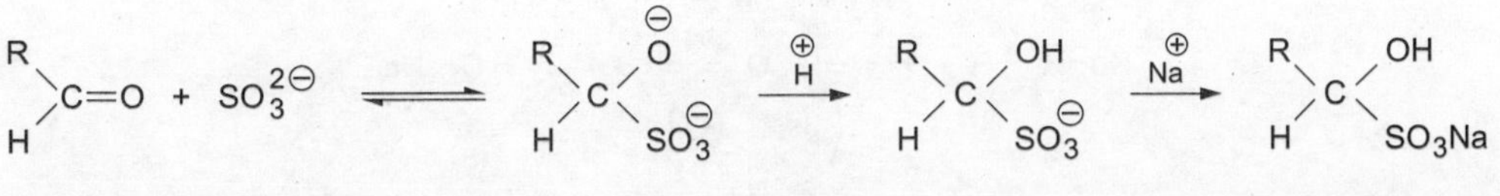

(iv) Carbanion addition A large number of carbanion addition reactions are known. Addition of Grignard reagent is given for illustration. Grignard reagent may be considered as a carbanion donor due to the polarized carbon–metal bond, $\overset{\delta-}{R}—\overset{\delta+}{MgX}$.

A straight forward reaction is then possible, e.g.,

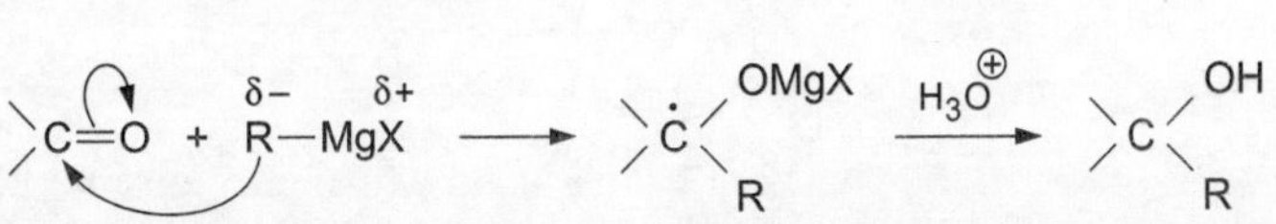

However, addition of $MgBr_2$ (Lewis acid) increases the rate of addition. From this and other evidence (complex of Mg with the carbonyl oxygen), it is suggested that one molecule of RMgX complexes with the oxygen to facilitate the attack of the other molecule to the carbonyl carbon.

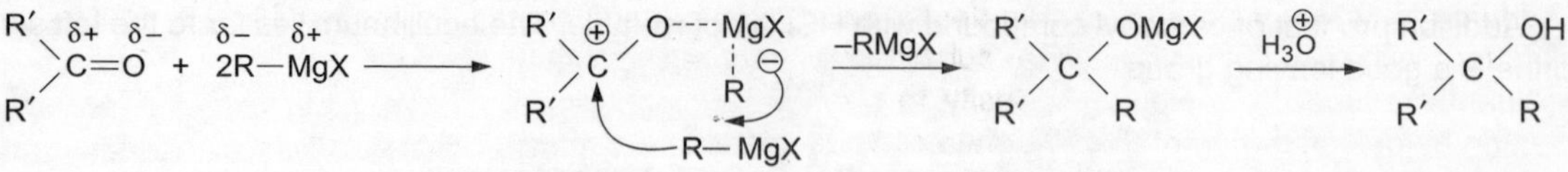

(v) Addition of derivatives of ammonia (Addition–elimination) Derivatives of ammonia add to the carbonyl group by donating the free electron pair on nitrogen to the carbonyl carbon. Subsequent migration of a proton from the nitrogen to the negatively charged oxygen gives a product which on protonation eliminates a molecule of water. The result is replacement of oxygen and formation of a stable product. Thus, hydroxylamine, hydrazine, phenylhydrazine, semicarbazide, etc., give respectively oxime, hydrazone, phenylhydrazone, semicarbazone, etc. The mechanisms of the reaction are generalised as given below.

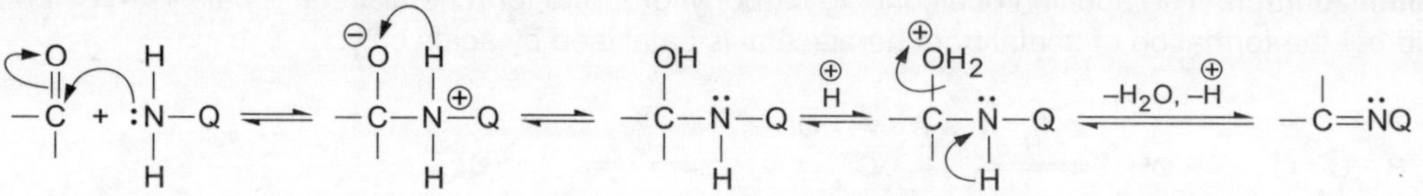

(where Q = OH, NH_2, PhNH, $NHCONH_2$, etc.)

Strong nucleophiles (e.g., NH_2OH) do not need acid catalysis for the first step but weaker nucleophiles need acid to aid the attack on carbon. Acid, however, is necessary for the dehydration step which is slow with base. Hence, the reactions are subject to general acid catalysis. Strong acids, however, reduce the concentration of nucleophiles $(Q\ddot{N}H_2 + \overset{\oplus}{H} \longrightarrow Q\overset{\oplus}{N}H_3)$.

Therefore, the reaction best proceeds at an optimum pH ($\approx$ 3–4).

Orientation of addition to carbonyl group– Since the carbon-hetero atom bond is polar, oxygen forming the negative end of the dipole, nucleophile is attached to the carbon and electrophile to the oxygen atom.

Stereochemistry of nucleophilic addition to carbonyl group– The molecule is flat as the carbon is sp^2-hybridized. Since both the sides are equivalent, the nucleophile is free to approach the carbon from either side of the plane to produce a racemic mixture.

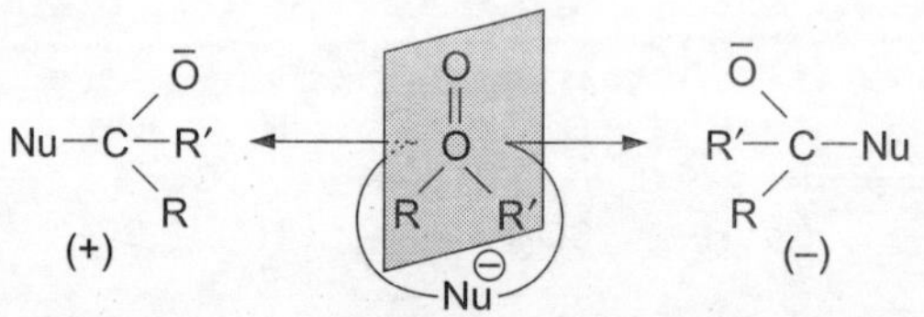

When the carbonyl group of ketones has an asymmetric α-carbon, the two sides of the flat carbonyl compound are no longer equivalent. The bulky oxygen atom orients itself so that it is farthest from the largest of the three groups on the α-carbon.

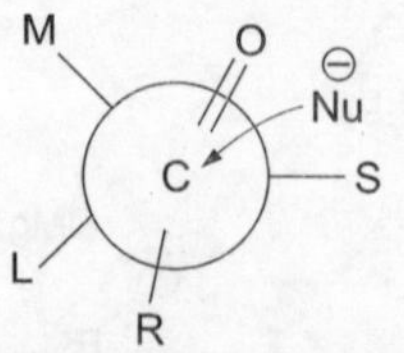

Preferential nucleophilic attack then occurs from the least crowded side resulting in the formation of unequal amounts of the diastereomers. This is the basis of Cram's rule for the prediction of the diastereomer that will be predominantly formed. The formation of unequal amounts of diastereomers when an asymmetric centre is created in the presence of another asymmetric centre is known as *asymmetric induction*.

(b) Addition to activated carbon–carbon double bond Compounds containing carbon–carbon double bond conjugated with electron-withdrawing substituents undergo nucleophilic addition. Electron-withdrawing substituents reduce the π-electron density to promote nucleophilic attack and stabilize the intermediate carbanion by delocalization of the –ve charge. Thus, nucleophilic additions are observed in αβ-unsaturated aldehydes, ketones, esters, nitriles, etc. The reactions are often catalysed by base. The base converts the nucleophile (HA) to a stronger nucleophile ($\overset{\ominus}{A}$).

(i) $R{-}CH{=}CH{-}CO{-}R' \xrightarrow{NH_3} R{-}CH(NH_2){-}CH_2{-}CO{-}R'$

(ii) $CH_2{=}CH{-}C(=O){-}OCH_3 \xrightarrow[MeONa]{C_6H_5SH} C_6H_5S{-}CH_2{-}CH_2{-}C(=O){-}OCH_3$ Methyl-β-phenylmercaptopropionate

$CH_2{=}CH{-}C(=O){-}OCH_3 \xrightarrow{C_2H_5OH,\ \overset{\oplus}{H}} C_2H_5O{-}CH_2{-}CH_2{-}C(=O){-}OCH_3$ Methyl-β-ethoxypropionate

(iii) $Ph{-}CH{=}CH{-}CO_2R + H_2C(COOR)_2 \xrightarrow{EtONa} Ph{-}CH(CH(COOR)_2){-}CH_2{-}CO_2R$

(iv) $RNH_2 + CH_2{=}CH{-}CN \longrightarrow RNH{-}CH_2{-}CH_2{-}CN$

Mechanism

The mechanism of the nucleophilic addition of HA to the substrate $-\overset{|}{C}=\overset{|}{C}-Z$ (where Z = CHO, COR, COOR, $CONH_2$, CN, NO_2, etc.) in the presence of a base is given below:

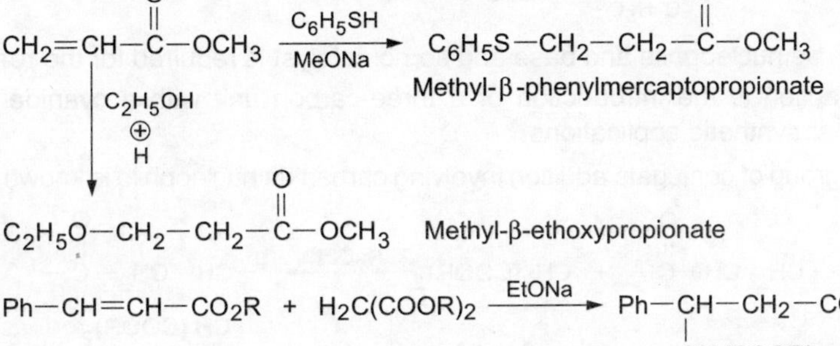

The nucleophile attacks the β-carbon. The negative charge in the resulting carbanion is delocalized by the carbonyl group. Subsequent protonation completes the addition. Protonation occurs chiefly on the oxygen because it is more negative than the carbon. Therefore, an overall 1, 4-addition occurs, which transforms into αβ-addition product. Considering the steric and electronic factors the electron-withdrawing effect decreases in the order CHO > COR > COOR > CN > NO_2, etc.

The most important nucleophilic addition reactions of synthetic importance are cyanoethylation and Michael reaction.

Cyanoethylation When acrylonitrile is treated with nucleophilic reagent in the presence of a base, 2-cyanoethyl group is attached to the nucleophile. The process is known as cyanoethylation. The nucleophilic reagent may be alcohol, phenol, 1° and 2° amines.

$$C_2H_5OH + CH_2{=}CH{-}CN \xrightarrow{\text{Base}} C_2H_5O{-}CH_2{-}CH_2{-}CN$$

β-Ethoxypropionitrile

The nucleophile, $C_2H_5\overset{\ominus}{O}$, attacks the β-carbon. The –ve charge on the resulting anion is stabilized by the cyano group. Subsequent abstraction of proton from the solvent completes the reaction.

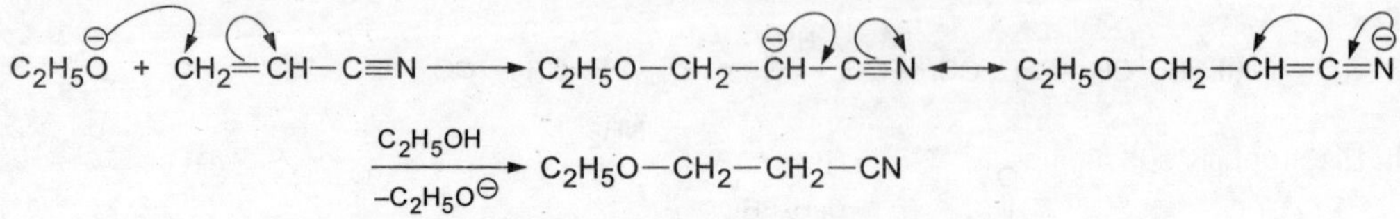

Amines function both as nucleophile and base and so no catalyst is required for the reaction.

The utility of the reaction is the introduction of a three-carbon unit with a cyanide group which can be manipulated for further synthetic applications.

Michael reaction A group of conjugate addition involving carbanion nucleophile is known as Michael reaction.

$$\text{(i)}\quad -CH{=}CH{-}\overset{O}{\overset{\|}{C}}- + CH_2(COOR)_2 \xrightarrow{\text{NaOEt}} -CH{-}CH_2{-}\overset{O}{\overset{\|}{C}}- \quad (\text{CH at C}\beta: CH(COOR)_2)$$

$$\text{(ii)}\quad CH_3{-}CH{=}CH{-}CO_2Et + CH_3NO_2 \xrightarrow{\text{NaOEt}} CH_3{-}\underset{CH_2NO_2}{\underset{|}{CH}}{-}CH_2{-}CO_2Et$$

Ethyl-3-methyl-4-nitrobutyrate

The attacking nucleophile, the enolate anion, is generated by the base NaOEt from a variety of active methylene compounds such as malonic ester, ethyl acetoacetate, ethyl cyanoacetate, nitroalkanes, etc. The mechanism of addition follows the general mechanism given earlier.

Since a large number of different substrates and different nucleophiles can be employed, the reaction has useful synthetic applications.

Addition of C = C vs C = O It is seen that the most common activating group is C = O which we have seen undergoing nucleophilic addition. When C = C and C = O groups are conjugated it is seen that the addition is usually to C = C. This may be explained on the stabilities of the products formed on addition to these bonds.

The product on addition to C = C has a residual C = O while the product on addition to C = O has a residual C = C.

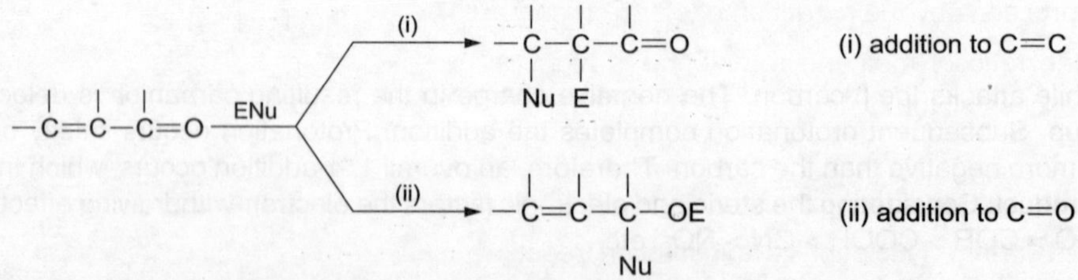

Since C = O is a stronger bond than C = C, the preferential addition is to C = C.

However, steric hindrance may be an important factor. Thus, PhMgBr adds to C = O in PhCH = CH— CHO while the addition is to C = C in PhCH = CH – $COCMe_3$. The inductive effect of Me group may also be a factor besides steric hindrance.

2. SUBSTITUTION REACTIONS

A reaction in which one group or atom is replaced by another is called a substitution reaction. The incoming group is bonded to the same carbon to which the leaving group was bonded. Substitution reaction has been classified according to the nature of the substituents involved. Thus—

I. Free radical substitution $A:B + \dot{Q} \longrightarrow A:Q + \dot{B}$

II. Nucleophilic substitution $A:B + :\overset{\ominus}{Q} \longrightarrow A:Q + :\overset{\ominus}{B}$

III. Electrophilic substitution $A:B + \overset{\oplus}{Q} \longrightarrow A:Q + \overset{\oplus}{B}$

It will be seen that in all types of substitutions the displaced species belong to the same class as the attacking species.

I. Free radical substitution

Radical substitution reactions are initiated by radicals in the gas phase or in non-polar solvents. Thus, methane and chlorine react in the presence of sunlight or heat to give methyl chloride.

$$CH_4 + Cl_2 \xrightarrow[300\,^{\circ}C]{h\nu\text{ or}} CH_3Cl + HCl$$

Light energy or heat causes homolytic fission of chlorine producing chlorine radicals which attack methane to form methyl chloride.

$$Cl:Cl \xrightarrow{h\nu\text{ or }300\,^{\circ}C} \dot{C}l + \dot{C}l \quad \text{... (i)}$$

$$H_3C:H + \dot{C}l \longrightarrow H_3\dot{C} + HCl \quad \text{... (ii)}$$

$$H_3\dot{C} + Cl:Cl \longrightarrow H_3C:Cl + \dot{C}l \quad \text{... (iii)}$$

The mechanism is supported by the fact that no reaction occurs in the dark, and in the presence of tetraethyl lead (0.02%) the reaction takes place at 140 °C. Tetraethyl lead decomposes at 140 °C to ethyl radical which produces chlorine radical from chlorine for the propagation of the reaction as given above.

$$Pb\,(C_2H_5)_4 \xrightarrow{140\,^{\circ}C} 4\dot{C}_2H_5 + Pb\,;\ \dot{C}_2H_5 + Cl:Cl \longrightarrow C_2H_5Cl + \dot{C}l$$

The reaction proceeds by the repetition of steps (ii) and (iii).

When the ratio of methane to chlorine is high, methyl chloride is formed predominantly and when chlorine is in excess all the hydrogens are replaced to give carbon tetrachloride.

II. Nucleophilic substitution

(a) At saturated carbon Nucleophilic substitution reaction involves the displacement of a nucleophile by another. These reactions have great synthetic importance. A classical example is the hydrolysis of alkyl halides.

$$H\overset{\ominus}{O}: + R:X \longrightarrow HO:R + :\overset{\ominus}{X}$$

The nucleophile furnishes an electron pair to the carbon from which the leaving group departs with the bonding pair of electrons. Investigations by Ingold and co-workers indicate that nucleophilic substitution reaction can proceed by two different paths which have been designated by Ingold as S_N1 and S_N2 depending on the nature of the substrate, the nucleophile, the leaving group and the solvent.

Mechanism

S_N1 mechanism Kinetic studies of the hydrolysis of *t*-butyl bromide indicate that the rate of the reaction is proportional to the concentration of the alkyl halide, i.e., rate $\propto [R_3CX]$.

Since the rate of reaction is dependent on one of the reactants, the reaction is a first-order reaction. Nucleophilic substitution reaction which follows first-order kinetics is designated S_N1 (*S*ubstitution *N*ucleophilic *U*nimolecular).

As the rate of reaction is independent of $[\overset{\ominus}{O}H]$, it is interpreted that the halide undergoes slow ionization in the first step producing carbocation intermediate. In the second step a rapid attack of $\overset{\ominus}{O}H$ on the carbocation completes the hydrolysis.

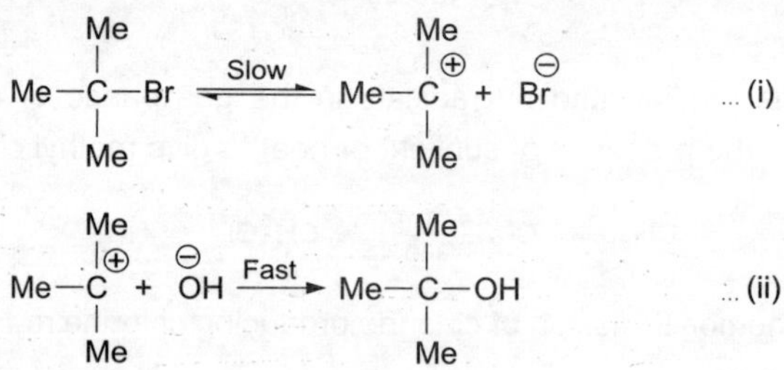

The energy required for the ionization of the halide is supplied by the energy of solvation of the ions. Since a carbocation is formed in the slowest step, the alkyl halide which can most easily form a stable carbocation will favour hydrolysis by S_N1 path. Hence, the order of hydrolysis of alkyl halides by S_N1 path is:

Allyl, Benzyl > 3° > 2° > 1° > CH_3X (cf. inductive effect and resonance effects)

Stereochemistry of S_N1 reaction Since a carbocation is flat (sp^2, trigonal planar) with the vacant 2p orbital vertical to the plane bearing the three groups, the attack of the reagent can occur from either side of the plane with equal probability, i.e., a racemic product should result if the alkyl halide is chiral.

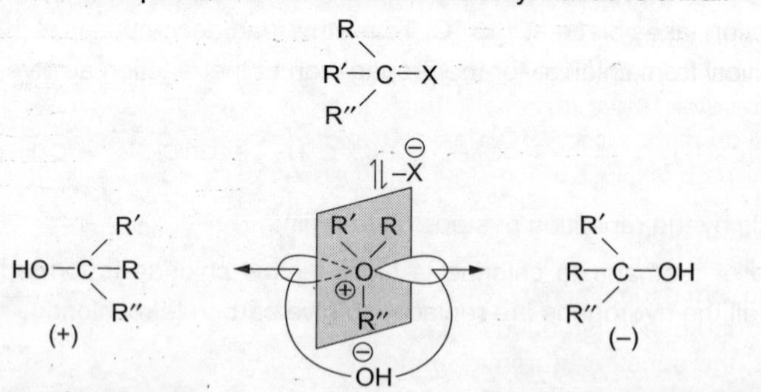

Inversion of configuration Retention of configuration

Pure racemization (50/50 mixture) is rarely observed. This is because the leaving group lies close to the carbocation shielding the side from the attack till it has sufficiently moved away. Thus, more attack of the reagent occurs from the opposite side to the leaving group. This causes more inversion than retention of configuration. Stable carbocations have longer life to permit solvation from either side of the plane of the carbocation resulting in greater proportion of racemization. Greater proportion of inversion is observed with more nucleophilic solvent due to faster attack from the opposite side to the leaving group.

S_N2 mechanism Nucleophilic substitution reactions which follow second-order kinetics is called S_N2 (*S*ubstitution *N*ucleophilic *B*imolecular) reaction. The rate of a second-order reaction depends upon the concentrations of both the reactants. Thus, the rate of hydrolysis of methyl bromide with NaOH has been found to be of second order, i.e.,

$$\text{the rate} \propto [CH_3Br][\overset{\ominus}{O}H].$$

Since the rate-determining step involves both CH_3Br and $\overset{\ominus}{O}H$, a collision between the two reactants resulting in the direct displacement of $\overset{\ominus}{Br}$ by $\overset{\ominus}{O}H$ occurs in such a way that while a new C – OH bond is being formed, the old C – Br bond starts breaking, i.e., the bond formation and the bond breaking are simultaneous. Hence, the reaction is a concerted one-step reaction without any intermediate.

During the collision an energetic hydroxide ion approaches the methyl bromide molecule from the side opposite to bromine to avoid repulsion, i.e., at 180° to the leaving group—a back-side attack. When the $\overset{\ominus}{O}H$ is sufficiently near the electron-deficient carbon of the substrate, it begins to form a bond with it and the C – Br bond starts stretching. At one stage of the reaction, a state is reached when the OH and Br are partially bonded to the central carbon and the non-participating groups lying in a plane perpendicular to the line HO...C...Br. This state is called the transition state. In the transition state partial negative charge of the hydroxide ion is transferred to bromine via the carbon atom. With further approach of hydroxide, a complete C – OH bond is formed and bromine departs with the bonding pair of electrons.

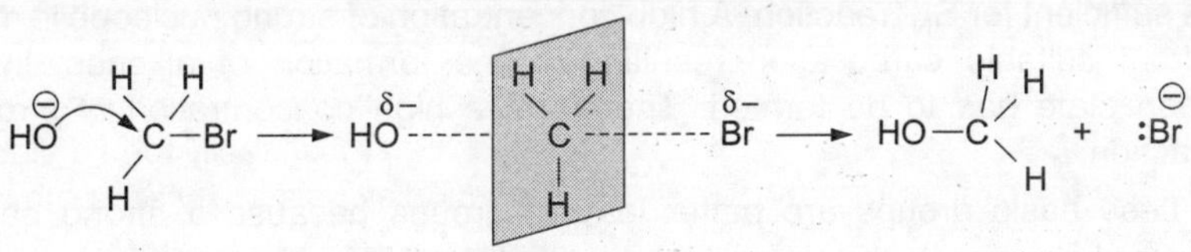

Transition state

In the transition state five groups or atoms are bonded to the α-carbon. As we go along the series from methyl bromide to *t*-butyl bromide, the increasing crowding of the carbon bearing the bromine atom progressively decreases the nucleophilic attack. Also, the increasing +I effect along the series makes the carbon bearing the bromine progressively less positively polarised and consequently less readily attacked by the nucleophile. The steric factor is, however, more important than the electronic factor. Hence, the E_{act} for the formation of the transition state will be highest for 3° halides and least for methyl halides. Therefore, the rate of hydrolysis of alkyl halides by S_N2 path is CH_3X > 1° > 2° > 3°, i.e., reverse of S_N1 path.

Stereochemistry of S_N2 reaction—From the course of the direct displacement reaction as shown above, it is seen that the molecule is turned inside out. A Walden inversion is therefore expected to take place. An optically active halide on hydrolysis by S_N2 path, therefore, should give an alcohol with inversion of configuration. The change of configuration can be established by observing the directions of optical rotation. In this case, however, the substrate (bromide) and the product (alcohol) are two different compounds. The directions of rotation and the configurations of two different compounds are not usually related. Hence, the configurations of the substrate and the product should be related to arrive at the conclusion.

An elegant method has been suggested (Huges and Ingold) to establish the inversion of configuration in S_N2 reaction. The method involves the conversion of (+)2 iodooctane with potassium radioiodide ($K^{128}I$) in acetone to (–)2-iodooctane. The reaction was found to be bimolecular (S_N2), i.e., rate $\propto [C_6H_{13}CHICH_3][\overset{\ominus}{I}{}^*]$. The exchange of ordinary iodide with the radioactive iodide was accompanied by the loss of optical activity.

This indicates the formation of (–) isomer from the (+) isomer to result in racemization.

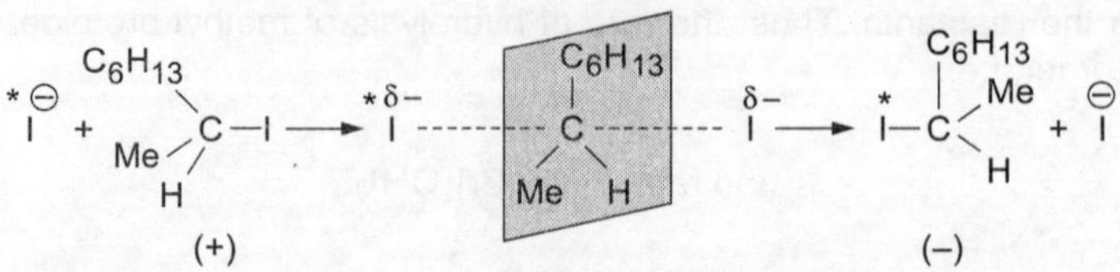

The rate of loss of optical activity (i.e., racemization) was found to be twice the rate of iodine exchange (i.e., inversion)—one (+) molecule is inverted and another (+) molecule pairs with it to form a (±) modification. The above formulated mechanism of S_N2 reaction is therefore established. Inversion of configuration is always indicative of S_N2 reaction.

Factors influencing S_N1 and S_N2 reactions

(i) Solvent Polar solvents help in the separation and stabilization of unlike charges, i.e., aid ionization. In S_N1 reaction ionization occurs in the rate-determining step. Hence, polar solvents promote S_N1 reaction. In S_N2 reaction, the charge brought in by the nucleophile is spread over a large part in the transition state. Hence polar solvents have little effect on the transition state. However, highly polar solvents form strong solvent layer around the nucleophile. Therefore, extra energy is required to break the solvent layer for the attack. Hence strongly polar solvents slightly slow down the S_N2 reaction.

(ii) Nucleophile In S_N1 reaction, a carbocation is attacked by the nucleophile. Hence, a low concentration of weak nucleophile is sufficient for S_N1 reaction. A high concentration of strong nucleophile may act as base by accepting proton from suitable carbocation resulting in the formation of alkenes. In S_N2 reaction, a high-energy transition state has to be formed. Therefore, a high concentration of strong nucleophile is required for S_N2 reaction.

(iii) Leaving group Less basic groups are better leaving groups because a strong base has a greater tendency for a backward direction in the reversible reaction $HA \rightleftharpoons H^{\oplus} + A^{\ominus}$.

Strong bases such as $\overset{\ominus}{O}H$, $\overset{\ominus}{O}R$, $R_2\overset{\ominus}{N}$, etc., are not good leaving groups. Thus, alcohols are resistant to substitution in non-acidic medium. In acidic medium, however, the hydroxyl group leaves as H_2O, which is a weak base.

$$R{-}OH \xrightarrow{\overset{\oplus}{H}} R{-}\overset{\oplus}{O}H_2 \xrightarrow{\overset{\ominus}{Br}} R{-}Br + H_2O$$

Increase in the ionic size of the elements of the same group in the periodic table causes decrease in the basicity as the charge to size ratio decreases. The basicity order of the halogens is $\overset{\ominus}{I} < \overset{\ominus}{Br} < \overset{\ominus}{Cl} < \overset{\ominus}{F}$. Therefore, the rate of hydrolysis of the alkyl halides is RI > RBr > RCl by either S_N1 or S_N2 path.

S_Ni mechanism Nucleophilic substitution reaction which follows second-order kinetics and yet with no change in the configuration of the product is identified as S_Ni, which means *S*ubstitution *N*ucleophilic *I*nternal. Thus, the esterification of chiral alcohols with thionyl chloride results in the retention of the configuration of the product.

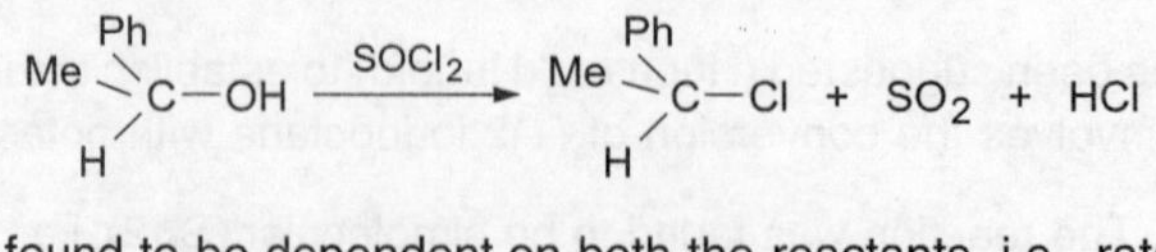

The rate of the reaction is found to be dependent on both the reactants, i.e., rate $\propto$ [PhCH(Me)OH][$SOCl_2$]. Thionyl chloride reacts with alcohol to furnish alkyl chlorosulphite (21) which has the same configuration as the alcohol. There is evidence to show that the transformation of (21) to product involves an ion pair (22). The chloride ion is then supplied by the chlorosulphite anion for the attack. The attack occurs from the front side since the chlorosulphite anion is held from the front side. Hence, no inversion of configuration is observed.

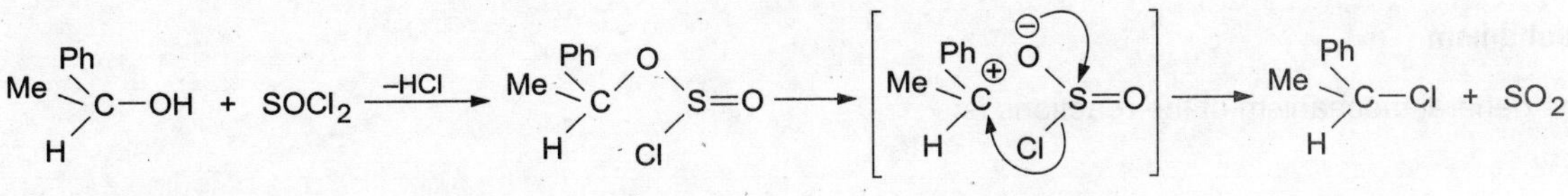

(21) (22)

The overall reaction may be considered as an internal attack.

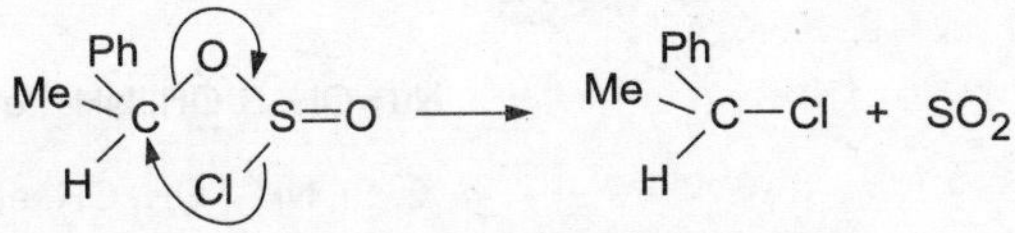

Hence, the reaction is designated as $S_N i$ to distinguish it from $S_N 2$.

When the reaction is carried out in the presence of pyridine, the pyridine hydrochloride formed in the reaction supplies the effective nucleophile, $\overset{\ominus}{Cl}$, for a back-side attack as in normal S_N2 reaction with inversion of configuration.

$$C_5H_5\ddot{N} + HCl \longrightarrow C_5H_5\overset{\oplus}{N}H\overset{\ominus}{Cl}$$

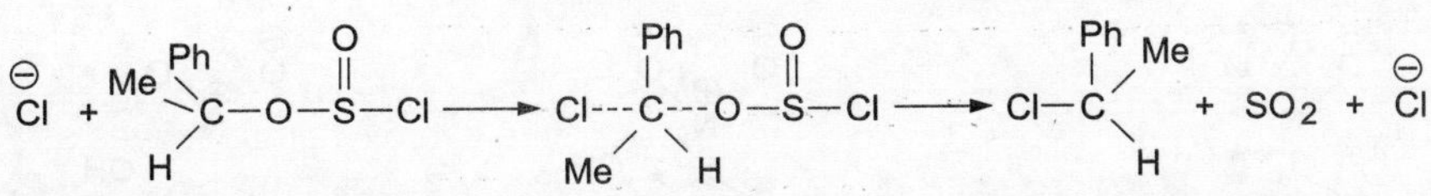

(b) At unsaturated carbon When a carbon atom multiply bonded to hetero atom (e.g., O, N, S, etc.), bears a good leaving group such as Cl, OH, OR, NH_2, etc., nucleophilic attack on the carbon results in substitution rather than addition. Some examples are given for illustration.

(i) Hydrolysis of acid chloride, acid amide and ester:

$$CH_3COCl + H_2O \longrightarrow CH_3COOH + HCl$$

$$CH_3CONH_2 + \overset{\ominus}{O}H \longrightarrow CH_3COOH + NH_3$$

$$CH_3COOC_2H_5 + \overset{\ominus}{O}H \longrightarrow CH_3COOH + C_2H_5OH$$

(ii) Formation of acid amide from acid chloride:

$$CH_3COCl + \ddot{N}H_3 \longrightarrow CH_3CO\ddot{N}H_2 + HCl$$

(iii) Ester from acid:

$$CH_3COOH + C_2H_5\ddot{O}H \xrightarrow{H^{\oplus}} CH_3COOC_2H_5 + H_2O$$

Mechanism

The general mechanism of the reactions is:

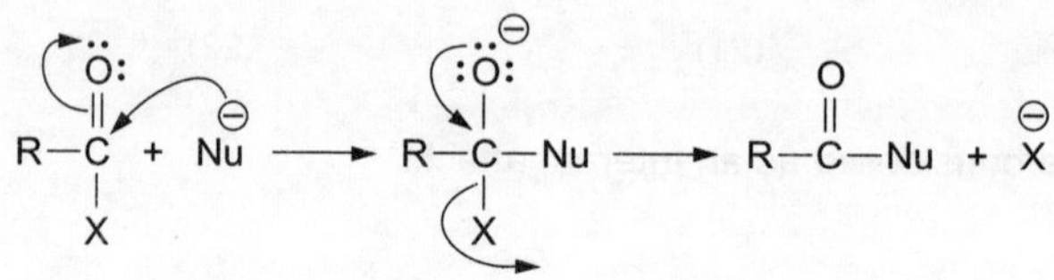

$Nu = \overset{\ominus}{O}H, R\ddot{O}H, \ddot{N}H_3$, etc.

$X = Cl, NH_2, OH, OR$, etc.

The nucleophilic attack on the unsaturated carbon displaces an electron pair to the oxygen atom in the transition state. When the electron pair reverts, the leaving group is displaced.

(c) Aromatic nucleophilic substitution— (i) Substitution of hydrogen of benzene Nucleophilic substitution of the hydrogen of benzene is difficult because (a) the π-electron cloud will repel the nucleophile and (b) it would be difficult for the ring to accommodate the negative charge brought in by the nucleophile. However, the presence of a strong electron-withdrawing group may overcome the difficulties and nucleophilic substitution then is possible. Thus, nitrobenzene gives *o*-nitrophenol on treatment with strong NaOH in the presence of oxidising agents such as KNO_3 or $K_3Fe(CN)_6$.

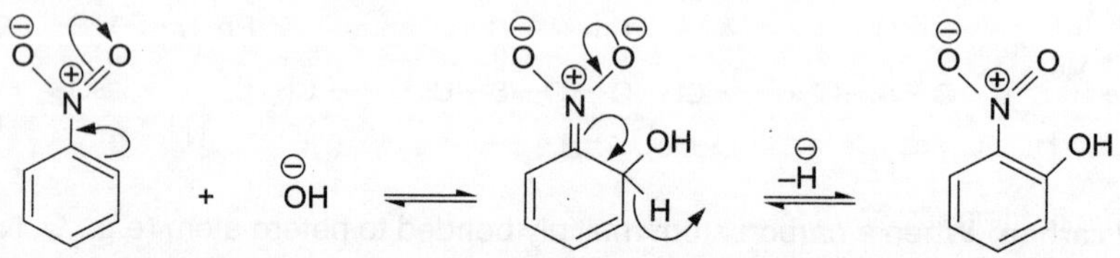

Since $\overset{\ominus}{O}H$ is a better leaving group than $H^{\ominus}$, the expulsion of $H^{\ominus}$ is aided by oxidation.

(ii) Substitution of groups other than hydrogen Nucleophilic substitution is observed in suitably substituted aromatic compounds. These reactions may be unimolecular (S_N1) or bimolecular (S_N2).

S_N1 type—A common example of aromatic nucleophilic substitution which resembles nucleophilic substitution at saturated carbon by S_N1 path is the decomposition of diazonium salts in polar medium and formation of mixed products in the presence of various nucleophiles.

The rate of reaction is found to be dependent on the concentration of $ArN_2^{\oplus}$ only, i.e., the reaction is unimolecular (S_N1). Hence, it is presumed that in the first slow, rate-determining step, heterolysis of C – N bond takes place with the formation of nitrogen and aryl cation. This is followed by a fast attack of the nucleophile in the second step. The aryl cation is very reactive and takes up any nucleophile present, even recombines with the eliminated N_2. Therefore, the reaction is reversible.

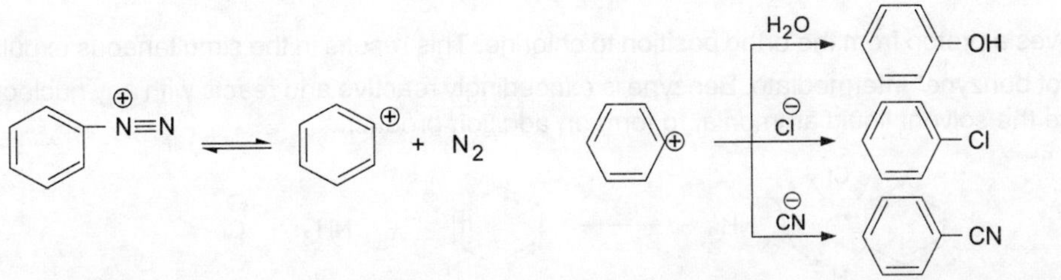

Although aryl cation is very unstable, the driving force for its formation is the elimination of very stable nitrogen (bond energy of $N \equiv N = 226$ kcal/mol).

S_N2 type—Halogens activated by strong electron-withdrawing groups from *o*- and *p*-positions undergo displacement by bimolecular mechanism.

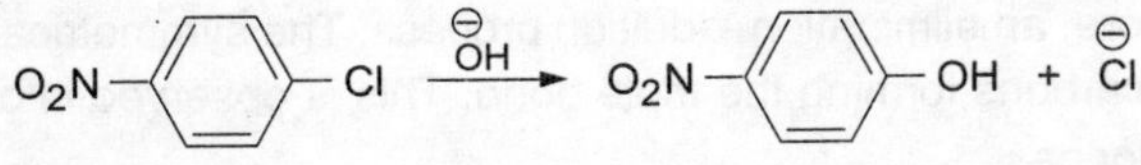

The rate of the reaction is proportional to the concentration of both the reactants, i.e., rate $\propto [ArX][\overset{\ominus}{Nu}]$. The reaction fails in the absence of the electron-withdrawing group, NO_2. Hence, activation of the halogen by the NO_2 group is suggested.

The carbon bearing the halogen is electron-deficient due to the electron withdrawal by the NO_2 and Cl groups. This promotes attack by the nucleophile. The intermediate formed on attack of the nucleophile is stabilized by delocalization of the negative charge by the NO_2 group. The intermediate then passes to more stable product by expulsion of the halogen.

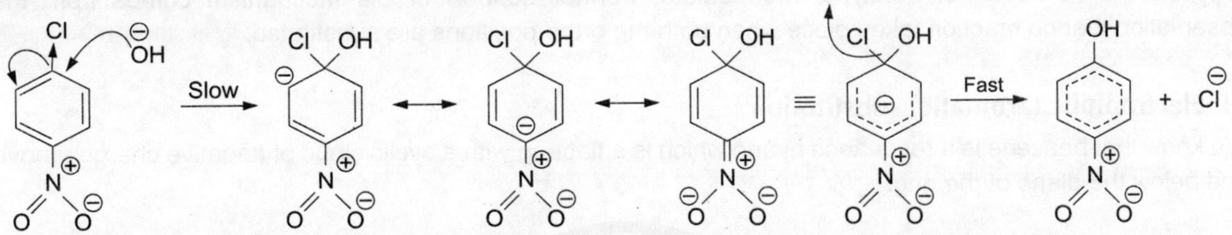

The reaction is not exactly analogous to aliphatic S_N2 reaction in the following matters:

(a) The attack of the nucleophile occurs from the side as the back-side attack is sterically hindered by the ring.

(b) The carbon bearing the leaving group forms four rather than five bonds as in normal S_N2 reaction.

(c) The bond to the attacking nucleophile is first formed and then the bond to the leaving group breaks, i.e., it is an addition–elimination process.

(d) An intermediate rather than a transition state is formed. Hence, the reaction is designated S_N2 (aromatic).

(iii) Substitution of unactivated halogens (Benzyne mechanism) Unactivated halogens in aromatic compounds undergo indirect nucleophilic displacement in the presence of very strong bases such as sodamide in liquid ammonia at low temperature (−33 °C) or strong NaOH at high temperature (340 °C).

$$C_6H_5Cl + \overset{\ominus}{N}H_2 \xrightarrow[-33\,°C]{\text{liq. } NH_3} C_6H_5NH_2 + \overset{\ominus}{Cl}$$

It has been observed that $\overset{\ominus}{N}H_2$ is able to remove a proton from the benzene ring. It is, therefore, suggested that

$\overset{\ominus}{N}H_2$ removes a proton from the ortho position to chlorine. This results in the simultaneous expulsion of $\overset{\ominus}{Cl}$ and formation of benzyne* intermediate. Benzyne is exceedingly reactive and reacts with any nucleophile present, in this case the solvent liquid ammonia, to form an addition product.

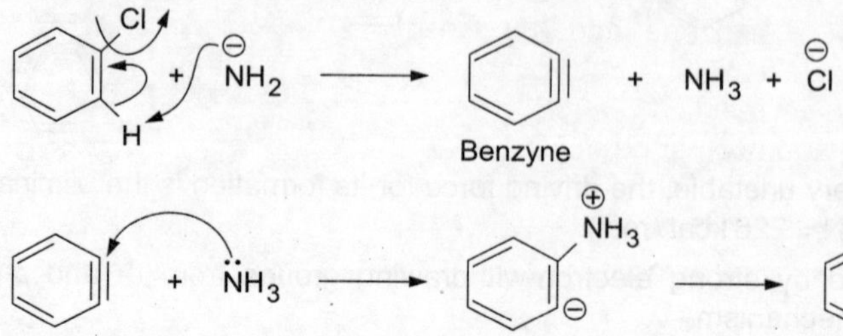

The reaction is, therefore, an elimination–addition process. The symmetrical benzyne intermediate can be attacked at either of the carbons forming the triple bond. This is observed in chlorobenzene with labelled carbon (^{14}C) bearing the chlorine.

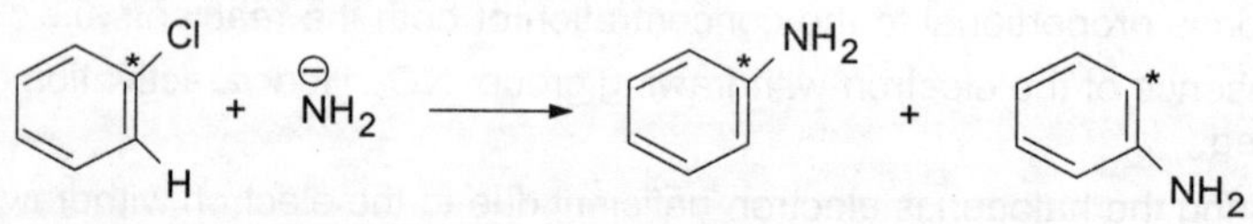

Thus, *p*-chlorotoluene on treatment with strong NaOH at 340 °C gives a mixture of *o*- and *p*-cresols.

This cine-substitution (aromatic nucleophilic substitution at a different position from the leaving group) supports the formation of benzyne intermediate. Further support of the mechanism comes from the observation that no reaction takes place when both the ortho positions are substituted.

III. Electrophilic (aromatic) substitution

We know that benzene is a resonance hybrid which is a flat ring with a cyclic cloud of negative charge, above and below the plane of the ring.

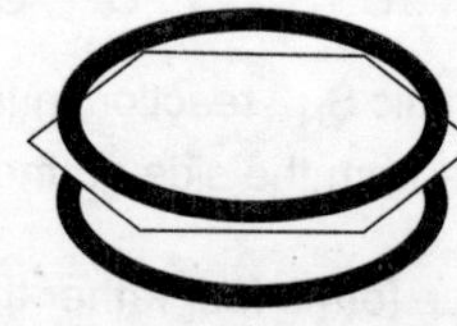

Benzene ring, therefore, discourages nucleophilic attack and encourages electrophilic attack. Alkenes also encourage electrophilic attack resulting in addition while the electrophilic attack on benzene results in substitution since addition would involve loss of resonance stabilization of benzene.

---

* Acetylenic bond in benzyne is unlikely since the ring will be greatly deformed with accompanying strain. It has been suggested that the third bond is formed by the overlap of the two sp^2 orbitals vacated by hydrogen and chlorine. The overlap of the two sp^2 orbitals will be poor and consequently benzyne will be very reactive.

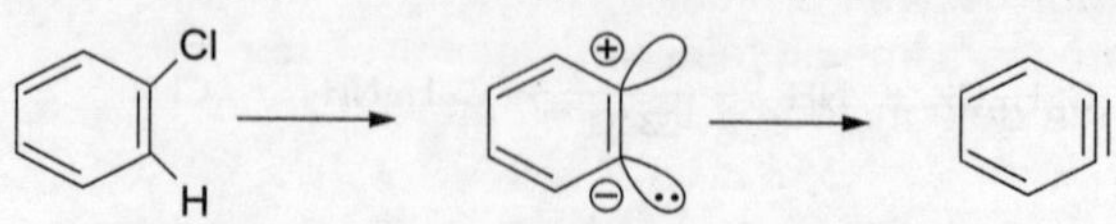

Its existence has been established by trapping experiment and spectroscopy.

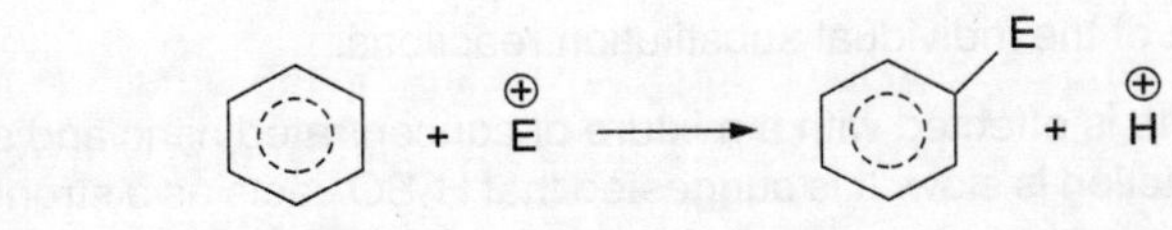

Hence, the typical reactions of benzene and its derivations are electrophilic substitution. Aromatic electrophilic substitution includes a wide variety of reactions, e.g., nitration, sulphonation, halogenation, Friedel–Crafts reactions, etc. The reaction permits the direct introduction of groups to the ring and their subsequent transformation to various other products.

$$ArH + HNO_3 \xrightarrow{H_2SO_4} ArNO_2 + H_2O$$

$$ArH + Cl_2 \xrightarrow{AlCl_3} ArCl + HCl$$

$$ArH + H_2SO_4 \xrightarrow{SO_3} ArSO_3H + H_2O$$

$$ArH + RCl \xrightarrow{AlCl_3} ArR + HCl$$

Mechanism

The various aromatic electrophilic substitutions follow the same mechanistic pattern which is generalised below.

The reagent and the catalyst (Lewis acids or proton acids) undergo acid–base reaction to produce the attacking electrophile which then attacks the ring to form a carbocation (σ complex) in the first slow step. In the second step the proton from the site of attack is rapidly removed by the base to complete the reaction.

$$E-Nu + Cat \rightleftharpoons \overset{\oplus}{E} + Nu-\overset{\ominus}{Cat} \quad \text{... (i)}$$

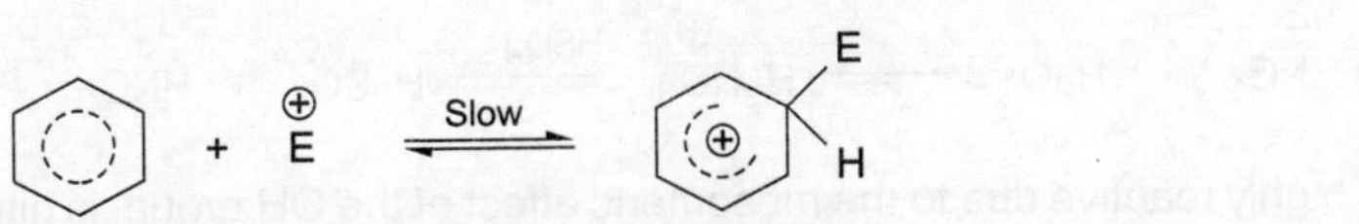

σ complex

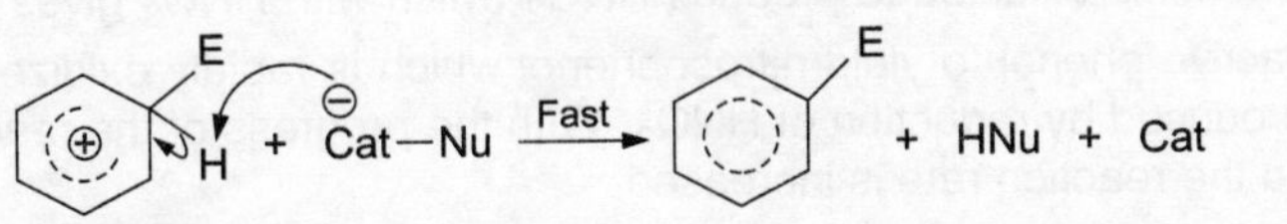

... (ii)

The energy gained in passing from the σ complex to the product (regain of aromaticity) provides the energy for breaking the strong C – H bond. It may seem that the formation of σ complex would involve high energy. This is, however, not so because the energy liberated by the formation of a C – E bond and the delocalization of the positive charge lowers the energy of the σ complex.

The rate of reaction does not involve the breaking of C – H bond. This has been established by *isotope effect.** The rates of reactions are the same on replacement of hydrogen by deuterium or tritium. Hence, the rate of the substitution reaction is determined by the slow attachment of the electrophile to the ring in the first step.

* A difference in reaction rate due to a difference in the isotope present in the substrate is called isotope effect.

Let us now consider some of the individual substitution reactions.

(a) Nitration Nitration of benzene is effected with a mixture of concentrated nitric and sulphuric acids. In the absence of sulphuric acid the reaction is slow. It is suggested that H_2SO_4 acts as a strong acid and protonates HNO_3 to generate nitronium ion, $\overset{\oplus}{N}O_2$. This has been confirmed by various methods.

$$HO{-}NO_2 + H_2SO_4 \rightleftharpoons H_2\overset{\oplus}{O}{-}NO_2 + \overset{\ominus}{HSO_4} \xrightleftharpoons{H_2SO_4} \overset{\oplus}{H_3O} + \overset{\oplus}{NO_2} + 2\overset{\ominus}{HSO_4}$$

Overall reaction is $HNO_3 + 2H_2SO_4 \rightleftharpoons \overset{\oplus}{NO_2} + 2\overset{\ominus}{HSO_4} + \overset{\oplus}{H_3O}$.

The nitronium ion then attacks the benzene ring to form a carbocation in the first step.

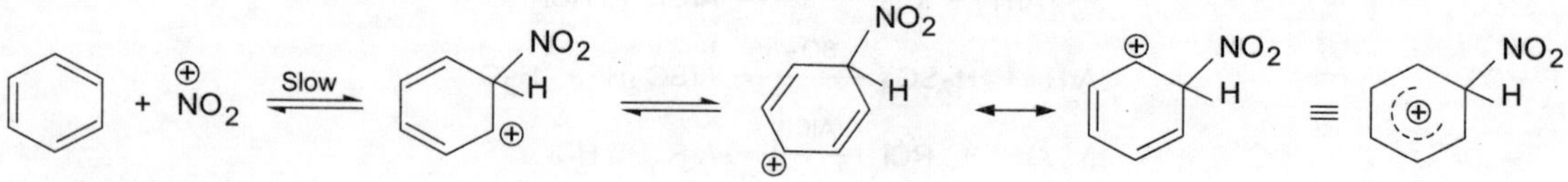

In the second step, a fast abstraction of hydrogen from the site of attack by the base ($HS\overset{\ominus}{O_4}$) completes the reaction.

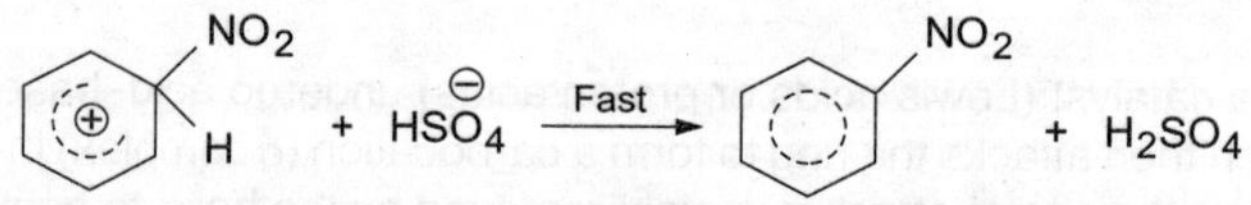

The presence of appreciable amount of water in the acid mixture is not desirable since it reduces the nitronium ion; hence, the use of concentrated acid mixture.

$$\overset{\oplus}{NO_2} + H_2O \rightleftharpoons H_2\overset{\oplus}{NO_3} \xrightleftharpoons{\overset{\ominus}{HSO_4}} H_2SO_4 + HNO_3$$

Phenol, which is highly reactive due to the mesomeric effect of the OH group, is nitrated even with dilute HNO_3. A small amount of phenol is oxidized to produce HNO_2 which with HNO_3 gives nitrosonium ion, $\overset{\oplus}{NO}$. The latter nitrosates the reactive phenol to yield nitrosophenol which is rapidly oxidized to nitrophenol with HNO_3 and nitrous acid is produced by reduction of HNO_3. With the progress of the reaction more and more nitrous acid is produced and the reaction rate is increased.

$$HNO_2 + 2HNO_3 \rightleftharpoons \overset{\oplus}{H_3O} + 2\overset{\ominus}{NO_3} + \overset{\oplus}{NO}$$

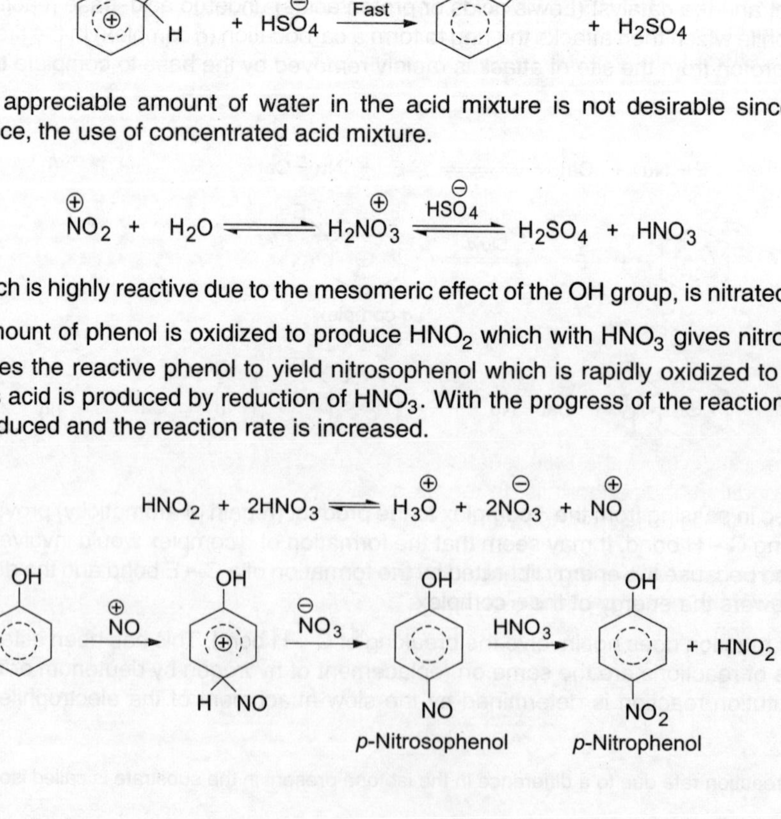

p-Nitrosophenol *p*-Nitrophenol

(b) Sulphonation Benzene on heating with concentrated or better with fuming sulphuric acid gives benzene sulphonic acid, $C_6H_5SO_3H$. Sulphonation can also be effected with $ClSO_3H$.

$$C_6H_6 + H_2SO_4 \rightleftharpoons C_6H_5SO_3H + H_2O$$

The reaction is slow with concentrated H_2SO_4 but rapid with oleum or SO_3 in inert solvent. The electrophile is SO_3 which is present in small amount in H_2SO_4.

$$2H_2SO_4 \rightleftharpoons SO_3 + H\overset{\ominus}{S}O_4 + H_3\overset{\oplus}{O}$$

The electrophile, SO_3, is neutral but has a powerful electrophilic sulphur which attacks the ring.

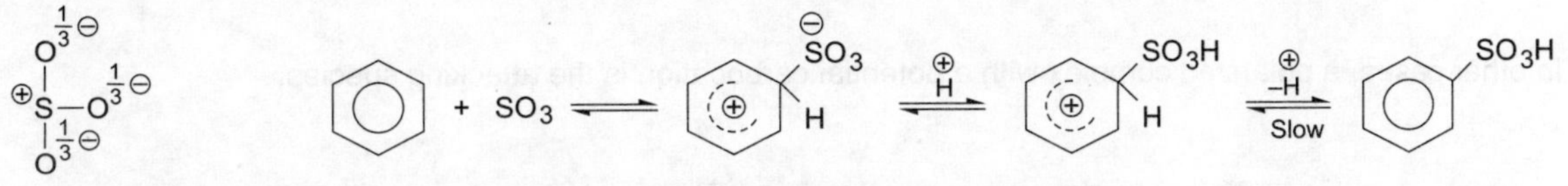

The rate-determining step involves the breaking of C – H bond since deuterated benzene is sulphonated more slowly (isotopic effect). The reaction is reversible. On treatment with steam, SO_3H group is replaced by hydrogen. The reversibility of the reaction has practical utility.

(c) Halogenation Free halogens can attack activated benzene rings but Lewis acid catalyst is required for benzene ring.

It is suggested that probably benzene first forms a π complex with the halogen molecule, e.g., Br_2. The Lewis acid ($FeBr_3$) then polarizes the Br – Br bond and helps in the formation of a σ complex between benzene carbon and the electrophilic end of the polarized bromine by removing the incipient bromide ion. Subsequent abstraction of hydrogen in the second step completes the reaction.

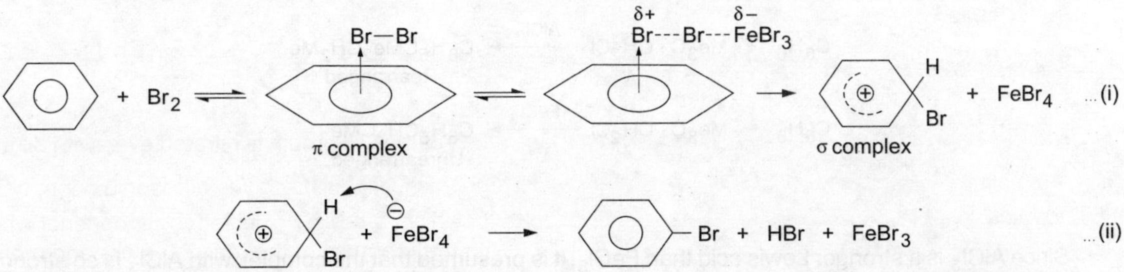

The order of reactivity of the halogens is $F_2 > Cl_2 > Br_2 > I_2$. Fluorine is too reactive for practical use. Under ordinary condition, iodination fails. In the presence of HNO_3 direct iodination has been effected. The attacking electrophile $I^{\oplus}$ is produced by HNO_3.

(d) Friedel–Crafts reaction Alkylation and acylation of aromatic rings with alkyl halides and acid chlorides or anhydrides respectively in the presence of Lewis acids, e.g., $AlCl_3$, $FeBr_3$, BF_3, BCl_3, etc., is known as Friedel–Crafts reaction.

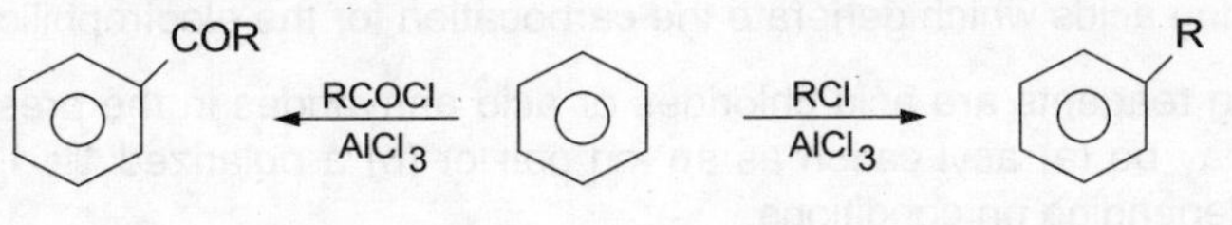

(i) Alkylation—The function of the catalyst is to provide a real or potential carbocation for the electrophilic attack. When the alkyl group can form a stable carbocation as in case of 3° halides, the attacking species is the real carbocation which forms an ion pair (23).

$$Me_3CBr + AlBr_3 \rightleftharpoons Me_3\overset{\oplus}{C}\ \overset{\ominus}{AlBr_4}$$

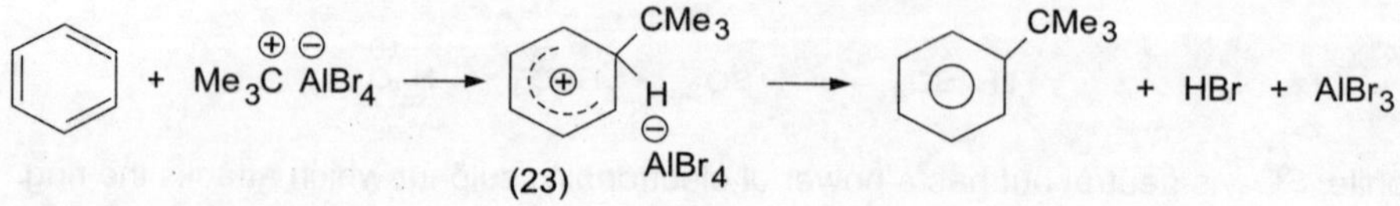

(23)

In other cases, a polarized complex with a potential carbocation is the attacking species.

$$R{-}Cl + AlCl_3 \rightleftharpoons \overset{\delta+}{R}{---}Cl{---}\overset{\delta-}{AlCl_3}$$

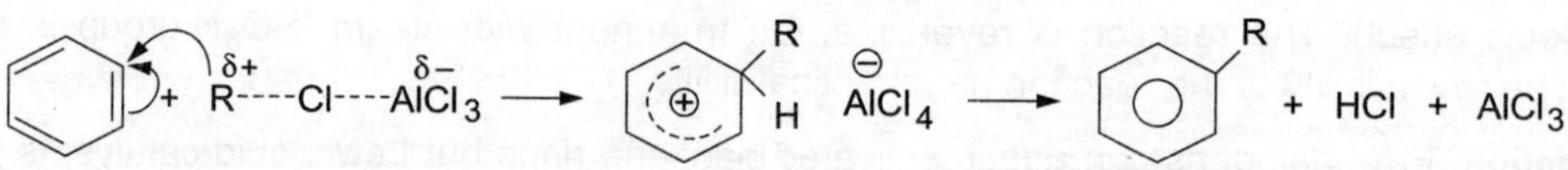

(24)

The intermediates (23) and (24) have been isolated in some cases. It has been observed that the same alkyl halide gives a rearranged and an unrearranged product with different Lewis acid catalysts.

$$C_6H_6 + Me_3C \cdot CH_2Cl \xrightarrow{AlCl_3} \underset{\text{Rearranged}}{C_6H_5CMe_2CH_2Me}$$

$$C_6H_6 + Me_3C \cdot CH_2Cl \xrightarrow{FeCl_3} \underset{\text{Unrearranged}}{C_6H_5CH_2CMe_3}$$

Since $AlCl_3$ is a stronger Lewis acid than $FeCl_3$, it is presumed that the complex with $AlCl_3$ is so strongly polarized that the alkyl group attains almost a free carbocation character to undergo rearrangement.

$$Me_3C{-}\overset{\delta+}{CH_2}{------}Cl{------}\overset{\delta-}{AlCl_3} \longrightarrow Me_2\overset{\delta+}{C} \cdot CH_2Me{------}Cl{------}\overset{\delta-}{AlCl_3}$$

The alkylating reagent besides alkyl halides may be aliphatic alcohols, alkenes, ethers, etc., in the presence of strong proton acids which generate the carbocation for the electrophilic attack.

(ii) Acylation—Acylating reagents are acid chlorides or acid anhydrides in the presence of Lewis acid. The electrophilic species may be (a) acyl cation as an ion pair or (b) a polarized 1 : 1 complex. Probably both mechanisms operate depending on conditions.

(i)

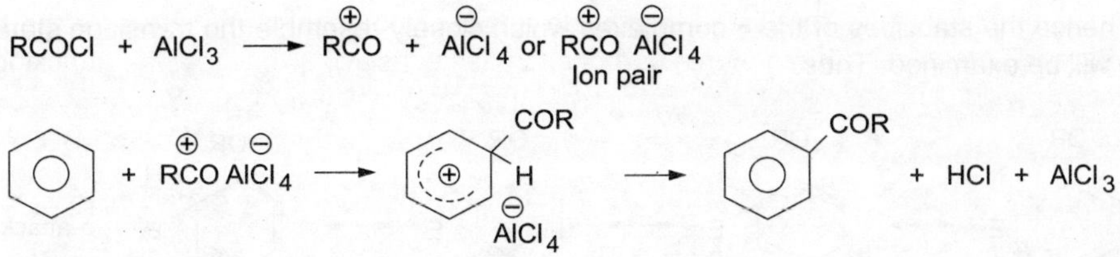

(ii)

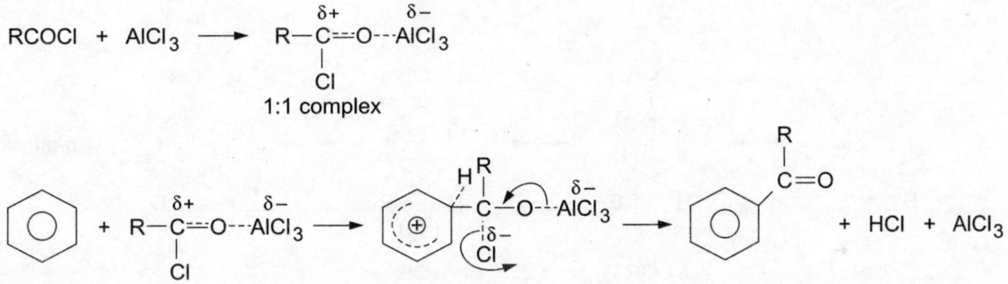

In both cases, one mole of the catalyst remains complexed with the product, ketone. Hence, slightly more than one mole of Lewis acid is required for acylation. Acylation may be effected with acid anhydrides also. The attacking species in this case may be a free $R\overset{\oplus}{C}O$ or RCOCl. (For further details see Friedel–Crafts reaction, Chapter 2.)

Effect of substituents in aromatic rings In planning syntheses based on substitution of mono-substituted benzenes, it is necessary to have prior knowledge to predict which position of the ring is most likely to be substituted and how readily the substitution will occur.

It has been observed that the group already present influences the orientation of substitution of the incoming group and the reactivity of the ring. Mono-substituted benzene on further substitution gives either *m*-isomer predominantly or a mixture of *o*- and *p*-isomers predominantly. Groups (substituents) which induce faster electrophilic attack than on benzene are called *activating* and in the reverse case (i.e., if slower) they are called *deactivating.*

On the basis of the above, groups have been divided into two classes, 'A' and 'B'. Thus,
'A' class of groups are *o*-/*p*-orienting with activation, e.g., NR_2, NH_2, OH, OR, NHCOR, OCOR, etc.
'B' class of groups are *m*-orienting with deactivation, e.g., NO_2, CHO, CO_2H, SO_3H, CN, $\overset{\oplus}{N}R_3$, CN, CCl_3, etc.

Let us now consider the electrophilic substitution in C_6H_5OR which has one 'A' class of groups. Benzene derivatives containing 'A' class of groups have in common an atom, adjacent to the ring, that has at least one electron pair. The electronic displacement by +M(mesomeric) effect of these groups increases the overall electron density of the ring. The electron density is more marked at *o*- and *p*-positions than at *m*-position.

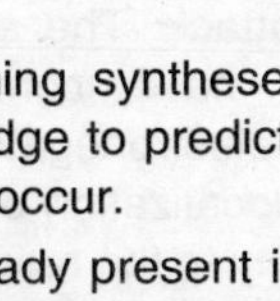

Hence, these groups cause facile (fast reaction) electrophilic substitution at *o*- and *p*-positions.

This effect of the group OR on the rates of attack at *o*-, *p*- and *m*-positions can be explained on the basis of the stabilities of the transition states formed on attack at these positions. This, however, is usually not possible and hence the stabilities of the σ complexes which closely resemble the transition states in energy and structure will be examined. Thus,

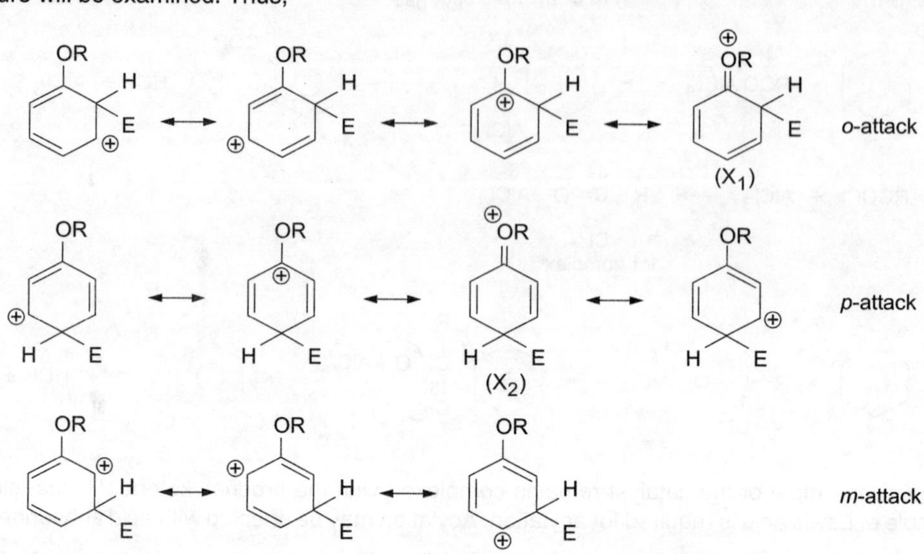

It is seen that the σ complexes formed on attack at *o*- and *p*-positions are both stabilized by four canonical structures relative to three for *m*-attack. The extra fourth structures (marked X_1 and X_2) are specially stable because all the atoms have complete octet. This factor overshadows the electron-withdrawing inductive effect of the electronegative oxygen atom. Thus, the unshared pair of electrons on oxygen atom helps in greater delocalization of the positive charge formed on attack at *o*- and *p*-positions. This gives added resonance stability to the respective carbocations.

As the more stable carbocations are expected to be formed more rapidly, the substitution products are nearly completely *o*-/*p*-isomers.

Substitution in chlorobenzene Chlorine is strongly electronegative. Its electron-withdrawing inductive effect deactivates the ring at all positions, yet chlorine aids *o*- and *p*-substitutions.

On drawing all the possible canonical forms of the σ complexes formed on attack at *o*-, *p*- and *m*-positions as for C_6H_5OR earlier, it will be seen that the extra fourth canonical forms (a) and (b) (cf X_1 and X_2 for C_6H_5OR) for the *o*- and *p*-σ complexes are specially stable since all the atoms in each have complete octet and the delocalization of the positive charge is beyond the ring.

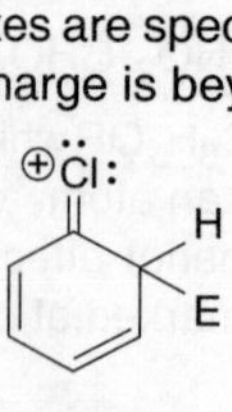

o-attack
(a)

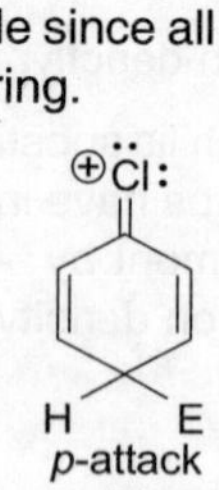

p-attack
(b)

Hence, these canonical forms make great contributions to the respective hybrids and strongly stabilize them relative to the σ complex for the meta-attack. Therefore, though C_6H_5Cl is less reactive than benzene, it undergoes *o*-/*p*-substitution. Substitution in C_6H_5Cl is, however, more difficult than in benzene due to overall deactivation. (To draw the resonance forms of all the σ complexes for C_6H_5Cl, substitute Cl for OR in the canonical forms given for C_6H_5OR.)

Substitution in toluene Although there is no unshared pair in CH_3 group, toluene undergoes *o*-/*p*-substitution. This is due to the +I effect in addition to hyperconjugative effect of the methyl group.

As before let us examine all the resonance forms of the σ complexes. It is seen that one of the resonance forms in each case of attack at *o*- and *p*-positions has a positive charge on a carbon adjacent to the CH_3 group.

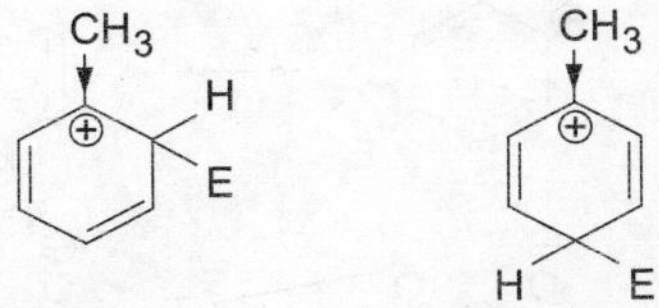

o-attack *p*-attack

These forms are specially stable being 3° carbocations. Such form is absent in case of attack at *m*-position. This outweighs the stability of the σ complexes formed on attack at *m*-position. Hence toluene undergoes *o*-/*p*-substitution.

In case of phenyl group substituted in benzene, an electron pair of the substituent (phenyl) group may stabilize the canonical forms of the σ complexes for *o*- and *p*-attacks.

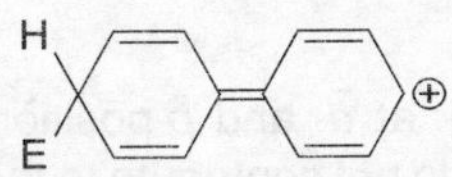

Hence, biphenyl undergoes faster electrophilic attack than benzene at *o*- and *p*-positions. It should be remembered that the effect of either activating or deactivating groups is reflected at *ortho* and *para* positions. Thus,

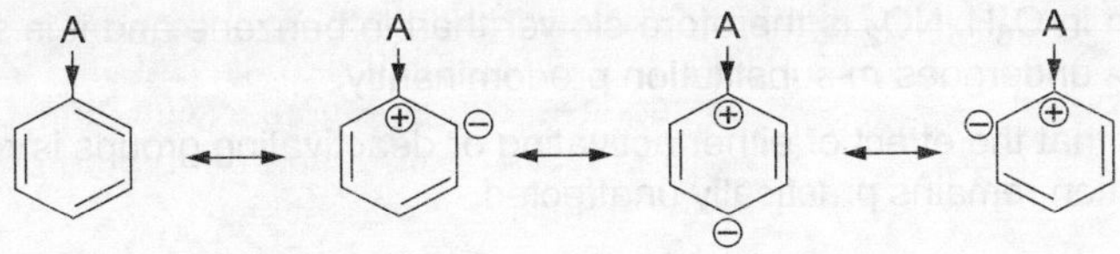

Activating

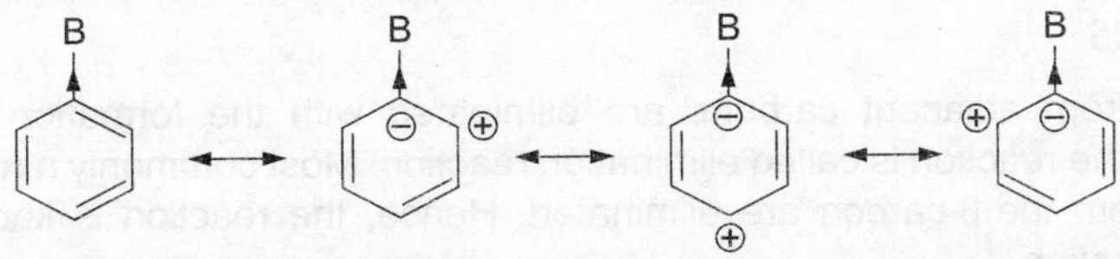

Deactivating

Substitution in benzene with 'B' class of substituents All the substituents of 'B' class are strongly electron-withdrawing due to a positively charged or positively polarized atom adjacent to the ring.

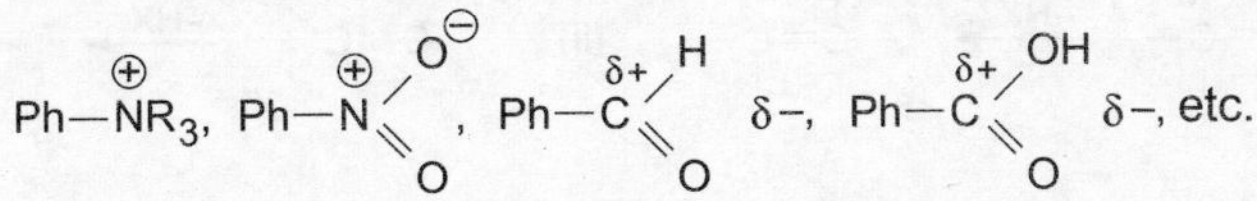

Hence, these groups overall deactivate the ring by electron withdrawal. The deactivation is more marked at *o*- and *p*-positions than at *m*-position. This can be seen from the stabilities of the σ complexes formed on attack at these positions, e.g., in $C_6H_5NO_2$.

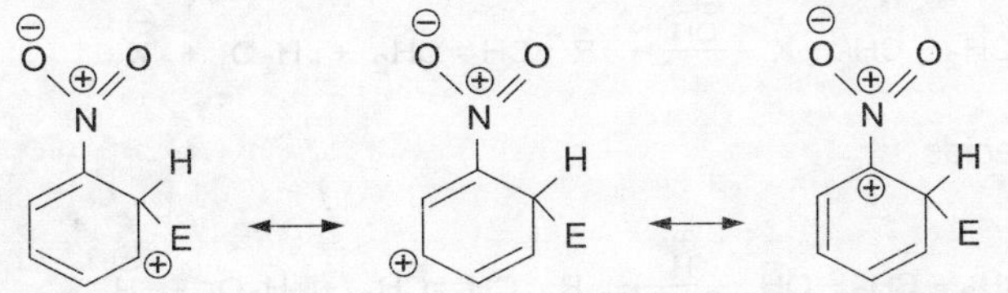

o-attack

(y_1) (High energy)

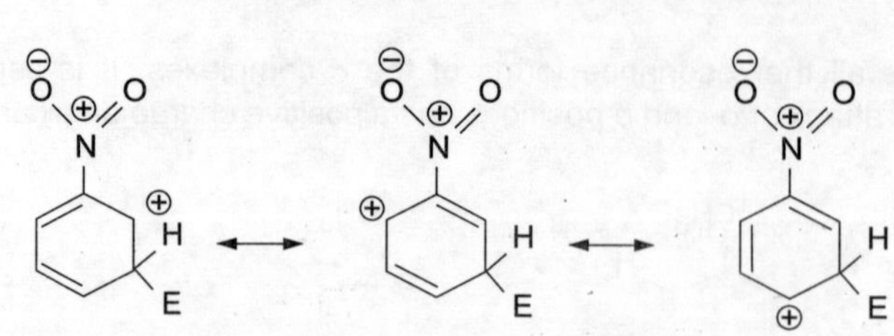

m-attack

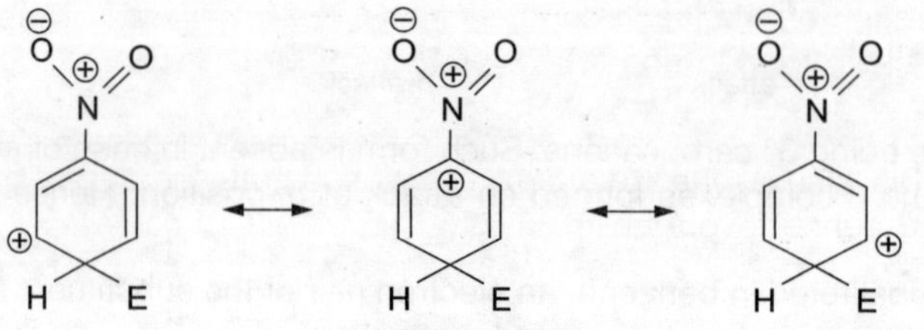

p-attack

(y_2) (High energy)

The canonical forms (Y_1) and (Y_2) on attack at *o*- and *p*-positions have each positive charges on adjacent atoms. These forms are of high energy and do not contribute to the hybrid. Consequently, the delocalization of the positive charge restricted in two canonical forms of the ring for *o*-/*p*-attack is less than for *m*-attack in which no such destabilizing forms are present. Thus, the NO_2 group does not aid the attack at any position and specially discourages the attack at *o*- and *p*-positions.

The attack at any position in $C_6H_5NO_2$ is therefore slower than in benzene and it is specially slow at *o*-/*p*-positions. Hence, $C_6H_5NO_2$ undergoes *m*-substitution predominantly.

From the above it is seen that the effect of either activating or deactivating groups is reflected at ortho and para positions while *m*-position remains practically unaffected.

3. ELIMINATION REACTIONS

When two groups or atoms from adjacent carbons are eliminated with the formation of unsaturated compounds (alkene or alkyne), the reaction is called elimination reaction. Most commonly a nucleophile (from the α-carbon) and a proton from the β-carbon are eliminated. Hence, the reaction is known as 1, 2- or αβ-elimination or simply β-elimination.

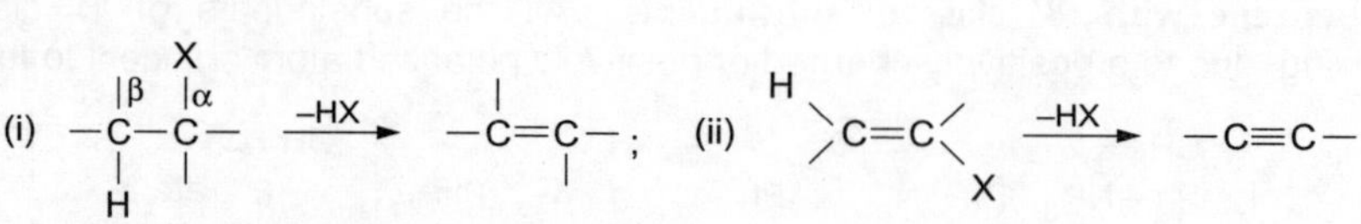

Some familiar elimination reactions are:

(i) Dehydrohalogenation of alkyl halides by base.

$$R-CH_2-CH_2-X \xrightarrow{\overset{\ominus}{OH}} R-CH{=}CH_2 + H_2O + \overset{\ominus}{X}$$

(ii) Dehydration of alcohols by acids.

$$R-CH_2-CH_2-OH \xrightarrow{\overset{\oplus}{H}} R-CH{=}CH_2 + H_2O + \overset{\oplus}{H}$$

(iii) Hofmann's degradation of quarternary bases by heat.

$$R-CH_2-CH_2-\overset{\oplus}{N}R_3\overset{\ominus}{O}H \xrightarrow{\Delta} R-CH=CH_2 + R_3N + H_2O$$

The presence of at least one hydrogen on the β-carbon is necessary for elimination. The driving forces for elimination are (a) stability of the olefin formed and (b) the relief from steric strain due to crowding in the substrate.

Branching at the β-carbon (as also at the α-carbon) of the substrate produces substituted olefins stabilized by hyperconjugation and hence favours elimination. Thus, Me_3CCl gives only 16% olefin while $Me_2CH-CMe_2Cl$ gives 62% olefin.

Strain in the substrate due to crowding by the substituents can be relieved on the formation of olefin since the bond angles increase from 109.5 in the substrate (sp^3-hybridized) to 120° in the product (sp^2-hybridized). Hence 3° halides favour elimination most and 1° halides the least, i.e., the order of elimination in halides is 3° > 2° > 1°.

The elimination reactions like S_N reactions may proceed by either unimolecular or bimolecular mechanisms. These elimination reactions have been designated E1 and E2 on their resemblance to S_N1 mechanism and S_N2 mechanism respectively.

(a) E1 mechanism The elimination reaction in which the rate of reaction is dependent on the concentration of the substrate only, i.e., kinetically of the first order, is designated E1. Since the rate of reaction is independent of the concentration of the reagent, it is interpreted, as in S_N1, that the first step of the reaction is the slowest step involving ionization of the substrate. This is followed by the rapid removal of a proton from the β-carbon by the reagent in the second step. This is illustrated below.

(i) Dehydrohalogenation of alkyl halides—The rate of elimination of a halacid from *t*-butyl bromide in basic medium is found to be proportional to $[Me_3CBr]$. Therefore, the halide undergoes slow ionization in the first step. This is followed by a rapid extraction of a proton from the carbocation by the base or solvent in the second step.

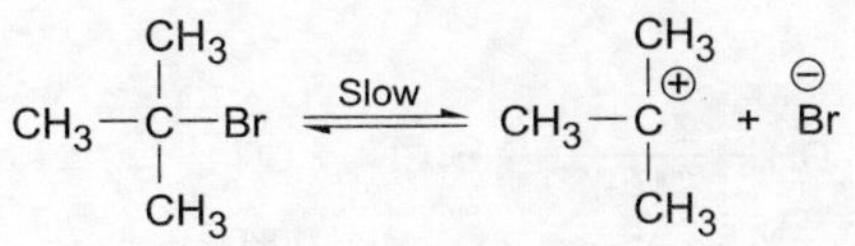

...(i)

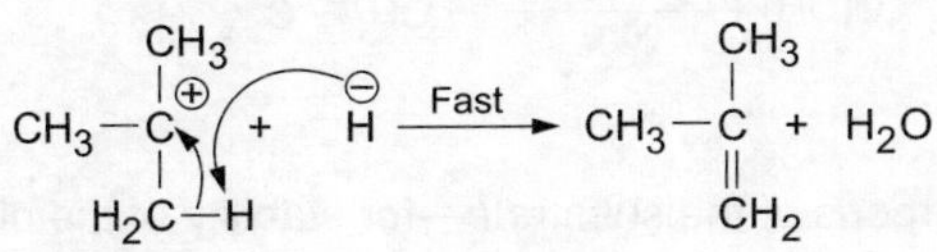

...(ii)

It is seen that a carbocation is formed in the first step in both E1 and S_N1 reactions. Hence, the reagent can attack the carbon to give substitution product and also can accept a proton to give elimination product. In practice both alcohol (substitution product) and alkene (elimination product) are obtained on hydrolysis of Me_3CBr.

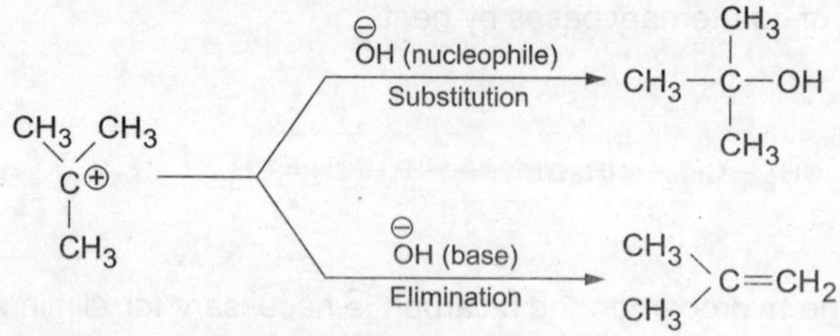

When more than one alkene can be formed, that alkene will predominate which has larger number of alkyl groups on the double-bonded carbons—this is Saytzev's rule. This is understandable since the substituted alkyl groups will stabilize the alkene by hyperconjugation.

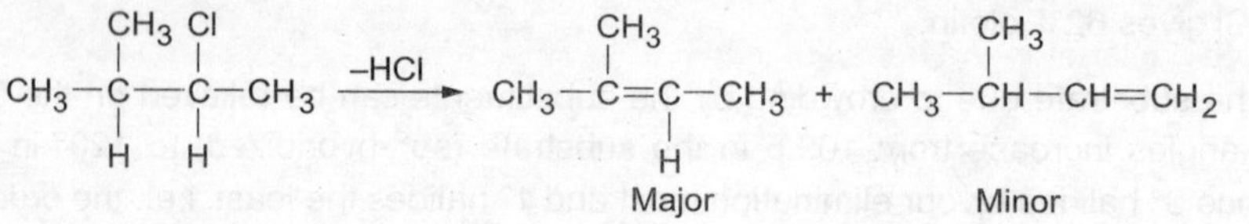

(ii) Dehydration of alcohols—Acid-catalysed dehydration of alcohols follows E1 mechanism. The dehydration is carried out at elevated temperature with sulphuric acid.

Alcohol is first protonated which weakens the C – O bond. Hence, water is eliminated from the protonated alcohol with generation of a carbocation. The latter then expels a proton to form a stable alkene.

$$Me_3C(OH) \xrightarrow{H_2SO_4} Me_3C-\overset{\oplus}{O}H_2 \xrightarrow{-H_2O} Me_3\overset{\oplus}{C}$$

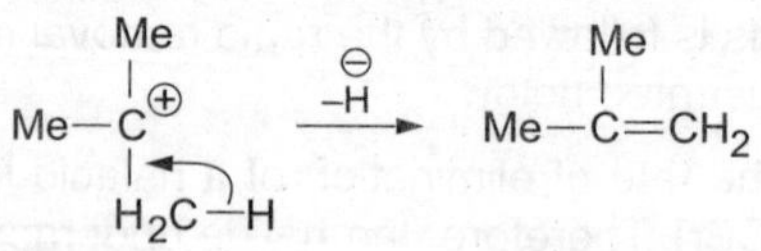

The concentration of acid depends upon how fast the carbocation is formed, i.e., on the stability of the carbocation. Primary alcohols generate unstable carbocations and hence require high temperature and high concentration of acid while 3° alcohols require lower temperature and lower concentration of acid for dehydration. Thus,

$$CH_3CH_2OH \xrightarrow[170°C]{Conc.\ H_2SO_4} CH_2{=}CH_2$$

$$(CH_3)_3C(OH) \xrightarrow[90°C]{20\%\ H_2SO_4} CH_3-C(CH_3){=}CH_2$$

E1 reaction is facilitated by

(i) branching at the α- and β-carbons of the substrate—for stability of the olefin,

(ii) strong polar solvent—to aid ionization,

(iii) low concentration of base—the greater stability of the alkene over the carbocation makes the extraction of proton easy.

(b) E2 mechanism When the rate of elimination reaction is dependent on both the substrate and the reagent, i.e., rate ∝ [substrate][reagent], the reaction is kinetically of the second order or bimolecular. Such bimolecular elimination reaction is designated E2 on its similarity with S_N2.

Since the reaction involves both the reactants in the rate-determining step, it is interpreted as in S_N2, that the reaction occurs in one step in which both the groups (proton and the leaving group) depart simultaneously through the intermediate transition state. It is visualized that as the base abstracts a proton from the β-carbon, simultaneous departure of the nucleophile takes place from the α-carbon. In the transition state the β C – H and α C – X bonds are stretched on the attack of the reagent with the incipient π-bond formation.

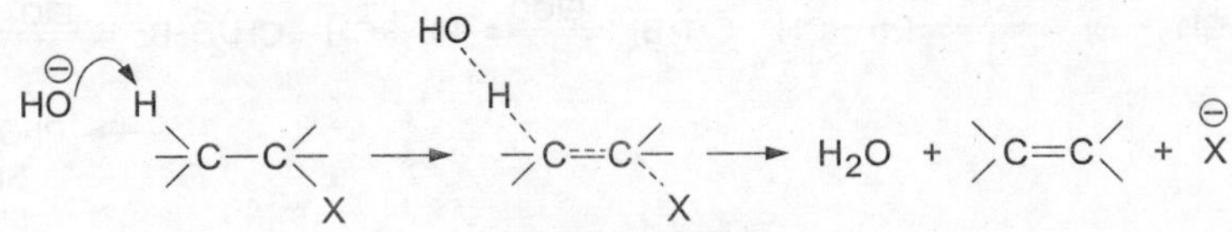

The energy of the transition state will be least when the two leaving groups, the α- and β-carbons and the attacking base are coplanar in the transition state. Also, the two leaving groups (H and X) should be *trans* to each other to effect π bond.

The two leaving groups orient themselves in the trans position when a σ bond exists between the α- and β- carbons. When, however, free rotation is not allowed as in the case of double bond, elimination is difficult when the two leaving groups are *cis* to each other. Thus, acetylene dicarboxylic acid is more easily formed from chlorofumaric acid (25) than from chloromaleic acid (26).

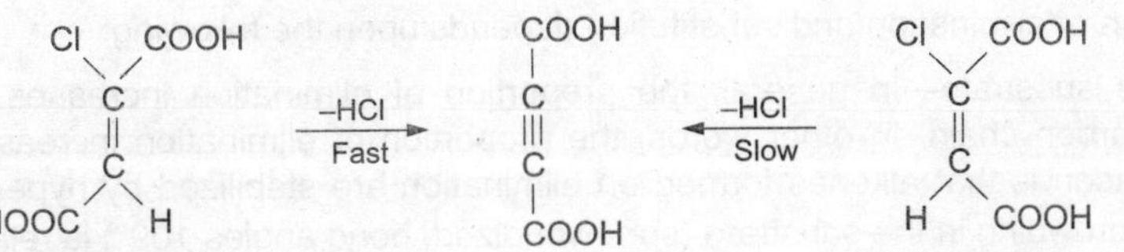

Leaving groups trans (25) — Leaving groups cis (26)

E2 reaction is facilitated by

(i) branching at α- and β-carbons—since more stable olefin is formed,

(ii) strong base of high concentration—since a strong C – H bond has to break,

(iii) solvent of low polarity—polar solvents form a strong solvent wall around the base restricting the attack. Hence DMF or DMSO are usually used as solvents.

(c) E1cB mechanism It may be argued that a second-order elimination reaction may as well proceed in two steps as in E1 reaction. The first step involves a fast and reversible removal of a proton from the β-carbon with the formation of a carbanion which then loses the leaving group in the second slow rate-determining step.

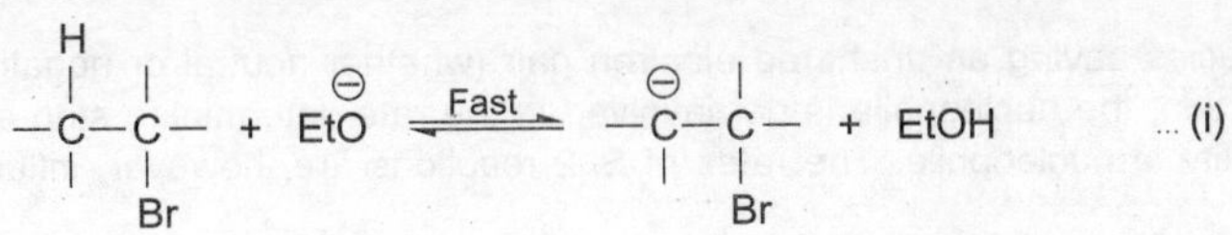

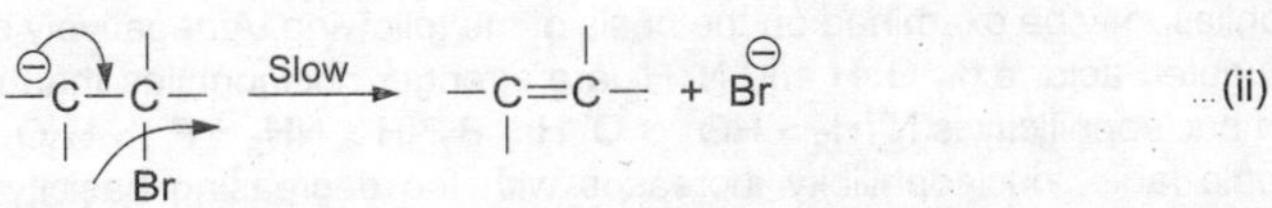

The overall rate of this reaction is thus dependent on the concentration of the conjugate base of the substrate (carbanion). Hence, this mechanism has been designated as E1cB (Elimination, Unimolecular from conjugate base).

To distinguish between E2 and E1cB mechanisms, deuterium exchange experiment was performed.

For this 2-phenylethyl bromide was treated with sodium ethoxide in EtOD. This substrate was selected because the Ph group is expected to increase the acidity of the β-hydrogen and also to stabilize the carbanion to exist long enough for incorporation of deuterium in the starting material from the solvent EtOD.

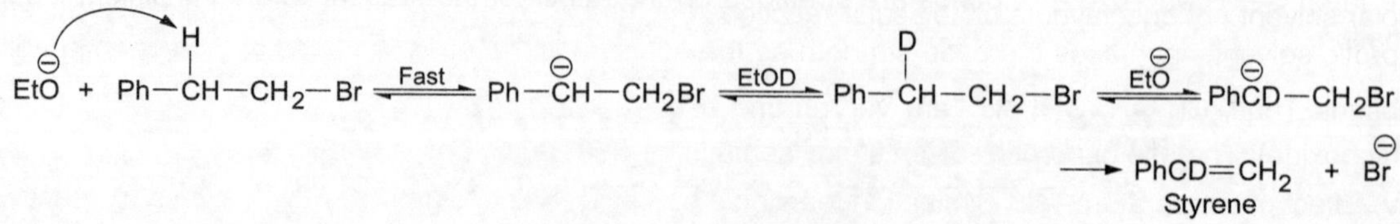

The reaction was interrupted before completion and analysed for deuterium content. No deuterium incorporation was found either in the substrate or in the styrene. Hence, no reversible carbanion was formed. The reaction followed E2 path. However, the E1cB mechanism does operate in substrates having strong electron-withdrawing groups, e.g., chlorine on β-carbon, and poor leaving groups, e.g., fluorine as in Cl_2CH-CF_3.

Elimination vs substitution Elimination reactions are usually accompanied by substitution reactions. When the reagent is a good base, it accepts protons to yield elimination products (alkenes) and if it is a good nucleophile* then it attacks the carbon to give substitution products.

The proportion of elimination and substitution depends upon the following:

(i) Structure of the substrate—In general, the proportion of elimination increases with increase in the branching of the carbon chain. In other words, the proportion of elimination increases from 1° → 2° → 3° substrates. The reason is that alkenes formed on elimination are stabilized by hyperconjugation. Also the steric strain due to crowding in the substrate (sp^3-hybridized, bond angles 109°) is relieved on the formation of alkene (sp^2-hybridized, bond angles 120°) whereas on substitution the strain is reintroduced. Suitably substituted groups, e.g., C=C and Ph, in the substrate that can stabilize the developing alkene favour elimination. Thus, ethyl bromide gives about 1% alkene while 2-phenylethyl bromide gives about 99% styrene.

(ii) Nature of the base—Strong bases promote elimination over substitution in general, and in particular E2 over E1. In low base concentration and in polar solvents S_N1 is favoured over E1. Higher concentration of base in non-polar solvents favours E2 over S_N2. Hence, alcoholic KOH favours elimination and aqueous KOH favours substitution. Strong nucleophiles but weak bases promote substitution over elimination whereas strong bases, but weak nucleophiles promote elimination over substitution. Though pyridine and R_3N are not strong bases they are poor nucleophiles because the branching at the nitrogen atom causes steric hindrance to nucleophilic attack on carbon. Hence, they act as base to accept the more exposed hydrogens of the

* Nucleophilicity—Any species having an unshared electron pair (whether neutral or negatively charged) may act as nucleophile. In S_N1 reaction, the nucleophile is not involved in the rate-determining step and so the S_N1 reaction is independent of the identity of nucleophile. The rates of S_N2 reactions are, however, influenced by the strengths of nucleophiles.

The identity of nucleophiles may be examined on the basis of the following. A negatively charged species is stronger nucleophile than its conjugated acid, e.g., $O^{\ominus}H$ and $N^{\ominus}H_2$ are stronger nucleophiles than H_2O and NH_3 respectively. The approximate order of nucleophilicity is $N^{\ominus}H_2 > RO^{\ominus} > O^{\ominus}H > R_2NH > NH_3 > F^{\ominus} > H_2O$.

Going down the periodic table, nucleophilicity increases with the decreasing basicity of the elements, e.g, the nucleophilicity order of the halides is $I^- > Br^- > Cl^- > F^-$. This is due to increasing charge to size ratios as we go along the series with progressive increase of the solvent layer by hydrogen bonding in protic solvents. This restricts nucleophilc attack on the substrate.1[2]

The order is reversed in aprotic solvents in which the solvent layer is absent. Thus, in DMF or DMSO the nucleophilicity order is $Cl^- > Br^- > I^-$.

substituent groups to afford alkene. A similar steric effect is observed with the size of the base or nucleophile. Elimination increases with increase in the size of the nucleophile.

(iii) Nature of solvent—For most reactions, increasing solvent polarity increases the rate of S_N1 reactions and decreases S_N2 reactions. Hence, the pathway can be changed with changing polarity of the solvent. A less polar solvent not only favours bimolecular reactions but also E2 over S_N2. Change of hydroxylic solvents to aprotic solvents increases the base strength as the solvent layer around the base by hydrogen bonding is absent. Thus, $\overset{\ominus}{Cl}$, $\overset{\ominus}{O}H$, $\overset{\ominus}{O}R$, etc., are very strong bases in DMF (dimethylformamide) or DMSO (dimethyl sulphoxide). The use of aprotic solvents may sometimes change the pathway from E1 to E2.

(iv) Effect of temperature— In elimination reaction a strong C – H bond has to break, hence a high-activation energy is required for elimination reaction rather than for substitution reaction.

In general, the proportion of elimination increases on using a strong base of high concentration and a solvent of low polarity. On the other hand the proportion of substitution increases by using a weak base of low concentration and a solvent of high polarity.

Orientation in elimination reactions Substrates having alternative β-hydrogens give a mixture of olefins on elimination.

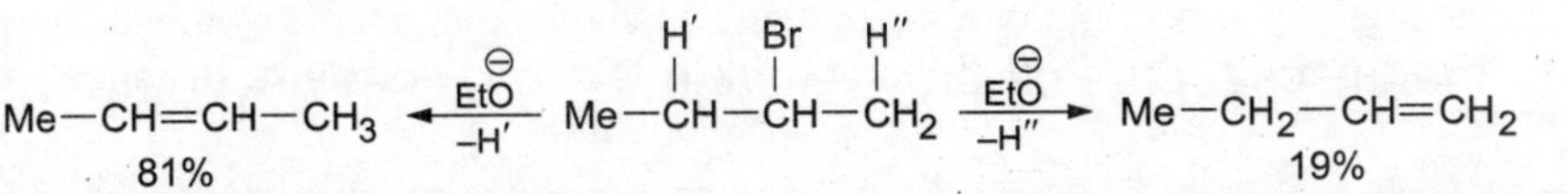

To help in forecasting the major product of elimination (alkene), there are two empirical rules: (i) Saytzev rule and (ii) Hofmann rule.

(i) Saytzev rule—The rule states that neutral substrates (alkyl halides, alkyl toluenesulphonates) lead predominantly to that alkene which is more highly substituted on the carbons of the double bond.

In E1 mechanism the leaving group is gone before the abstraction of proton. Hence the direction of elimination depends wholly on the relative stabilities of the olefins. Therefore, Saytzev rule governs the orientation of E1 reaction.

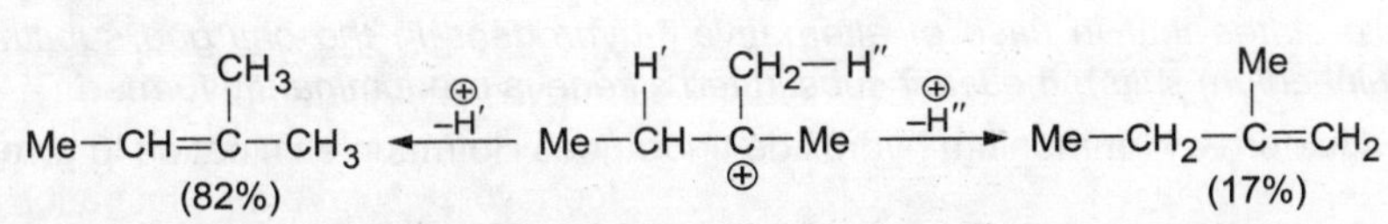

In suitable substrates the rearrangement of the carbocation before elimination may give different alkenes. For steric reasons the non-Saytzev product may be the major product in suitable substrates.

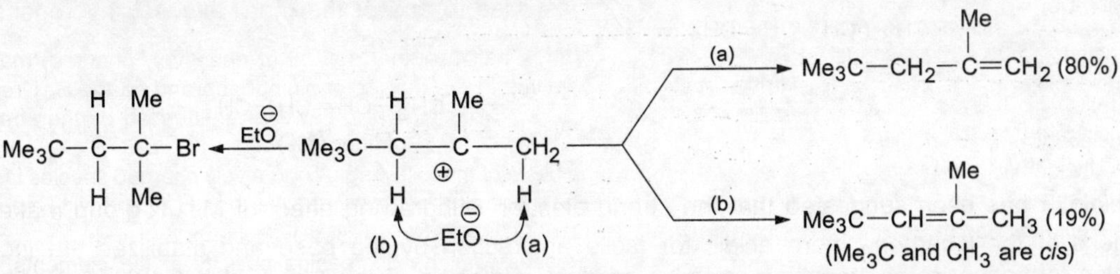

The olefin obtained through path (b) is minor due to steric hindrance. In E2, it is suggested that the incipient olefinic bond formation in the transition state is being stabilized by the inductive effect of the alkyl groups, thereby lowering the energy of the transition state. Therefore, with the increasing number of alkyl groups there will be increasing stability of the transition state with progressive lowering of energy of the transition state.

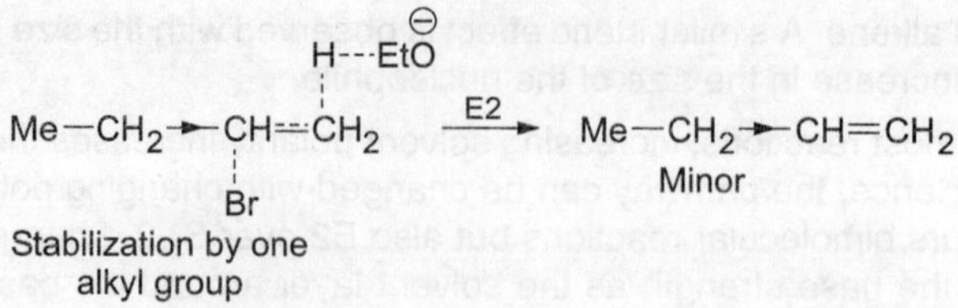

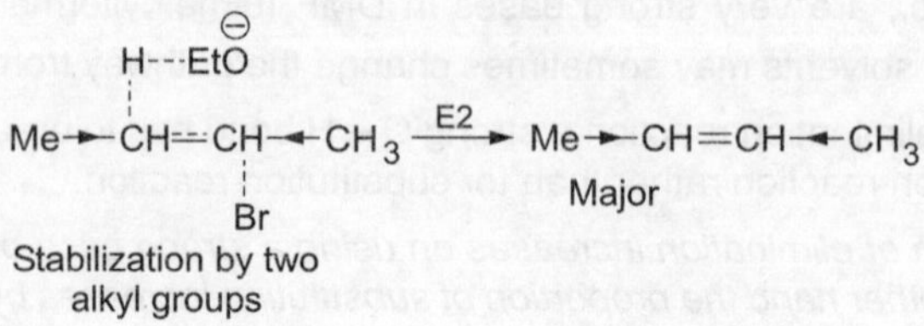

(ii) Hofmann rule—When a quaternary ammonium hydroxide is strongly heated (<125 °C) it decomposes to yield a tertiary amine, water and alkene.

$$Me_3\overset{\oplus}{N}-CH_2-CH_2-CH_3\overset{\ominus}{O}H \xrightarrow{\Delta} Me_3N: + CH_2=CH-CH_3 + H_2O$$

This is known as Hofmann elimination or β-elimination. The reaction involves abstraction of a proton from β-carbon with the simultaneous expulsion of the leaving group.

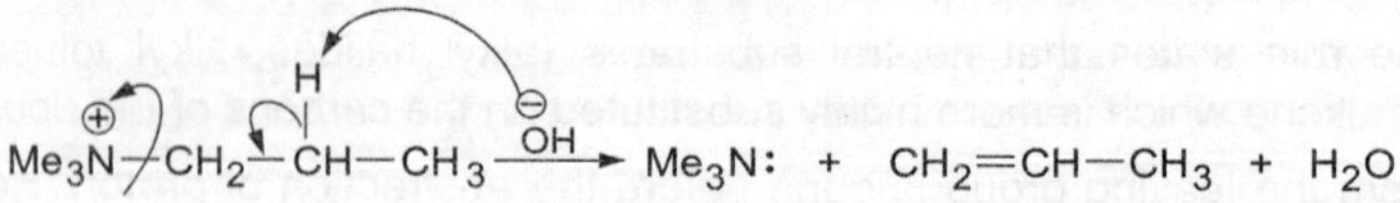

When there are alternative β-hydrogens in the quaternary ammonium salts, a mixture of alkenes is formed.

Hofmann rule states that in case of alternative β-hydrogens in the charged substrates (quaternary ammonium and sulphonium salts), the least substituted alkene is predominantly formed.

Thus, 2-butylquaternary ammonium hydroxide undergoes Hofmann elimination to give 1-butene as the major product.

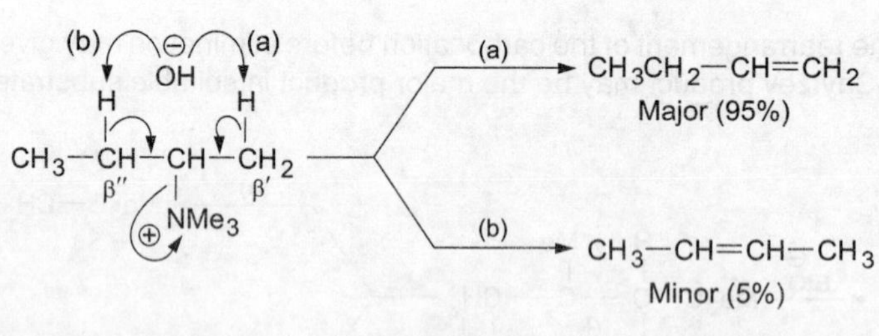

To explain, it has been suggested that the strong electron-withdrawing effect of $Me_3\overset{\oplus}{N}$ group makes the hydrogens of the β-carbons more acidic for facile abstraction by the base and stabilizes the incipient carbanion formation in the transition state on gradual stretching of the β C – H bond. In this particular compound with alternative β-hydrogens, the β′′-hydrogens are less acidic due to +I effect of the adjacent methyl group. Hence, β′-hydrogen which is relatively more acidic is removed to give predominantly l-butene.

Hofmann product increases on increasing branching in the base. Steric effect due to crowding in the leaving group or in the substrate promotes Hofmann elimination.

In general the proton acidity and for that matter the inductive effect is the more important factor for Hofmann elimination. Whatever be the conditions, that alkene is formed in which its double bond is conjugated with Ph or C = C groups, e.g.,

$$PhCH_2CH_2-\overset{\oplus}{N}(Me)_2-CH_2-CH_3\overset{\ominus}{O}H \xrightarrow{150\,^{\circ}C} \underset{\text{Styrene (93 \%)}}{PhCH=CH_2} + Me_2NEt$$

Hofmann elimination has been very useful in the degradation of nitrogeneous heterocyclics for structure determination. Thus,

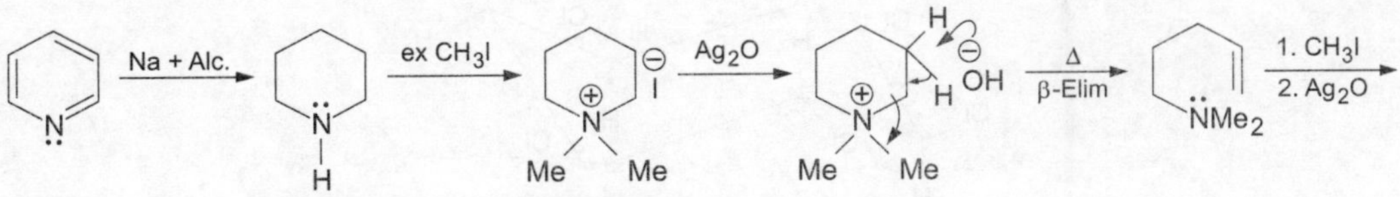

Pyridine Piperidine *N, N*-Dimethylpiperidinium iodide

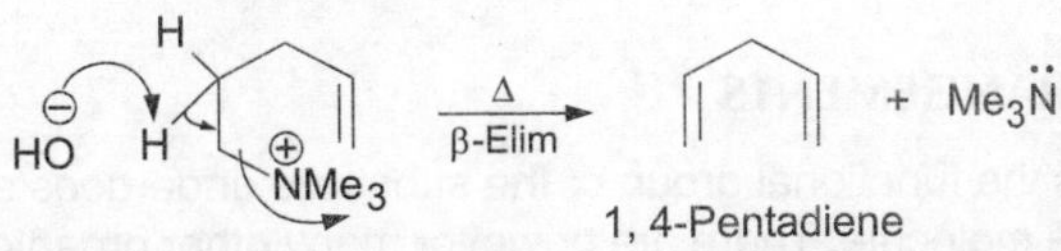

1, 4-Pentadiene

Stereochemistry of E2 Elimination results in π-bond formation. In E2 reaction the p orbitals which develop on the α- and β-carbons with the departure of the leaving groups should be parallel for maximum overlap. For this both the leaving groups and the carbons bearing them should be in one plane.

When the two leaving groups are planar there can be two extreme conformations: (a) anti-periplanar (27), i.e., the two groups are in trans position and (b) syn-periplanar (28), i.e., the two groups are in cis position.

The elimination then may proceed as given below.

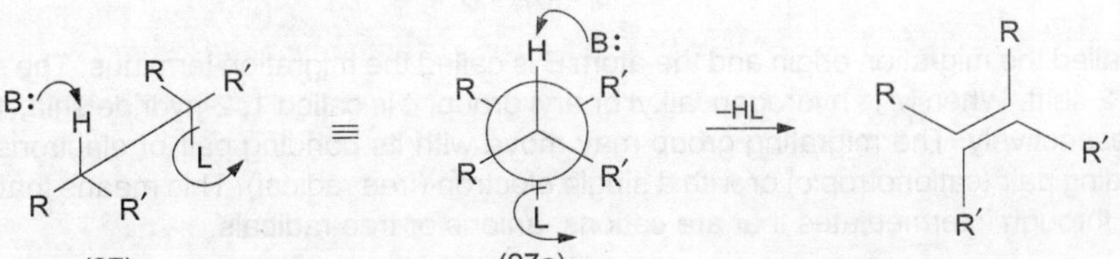

(27) (27a)

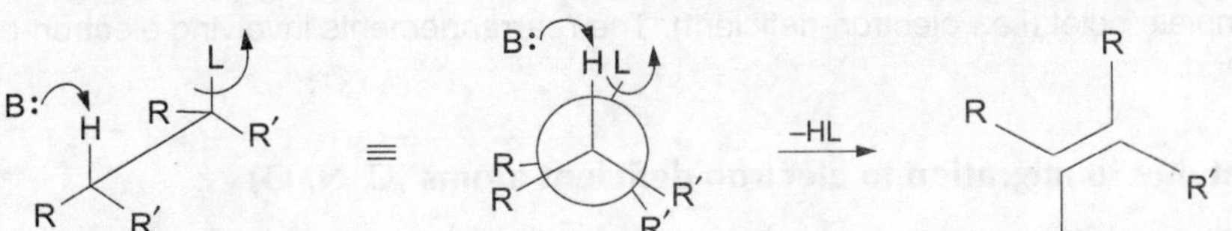

(28) (28a)

From the Newman projections of the trans and cis conformations the elimination is expected to be more facile from the trans conformation (27a) than from the cis conformation (28a). This is because (i) in (27a) the attacking base approaches from the farthest side of the leaving group while in (28a) the attack is from the same side of the leaving group which causes repulsion, (ii) the developing charge on the β-carbon displaces the leaving group with its bonding pair from the back side (as in S_N2), a path of least energy, and what is most important is (iii) the elimination occurs from the lower-energy staggered conformation (27a) than from the higher-energy eclipsed conformation (28a).

Hence, the transition state and consequently the pathway for elimination is of lower energy when the leaving groups are *trans* (27) than when they are *cis* (28).

Therefore, most E2 reactions proceed faster when the leaving groups are *trans* (25) than when they are *cis* (26). The β-isomer of hexachlorocyclohexane has all the six chlorines in the equatorial bonds so that they are all *trans* to each other and no hydrogen is available in the trans position. The result is that the elimination of HCl is slower by 7000–24000 times in β-isomer than in other isomers.

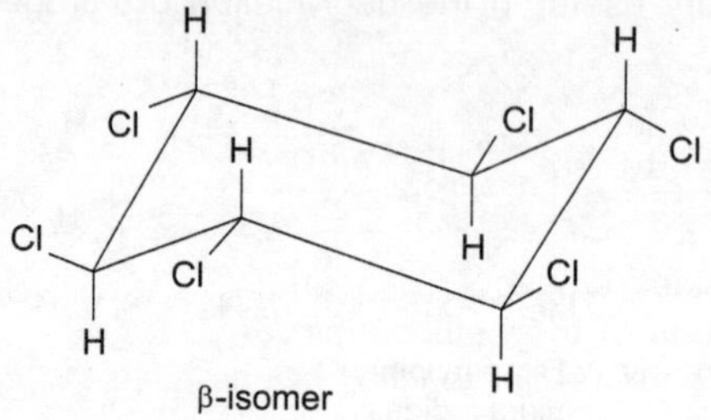

β-isomer

4. MOLECULAR REARRANGEMENTS

In most organic reactions the functional group of the substrate undergoes structural change without affecting the carbon skeleton of the molecule. There are however many other organic reactions in which atoms, groups (alkyl or aryl), double bonds or functional groups migrate within the molecule. The latter types of reactions are known as rearrangement reactions or molecular rearrangement. Thus, molecular rearrangement involves modification in the sequence of atoms or groups in a molecule resulting in a new structure.

Migration of atoms or groups occurs from one atom to another (usually adjacent) within the same molecule by Whitmore 1, 2-shift.

$$\overset{\displaystyle M}{\underset{|}{A}}\!-\!B \longrightarrow A\!-\!\overset{\displaystyle M}{\underset{|}{B}}$$

The atom A is called the migration origin and the atom B is called the migration terminus. The shift of M from A to B is called 1, 2-shift. When M is hydrogen, alkyl or aryl group, it is called 1, 2-hydride shift, 1, 2-alkyl shift or 1, 2-aryl shift respectively. The migrating group may move with its bonding pair of electrons (anionotropic), without the bonding pair (cationotropic) or with a single electron (free radical). This means that rearrangement may take place through intermediates that are cations, anions or free radicals.

A large number of molecular rearrangements involve anionotropic migration of a group to an adjacent atom with incomplete octet (i.e., electron-deficient). The rearrangements involving electron-deficient species are more common.

Rearrangement due to migration to electron-deficient atoms (C, N, O)

During a reaction an electronegative group may depart with its bonding pair of electrons leaving behind an electron-deficient atom with six electrons. This results in the migration (1, 2-shift) of a group with its bonding pair from the adjacent atom to the electron-deficient atom. The migrating group may be hydrogen, carbon, nitrogen, oxygen, sulphur or halogens.

The migrating group may either (i) detach from the migration origin and then form bond with the migration terminus (electron-deficient atom) or (ii) may remain partly bonded to both migration origin and terminus to form a bridged ion intermediate or transition state. The general mechanistic possibilities by 1, 2-shift are given below.

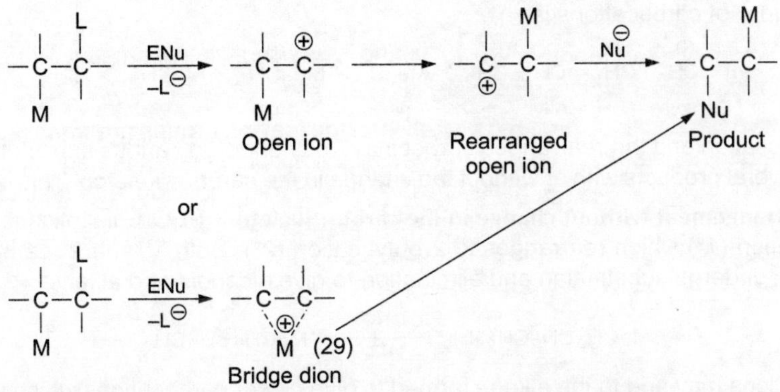

When M is a hetero atom, besides crossover experiments there is stereochemical evidence that (29) is formed. The nonbonding electrons of the hetero atom are said to be involved in the neighbouring group participation in forming (29) since the rate of reaction is increased by anchimeric* assistance. Alkyl group or hydrogen has no non-bonding electrons. It is quite possible that those groups first leave the migration origin to form open ion and then form the bridged ion because the rearrangements do not show the increased rate expected from anchimeric assistance.

The corresponding rearrangements with radical and anion intermediates are seldom encountered because of unfavourable distribution of electrons in the molecular orbital encompassing the three atoms in the bridged ion. Rearrangements to electron-deficient carbon, nitrogen and oxygen will be separately studied.

Rearrangements to electron-deficient carbon (Carbocation rearrangement)

Carbocation intermediates are generated in the course of various types of reactions, e.g., (i) solvolytic substitution and elimination reactions (ii) protonation of alcohols, ethers, alkenes, alkynes, etc., (iii) decomposition of diazonium salts, etc. If the carbocation generated in a reaction is unstable, it rearranges to a more stable carbocation by 1,2 shift so that rearrangement is observed in the product. Thus, the driving force of the rearrangement is the stability of the carbocation which depends on the dispersal of the positive charge on the carbon. The dispersal of the charge increases with increased substituents on the cationic carbon by inductive and hyperconjugative effects. Conjugation of cationic carbon with π electrons increases the stability further. This may reverse the rearrangement, e.g.,

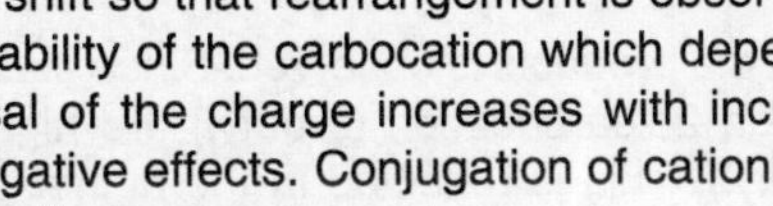

* When a group with an unshared electron pair and β to the leaving group is present, the rate of substitution is greater than expected. This is due to neighbouring group participation. The first step is intramolecular nucleophilic substitution by the neighbouring group forming a bridged ion. In the second step the external nucleophile pushes out the neighbouring group, i.e., the molecule undergoes two S_N2 substitutions, so that the configuration is retained. Thus, the neighbouring group aids the nucleophilic attack and consequently increases the rate.

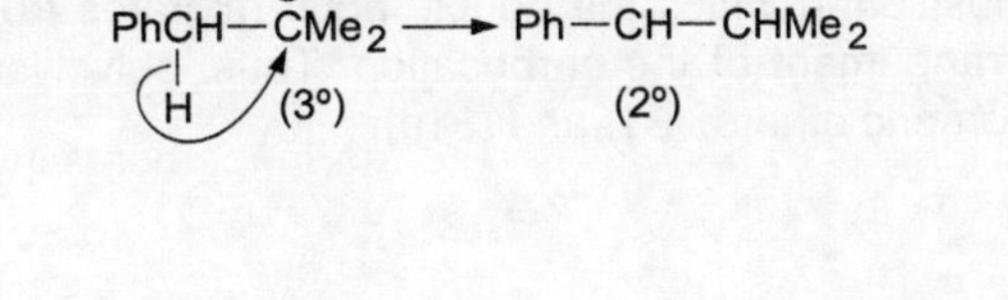

Thus, the stability order of carbocations is:

$$\underset{\text{Benzyl}}{Ph-\overset{\oplus}{C}H_2},\ \underset{\text{Allyl}}{CH_2{=}CH-\overset{\oplus}{C}H_2} > \underset{3°}{Me_3\overset{\oplus}{C}} > \underset{2°}{Me_2\overset{\oplus}{C}H} > \underset{1°}{Me\overset{\oplus}{C}H_2} > \overset{\oplus}{C}H_3$$

Initially formed carbocation and the rearranged carbocation may undergo various substitution and elimination reactions to yield several products with or without the change in the carbon skeleton. This is illustrated below.

(a) Carbocation rearrangement without change in the carbon skeleton (i) On diazotisation, 1-amino butane produces 1-butyl cation (1°) which rearranges to 2-butyl cation (2°). Both 1° and 2° carbocations under the condition of reaction undergo substitution and elimination to give alcohols and alkene.

$$MeCH_2CH_2CH_2NH_2 \xrightarrow[HCl]{NaNO_2} MeCH_2CH_2\overset{\oplus}{C}H_2$$

Further, both the cations may add to the alkene formed to give newer carbocations which may again undergo the whole series of reactions. Thus, a plethora of products may be formed.

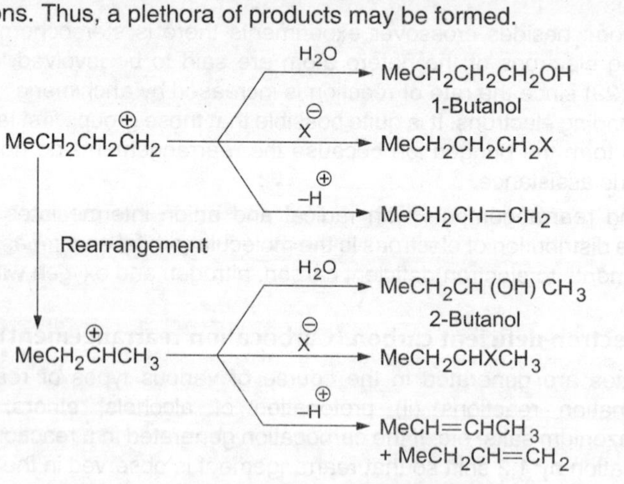

No change in the carbon skeletons in the products is observed. Since stable carbocations have longer life, the yields of the products formed through 2° carbocation (2-butyl) are higher than those from the less stable initially formed 1° carbocation (1-butyl). This is reflected in the higher percentage yields of 2-butanol over 1-butanol.

(ii) Allylic rearrangement—Another most widely recognized example of this class of rearrangement occurs in the substitution at the allylic position in which the double bond migrates from one position to an adjacent position with consequent rearrangement of the carbocation. Thus, solvolysis of 3-chlorobut-1-ene (30) in EtOH by S_N1 path gives two isomeric ethers, (31) and (31a).

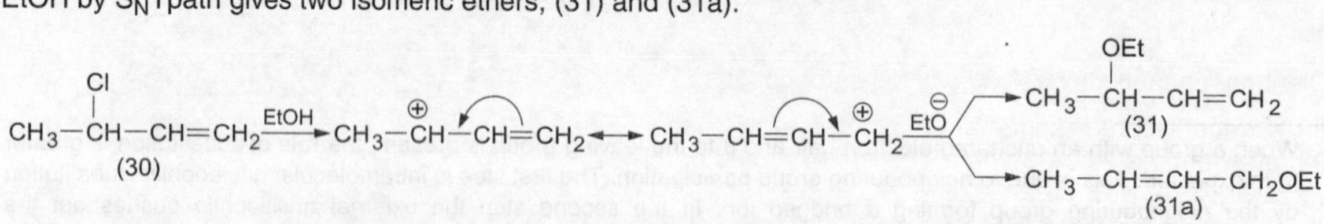

With NaOEt in high concentration, the reaction follows S_N2 path with no rearrangement.

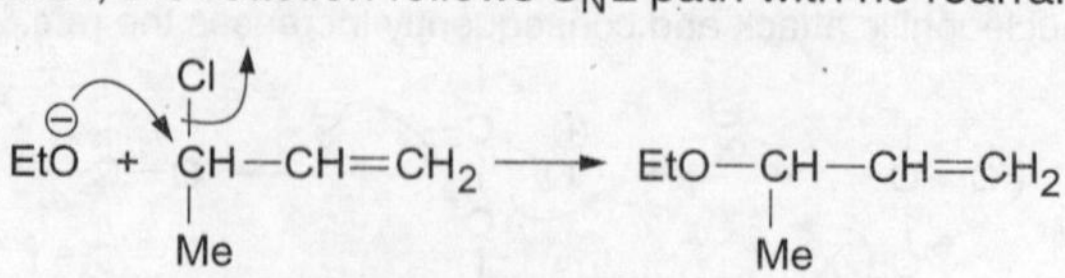

When, however, the alpha carbon is substituted with bulky groups, direct S_N2 displacement with allylic rearrangement is observed.

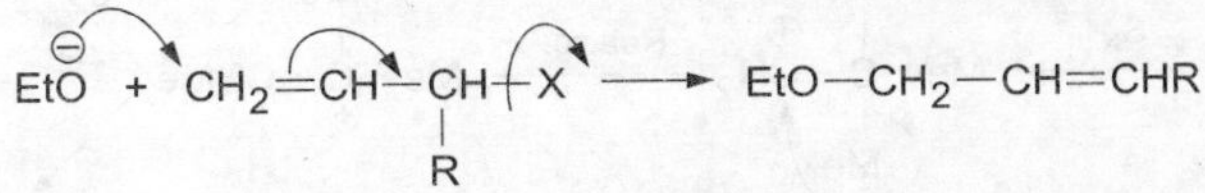

Bimolecular displacement reaction with allylic rearrangements are designated S_N2'.

(b) Carbocation rearrangement with change in the carbon skeleton (i) Hydrocarbon rearrangement—During the cracking of petroleum hydrocarbons in the presence of Lewis acids, carbocations are generated from straight-chain hydrocarbons. These carbocations undergo rearrangements to form branched-chain products. The process has been commercially utilized for producing anti-knock fuels for automobiles.

$$\text{(i)}\ \underset{(20\ \%)}{CH_3CH_2CH_2CH_3} \underset{(150\ ^\circ C)}{\overset{AlBr_3}{\rightleftharpoons}} \underset{(80\ \%)}{(CH_3)_3CH}$$

Another example is the interconversion of methylcyclopentane and cyclohexane.

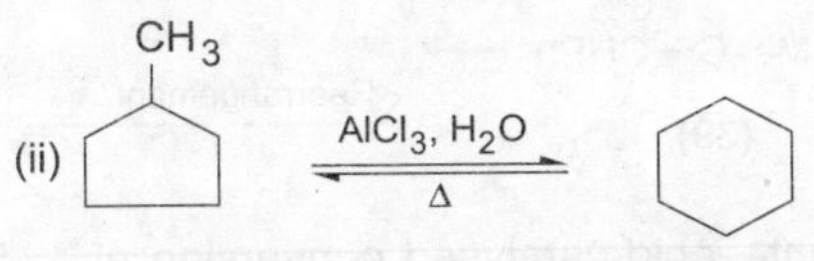

(12.5 %) (87.5 %)

In the presence of acids, carbocations generated from alkenes readily undergo rearrangement to form products with change in the carbon skeleton.

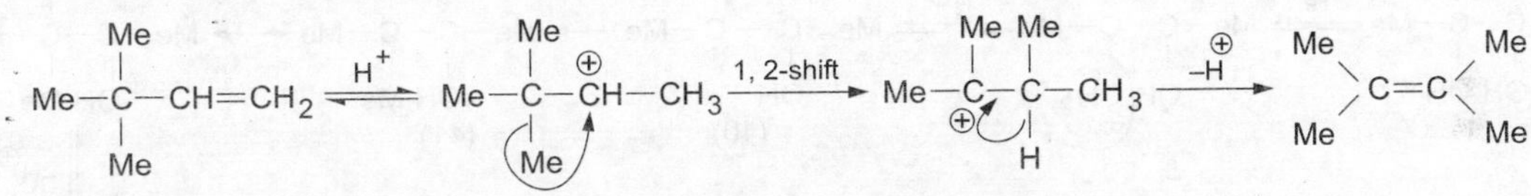

In the Friedel–Crafts alkylation, the alkyl cations rearrange before attacking.

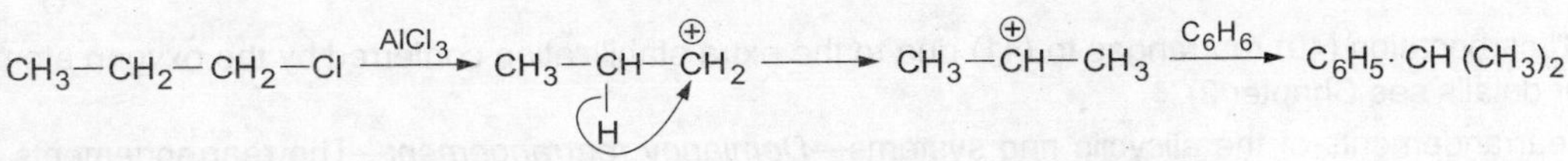

Dienone–phenol conversion involves carbocation rearrangement (see Chapter 2).

(ii) Neopentyl rearrangement—Hydrolysis of neopentyl bromide (32) under S_N1 conditions gives 2-methyl-butane-2-ol (33) instead of the expected neopentyl alcohol (34).

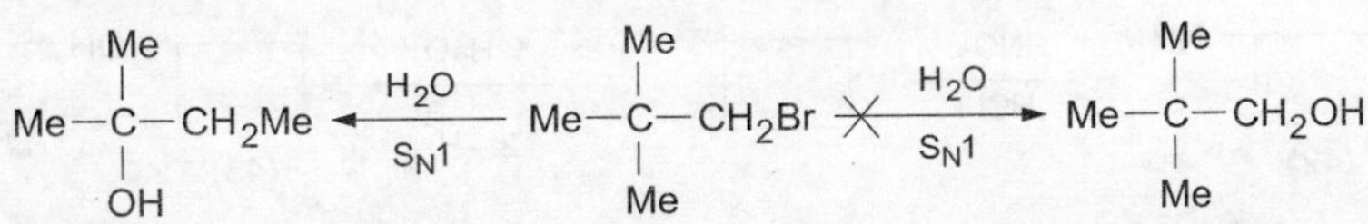

(33) (32) (34)

Along with (33), 2-methylbutene-2 (36) is also obtained. This is explained due to the rearrangement of the first formed 1° carbocation to 3° carbocation (35).

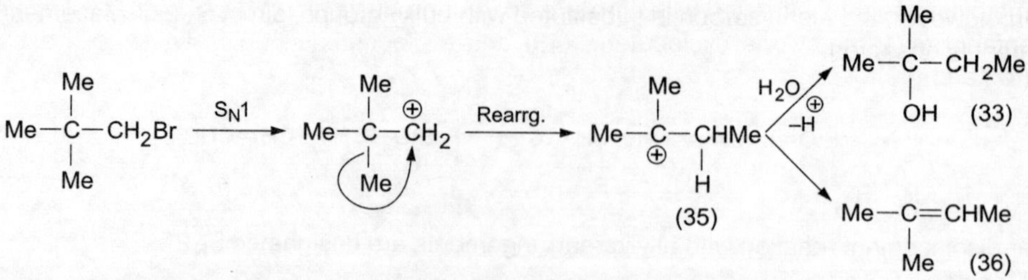

Reaction under S_N2 conditions is slow due to steric factors. However, (32) forms neopentyl ethyl ether (37) by S_N2 path on treatment with sodium ethoxide without rearrangement.

$$Me_3C{-}CH_2Br \xrightarrow[S_N1]{\overset{\ominus}{Et O}} Me_3C{-}CH_2OEt$$

(37)

Hence, in the absence of other information rearrangement is often taken as an evidence of S_N1 reaction and for that matter carbocation formation. However, the phenyl analogue (38) of neopentyl-type bromide does not rearrange due to the greater stability of the benzyl cation (39) over 3° carbocation.

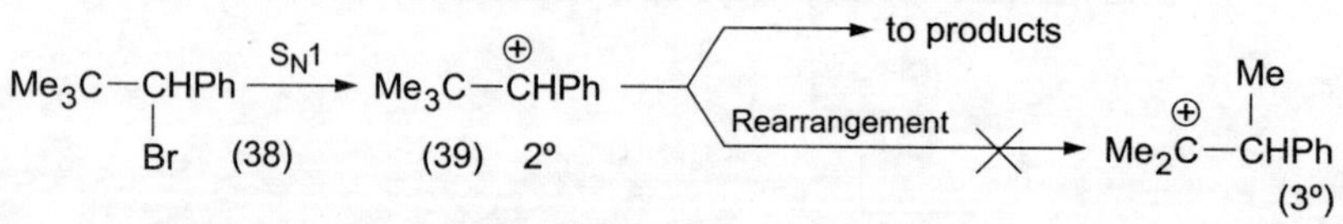

(iii) Pinacol–pinacolone rearrangement—Acid-catalysed conversion of 1, 2-diols (e.g., pinacol) to ketones (e.g., pinacolone) is another example of the rearrangement of carbocation with change in the carbon skeleton. The rearrangement involves 1, 2-methyl shift.

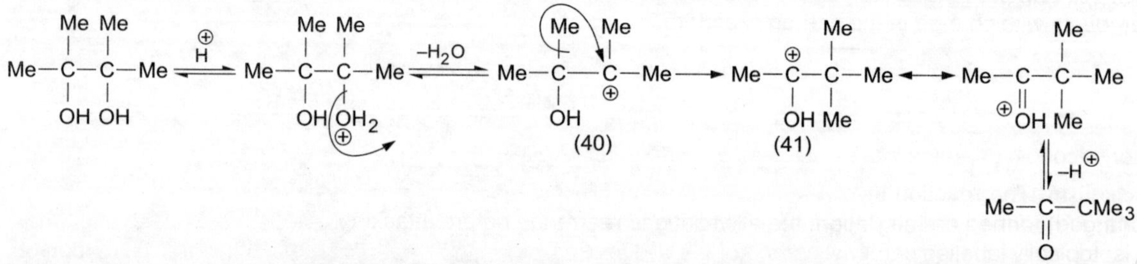

The 3° carbocation (40) rearranges to (41) due to the extra stabilization conferred by the oxygen atom. (For further details see Chapter 2).

(iv) Rearrangements of the alicyclic ring systems—*Demjanov rearrangement*—The rearrangements of the carbocations generated during the deamination of alicyclic primary amines is known as Demjanov rearrangement. The rearrangement results in substitution, elimination and ring contraction or expansion. Thus, cyclobutylamine (42) on treatment with nitrous acid gives a mixture of cyclobutanol (43) and cyclopropylcarbinol (44), the latter with ring contraction.

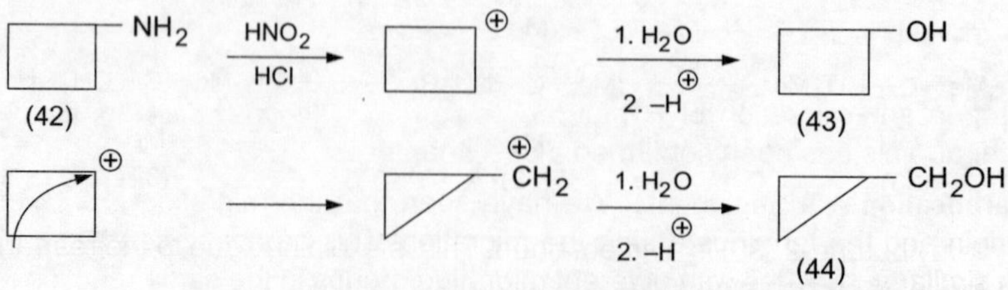

If cyclobutyl methylamine (45) is treated with nitrous acid, four products are obtained, viz., cyclobutylcarbinol (46), cyclopentanol (47), methylene cyclobutene (48) and cyclopentene (49) in which ring expansion is observed in (47) and (49).

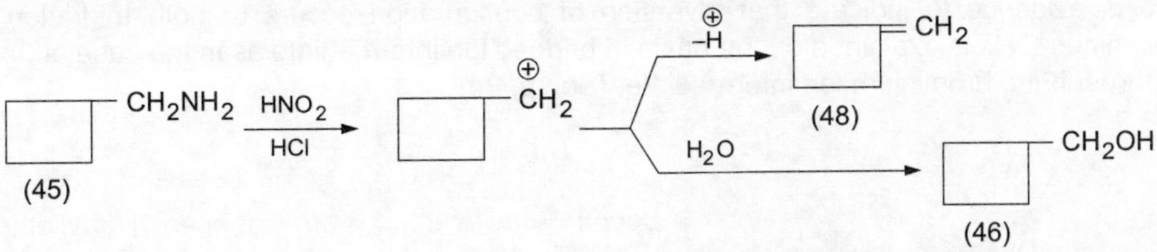

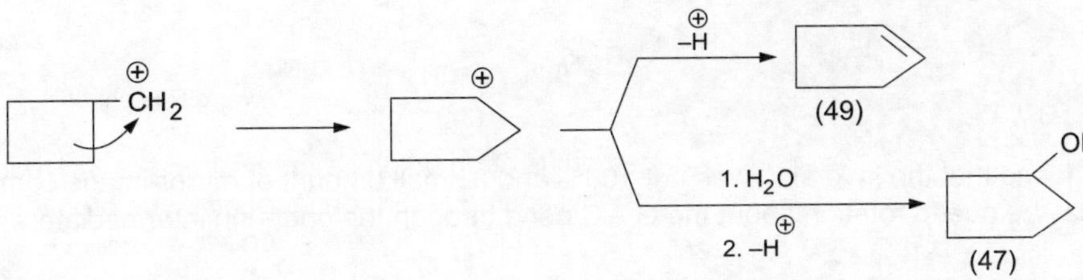

It will be seen that when the positive charge is on the alicyclic ring, the migration of ring methylene group causes ring contraction (44). When the positive charge is placed on the carbon α to the alicyclic ring, expansion of the ring occurs (47) & (49).

By this rearrangement, seven- and eight-membered rings may be prepared.

(v) Wolff rearrangement—This rearrangement does not involve carbocations. It involves rearrangement to electron-deficient carbon but without any charge on the carbon, i.e., a carbene. Thus, α-diazoketones rearrange to ketenes with loss of nitrogen in the presence of solid Ag_2O or on irradiation or heating.

$$RCOCHN_2 \xrightarrow{Ag_2O} R-CH=C=O + N_2$$

Ketenes are very reactive and react with the nucleophiles present. Thus, the reaction in the presence of water, alcohols or amines gives acids and their derivatives.

Mechanism The reaction involves migration of the group, R, to the adjacent electron-deficient carbon (but uncharged) formed on the departure of nitrogen molecule. This has been suggested on the observation that the isotopically labelled carbonyl carbon of the α-diazoketone is found to be present in the carboxyl carbon of the resulting acid when the reaction is carried out in the presence of water.

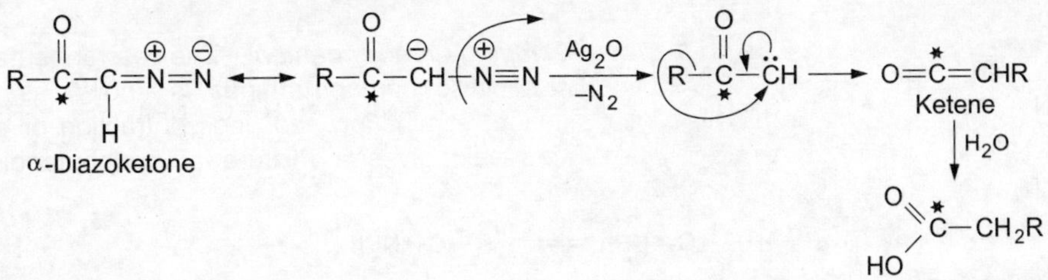

Splitting of nitrogen and migration of R may be concerted. The group R migrates with retention of configuration if R is chiral. This has been confirmed. (See Chapter 2.)

Stereochemistry of carbocation rearrangements We have seen that the migrating group remains joined to both the migration origin and the terminus during the migration. This has been confirmed by the crossover experiments with two similar substrates with different migrating groups in the same reaction mixture when no crossover products were obtained. In case of hydrogen migration, the reaction was conducted in D_2O or EtOD but no deuterium was incorporated in the product. The rearrangement is therefore intramolecular. Hence, when the migrating group is chiral, we can expect no change in configuration of the migrating group.

There is evidence to indicate that inversion of configuration occurs at both migration origin and migration terminus. This is explained on the basis of bridged ion intermediate as in the case of trans-addition to alkenes through the brominium ion intermediate. (See p. 34)

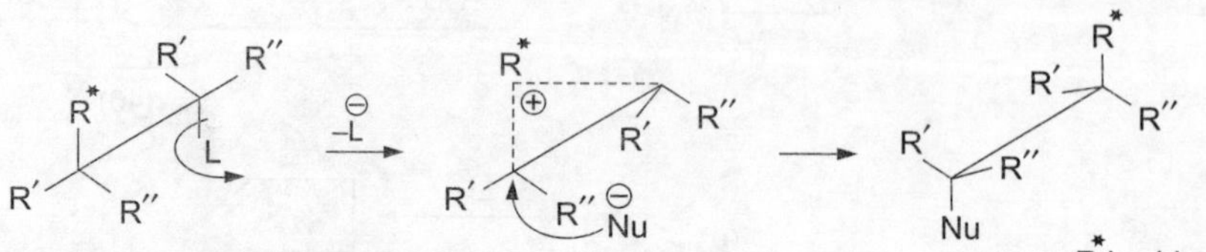

were $\overset{*}{R}$ is chiral

It was, however, found that the inversion was not 100% and a small amount of mirror-image compound was obtained. This may be due to rotation about the C – C bond through the open-ion intermediate.

Rearrangements to electron-deficient nitrogen

Similar to the electron-deficient carbons such as carbocation and carbene intermediates, electron-deficient nitrogen species are known in which the nitrogen bears a positive charge, $R_2\overset{\oplus}{N}$: (cf carbocation) or the nitrogen has an open sextet of electrons, $R\ddot{N}$: a nitrene (cf. carbene). Hence, as in the case of electron-deficient carbons, migration of alkyl or ary groups with their bonding pair of electrons takes place to the electron-deficient nitrogen with consequent rearrangement.

Some well-known examples of rearrangements to electron-deficient nitrogen are Hofmann, Curtius, Schmidt, Beckmann rearrangements, etc. The general pattern of the rearrangement of this group of reactions is shown below:

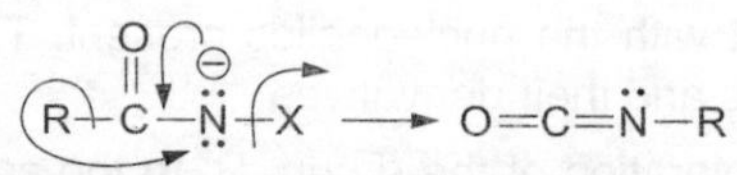

Beckmann rearrangement involves the conversion of ketoximes to amides while the rest involves the transformation of acids into an amine with one carbon less than the starting acid. Thus:

Beckmann

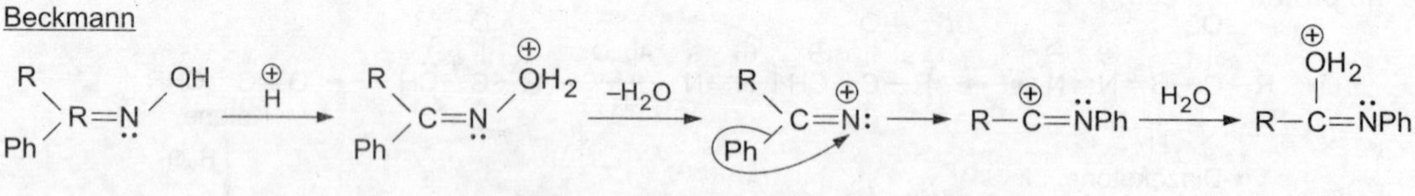

Curtius

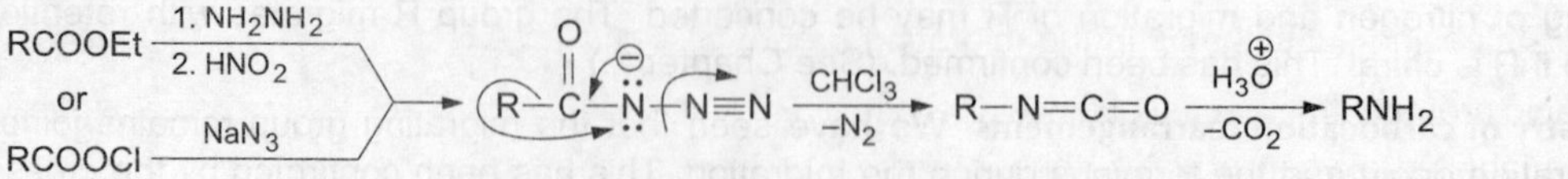

Hofmann

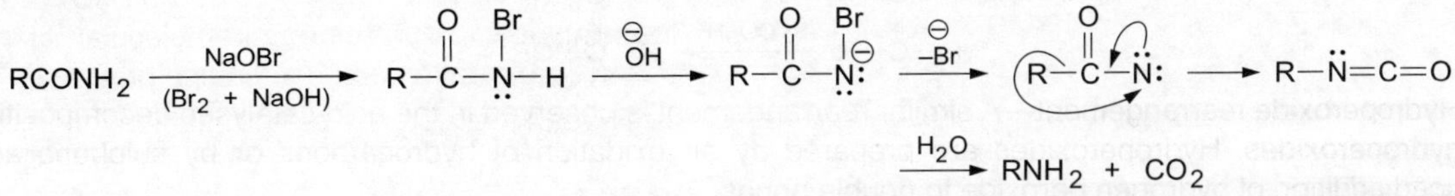

Schmidt

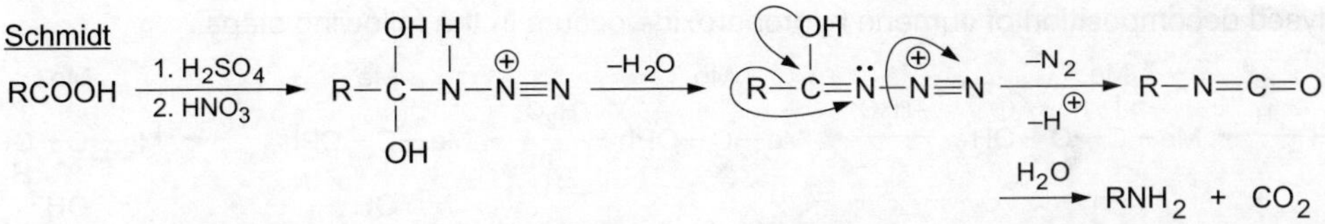

The configuration of the migrating group is retained in all the rearrangements of electron-deficient nitrogen. This has been confirmed by correlating the configurations of the chiral acid and the resulting chiral amine in Hofmann rearrangement. Both have the same relative configurations.

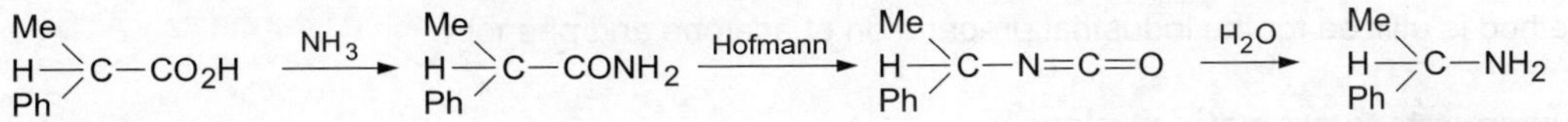

(+)-2-Phenylpropionic acid (–)-1-Phenylmethylamine

Rearrangements to electron-deficient oxygen

From the foregoing rearrangements to electron-deficient carbons and nitrogens, it is logical to expect similar rearrangements to electron-deficient oxygen. Such rearrangements are indeed observed in Baeyer–Villiger oxidation and hydroperoxide rearrangement.

(i) Baeyer–Villiger oxidation—The reaction involves the oxidation of ketones to esters by reaction with hydrogen peroxide or peracids

$$R_2CO + R'CO_3H \longrightarrow RCOOR + R'COOH$$

Cyclic ketones are converted to lactones with ring expansion.

Mechanism Acid-catalysed addition of peracid to ketones gives an adduct, peroxide intermediate (50). The adduct then undergoes loss of carboxylate anion and migration of a group to the electron-deficient oxygen to give the protonated ester.

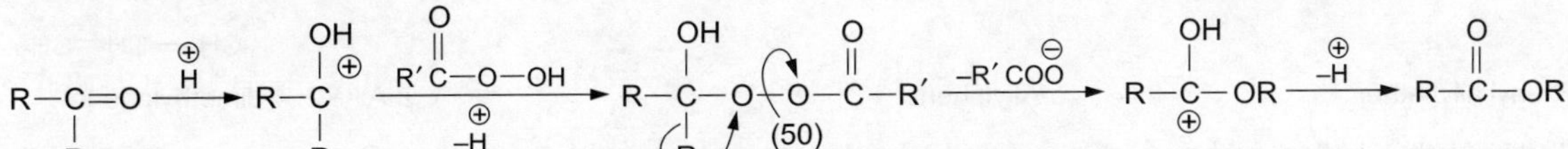

(50) Adduct

The key step of the reaction is the heterolytic fission of the O – O bond of the adduct to generate an electron-deficient oxygen to which the migration occurs.

Electron-releasing substituents in the migrating group, R, and electron-withdrawing substituents in R′ group of the acid promote the reaction. Hence, the loss of $R'COO^{\ominus}$ and migration of R is concerted. It has been found that the labelled oxygen of the ketone is entirely present as the carbonyl oxygen of the ester which supports the mechanism.

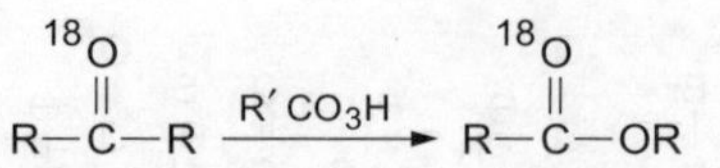

(ii) Hydroperoxide rearrangement—A similar rearrangement is observed in the acid-catalysed decomposition of hydroperoxides. Hydroperoxides are prepared by air oxidation of hydrocarbons or by sulphuric acid induced addition of hydrogen peroxide to double bonds.

Thus, acid-catalysed decomposition of cumene hydroperoxide occurs in the following steps.

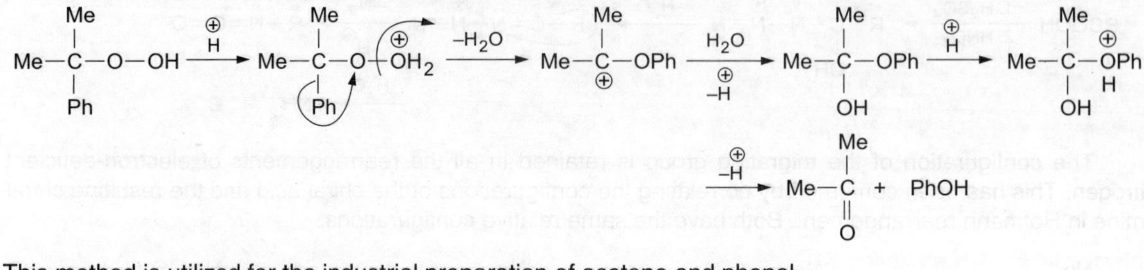

This method is utilized for the industrial preparation of acetone and phenol.

Rearrangements to aromatic nucleus

These rearrangements involve the migration of a group, X, from a substituted hetero atom Z to the activated positions of the aromatic nucleus, e.g., ortho and para positions of benzene ring.

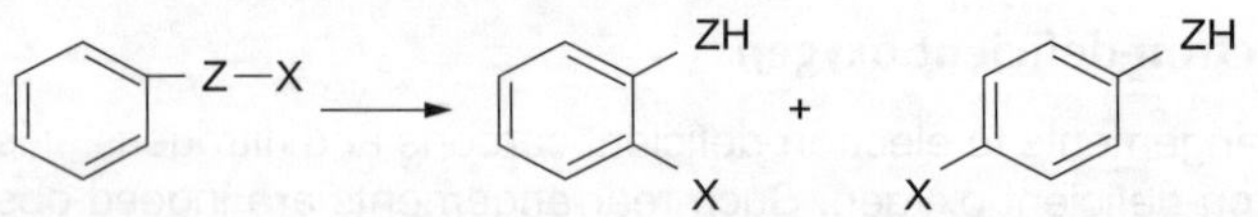

The rearrangements may be classified on the basis of hetero atoms bearing the migrating groups.

(a) Rearrangements of phenol derivatives Claisen and Fries rearrangements are examples of this class of rearrangements (see Chapter 2).

(i) Claisen rearrangement—The reaction involves the migration of allyl group from oxygen to the ortho position. When both the ortho positions are substituted, migration occurs at the para position.

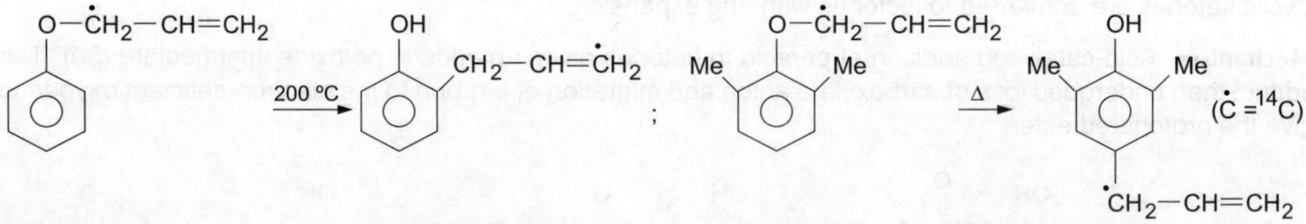

Phenyl allyl ether o-Allylphenol *p*-Allyl-2, 4-dimethylphenol

Studies with labelled carbon indicates end-interchange during ortho migration. During para migration the end-interchange occurs twice so that there is no rearrangement in the final product.

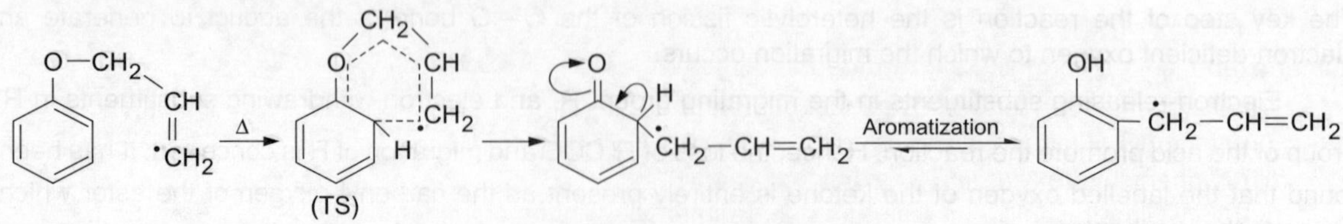

Similar rearrangement is observed in aliphatic allyl ethers.

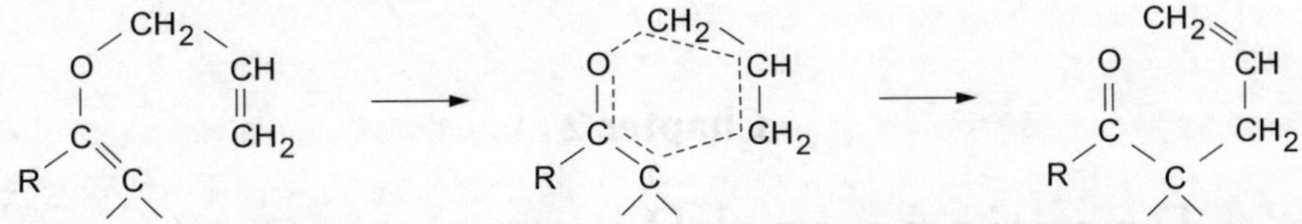

(ii) Fries rearrangement—Phenolic esters on heating in the presence of $AlCl_3$ give *o*- and *p*-acyl phenols. The rearrangement involves migration of acyl group from the oxygen to the aromatic ring, i.e., the reaction is a self- acylation.

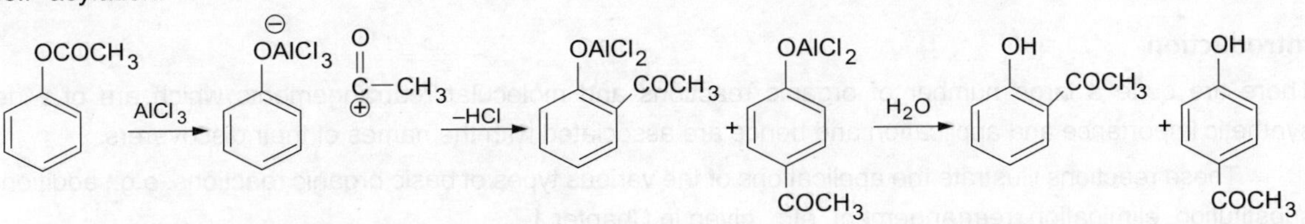

(b) Rearrangement of aniline derivatives A group of rearrangements involves the migration of groups from nitrogen to the aromatic ring on treatment with mineral acids. These rearrangements are either intramolecular or intermolecular. Thus—

Intramolecular rearrangement:

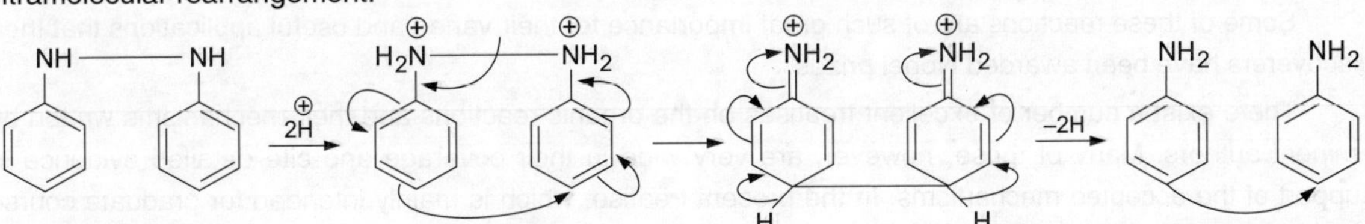

Hydrazobenzene Paramigration Benzidine

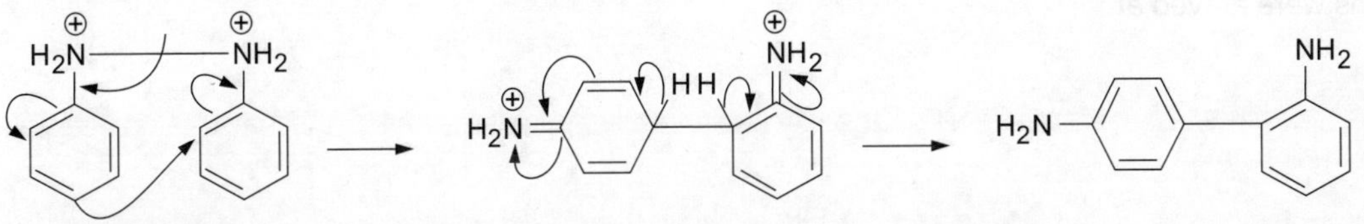

Ortho migration

Other examples are the conversion of phenylnitramine to *o*- and *p*-nitroanilines and phenylsulphamic acid to sulphanilic acid and orthanilic acid.

Intermolecular rearrangement:

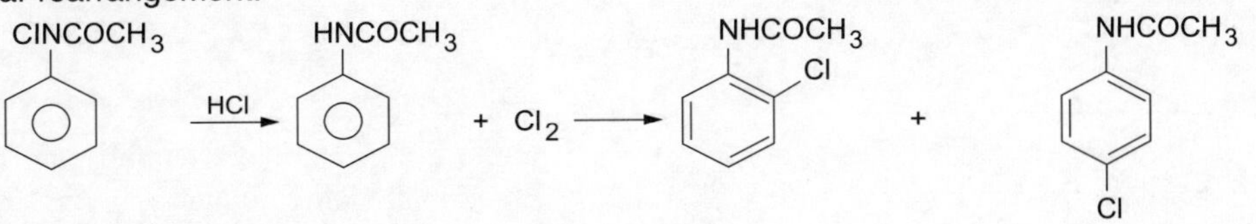

n-chloroacetanilide *o*-and *p*-chloroacetanilides

Other examples of intermolecular rearrangements are the conversion of

(i) Diazoaminobenzene to *p*-aminoazobenzene

(ii) *N*-methyl-*N*-nitrosoaniline to *p*-nitroso-*N*-methylaniline

(iii) *N*-phenylhydroxylamine to *p*-aminophenol

(iv) *N, N*-Dimethylanilinium chloride to 2, 4-dimethylanilinium chloride, etc.

Chapter 2

Reactions and Rearrangements

Introduction

There are quite a large number of organic reactions and molecular rearrangements which are of wide synthetic importance and application and hence are associated with the names of their discoverers.

These reactions illustrate the applications of the various types of basic organic reactions, e.g., addition, substitution, elimination, rearrangement, etc., given in Chapter 1.

By the dexterous application of these named reactions and rearrangements, it has been possible to produce useful materials for civil and military use—medicines, fuels, lubricants, paints, fabrics, polymers, building materials, explosives, etc.

Some of these reactions are of such great importance for their varied and useful applications that their discoverers have been awarded Nobel prizes.

There exist a number of excellent treatises on the organic reactions and their mechanisms written by eminent authors. Many of those, however, are very wide in their coverage and cite detailed evidence in support of the accepted mechanisms. In the present treatise, which is mainly intended for graduate course students, accepted mechanisms have been taken for granted without going too deep in the logic as to how the mechanisms were arrived at.

ACYLOIN CONDENSATION

When carboxylic acid esters are refluxed with metallic sodium in aprotic solvents such as ether, benzene, toluene or xylene, free from oxygen, α-hydroxy ketones called acyloins are formed. This is called acyloin condensation.

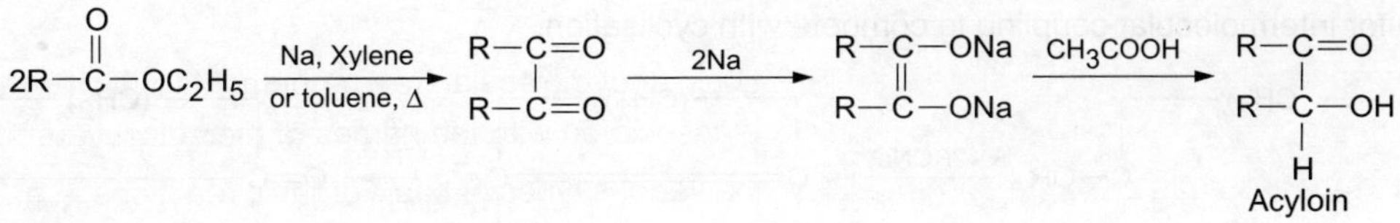

The yield of acyloin is good when R = alkyl group. With diesters, cyclic acyloins have been prepared.

Mechanism

The mechanism of the condensation is not clearly known but it is suggested that the reaction proceeds through a diketone intermediate, since diketone has been isolated in small amounts as a side product.

As the reaction occurs in the presence of metallic sodium, a direct transfer of electron, i.e., a radical mechanism is suggested.

The metallic sodium donates its electron to the carbonyl carbon to give (i) which subsequently dimerizes to yield (ii). Loss of both the alkoxy groups from (ii) produces 1, 2-diketone (iii). Further reduction gives sodium salt of enediol (iv). Finally, addition of acid yields 1, 2-diol which tautomerizes to the stable acyloin (v).

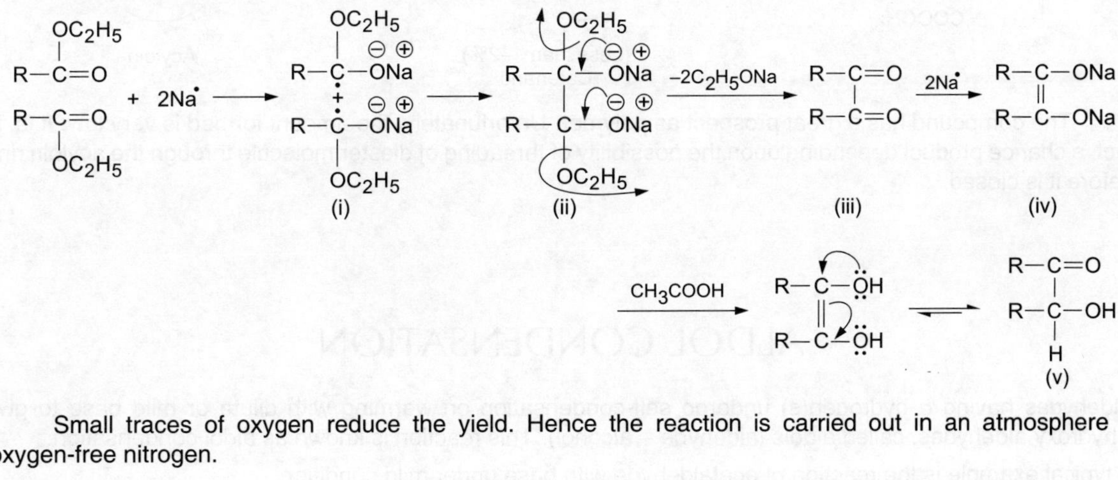

Small traces of oxygen reduce the yield. Hence the reaction is carried out in an atmosphere of oxygen-free nitrogen.

Applications

The condensation has considerable preparative value.

1. Preparation of cyclic acyloins The condensation has been employed with great success for the preparation of cyclic acyloins. Long-chain dicarboxylic esters have been converted to large-ring compounds without high dilution technique. The method is the best for closing rings of ten members or more.

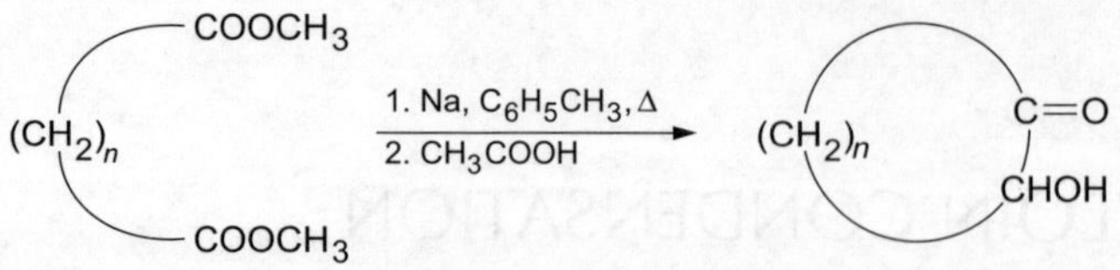

, where n = 10 to 20 or more

The yields are as high as 60–95% for 10 to 20 membered rings.

To account for the ready formation of large rings, it is suggested that the two ends of the ester are adsorbed, albeit weakly, to nearby sites on the surface of the sodium metal. Thus, the reactive ends are not available for intermolecular coupling to compete with cyclisation.

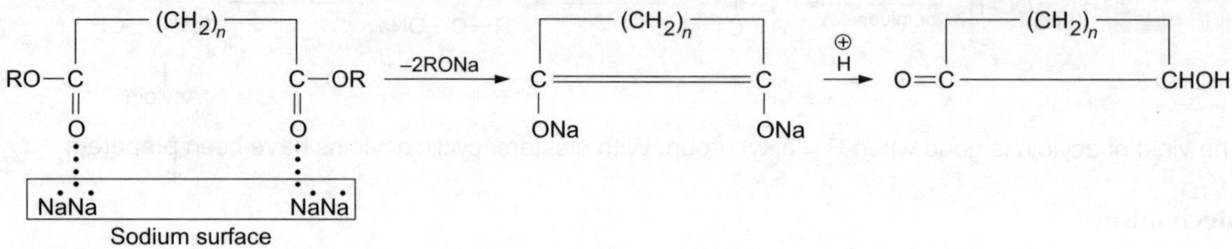

2. Preparation of catenane An interesting and unique compound called catenane, a compound with interlocking rings, was formed when acyloin condensation was employed for ring closure with ester of 34-carbon dicarboxylic acid.

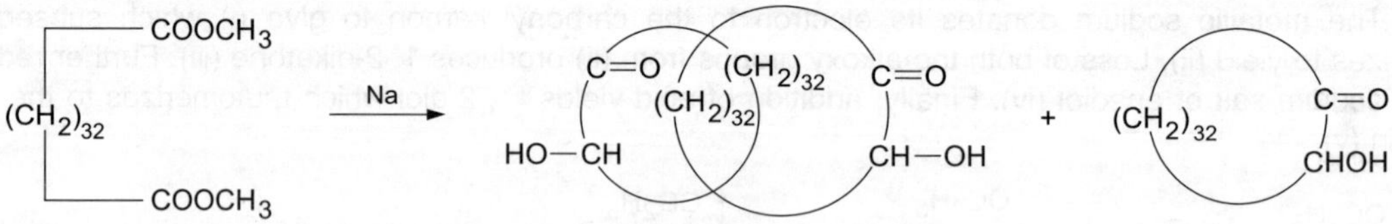

(Less than 1–2%) Catenane — Acyloin

The compound has a great prospect as polymer. Unfortunately, the amount formed is very low. It is, in fact, a chance product depending upon the possibility of threading of diester molecule through the acyloin ring before it is closed.

ALDOL CONDENSATION

Aldehydes having α-hydrogen(s) undergo self-condensation on warming with dilute or mild base to give β-hydroxy aldehydes, called aldols (<u>ald</u>ehyde + alcoh<u>ol</u>). This reaction is known as aldol condensation.

A typical example is the reaction of acetaldehyde with base under mild condition.

$$CH_3CHO + CH_3CHO \underset{}{\overset{\overset{\ominus}{OH}}{\rightleftharpoons}} \underset{\text{Acetaldol}}{CH_3CH(OH)CH_2CHO}$$

Various basic reagents such as dilute sodium hydroxide, aqueous alkali carbonate, alkali metal alkoxides, etc., may be used. The reaction is not favourable for ketones.

Aldol condensation has broad scope. It can occur between

(i) two identical or different aldehydes,

(ii) two identical or different ketones and

(iii) an aldehyde and a ketone.

When the condensation is between two different carbonyl compounds, it is called crossed aldol condensation.

Mechanism

The first step involves the formation of a resonance-stabilized enolate anion by the removal of an α-hydrogen from the aldehyde by the base. In the second step the enolate anion attacks the carbonyl carbon of the second molecule of the aldehyde to form an alkoxide ion. The latter then takes up a proton from the solvent to yield aldol in the third step.

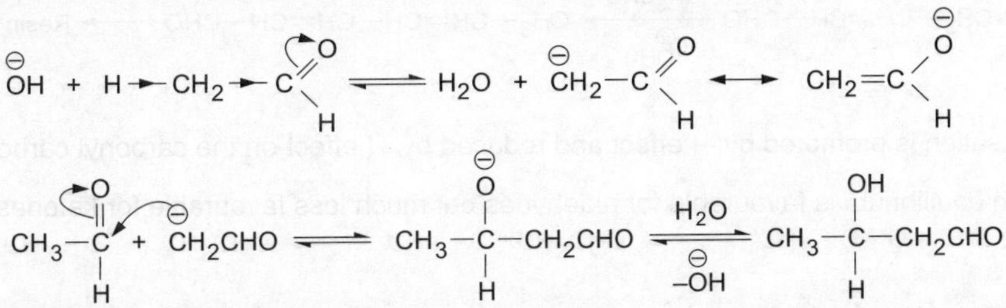

Thus, the overall reaction is an addition of enolate anion to the carbonyl double bond. [Recall that Michael reaction involves addition to an activated carbon–carbon double bond.]

Usually aldol as such is not isolated, e.g., acetaldol is isolated as a cyclic hemiacetal.

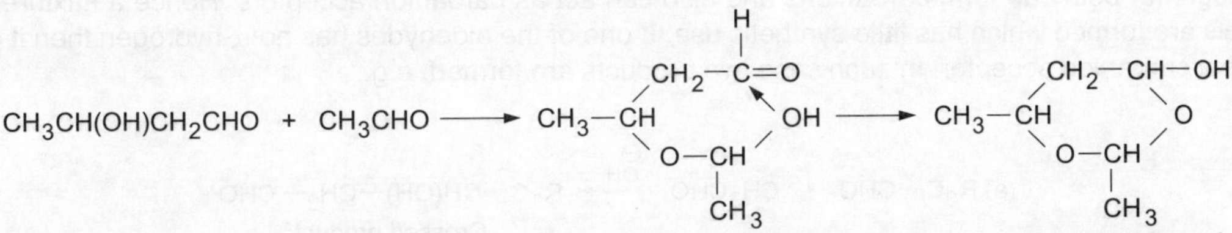

Cyclic hemiacetal

Aldol is isolated under reasonable mild condition, i.e., using aqueous K_2CO_3 as base.

The reaction between two ketones is not very successful. The equilibrium is not favourable and lies far to the left.

$$2CH_3COCH_3 \overset{\ominus OH}{\rightleftharpoons} CH_3-\underset{\underset{CH_3}{|}}{C}(OH)-CH_2-CO-CH_3$$

This is because the carbonyl carbon of ketone is less positive (due to +I effect) and more sterically hindered relative to aldehydes. This reduces the nucleophilic attack on the carbonyl carbon. However, it is possible to prepare diacetone alcohol in reasonable good yield by boiling acetone with solid $Ba(OH)_2$ in a specially devised apparatus.

Salient features of aldol condensation

(a) Aldols are easily dehydrated to α,β-unsaturated compounds on heating alone or with acid or base.

$$\underset{\beta\text{-Hydroxy butyraldehyde}}{CH_3-CH(OH)-CH_2CHO} \xrightarrow[\Delta]{\overset{\oplus}{H} \text{ or } \overset{\ominus}{OH}} \underset{\text{Crotonaldehyde}}{CH_3-CH=CH-CHO}$$

$$\underset{\text{Diacetone alcohol}}{(CH_3)_2C(OH)CH_2COCH_3} \xrightarrow[\Delta]{\overset{\oplus}{H} \text{ or } \overset{\ominus}{OH}} \underset{\text{Mesityl oxide}}{(CH_3)_2C=CH-CO-CH_3}$$

(b) When aldol condensation is carried out in the presence of strong alkali, repeated condensation and dehydration results in the formation of resins.

$$CH_3-CH=CH-CHO \xrightarrow[\overset{\ominus}{OH}]{CH_3CHO} CH_3-CH=CH-CH=CH-CHO \longrightarrow \text{Resin}$$

(c) The condensation is promoted by –I effect and reduced by +I effect on the carbonyl carbon.

(d) The reaction equilibrium is favourable for aldehydes but much less favourable for ketones.

Crossed aldol condensation

When the condensation is between two different carbonyl compounds, it is called crossed aldol condensation.

(i) Crossed aldol condensation between two different aldehydes When both the aldehydes have α-hydrogen(s) both can form carbanions and also can act as carbanion acceptors. Hence a mixture of four products are formed which has little synthetic use. If one of the aldehydes has no α-hydrogen then it can act only as a carbanion acceptor. In such case two products are formed, e.g.,

$$\text{(a) } R_3C-CHO + CH_3CHO \xrightarrow{\overset{\ominus}{OH}} \underset{\text{Crossed product}}{R_3C-CH(OH)-CH_2-CHO}$$

$$\text{(b) } CH_3CHO + CH_3CHO \xrightarrow{\overset{\ominus}{OH}} \underset{\text{Simple product (normal)}}{CH_3CH(OH)CH_2CHO}$$

However, a good yield of the crossed product is obtained by slowly adding the aldehyde having α-hydrogen to a mixture of the aldehyde having no α-hydrogen and the catalyst, e.g.,

$$C_6H_5CHO + \overset{\ominus}{OH} \xrightarrow[\text{Slow addition}]{CH_3CHO} C_6H_5CH(OH)CH_2CHO \xrightarrow{-H_2O} \underset{\text{Cinnamaldelyde}}{C_6H_5CH=CH-CHO}$$

Formaldehyde having no α-hydrogen is a reactive carbanion acceptor due to the absence of steric hindrance and +I effect. Hence, when acetaldehyde is treated with excess of formaldehyde in the presence of Ca $(OH)_2$, crossed aldol condensation continues (three times) until trihydroxymethyl acetaldehyde, $(HOCH_2)_3CCHO$ (I) is formed. The latter having no α-hydrogen undergoes crossed Cannizzaro reaction to form pentaerythritol.

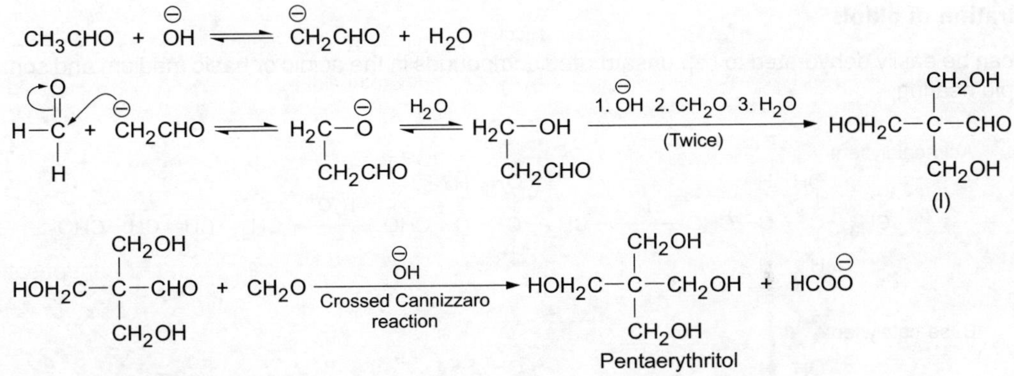

(ii) Crossed aldol condensation between two different ketones Due to poor reactivity of carbonyl carbons (+I effect and crowding) of ketones, a poor yield is obtained and so it is rarely attempted.

(iii) Crossed aldol condensation between an aldehyde and a ketone (a) When an aldehyde and a ketone both having α-hydrogens are condensed, two products are obtained. This is because ketones are poor carbanion acceptors and so cannot undergo self-condensation. Aldehydes being more reactive than ketones act as carbanion acceptors and the ketones provide the carbanions.

$$CH_3CHO + CH_3COCH_3 \overset{\ominus}{\underset{OH}{\rightleftharpoons}} CH_3-CH(OH)-CH_2-COCH_3$$

4-Hydroxypentan-2-one(crossed product)

$$CH_3CHO + CH_3CHO \overset{\ominus}{\underset{OH}{\rightleftharpoons}} CH_3-CH(OH)-CH_2-CHO$$

Acetaldol(normal product)

Usually, the crossed product is the predominant product. The formation of acetaldol can be minimized by slowly adding the aldehyde to the mixture of ketone and the catalyst base.

(b) When the addition is between a ketone and an aldehyde with no α-hydrogen, only one product is obtained. This is because the ketones are less reactive and cannot undergo self-condensation and the aldehyde does not undergo Cannizaro reaction which is slower than aldol condensation. Hence, the ketone provides the carbanion and the aldehyde acts as the carbanion acceptor. Thus,

$$\text{(i) } C_6H_5CHO + CH_3COCH_3 \xrightleftharpoons{\overset{\ominus}{OH}} C_6H_5-CH=CH-CO-CH_3$$

Benzylideneacetone

$$\text{(ii) } C_6H_5CHO + CH_3COC_6H_5 \xrightarrow{\overset{\ominus}{OH}} C_6H_5-CH=CH-CO-C_6H_5$$

Benzylideneacetophenone

$$\text{(iii) } CH_3COCH_3 + HCHO \xrightarrow{\overset{\ominus}{OH}} CH_3-CO-CH_2-CH_2OH$$

4-Hydroxybutanone-2

The reaction (iii) is difficult to stop at this stage and proceeds further till all the hydrogens of the ketone have been replaced by hydroxymethyl group to give $(HOCH_2)_3C-CO-C(CH_2OH)_3$.

Dehydration of aldols

Aldols can be easily dehydrated to α,β-unsaturated compounds in the acidic or basic medium and sometimes on simple heating.

Acid-catalysed:

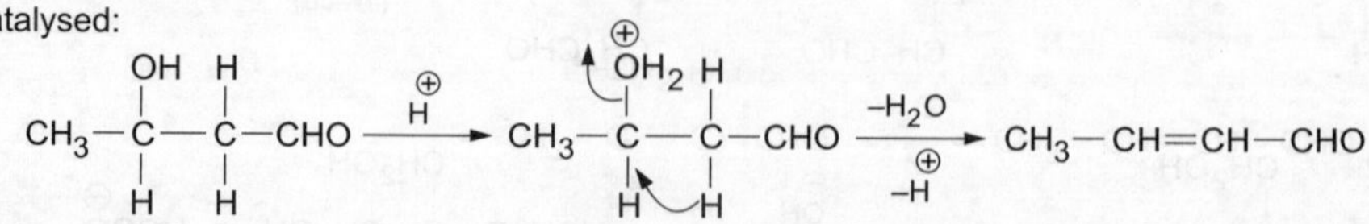

Base-catalysed:

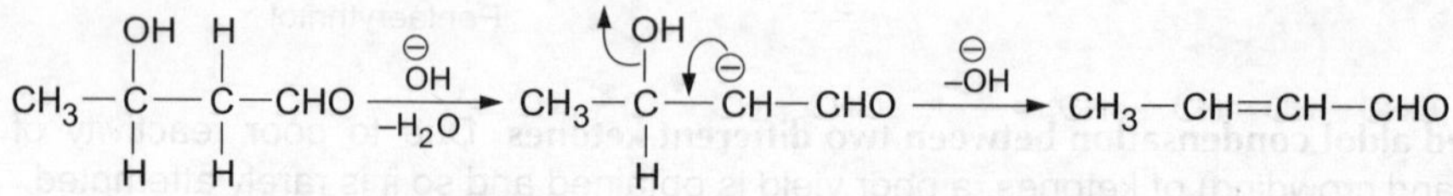

Applications

Several synthetic preparations are based on simple and crossed aldol condensations. Saturated and unsaturated aldehydes, ketones and alcohols of synthetic importance may be prepared.

(i) $2CH_3CHO \xrightarrow{\overset{\ominus}{O}H} CH_3CH(OH)CH_2CHO \xrightarrow[-H_2O]{\Delta} \underset{\text{Crotonaldehyde}}{CH_3CH{=}CHCHO} \xrightarrow{H_2/Ni} \underset{n\text{-Butanol}}{CH_3CH_2CH_2CH_2OH}$

(ii) $2C_3H_7CH_2OH \xrightarrow[250\ ^\circ C]{Cu} 2C_3H_7CHO \xrightarrow{\overset{\ominus}{O}H} C_3H_7CH(OH)CH(C_2H_5)CHO \xrightarrow[\Delta]{\overset{\oplus}{H}} C_3H_7CH{=}C(C_2H_5)CHO \xrightarrow{H_2/Ni}$

$\underset{\text{2-Ethylhexanol-1}}{C_3H_7CH_2CH(C_2H_5)CH_2OH}$

(iii) The intermediate β-ionone required for the synthesis of vitamin A is prepared by the condensation of citral with acetone and subsequent treatment with boron trifluoride.

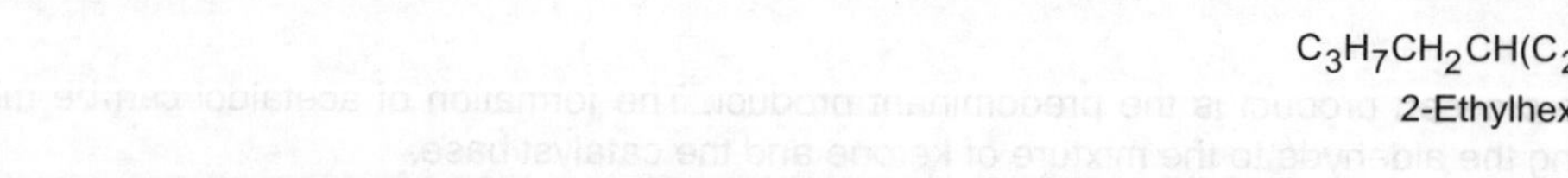

Citral ψ-Ionone β-Ionone

(iv) Aldol condensation is also effected in the presence of acid. Acetone with dry hydrochloric acid gas slowly gives mesityl oxide and phorone.

$2CH_3COCH_3 \xrightarrow{\text{Dry HCl gas}} \underset{\text{Mesityl oxide}}{(CH_3)_2C{=}CHCOCH_3} \xrightarrow[\text{HCl gas}]{CH_3COCH_3} \underset{\text{Phorone}}{(CH_3)_2C{=}CH{-}CO{-}CH{=}C(CH_3)_2}$

Mesitylene is obtained on distilling acetone with sulphuric acid.

(v) Aldol condensation of glycolaldehyde gives monosaccharides.

$$\underset{\text{Glycolaldehyde}}{3CH_2OHCHO} \xrightarrow{NaOH} \underset{\text{Formose}}{C_6H_{12}O_6}$$

(vi) Pyridine and quinoline having methyl groups at positions –2 and –4 undergo aldol type of condensation with aldehydes. The process forms the basis for the preparation of an important class of dyes, e.g., cyanine dyes (photographic sensitisers).

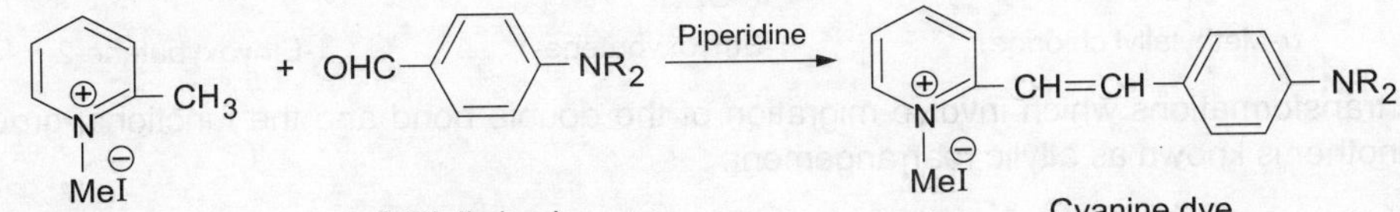

α-Picoline methiodide β-Dialkylamino benzaldehyde Cyanine dye

(vii) A number of compounds which have acidic C – H bonds undergo aldol-type condensation with aldehydes and ketones to produce valuable synthetic intermediates.

Thus, condensation of acetylene with aldehydes or ketones gives acetylenic alcohol, a valuable commercial product.

$$2CH_2O + HC{\equiv}CH \xrightarrow{Cu_2C_2} \underset{\text{2-Butyne-1, 4-diol.}}{HOH_2C{-}C{\equiv}C{-}CH_2OH}$$

The process is known as **ethynylation.**

Pentaerythritol (see above) is a valuable chemical. It is a medicine for heart trouble. Its nitroderivative, penterythritol tetra nitrate (PENT) is a valuable explosive. It is also used as a surface-coating agent. Reactions closely related to aldol condensation are: Perkin, Claisen, Knoevenagel, Dieckmann, Doebner, etc.

ALLYLIC REARRANGEMENT

Allylic compounds are those which have a functional group on a carbon atom α to an olefinic bond, e.g.,

$$-\overset{|}{C}{=}\overset{|}{\underset{|}{C}}{-}\overset{|}{\underset{|}{C}}{-}X$$

The double bond (and the functional group) in these compounds undergo acid- or base-catalyzed migration to form a new compound.

$$R{-}\overset{|}{C}{=}\overset{|}{\underset{|}{C}}{-}\overset{|}{\underset{|}{C}}{-}OH \xrightarrow{\overset{\oplus}{H} \text{ or } \overset{\ominus}{OH}} R{-}\overset{|}{\underset{OH}{C}}{-}\overset{|}{C}{=}\overset{|}{C}{-}$$

Examples:

$$\text{(a) } \underset{\text{2-Methyl-3-butenol-2}}{CH_2{=}CH{-}\overset{CH_3}{\underset{CH_3}{C}}{-}OH} \xrightarrow{\overset{\oplus}{H}} \underset{\text{3-Methyl-2-butenol-1}}{HOCH_2{-}CH{=}\overset{CH_3}{C}{-}CH_3}$$

$$\text{(b) } CH_3-CH=CH-CH_2OH \xrightarrow{H^{\oplus}} CH_3-CH(OH)-CH=CH_2$$

Crotyl alcohol α-Methylallyl alcohol

The incoming and outgoing nucleophiles may not be the same.

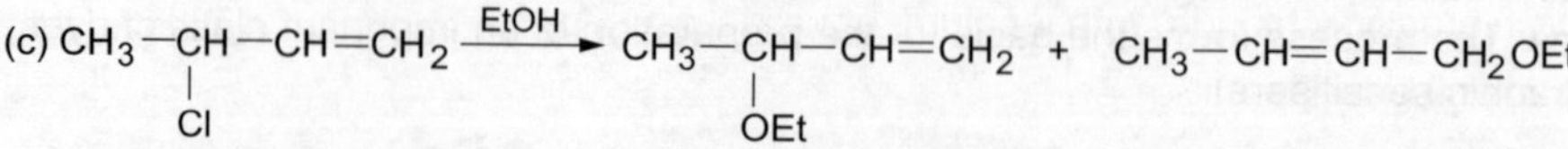

α-Methylallyl chloride α-Ethyoxybutene-1 1-Ethyoxybutene-2

Such transformations which involve migration of the double bond and the functional group from one carbon to another is known as allylic rearrangement.

Mechanism

Allylic rearrangement is observed generally in nucleophilic substitution reactions which may be S_N1 or S_N2 type.

S_N1 type Unimolecular nucleophilic substitution (S_N1) reaction in allylic compounds is almost always accompanied with rearrangement resulting in the formation of two products—one normal and the other rearranged. Thus, solvolysis of α-methylallyl chloride with alcohol gives two products [see eq.(c)]. This is understandable. The delocalisation of the positive charge in the first-formed carbocation (i) indicates partial positive charge on both C_1 and C_3. The nucleophilic attack can thus occur at both C_1 and C_3 to yield two products which are indeed obtained.

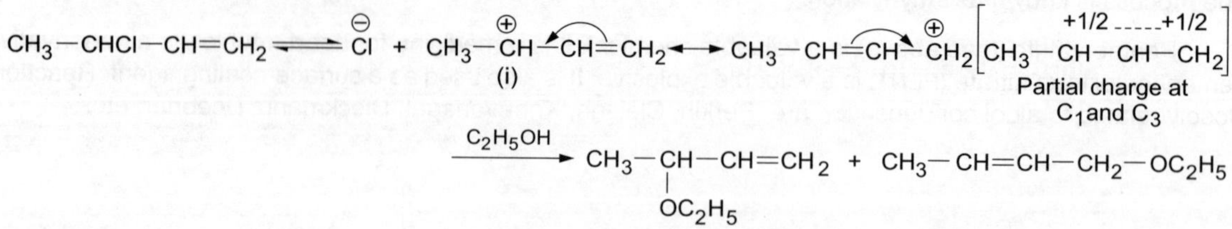

Normal (S_N1) product Rearranged (S_N1') product

The S_N1 reaction in which a rearranged product is obtained has been designated S_N1' to distinguish it from the normal S_N1 reaction.

S_N2 type When the substitution in allylic compounds is carried out under S_N2 conditions, i.e., in the presence of sodium ethoxide and alcohol, the reaction proceeds as normal S_N2 reaction to yield only one product.

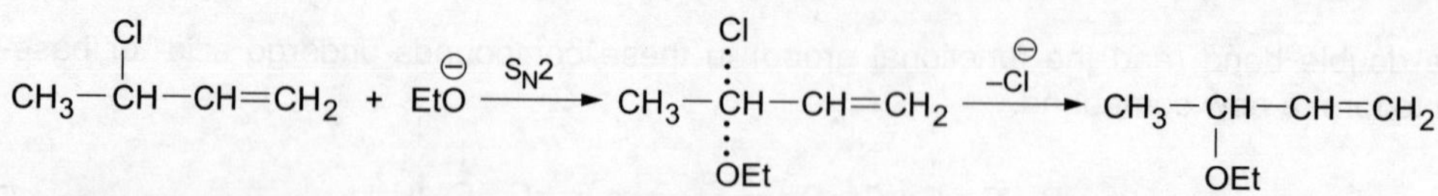

α-Methylallyl chloride Transition state 3-Ethyoxybutene-1

However, allylic rearrangements in bimolecular substitution reactions have also been observed in some cases. Such reactions are designated as S_N2'.

In S_N2' reaction, the nucleophile attacks the unsaturated γ-carbon rather than the α-carbon to give the rearranged product, e.g.,

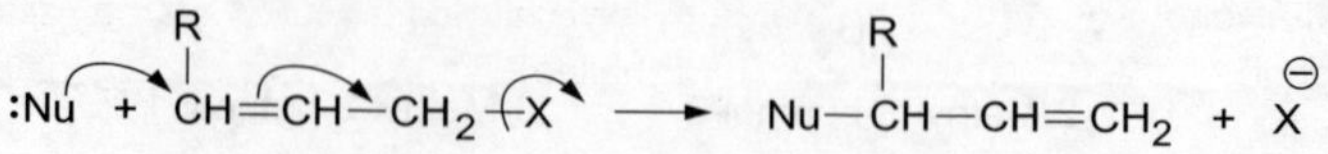

Generally the S_N2 reaction is much faster than the S_N2' reaction.

However, the S_N2' reaction may proceed concurrently with S_N2 or even to the exclusion of S_N2 when the α-carbon is crowded with substituents. The crowding in the α-carbon restricts the direct approach of the nucleophile to the α-carbon so that S_N2' reaction becomes significant.

Thus, α-chloroallyl chloride with sodium ethoxide in ethanol gives a normal S_N2 product and a rearranged S_N2' product as well.

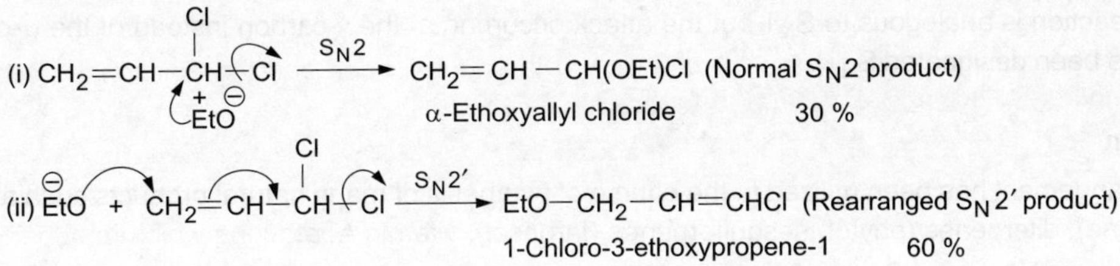

With highly substituted α-carbon, the S_N2 attack is completely inhibited and only the rearranged product is obtained (S_N2').

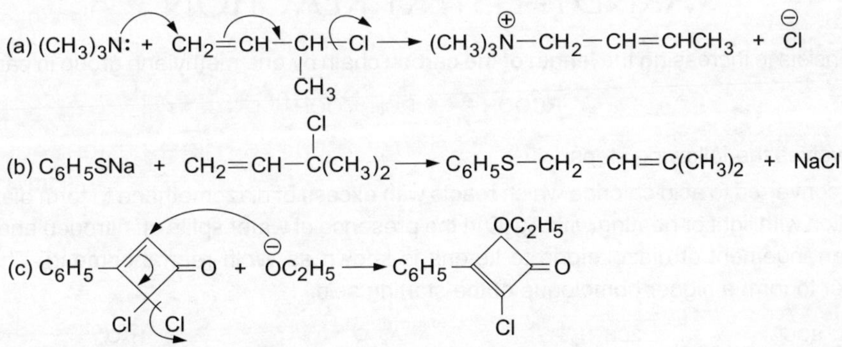

The S_N2' reaction is stereospecific. The nucleophile attacks from the same side of the molecule as the leaving group producing the same stereoisomer.

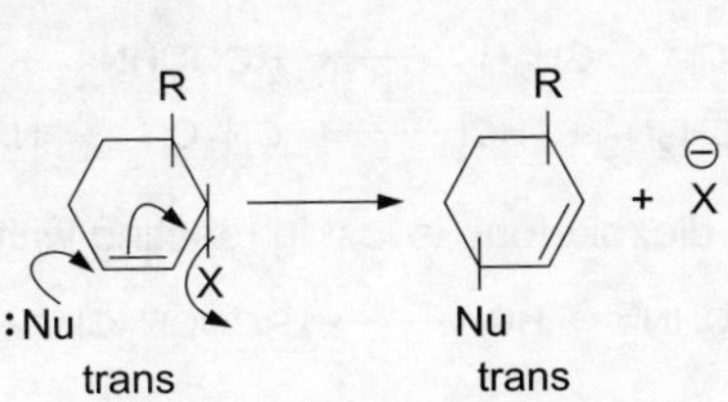

S_Ni type A suitably substituted allyl alcohol on treatment with $SOCl_2$ gives two halides.

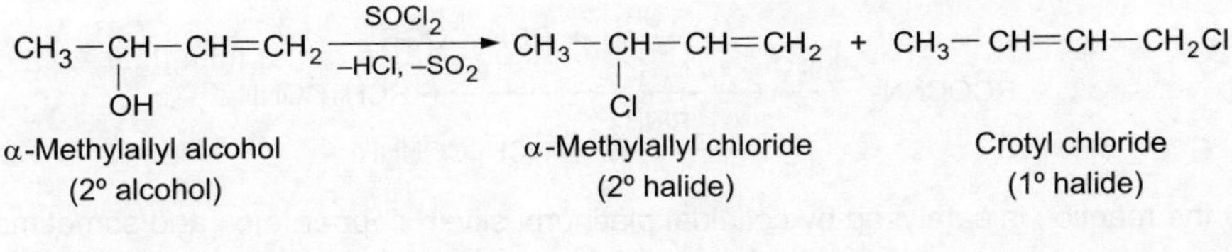

The formation of 2° halide with retention of configuration indicates a normal $S_N i$ reaction. The formation of 1° halide can be explained on the basis of the internal attack of Cl^- on the γ-carbon with consequent shift of the double bond.

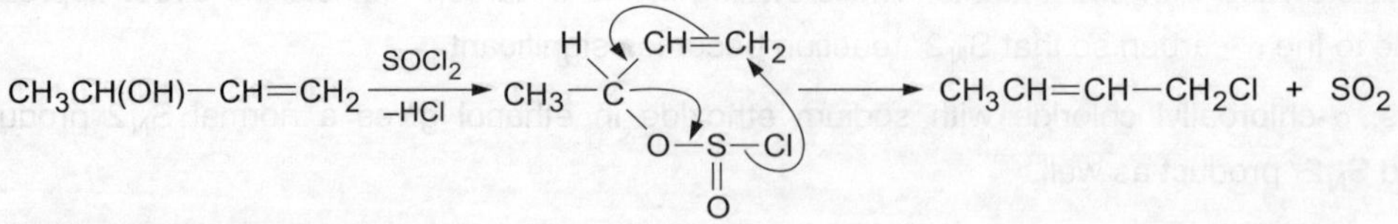

Since the reaction is analogous to $S_N i$, but the attack occurring at the γ-carbon instead of the α-carbon, the reaction has been designated $S_N i'$.

Application

Allylic rearrangement has been utilized in the course of synthesis of many natural products such as terpenes (citral, α-irone), diterpenes (phytol),sesquiterpenes (farnesol), vitamin A, etc.

ARNDT–EISTERT REACTION

The reaction consists in increasing the length of the carbon chain by one methylene group in carboxylic acids.

$$RCOOH \longrightarrow RCH_2COOH$$

The reaction involves the following steps:

The acid is first converted to acid chloride which reacts with excess of diazomethane to form diazoketone. The latter on irradiation with light or heating with Ag_2O in the presence of water splits off nitrogen and rearranges to ketene (this rearrangement of diazoketone to ketene is known as Wolff rearrangement). The ketene then reacts with water to form a higher homologue of the starting acid.

$$RCOOH \xrightarrow{SOCl_2} RCOCl \xrightarrow[-CH_3Cl,\ -N_2]{2CH_2N_2} RCOCHN_2 \xrightarrow{Ag_2O} R{-}CH{=}C{=}O \xrightarrow{H_2O} RCH_2COOH$$

Excess of diazomethane is used to consume the liberated hydrochloric acid.

$$RCOCl + CH_2N_2 \longrightarrow RCOCHN_2 + HCl$$
$$CH_2N_2 + HCl \longrightarrow CH_3Cl + N_2$$

In absence of excess diazomethane, diazoketone is lost in reacting with HCl to form chloromethyl ketone.

$$RCOCHN_2 + HCl \longrightarrow RCOCH_2Cl + N_2$$

If alcohol, ammonia or amine is present in place of water then ester, amide or substituted amide respectively is formed.

$$RCOCHN_2 \xrightarrow{Ag_2O} \begin{cases} \xrightarrow{R'OH} RCH_2COOR' \\ \xrightarrow{NH_3} RCH_2CONH_2 \\ \xrightarrow{R'NH_2} RCH_2CONHR' \end{cases}$$

Besides Ag_2O, the reaction is catalysed by colloidal platinum, silver, copper, etc., and sometimes heat.

The group R may be alkyl, aryl, heterocyclic or alicyclic and may contain reducible groups which remain unaffected. Acidic groups react with diazomethane and diazoketone.

Mechanism

Nucleophilic attack of diazomethane on the carbonyl carbon of the acid chloride gives an intermediate (i) which eliminates a molecule of HCl to give diazoketone (ii). Diazoketone then splits off a molecule of nitrogen to form a carbene (iii), which rearranges to ketene. The highly reactive ketene readily reacts with the nucleophile present (H_2O) to form the next higher acid.

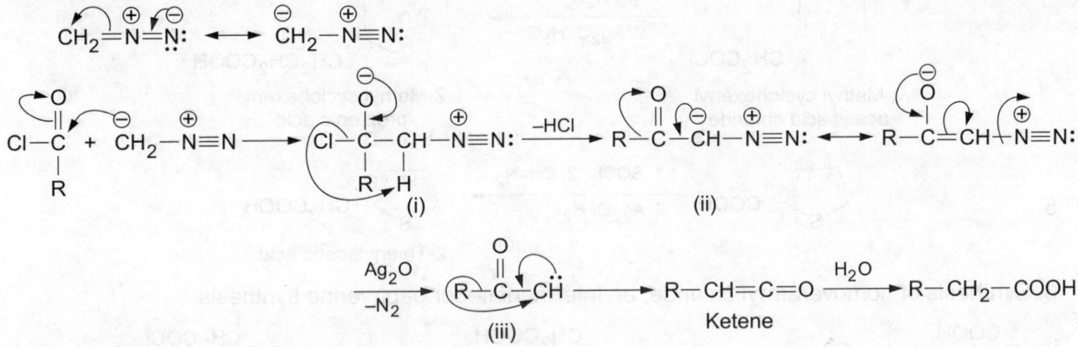

The presence of carbene (iii) has not been detected and therefore the two steps—splitting of nitrogen and migration of R group—may be concerted.

The mechanism has been supported by the fact that ketenes have been isolated or trapped. Further, isotopic labelling experiment has shown that the carbonyl carbon of diazoketone is present in the resulting acid as the carboxyl carbon.

$$R\overset{13}{C}OCHN_2 \xrightarrow[H_2O]{Ag_2O} RCH_2\overset{13}{C}OOH$$

The group R migrates with retention of configuration, for an optically active acid on conversion to its higher homologue and subsequent Barbier-Weiland degradation gives the original acid with the same configuration.

Mild reaction conditions permit this synthesis without affecting complex or reducible groups in the substrate. The yield is high. It has, therefore, many synthetic applications, especially in the field of natural products.

Applications

1. 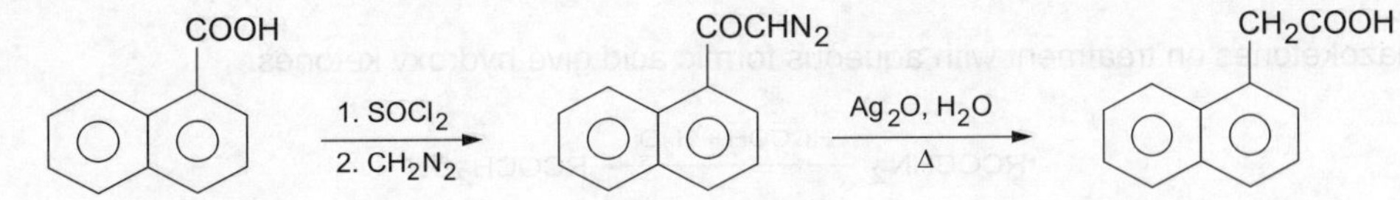

α-Naphthoic acid — Diazo-α-acetonaphthone — α-Naphthylacetic acid (80%)

2. 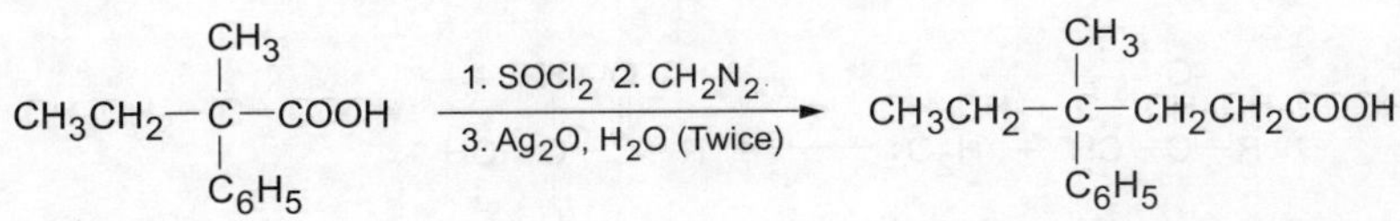

4-Methyl-4-phenylcaproic acid

3. 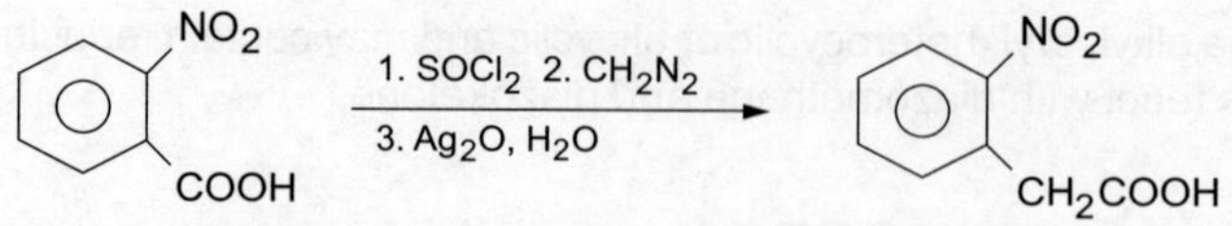

o-Nitrobenzoic acid — 2-Nitrophenylacetic acid

4. Double bond in the substrate remains unaffected.

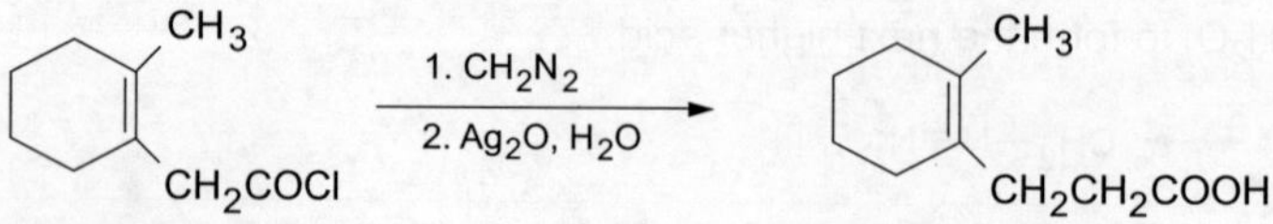

2-Methyl cyclohexenyl acetic acid chloride — 2-Methyl cyclohexenyl propionic acid

5. 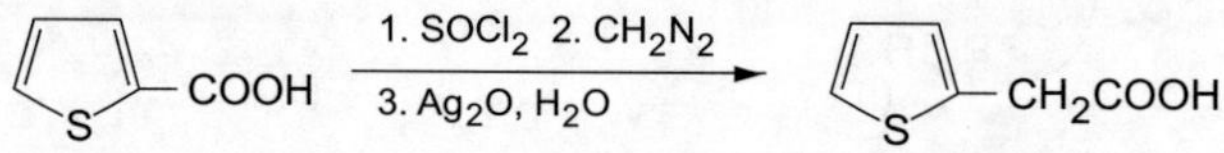

2-Thienylacetic acid

6. Synthesis of homoveratroyl chloride, an intermediate for papaverine synthesis.

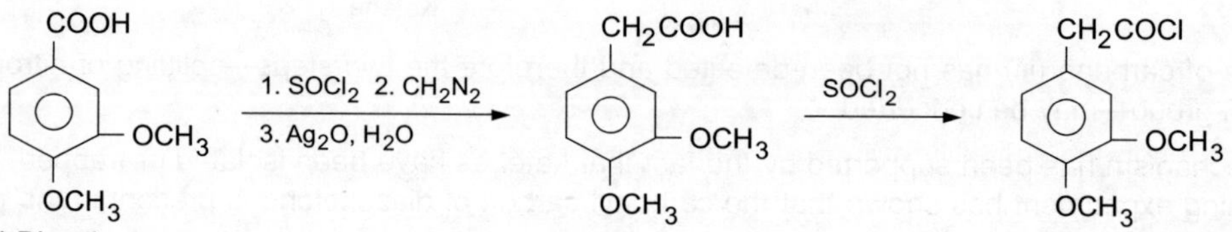

3,4-Dimethoxy benzoic acid — Homoveratroyl chloride

7. Synthesis of mescaline.

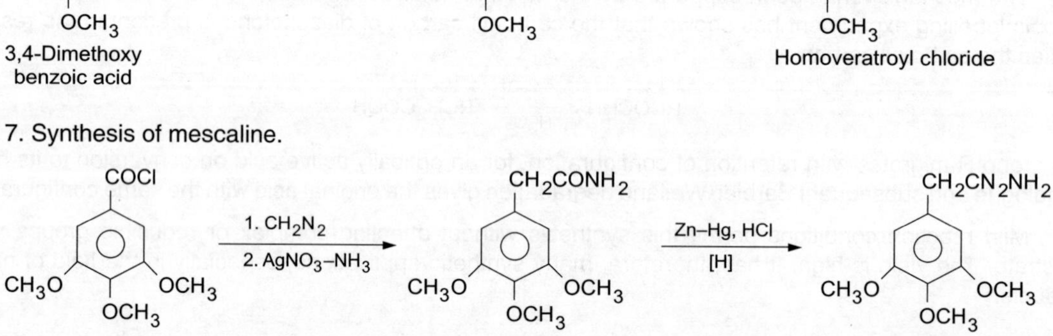

Mescaline (produces euphoria)

8. Diazoketones on treatment with aqueous formic acid give hydroxy ketones.

$$RCOCHN_2 \xrightarrow{HCOOH\,+\,H_2O} RCOCH_2OH$$

Probably in the absence of the catalyst, the species (iii) behaves as a carbocation and combines with the nucleophile, H_2O to form hydroxy ketone.

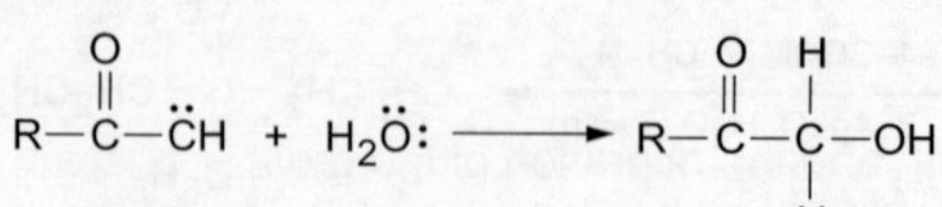

BAEYER–VILLIGER REARRANGEMENT

Baeyer–Villiger rearrangement is an example of the migration of a group from carbon to electron-deficient oxygen.

The reaction involves the oxidation of ketones to esters by the treatment with peracids such as peracetic acid, perbenzoic acid, pertrifluoroacetic acid, permonosulphuric acid, etc.

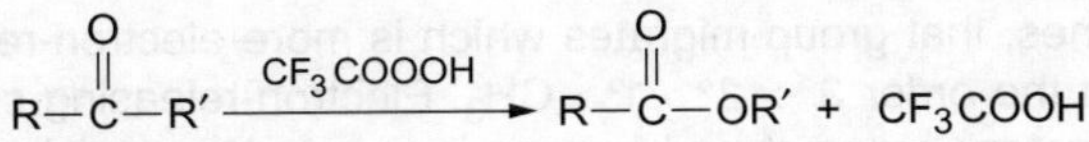

Cyclic ketones are converted to lactones with ring expansion.

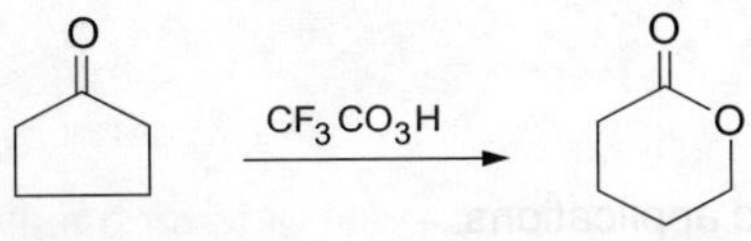

Cyclopentanone Lactone

The overall reaction is an insertion of oxygen atom between the carbonyl group and the adjacent carbon in ketone. Organic solvents which are inert under the conditions of reaction may be used. The choice of solvent depends upon the solubility of the reactants. Commonly used solvents are glacial acetic acid and chloroform.

Mechanism

Nucleophilic attack of the peracid on the protonated ketone gives an intermediate peroxide (i). The peroxide then undergoes loss of carboxylate anion and migration of a group from carbon to electron deficient oxygen to yield the protonated ester (ii). Finally the loss of proton gives the ester.

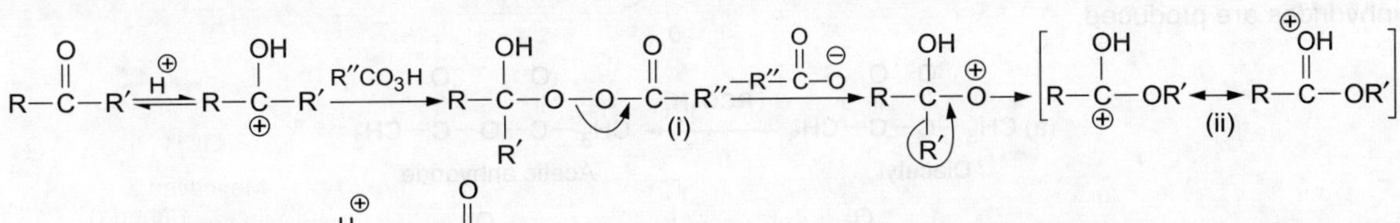

; where R′ is equal to CH_3, C_6H_5, CF_3, etc.

The reaction is catalysed by acids. Electron-releasing groups in the ketone and electron-withdrawing groups in peracids promote the reaction rate. Pertrifluoroacetic acid is very effective because trifluoroacetate ion is a good leaving group.

The mechanism is supported by the fact that the labelled oxygen atom of the ketone is entirely present in the carbonyl oxygen of the ester.

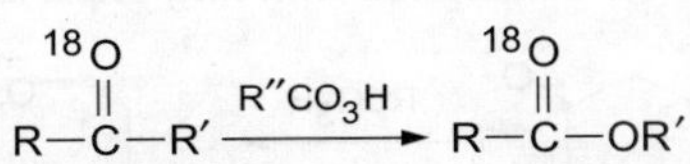

The loss of carboxylate anion and the migration of the group may be concerted. Syrkin has suggested that the peroxide (i) transforms into products by a cyclic mechanism, which shows that the last three steps may be concerted.

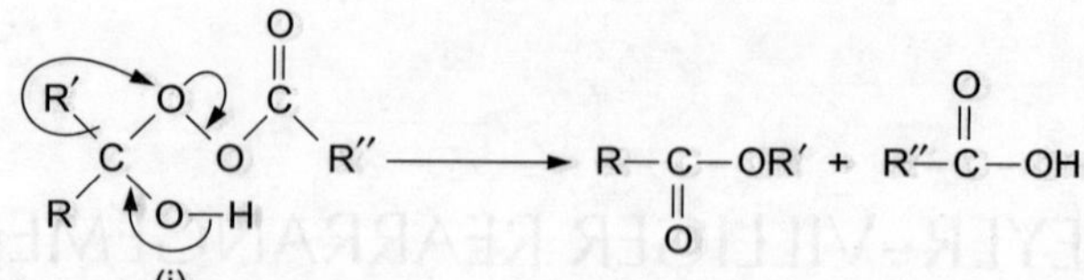

(i)

The migrating group retains its configuration as in other concerted reactions. For acylic compounds the migrating group, R′, must be 2°, 3° or vinylic. However, migration of 1° alkyl group may be brought about by using CF_3CO_3H or $BF_3-H_2O_2$ as reagent.

Baeyer–Villiger oxidation can be brought about with H_2O_2 and base also in some cases.

In unsymmetrical ketones, that group migrates which is more electron-releasing. Thus, the migratory aptitude of alkyl groups is in the order $3° > 2° > 1° > CH_3$. Electron-releasing substituents in the aryl group facilitate migration. The migratory order of aryl groups is *p*-anisyl > *p*-tolyl > phenyl > *p*-chlorophenyl > *p*-nitrophenyl, etc. In case of alkyl aryl ketones, it is the aryl group which migrates (except in case of *t*-butyl group).

Applications

The reaction has valuable synthetic applications.

1. Esters Esters, which are difficult to synthesize, can be prepared by this method.

$$\text{(a) } \underset{\text{Acetophenone}}{C_6H_5-CO-CH_2} \xrightarrow{CF_3CO_3H} \underset{\text{Phenylacetate}}{CH_3-\overset{O}{\overset{\|}{C}}-OC_6H_5}$$

$$\text{(b) } \underset{\text{Pinacolone}}{CH_3-CO-C(CH_3)_3} \xrightarrow{CF_3CO_3H} \underset{t\text{-Butylacetate}}{CH_3-\overset{O}{\overset{\|}{C}}-OC(CH_3)_3}$$

2. Anhydrides When 1, 2-diketones or *o*-quinones are subjected to Baeyer–Villiger rearrangement, anhydrides are produced.

$$\text{(a) } \underset{\text{Diacetyl}}{CH_3-\overset{O}{\overset{\|}{C}}-\overset{O}{\overset{\|}{C}}-CH_3} \xrightarrow{RCO_3H} \underset{\text{Acetic anhydride}}{CH_3-\overset{O}{\overset{\|}{C}}-O-\overset{O}{\overset{\|}{C}}-CH_3}$$

(b) 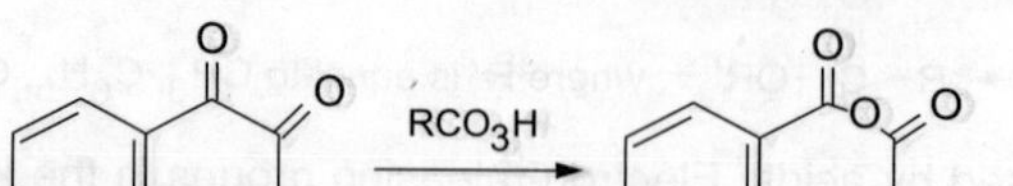

α-Naphthaquinone

The products can be converted to various types of compounds.

3. Lactones Cyclic ketones are converted to lactones with ring expansion.

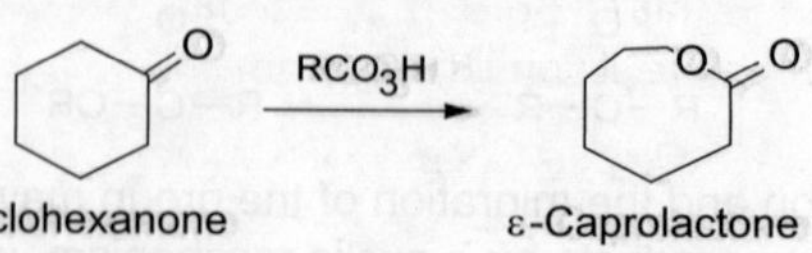

Cyclohexanone ε-Caprolactone

Long-chain hydroxyesters can be prepared from large ring-size ketones.

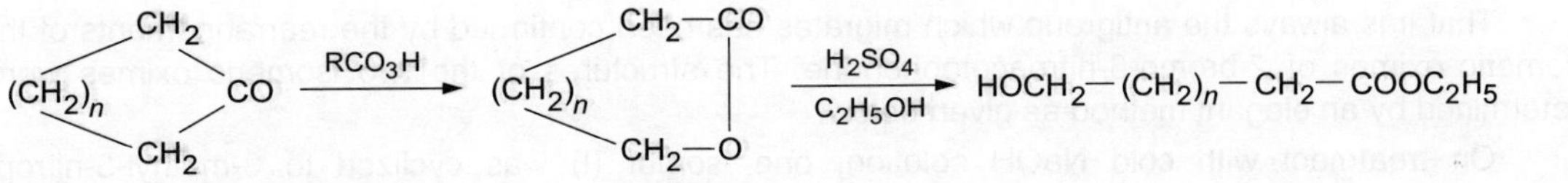

Lactone

With some condensed cyclic ketones, two lactones in varying proportions are formed. For example, camphor gives two lactones (I) and (II).

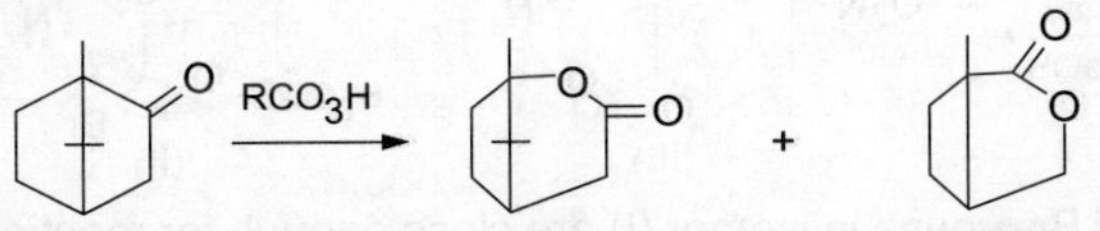

I (75%) II (25%)

Lactone (I) is the normal product formed by the migration of the tertiary bridgehead carbon while lactone (II) has been formed by the migration of the methylene group. The reason for the formation of two lactones in different proportions is steric factor.

4. Elucidation of structure The ester obtained as a result of the rearrangement may be hydrolysed to acid and alcohol from which the structure of the substrate can be determined.

The reaction is not successful with aldehydes. Aliphatic aldehydes are oxidized to acids by the migration of the hydrogen.

$$R{-}\overset{O}{\overset{\|}{C}}{-}H \xrightarrow{R''CO_3H} R{-}\overset{O}{\overset{\|}{C}}{-}OH$$

A few aromatic aldehydes have been converted to formates by the migration of the aryl group.

$$Ar{-}\overset{O}{\overset{\|}{C}}{-}H \xrightarrow{R''CO_3H} \underset{\text{Aryl formate}}{H{-}\overset{O}{\overset{\|}{C}}{-}OAr}$$

BECKMANN REARRANGEMENT

The acid-catalyzed conversion of ketoximes to *N*-substituted amides is known as Beckmann rearrangement. The reaction is catalysed by acidic reagents such as, H_2SO_4, $SOCl_2$, SO_3, P_2O_5, PCl_5, $C_6H_5SO_2Cl$, etc.

The reaction involves the migration of a group from carbon to electron-deficient nitrogen.

$$RR'C{=}NOH \xrightarrow{\overset{\oplus}{H}} RCONHR' \text{ or } R'CONHR$$

Some aldoximes undergo the rearrangement in the presence of polyphosphoric acid (PPA) but the reaction is not a general one. The migration of the group depends not on the migrational aptitude but upon the orientation of the group in relation to the OH group. It is found that the migrating group is always *anti* (i.e., *trans*) to the hydroxyl group. Thus, the reaction is stereospecific.

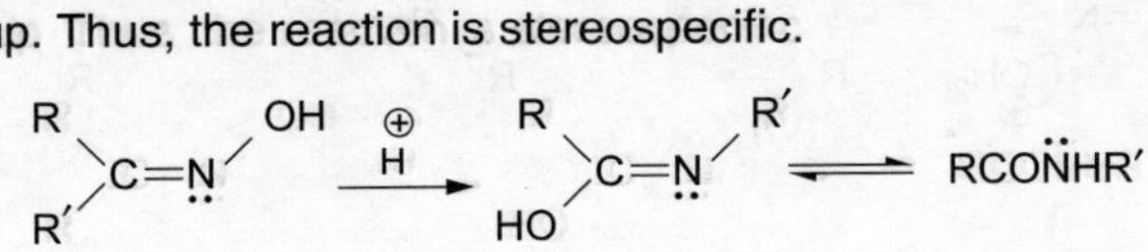

That it is always the antigroup which migrates has been confirmed by the rearrangements of the two isomeric oximes of 2-bromo-5-nitroacetophenone. The structures of the two isomeric oximes were first determined by an elegant method as given below.

On treatment with cold NaOH solution, one isomer (I) was cyclized to 3-methyl-5-nitrophenyl isooxazole (III) while the other isomer (II) remained unaffected even under drastic conditions.

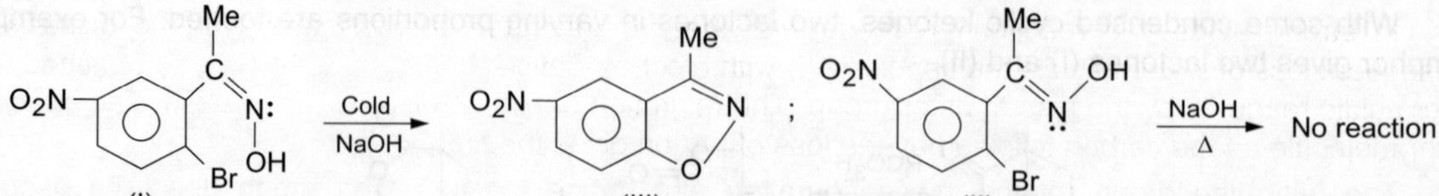

(I) (III) (II)

Obviously, the OH and Br groups in isomer (I) are close enough for reaction and cyclization. Hence, the Me and OH groups are *anti* (i.e., *trans*) to each other. In isomer (II), the OH and Br groups are far apart for reaction, i.e., the Me and OH groups are *syn* (i.e., *cis*) to each other. Thus, the structures of isomers (I) and (II) are confirmed.

Now, on subjecting the two isomers to Beckmann rearrangement it is found that (a) isomer (I) gives *N*-methyl-2-bromo-5-nitrobenzamide (IV) indicating the migration of the antigroup Me to the nitrogen atom and (b) isomer (II) gives *N*-(2-bromo-5-nitrophenyl)- acetamide (V) due to the migration of the *anti*-aryl group to the nitrogen atom.

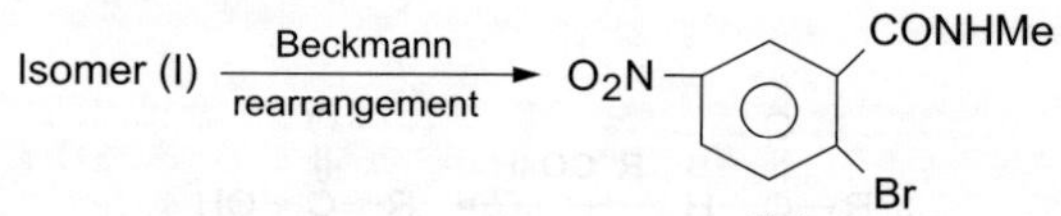

(IV)

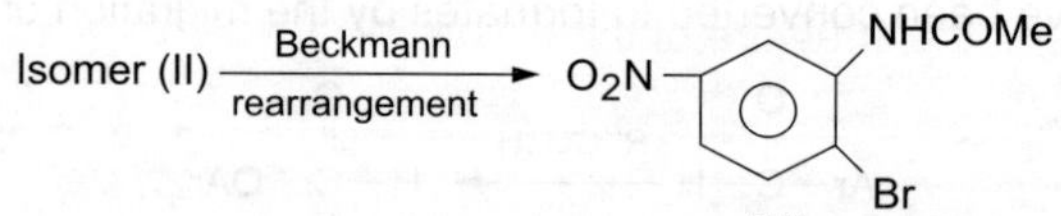

(V)

Oxime esters and ethers also undergo Beckmann rearrangement. The acidic reagents convert the OH group to a better leaving group—acids convert OH to H_2O, other reagents convert OH to an ester-leaving group, e.g., $OPCl_4$ from PCl_5, $OSO_2C_6H_5$ from $C_6H_5SO_2Cl$, etc. The reaction is facilitated by heat, polar solvents or an increase in the acid strength.

That direct interchange of the migrating group and OH does not occur is proved by the fact that ^{18}O is incorporated in the product in the presence of $H_2{}^{18}O$.

$$RR'C{=}NOH \xrightarrow[\overset{\oplus}{H}]{H_2{}^{18}O} R{-}\overset{\overset{^{18}O}{||}}{C}{-}NHR'$$

Mechanism

The mechanism of the reaction has been suggested as given below.

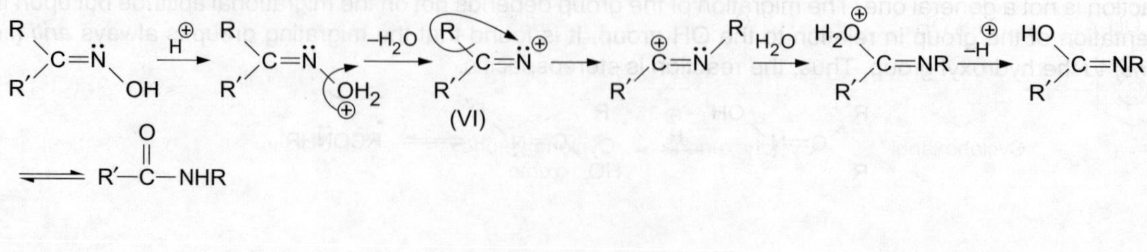

With other acidic reagents, e.g., $PhSO_2Cl$, the same intermediate (VI) is obtained.

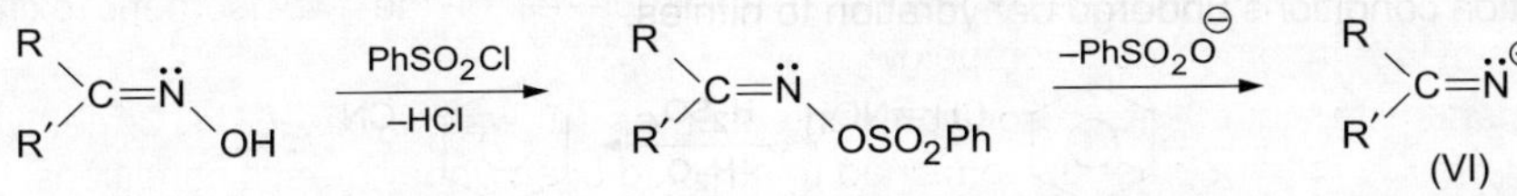

In strong acids, the reaction proceeds with the protonation of the OH group of the oxime with subsequent loss of water to yield the species (VI) with electron-deficient nitrogen which is also obtained with other acidic reagents by the loss of ester group. The migration of R then gives a carbocation. The attack of water molecule on the carbon followed by the loss of proton gives the amide.

The migrating group retains its configuration and hence the migrating group does not become completely free during the migration, otherwise the reaction cannot be stereospecific. Thus, the migration and the breaking of N–O bond may be concerted or at least very rapid. This has been supported by crossover experiments.

Applications

1. Configuration of ketoximes can be assigned A ketoxime gives an amide on Beckmann rearrangement. From the products of hydrolysis of the amide, the structure of the amide is known and for that matter, the configuration of the oxime is known.

Thus,

$$RR'CNOH \xrightarrow{H^{\oplus}} R'CONHR \xrightarrow{H_2O} RNH_2 + R'COOH$$

Formation of RNH_2 indicates the migration of the group R to the nitrogen atom. The groups R and OH are, therefore, *anti* to each other, i.e., the structure of the oxime is

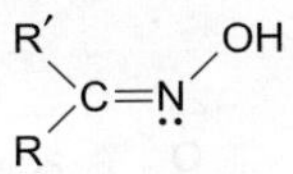

2. Synthesis of isoquinoline

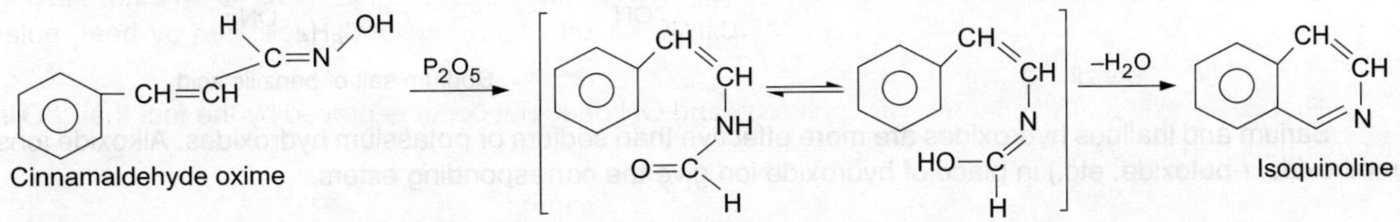

Cinnamaldehyde oxime → Isoquinoline

3. Synthesis of lactams Alicyclic ketones of all ring sizes undergo the Beckmann rearrangement of their oximes to yield lactams.

A product of considerable industrial importance is perlon (valuable textile polymer) which is prepared from ε-caprolactam. This is obtained by the Beckmann rearrangement of cyclohexanone oxime. It is synthesized from phenol as below.

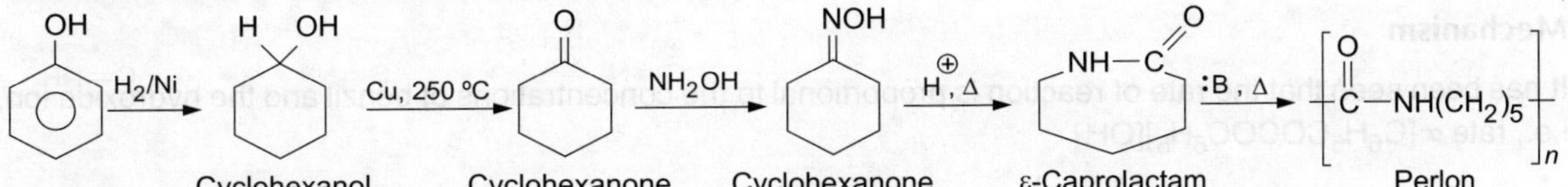

Cyclohexanol Cyclohexanone Cyclohexanone oxime ε-Caprolactam Perlon

Similarly, cyclopentanone oxime gives 2-piperidone under Beckmann condition. Aldoximes under the Beckmann reaction conditions undergo dehydration to nitriles.

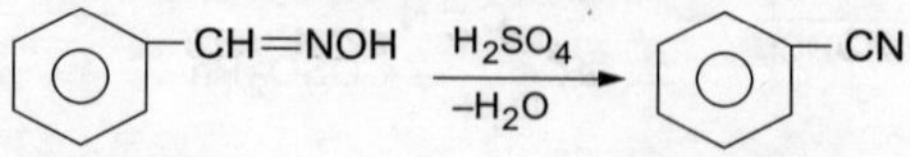

Benzaldoxime   Benzonitrile (Phenyl cyanide)

BENZILIC ACID REARRANGEMENT

The addition of a strong base to a carbonyl group results in the formation of an anion. The reversal of the anionic charge may cause expulsion of the attached group, X, e.g.,

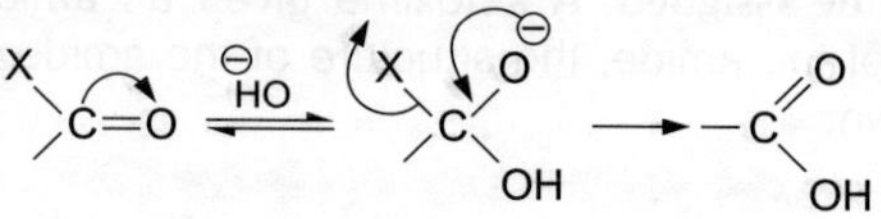

(cf.Hydrolysis of esters when X = OR)

However, in a 1, 2-diketone the group X may migrate to the adjacent electron-deficient carbonyl carbon forming α-hydroxy acid.

Thus, benzil on treatment with a strong base forms benzilic acid (salt), whence the name benzilic acid rearrangement.

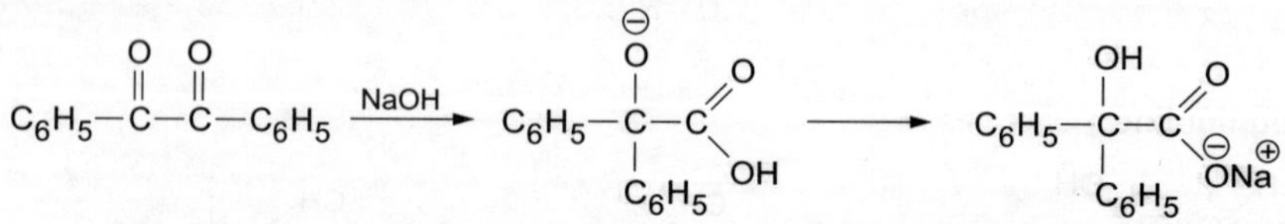

Benzil   Sodium salt of benzilic acid

Barium and thallous hydroxides are more effective than sodium or potassium hydroxides. Alkoxide ions (methoxide, *t*-butoxide, etc.) in place of hydroxide ion give the corresponding esters.

$$C_6H_5\cdot CO-CO-C_6H_5 \xrightarrow{CH_3ONa} (C_6H_5)_2C(OH)COOCH_3$$

Benzilic acid methyl ester

Phenoxide ions are too weak a nucleophile to attack. Besides aromatic 1, 2-diketones, aliphatic and heterocyclic diketones as also *o*-quinones undergo this rearrangement.

Mechanism

It has been seen that the rate of reaction is proportional to the concentrations of benzil and the hydroxide ion, i.e., rate $\propto [C_6H_5COCOC_6H_5][\bar{O}H]$

It has also been found that when the reaction is carried out in the presence of $H_2{}^{18}O$, benzil exchanges ^{18}O faster than it rearranges.

On the basis of the above observations, it has been suggested that a fast reversible nucleophilic attack occurs at the carbonyl carbon in the first step. The second step is the rate-determining step in which the migration occurs. Finally, a rapid proton transfer completes the process.

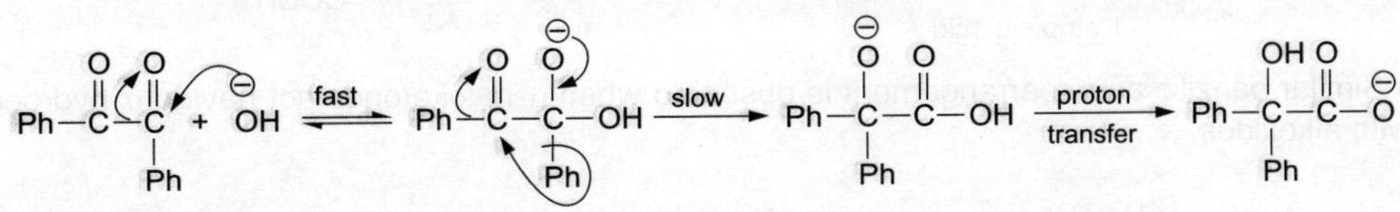

The rearrangement is analogous to intramolecular Cannizzaro reaction of glyoxal.

The carbonyl group which is attached to the less electron releasing of the two aryl groups is relatively more positively charged and, hence, is attacked by $\bar{O}H$. Consequently, the less electron-donating aryl group migrates to the other carbonyl group.

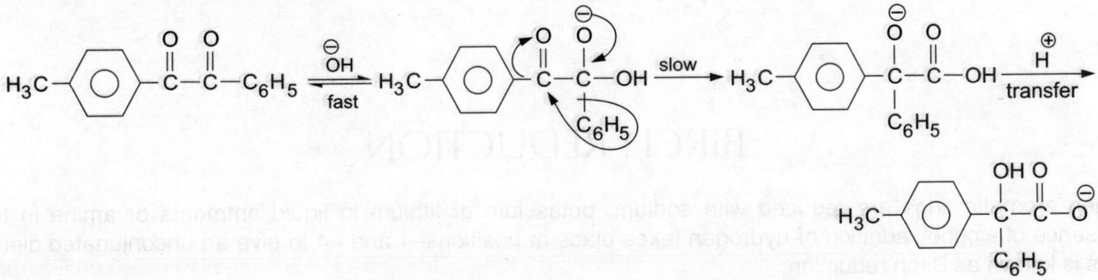

(*p*-Tolyl group is more electron-releasing than phenyl group)

Applications

The reaction is a general one and can take place with aromatic, heterocyclic, alicyclic, and aliphatic 1, 2-diketones as also 1, 2-quinones.

(i)

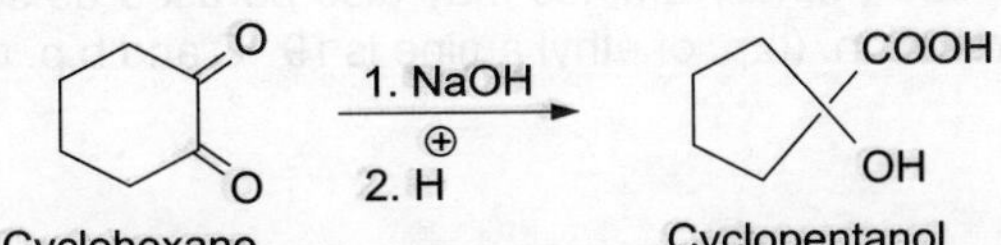

Cyclohexane -1, 2-dione → Cyclopentanol -1, -carboxylic acid

(ii)

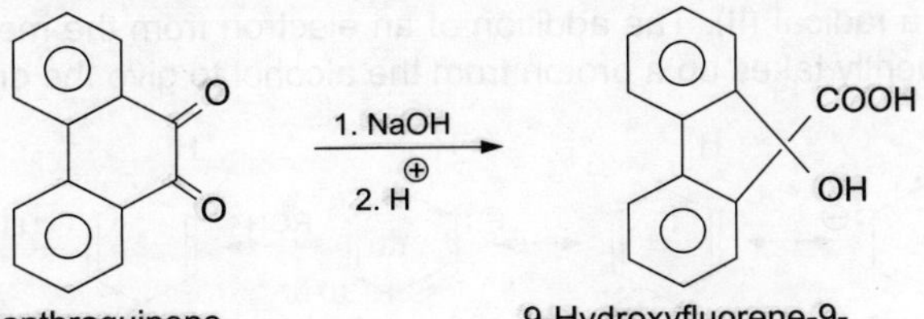

Phenanthraquinone → 9-Hydroxyfluorene-9-carboxylic acid

(iii)

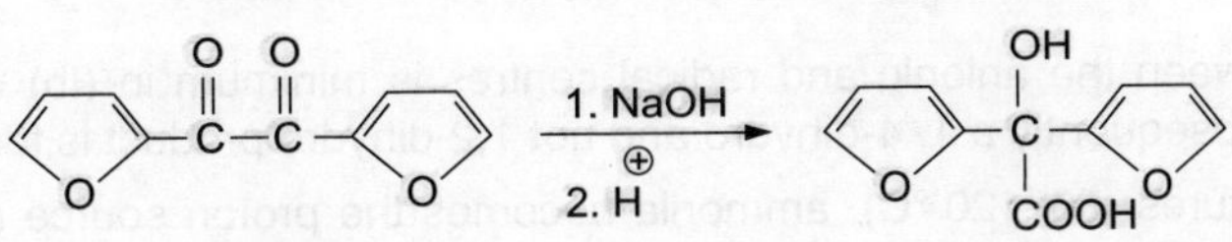

Furil → Furilic acid

(iv) 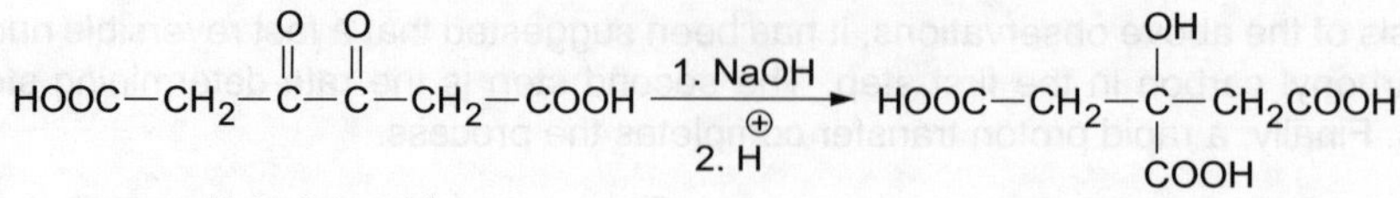

Ketopinic acid Citric acid

(v) Similar benzilic acid rearrangement is observed when α-haloketones not having α-hydrogens are treated with alkoxides.

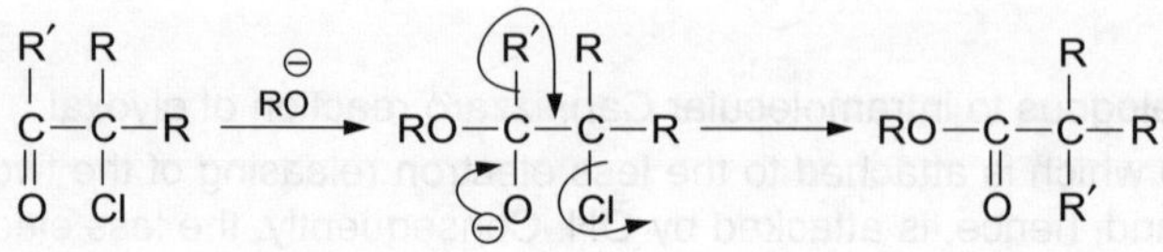

This reaction is known as semibenzilic rearrangement.

BIRCH REDUCTION

When aromatic rings are reduced with sodium, potassium or lithium in liquid ammonia or amine in the presence of alcohol, addition of hydrogen takes place at positions–1 and –4 to give an unconjugated diene. This is known as Birch reduction.

Thus, benzene gives 1, 4-dihydrocyclohexadiene and naphthalene gives 1, 4-dihydronaphthalene.

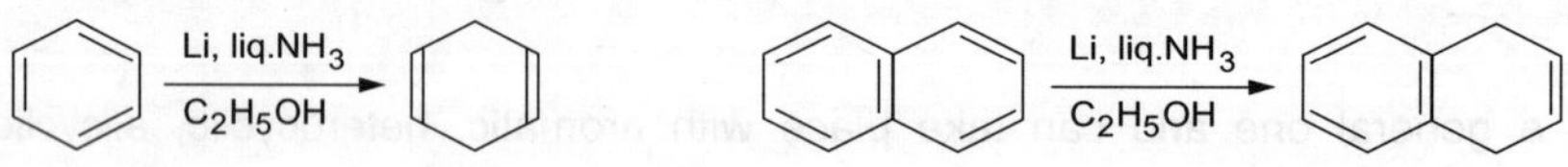

Liquid ammonia serves as solvent. Primary amines may also be used as solvent with advantage, since it permits higher temperature of reaction. (b.p. of ethyl amine is 19 °C and b.p. of liquid ammonia is −33 °C.)

Mechanism

The accepted mechanism of reduction involves the following sequential steps: The metal transfers one electron to the benzene ring to produce a resonance-stabilized anion radical (Ia–Ic) which accepts a proton from the alcohol to form a radical (II). The addition of an electron from the metal to the radical produces an anion (III) which subsequently takes up a proton from the alcohol to give the dihydro product.

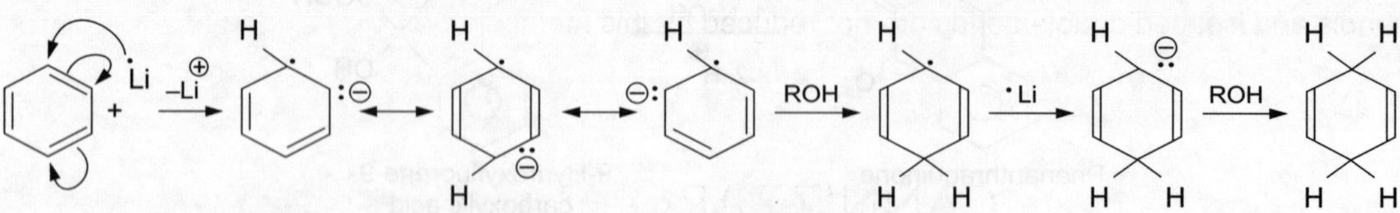

(Ia) (Ib) (Ic) (II) (III)

The repulsion between the anionic and radical centres is minimum in (Ib) which, therefore, adds a proton to give (II) and subsequently a 1, 4-dihydro and not 1,2-dihydro product is formed.

At higher temperatures (50–120 °C), ammonia becomes the proton source and alcohol need not be used. The amide ion thus formed is a strong base and isomerizes the 1, 4-dihydro product to 1,2-dihydro product.

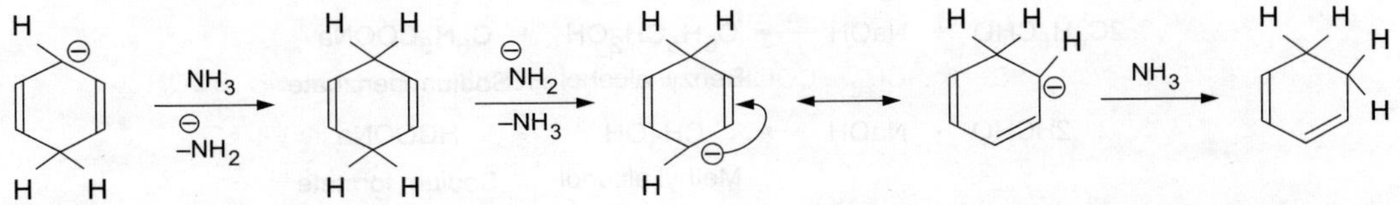

The 1, 2-dihydro product has a conjugated double bond and hence undergoes further reduction to form a tetrahydro derivative.

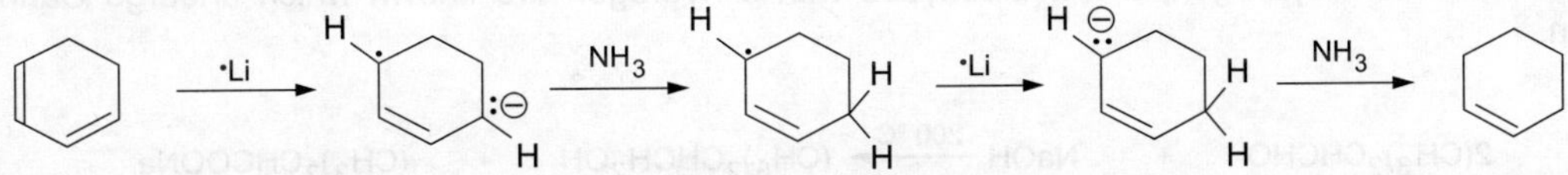

Cyclohexene has a single olefinic bond which is unaffected by the reagent. The presence of electron-withdrawing groups in the aromatic rings makes the rings more electron-accepting and hence the reaction is facilitated. The presence of electron-releasing groups have the reverse effect.

With substituted benzene the electron-donating group remains on the unsaturated carbon and the electron-withdrawing group remains on the saturated carbon in the products.

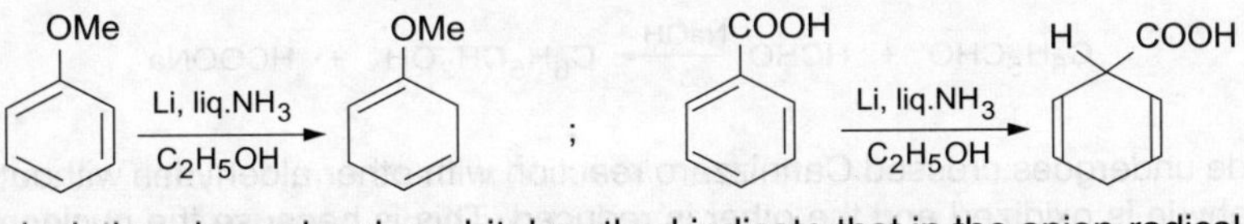

This is because, calculations by molecular orbital method indicate that in the anion-radical

(a) the electron density is the greatest at the ortho or meta positions with respect to the electron-releasing substituent in benzene and

(b) the electron density is the greatest at the para position with respect to the electron-withdrawing substituent in benzene.

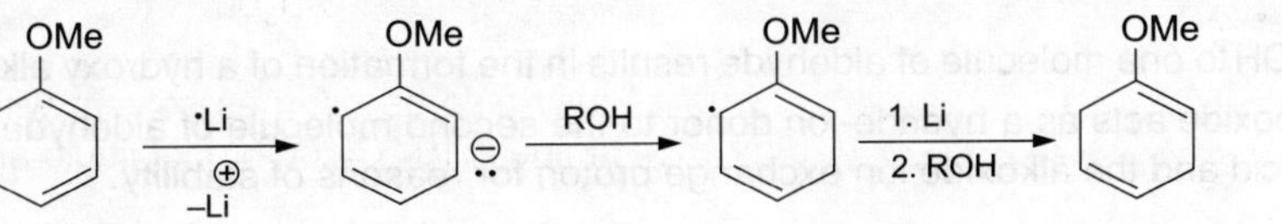

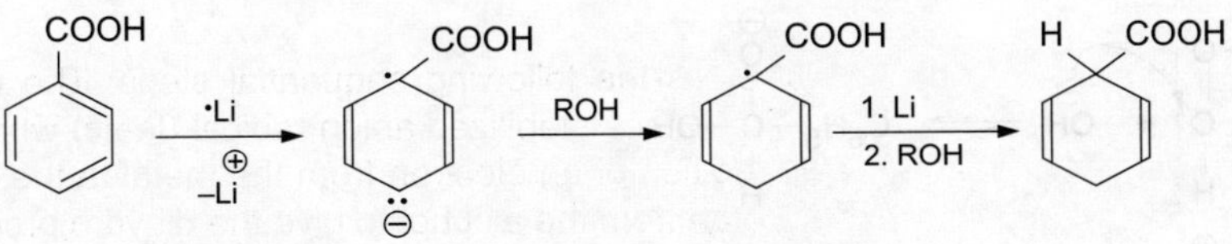

Phenols and isolated double bonds are not reduced by this method.

CANNIZZARO REACTION

In the presence of a strong base, aldehydes without α-hydrogens, i.e., nonaldolizable aldehydes undergo self-oxidation–reduction i.e., disproportionation reaction, This is known as Cannizzaro reaction. Thus, aromatic aldehydes (ArCHO), formaldehyde (HCHO), trialkyl acetaldehydes (R_3CCHO), heterocyclic aldehydes, 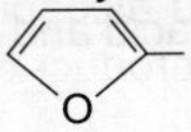 CHO etc., undergo Cannizzaro reaction, e.g.,

$$2C_6H_5CHO + NaOH \xrightarrow{\Delta} \underset{\text{Benzyl alcohol}}{C_6H_5CH_2OH} + \underset{\text{Sodium benzoate}}{C_6H_5COONa}$$

$$2HCHO + NaOH \xrightarrow{\Delta} \underset{\text{Methyl alcohol}}{CH_3OH} + \underset{\text{Sodium formate}}{HCOONa}$$

The reaction best proceeds with aromatic aldehydes. Although the reaction is characteristic of aldehydes without α-hydrogen, a few aldehydes with α-hydrogen are known which undergo Cannizzaro reaction.

$$\underset{\text{Dimethyl acetaldelyde}}{2(CH_3)_2CHCHO} + NaOH \xrightarrow{200\ ^\circ C} \underset{\text{2-Methylpropanol-1}}{(CH_3)_2CHCH_2OH} + \underset{\text{Sodium-2-methyl propanoate}}{(CH_3)_2CHCOONa}$$

The reaction can also occur between two different aldehydes having no α-hydrogens when it is called crossed Cannizzaro reaction.

$$C_6H_5CHO + HCHO \xrightarrow[\Delta]{NaOH} C_6H_5CH_2OH + HCOONa$$

When formaldehyde undergoes crossed Cannizzaro reaction with other aldehydes without α-hydrogens, it is seen that formaldehyde is oxidized and the other is reduced. This is because the nucleophilic attack occurs more readily on formaldehyde than on other aldehydes.

Mechanism

Rapid addition of $\overset{\ominus}{O}H$ to one molecule of aldehyde results in the formation of a hydroxy alkoxide ion which like aluminium-isopropoxide acts as a hydride-ion donor to the second molecule of aldehyde. In the final step of the reaction, the acid and the alkoxide ion exchange proton for reasons of stability.

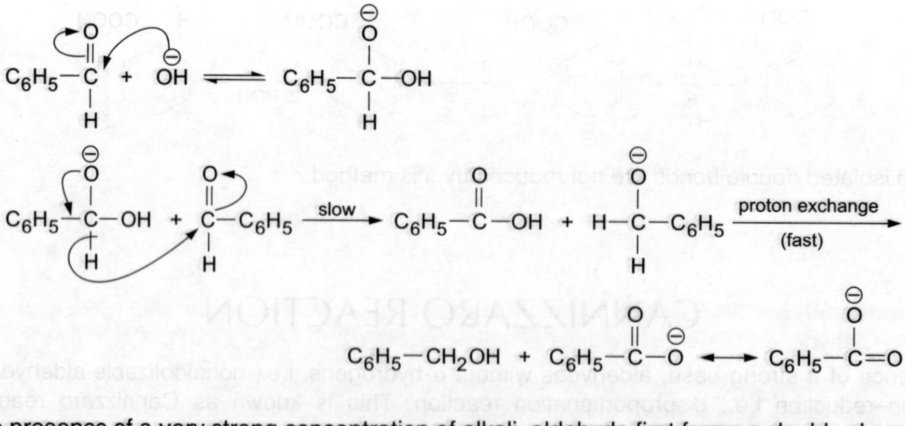

In the presence of a very strong concentration of alkali, aldehyde first forms a doubly charged anion (I) from which a hydride anion is transferred to the second molecule of the aldehyde to form acid and an alkoxide ion. Subsequently, the alkoxide ion acquires a proton from the solvent.

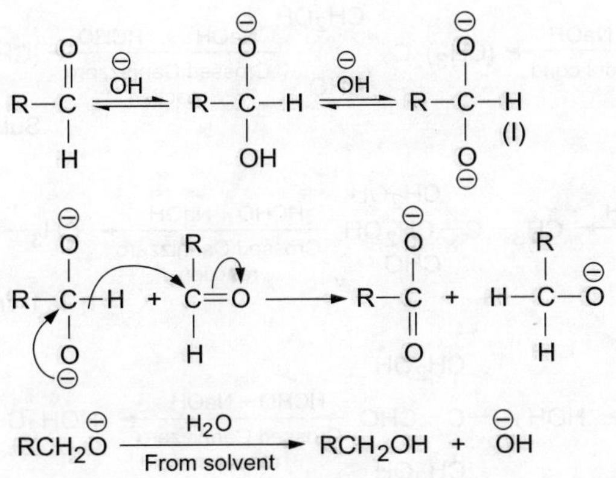

Evidence in support of the mechanism

(i) The reaction follows third-order law (second order in aldehyde and first order in base), i.e., rate $\propto [Ald]^2[OH]$. This suggests the reaction between the first-formed anion (from base and aldehyde) and another molecule of aldehyde in the rate-determining step.

In the presence of a high concentration of base, the reaction follows fourth-order law (second order in both the aldehyde and base), i.e., rate $\propto [Ald]^2 [\overset{\ominus}{O}H]$. This suggests the reaction between the doubly charged anion (formed from one molecule of aldehyde and two molecules of base) and another molecule of aldehyde.

(ii) That the hydride ion is directly transferred from one molecule of the aldehyde to the other, and does not become free in solution has been proved by the observation that the recovered alcohol does not contain deuterium when the reaction is performed in the presence of D_2O.

It is seen that the reaction depends on the nucleophilic attack on the carbonyl carbon. Hence, factors which reduce the positive charge of the carbonyl carbon retard the reaction. In extreme cases the reaction may not occur, e.g., *p*-dimethylaminobenzaldehyde does not undergo Cannizzaro reaction.

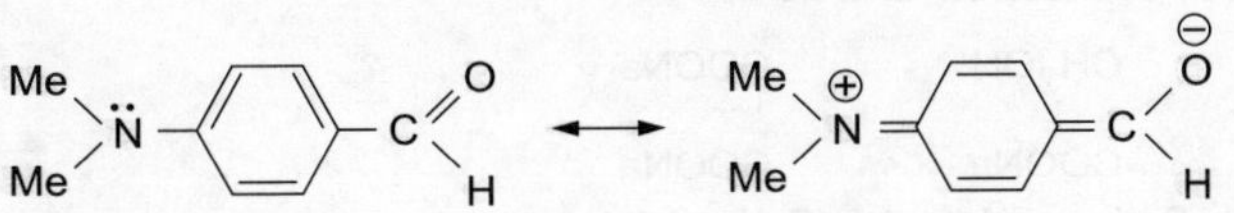

Similarly, sterically hindered aldehydes do not undergo the reaction.

Applications

1. Crossed Cannizzaro reaction One of the most important applications is the crossed Cannizzaro reaction between formaldehyde and other aldehydes having α-hydrogens.

During the reaction, the α-hydrogens are replaced by hydroxymethyl groups $-CH_2OH$ through aldol condensation and then the product, β-hydroxyaldehyde, undergoes crossed Cannizzaro reaction with formaldehyde.

Thus, aldehydes containing one, two or three α-hydrogens react as given below.

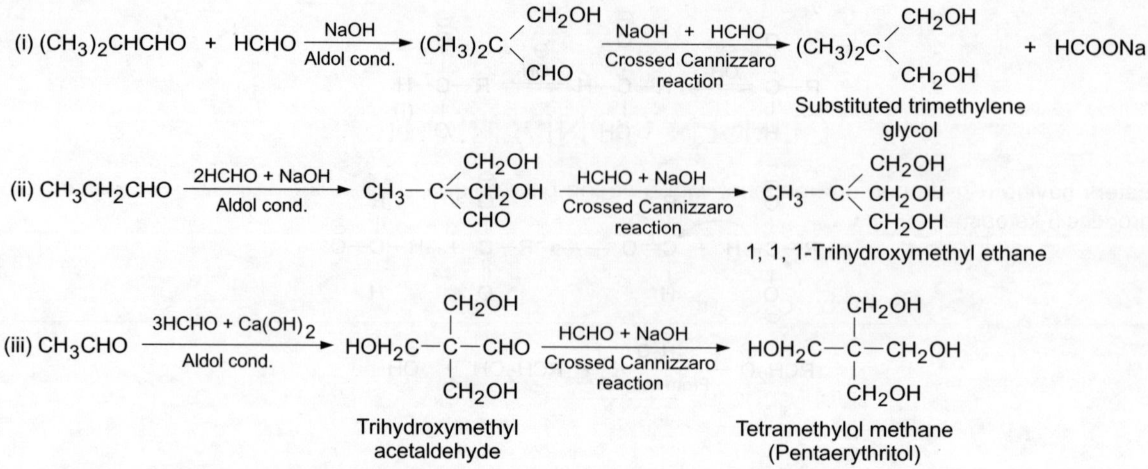

Pentaerythritol is an important industrial product. Its ester with polybasic acids gives resin polymers used for surface coating. Its tetranitro derivative (PETN) is a useful explosive.

2. Intramolecular Cannizzaro reaction Dialdehydes and α-keto aldehydes undergo intramolecular Cannizzaro reaction giving various valuable products.

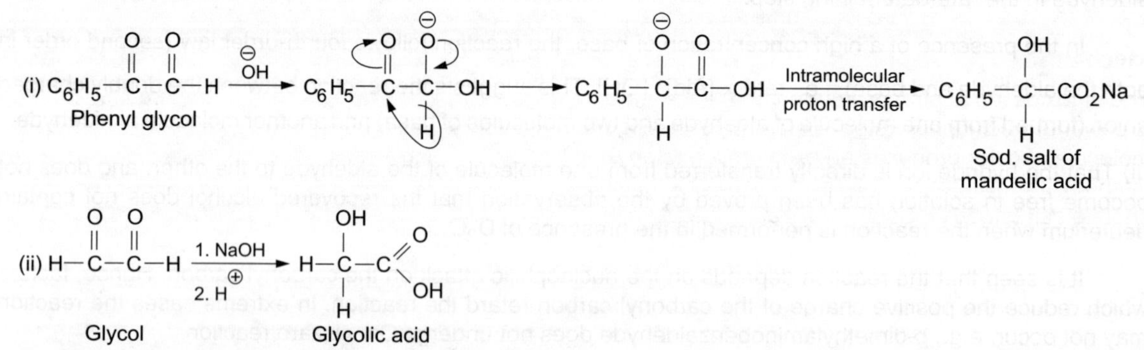

3. Synthesis of various types of alcohols and acids

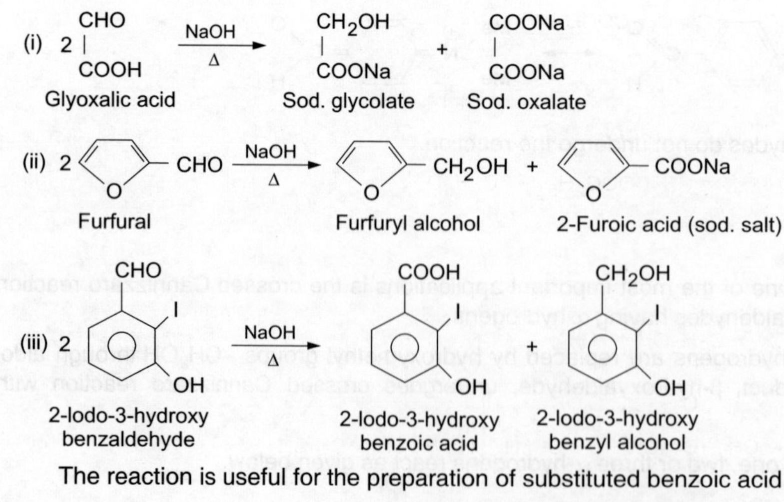

The reaction is useful for the preparation of substituted benzoic acid and benzyl alcohol.

CLAISEN CONDENSATION

Esters having α-hydrogen on treatment with a strong base, e.g., C_2H_5ONa, undergo self-condensation to produce β-ketoesters

$$2CH_3COOC_2H_5 \xrightarrow[2.\ H^{\oplus}]{1.\ C_2H_5ONa} \underset{\text{Ethyl acetoacetate}}{CH_3COCH_2COOC_2H_5}$$

$$2R'CH_2COOC_2H_5 \xrightarrow[2.\ H^{\oplus}]{1.\ C_2H_5ONa} R'CH_2COCH(R')COOC_2H_5$$

This reaction is called Claisen condensation although there are several closely related reactions which follow the same mechanistic pattern.

Mixed or crossed Claisen condensation also occurs between two different esters or between an ester and a ketone.

Mechanism

The ethoxide ion abstracts a proton from the α-carbon of the ester to produce the anion (of the ester) which is a powerful nucleophile (step I). The nucleophilic attack of the anion on the carbonyl carbon of a second molecule of ester produces an oxonium ion (step II), which eliminates an ethoxide ion to give the β-ketoester (step III). The β-ketoester having an active methylene group is acidic and reacts with sodium ethoxide to form enolate salt (step IV). Subsequent acidification with acetic acid (1 : 1) regenerates the β-ketoester.

$$C_2H_5\overset{\ominus}{O} + H{-}CH_2COOC_2H_5 \rightleftharpoons C_2H_5OH + :\overset{\ominus}{C}H_2COOC_2H_5 \quad \ldots \text{(I)}$$

$$CH_3{-}\underset{OC_2H_5}{\underset{|}{\overset{O}{\overset{\|}{C}}}} + \overset{\ominus}{C}H_2COOC_2H_5 \rightleftharpoons CH_3{-}\underset{OC_2H_5}{\underset{|}{\overset{\overset{\ominus}{O}}{\overset{|}{C}}}}{-}CH_2COOC_2H_5 \quad \ldots \text{(II)}$$

$$CH_3{-}\underset{OC_2H_5}{\underset{|}{\overset{\overset{\ominus}{O}}{\overset{|}{C}}}}{-}CH_2COOC_2H_5 \rightleftharpoons CH_3{-}\overset{O}{\overset{\|}{C}}{-}CH_2COOC_2H_5 + C_2H_5\overset{\ominus}{O} \quad \ldots \text{(III)}$$

$$CH_3{-}\overset{O}{\overset{\|}{C}}{-}CH_2COOC_2H_5 + C_2H_5\overset{\ominus}{O} \longrightarrow C_2H_5OH + \left[CH_3{-}\overset{O}{\overset{\|}{C}}{-}\overset{\ominus}{C}H{-}\overset{O}{\overset{\|}{C}}{-}OC_2H_5 \longleftrightarrow CH_3{-}\overset{O}{\overset{\|}{C}}{-}CH{=}\overset{\overset{\ominus}{O}}{\overset{|}{C}}{-}OC_2H_5\right.$$

$$\left.\longleftrightarrow CH_3{-}\overset{\overset{\ominus}{O}}{\overset{|}{C}}{=}CH{-}\overset{O}{\overset{\|}{C}}{-}OC_2H_5\right]\overset{\oplus}{Na} \equiv \left[CH_3{-}\overset{O}{\overset{\|}{C}}{-}CH{-}\overset{O}{\overset{\|}{C}}{-}OC_2H_5\right]^{\ominus}\overset{\oplus}{Na} \quad \ldots \text{(IV)}$$

$$\left[CH_3-\overset{O}{\overset{\|}{C}}-CH-\overset{O}{\overset{\|}{C}}-OC_2H_5\right]^{\ominus}\overset{\oplus}{Na} \xrightarrow{CH_3COOH} CH_3-CO-CH_2-COOC_2H_5 + CH_3COONa$$

The first three steps are in unfavourable equilibrium state. Hence, excess sodium ethoxide is used to force the equilibrium to shift in the forward direction by the formation of a resonance-stabilized enolate anion (step IV). This is substantiated by the fact that esters having only one α-hydrogen do not undergo Claisen condensation with C_2H_5ONa. This is because the ketoester formed (analogous to step III) cannot be converted to its enolate anion due to the absence of a second α-hydrogen, with the result that the equilibrium does not shift to the right.

However, in the presence of a very strong base such as triphenylmethyl sodium, such esters, e.g., ethyl isobutyrate, undergo Claisen condensation to give β-ketoesters. This is because the very strong base, $(C_6H_5)_3CNa$ acts in two ways.

(i) It withdraws the weakly acidic α-hydrogen irreversibly from the ester (analogous step I is highly reversible).

$$\underset{\text{Ethyl isobutyrate}}{CH_3-\overset{CH_3}{\overset{|}{C}H}-COOC_2H_5} + (C_6H_5)_3\overset{\ominus}{C} \rightleftharpoons CH_3-\underset{\ominus}{\overset{CH_3}{\overset{|}{C}}}-COOC_2H_5 + (C_6H_5)_3CH$$

(ii) It completely removes one of the equilibrium products, i.e., ethyl alcohol, so that the equilibrium shifts to the right. (Compare step III.)

$$\underset{\text{Ethyl isobutyrate}}{2(CH_3)_2CH-COOC_2H_5} \xrightleftharpoons{(C_6H_5)_3\overset{\ominus}{C}} \underset{\text{Ethyl isobutylisobutyrate}}{(CH_3)_2CH-\overset{O}{\overset{\|}{C}}-\underset{CH_3}{\underset{|}{\overset{CH_3}{\overset{|}{C}}}}-COOC_2H_5} + C_2H_5OH$$

$$(C_6H_5)_3CNa + C_2H_5OH \rightleftharpoons (C_6H_5)_3CH + C_2H_5ONa$$

Applications

Simple and crossed Claisen condensations have been extensively used in the synthesis of a wide variety of organic compounds, e.g., vitamins, sex hormones, alkaloids, terpenes, flavones, etc.

Crossed Claisen condensations between two different esters (both having α-hydrogens) have little synthetic value, for a mixture of four products are obtained. However, if one of the esters has no α-hydrogen, it acts as a carbanion acceptor and the self-condensation of the other ester is minimized. Commonly used esters with no α-hydrogen are ethyl benzoate, ethyl formate, ethyl oxalate, ethyl carbonate, etc. These esters are good carbanion acceptors.

Ketones are generally more acidic than esters and the rate of their base-catalyzed condensation (aldol) is very slow. Hence, ketones serve as nucleophiles in mixed Claisen condensation to give a large variety of products.

Some of the examples of crossed Claisen condensation and their applications are given below.

1. Condensation with ethyl benzoate

(a) $$\underset{\text{Ethyl benzoate}}{C_6H_5COOC_2H_5} + CH_3COOC_2H_5 \xrightarrow[2.\ \overset{\oplus}{H}]{1.\ C_2H_5ONa} \underset{\text{Ethyl benzoylacetate}}{C_6H_5COCH_2COOC_2H_5} + C_2H_5OH$$

(b) Synthesis of flavones (chrysin)

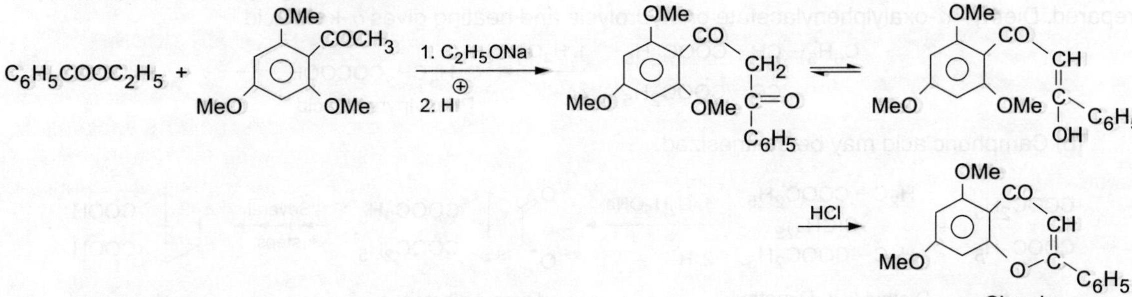

Chrysin

(c) Synthesis of nicotine from ethyl nicotinate.

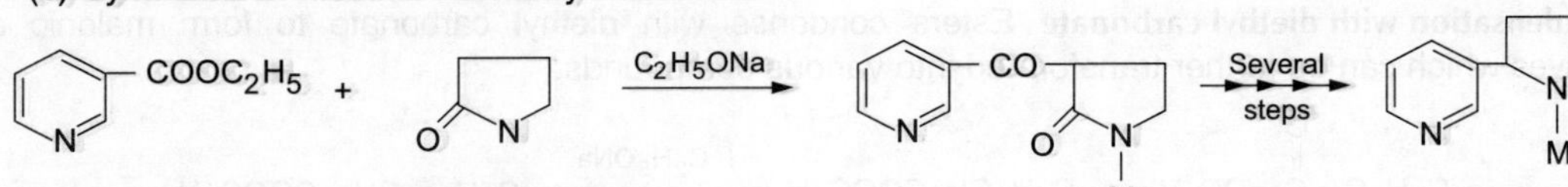

Ethyl nicotinate N-Methylpyrrolidone Nicotine

2. Condensation with ethyl formate

(a) Formylation

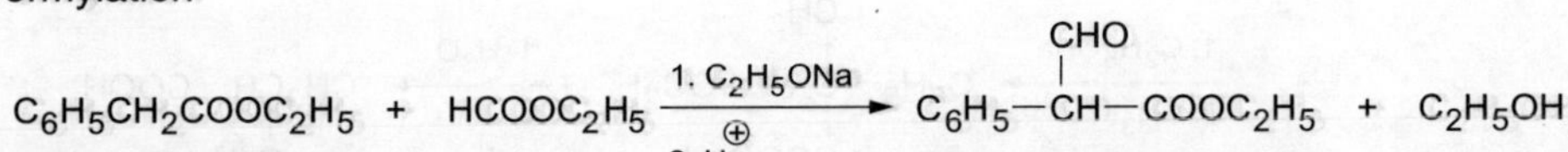

Ethyl phenylacetate Ethyl formylphenylacetate

The reaction is utilized for formylation during the synthesis of various natural products, e.g., equilenine, thiamin (vitamin B1), isoflavones, etc.

(b) Synthesis of daidzein (isoflavone)

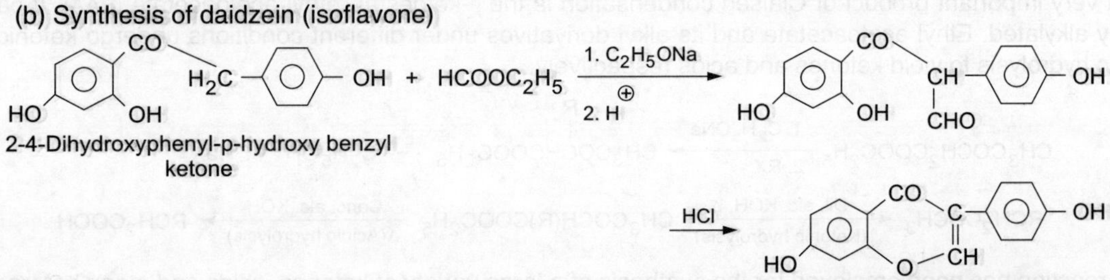

2-4-Dihydroxyphenyl-p-hydroxy benzyl ketone

Daidzein(isoflavone)

3. Condensation with diethyl oxalate (a) Ketones and esters condense with diethyl oxalate to give oxalyl derivatives which have synthetic utility since they lose carbon monoxide on heating to give malonic ester derivatives which may be used for the preparation of aryl-substituted dibasic acid derivatives and α-keto acids.

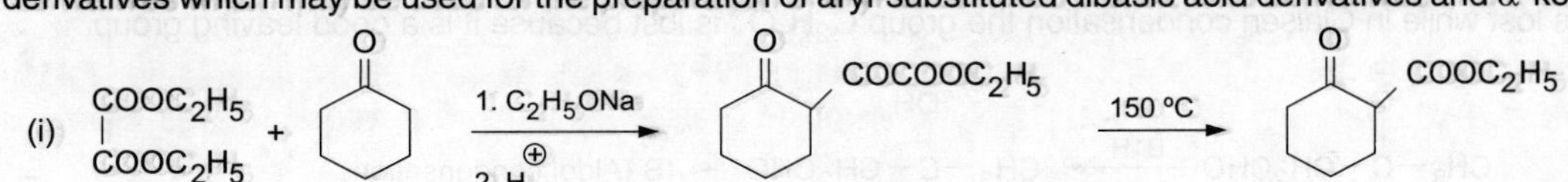

2-(Ethyl oxalyl)-cyclohexanone 2-Carbethoxy cyclohexanone

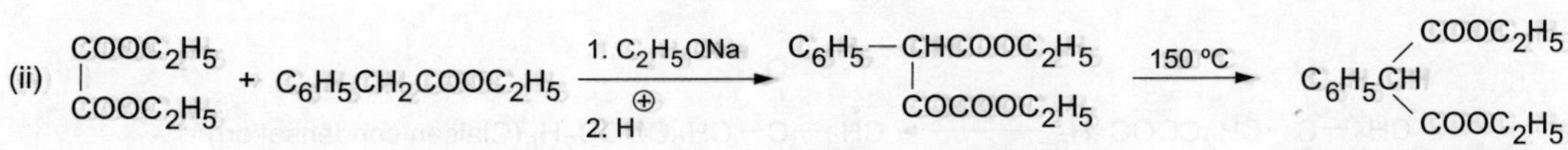

Diethyl-α-oxalylphenyl acetate Diethyl phenylmalonate

Phenyl-substituted malonic ester has important synthetic applications, e.g., phenobarbitone may be prepared. Diethyl- α-oxalylphenylacetate on hydrolysis and heating gives α-keto acid.

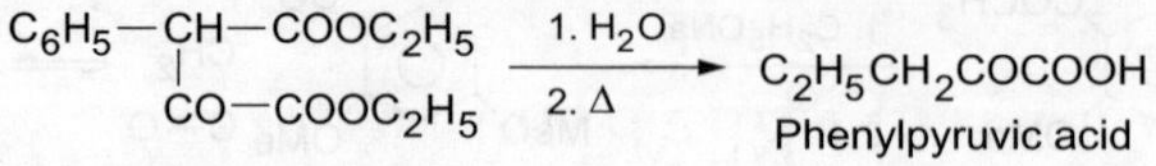

(b) Camphoric acid may be synthesized.

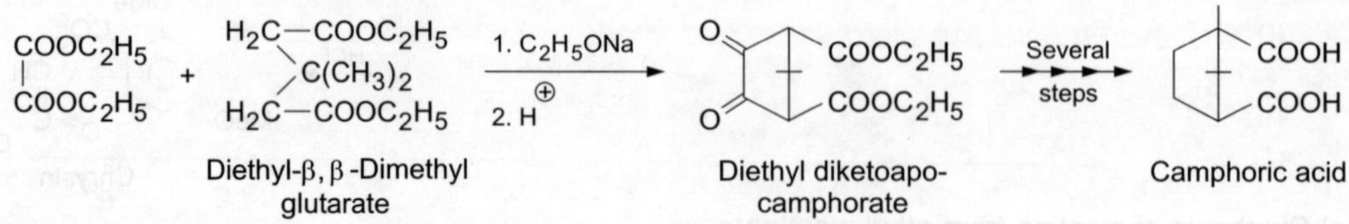

4. Condensation with diethyl carbonate Esters condense with diethyl carbonate to form malonic ester derivatives which can be further transformed into various compounds.

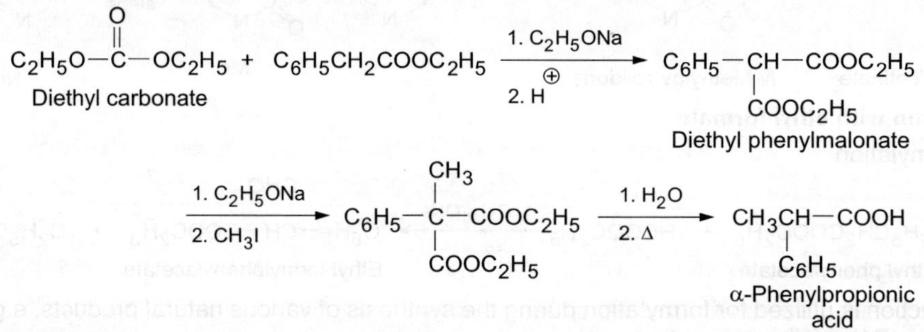

5. A very important product of Claisen condensation is the β-ketoester, ethyl acetoacetate (EAA). It can be easily alkylated. Ethyl acetoacetate and its alkyl derivatives under different conditions undergo ketonic and acidic hydrolysis to yield ketones and acids respectively.

$$CH_3COCH_2COOC_2H_5 \xrightarrow[2.\ RX]{1.\ C_2H_5ONa} CH_3CO\overset{R}{\overset{|}{C}}HCOOC_2H_5 + C_2H_5OH + NaX$$

$$RCH_2COCH_3 \xleftarrow[\text{(Ketonic hydrolysis)}]{\text{Dil. alc. KOH, }\Delta} CH_3COCH(R)COOC_2H_5 \xrightarrow[\Delta\text{(Acidic hydrolysis)}]{\text{Conc. alc. KOH}} RCH_2COOH$$

This reaction has been employed for the synthesis of a large variety of ketones, acids and many heterocyclic compounds. Intramolecular Claisen condensation in dibasic esters of six to eight carbons is called Dieckmann reaction. The product is a cyclic ketone derivative.

Claisen condensation is very similar to aldol condensation. The only difference is that, in aldol condensation no group is lost while in Claisen condensation the group $C_2H_5O^-$ is lost because it is a good leaving group.

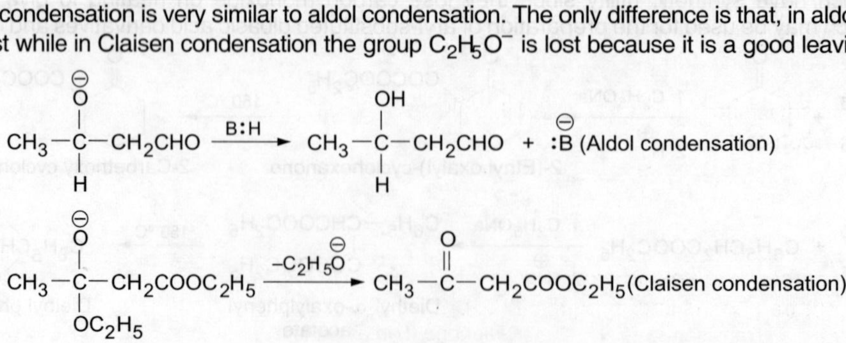

CLAISEN REARRANGEMENT

Claisen rearrangement involves the shift of a group from oxygen to carbon. Thus, when aryl allyl ethers are heated (ca 200 °C) they rearrange to *o*-allylphenols.

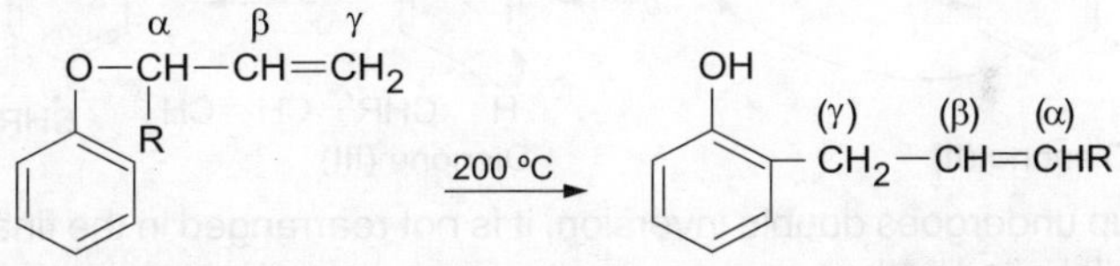

The group migrates to the ortho position, although some para product has been obtained in some cases. In general, when both ortho positions are free, the product is ortho compound and when both ortho positions are occupied, the product is para compound.

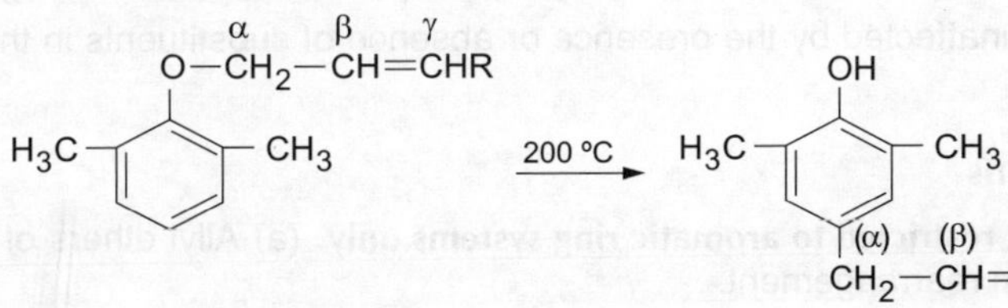

When both ortho positions and the para position are occupied, there is no reaction. Migration to the *m*-position has not been observed.

During the ortho migration, the allyl group undergoes allylic shift, i.e., the carbon atom α- to the oxygen atom in the substrate becomes γ- to the ring in the product. However, in the para migration no change of attachment of the allyl group in the product is observed. This has been confirmed by ^{14}C labelling in the allyl group.

No catalyst is required, for the reaction follows first-order kinetics, i.e., one molecule is involved in the rearrangement. Further, when a mixture of allyl ethers is heated, no crossover products are formed.

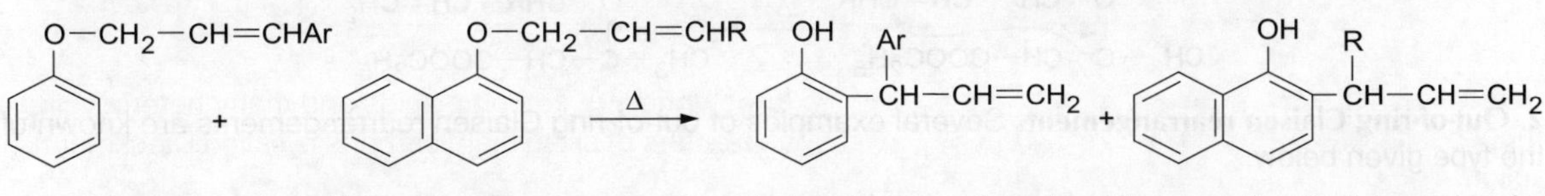

Therefore, the allyl group never separates during the reaction, i.e., the reaction is intramolecular rearrangement. This indicates that the reaction proceeds through a cyclic transition state in which the breaking of oxygen-allyl bond and the formation of carbon–carbon bond with the ring are concerted.

On the basis of the above considerations, the following mechanism of the rearrangement has been suggested:

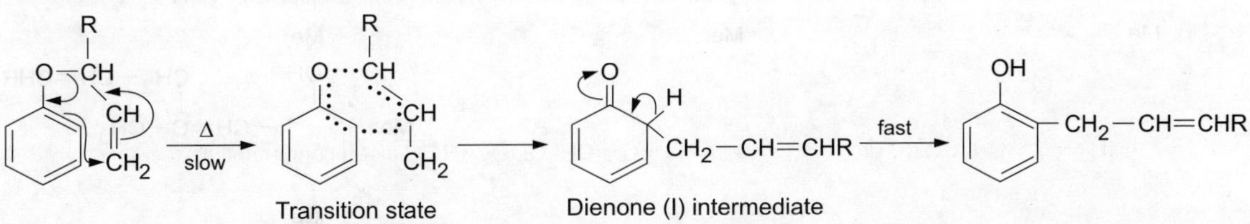

The cyclohexadienone (I) intermediate is converted rapidly into phenol for reasons of aromatic stability.

Para-migration Even when the ortho positions are substituted, the migration still occurs at the ortho position to form ortho-substituted dienone (II). However, the absence of hydrogen at the ortho position prevents enolization, i.e., aromatization. Hence the allyl group undergoes a second migration through a similar cyclic transition state to form a dienone (III) which aromatizes to a phenol with allyl group at position-4.

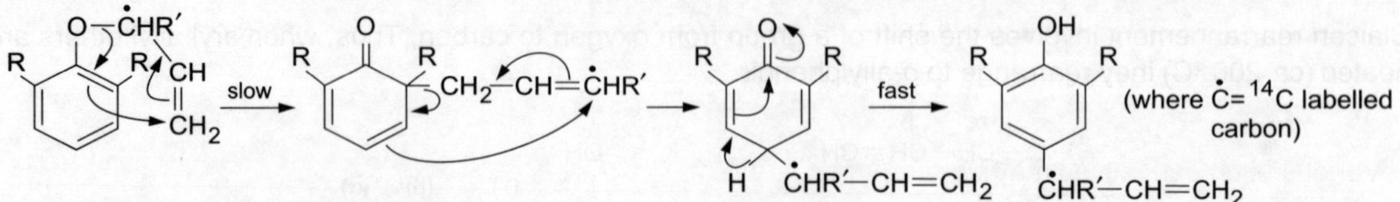

Dienone (II) Dienone (III)

Since the allyl group undergoes double inversion, it is not rearranged in the final product. This has been confirmed by isotopically labelled carbon.

There are enough evidence in support of this mechanism. The double inversion of the allyl group is proved by trapping the dienone (II) intermediate with maleic anhydride in a Diels–Alder reaction. Further, the dienone (II) prepared separately was found to give rapidly the para product on heating.

The reaction rate is unaffected by the presence or absence of substituents in the aromatic ring, since the reaction is not ionic.

Extension and Applications

1. The rearrangement is not restricted to aromatic ring systems only (a) Allyl ethers of enols, e.g., allyl vinyl ethers also undergo Claisen rearrangement.

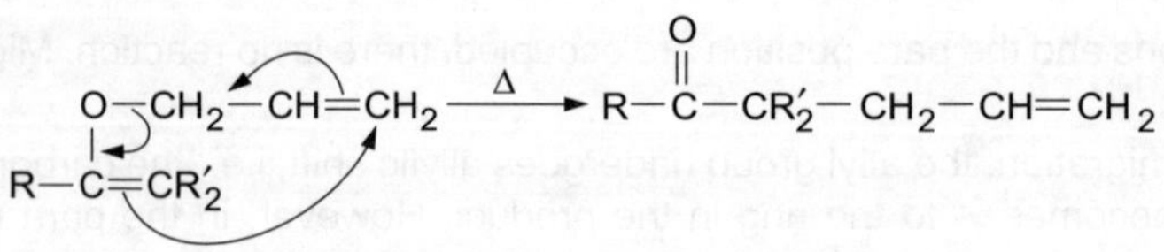

The product does not enolize (even when R or R′ = H) because ketones are more stable than enols.

(b) The *o*-allyl acetoacetic esters also rearrange similarly.

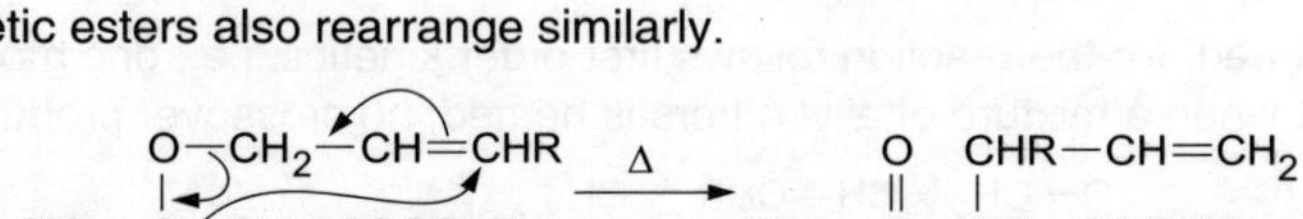

2. Out-of-ring Claisen rearrangement Several examples of out-of-ring Claisen rearrangements are known of the type given below.

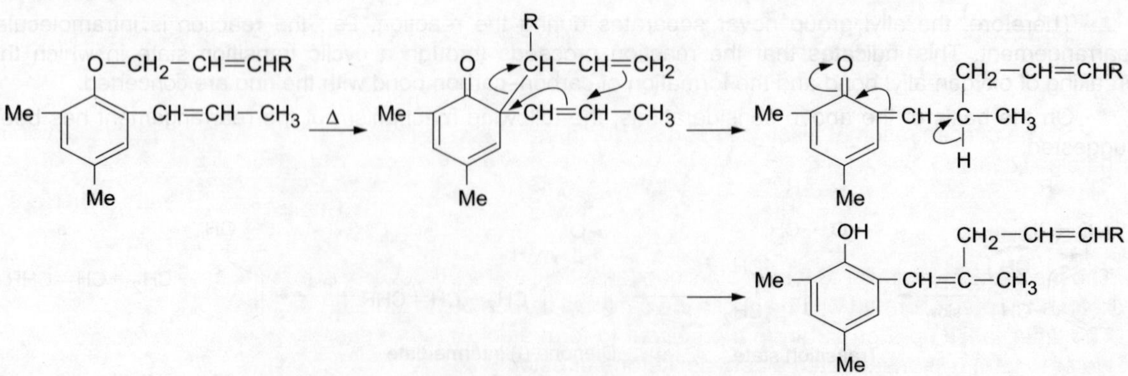

There is no rearrangement of the allylic group in the final product due to double inversion.

3. Synthetic applications Since aryl allyl ethers can be easily prepared, the rearrangement is employed to prepare various kinds of compounds, e.g.,

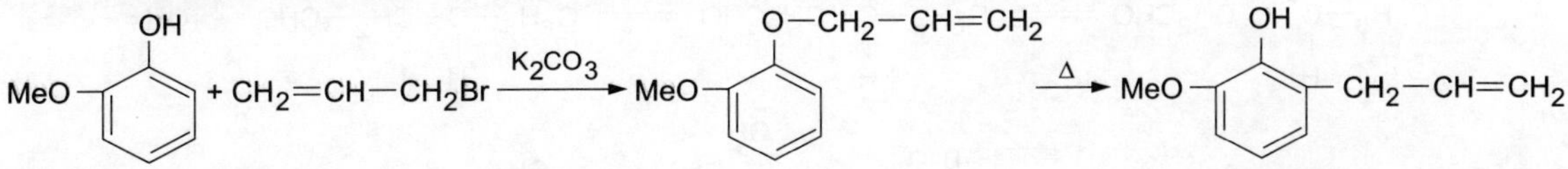

o-eugenol

Various such derivatives may be prepared.

Allyl aryl thioethers, e.g., $ArSCH_2—CH = CH_2$, do not ordinarily give orthoallyl thiophenols.

CLAISEN-SCHMIDT REACTION

When aromatic aldehydes react with aliphatic aldehydes or ketones in the presence of a strong base, three reactions are possible, e.g.,

(i) Cannizzaro reaction of the aldehyde having no α-hydrogen,

(ii) aldol condensation of the aliphatic aldehyde or ketone and

(iii) crossed aldol condensation between the aromatic aldehyde and the aliphatic aldehyde or ketone.

However, when aromatic aldehydes or ketones react with aliphatic aldehydes, ketones or esters having α-hydrogens under mild conditions, i.e., weak base (10% NaOH) and low temperature, a crossed aldol condensation with subsequent dehydration occurs predominantly, with the formation of α, β-unsaturated aldehydes, ketones or esters. This is known as Claisen–Schmidt reaction or simply Claisen reaction.

$$C_6H_5CHO + CH_3CHO \xrightarrow[\text{8-10 days}]{\text{10\% NaOH, room temp.}} \underset{\text{Cinnamaldehyde}}{C_6H_5CH{=}CH{-}CHO}$$

$$C_6H_5CHO + CH_3COCH_3 \xrightarrow[\text{2-3 days}]{\text{10\% NaOH, 30 °C}} \underset{\text{Benzylidene acetone}}{C_6H_5CH{=}CHCOCH_3}$$

$$C_6H_5CHO + CH_3COC_6H_5 \xrightarrow[\text{Below 30 °C}]{\text{10\% NaOH}} \underset{\text{Benzylidene acetophenone}}{C_6H_5CH{=}CHCOC_6H_5}$$

$$C_6H_5CHO + CH_3COOC_2H_5 \xrightarrow[\text{30 °C}]{\text{10\% NaOH}} \underset{\text{Ethyl cinnamate}}{C_6H_5CH{=}CH{-}COOC_2H_5}$$

The concentration of alkali is important, for in the presence of a strong base, Cannizzaro reaction may be significant.

Mechanism

The mechanism is similar to that of aldol condensation. In the presence of the base, an anion of the aldehyde, ketone or ester is formed which attacks the carbonyl carbon of the aromatic aldehyde to form an oxonium ion. The latter takes up a proton from the solvent to form aldol (I) which subsequently eliminates a molecule of water to form α,β-unsaturated aldehyde, ketone or ester.

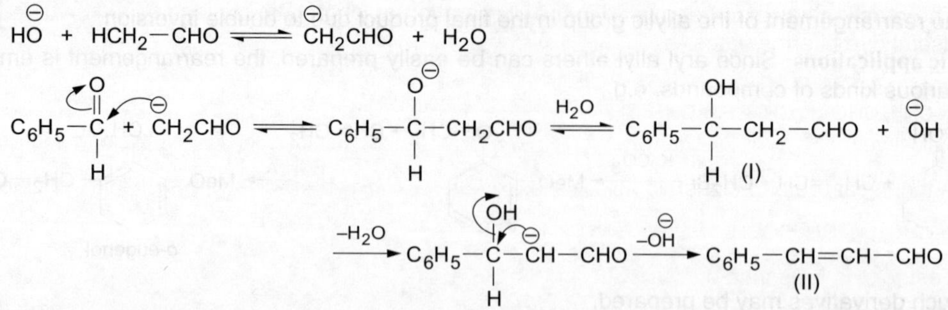

The aliphatic aldehyde may also undergo aldol condensation and dehydration but (II) predominates. This is because the aldol (I) loses water irreversibly due to conjugation of the double bond with the benzene ring.

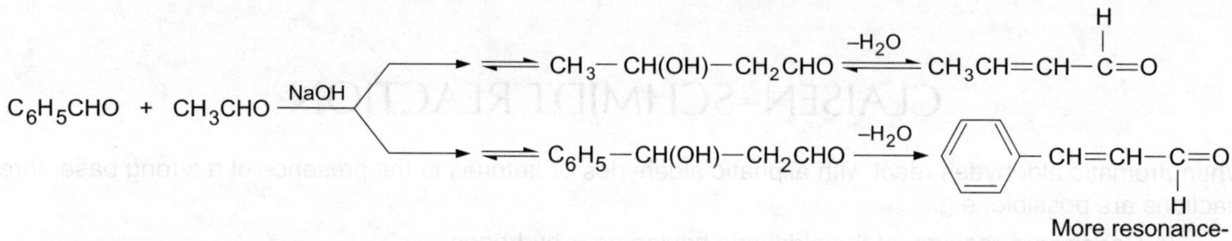

Electron-releasing groups in the aromatic ring at *o*- and *p*-positions to the carbonyl group retard the reaction by reducing the positive charge on the carbonyl carbon which is the point of attack of the carbanion. Electron-withdrawing groups have opposite effect.

Applications

1. The α,β-unsaturated carbonyl compounds obtained by this reaction are useful commercial products, e.g., cinnamaldehyde and benzylidene acetone are used in perfumery.
2. This reaction has been utilized in the synthesis of various natural products, e.g., β-ionone, piperine, flavones, flavonols, etc.

(i) In the synthesis of β-ionone

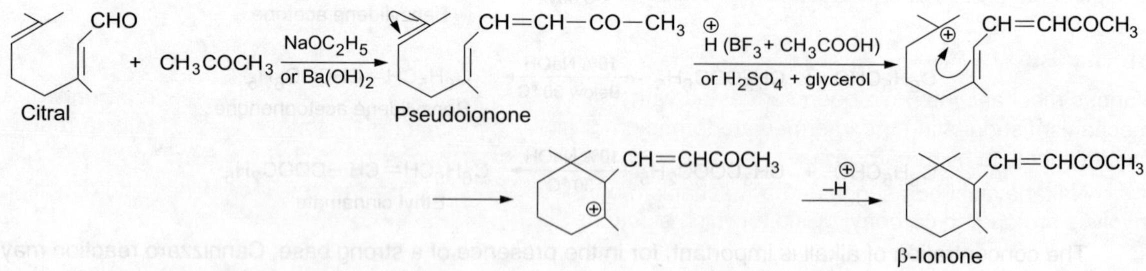

(ii) In the synthesis of flavones

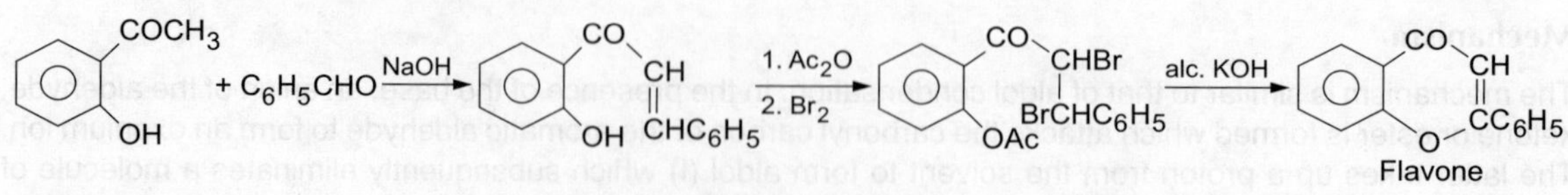

3. The reaction has also been used in the preparation of long-chain conjugated aldehydes, which are useful dye intermediates.

$$\underset{\text{Cinnamaldehyde}}{C_6H_5CH{=}CH{-}CHO} + \underset{\text{Crotonaldehyde}}{CH_3CH{=}CH{-}CHO} \xrightarrow[\text{+alcohol}]{\text{Piperidine acetate}} \underset{\text{7-Phenyl heptatrienal}}{C_6H_5{-}(CH{=}CH)_3{-}CHO} + \underset{\text{11-Phenyl undecapentenal}}{C_6H_5{-}(CH{=}CH)_5{-}CHO}$$

4. A technical route to cinnamic acid is the oxidation of benzalacetone with sodium hypochlorite.

$$C_6H_5CHO + CH_3COCH_3 \xrightarrow[30\ ^\circ C]{10\ \%\ NaOH} C_6H_5{-}CH{=}CH{-}CO{-}CH_3 \xrightarrow{NaOCl} C_6H_5CH{=}CHCOOH$$

5. Test for the presence of $-CH_2CO-$ group

The reaction has been used to detect the presence of $-CH_2CO-$ group in the natural products, for only if a compound contains $-CH_2CO-$ group, it will undergo the condensation.

$$C_6H_5{-}CH{=}O + H_2C(H){-}CO{-}CH_3 \xrightarrow{\overset{\ominus}{O}H} C_6H_5CH{=}CHCOCH_3$$

CLEMMENSEN REDUCTION

The reduction of carbonyl groups of aldehydes and ketones to methylene groups with amalgamated zinc and concentrated hydrochloric acid is known as Clemmensen reduction.

$$\underset{\text{Acetophenone}}{C_6H_5COCH_3} \xrightarrow[\text{Reflux}]{\text{Zn–Hg, HCl}} \underset{\text{Ethyl benzene}}{C_6H_5CH_2CH_3}$$

The reduction consists in refluxing the carbonyl compounds with amalgamated zinc and excess of concentrated hydrochloric acid. The reduction is useful especially for ketones containing phenolic or carboxylic groups which remain unaffected. Ketones are reduced more often than aldehydes. Such reduction is also observed in Wolff–Kishner reduction but Clemmensen reduction is easier to perform. The reduction, however, fails with acid-sensitive and high molecular weight substrates. The α, β-unsaturated ketones undergo reduction of both the olefinic and carbonyl groups. However, the reduction is specific for carbonyl groups of aldehydes and ketones containing other functional and reducible groups.

Mechanism

Various mechanisms have been suggested which are so contradictory that no conclusion can be drawn. A mechanism suggesting the intermediate formation of alcohol was rejected since the reagent fails to reduce most alcohols to hydrocarbons.

Nakabayaski has suggested a mechanism on the assumption that the reduction under acid condition involves protonated carbonyl group to which electrons are transferred from the metal.

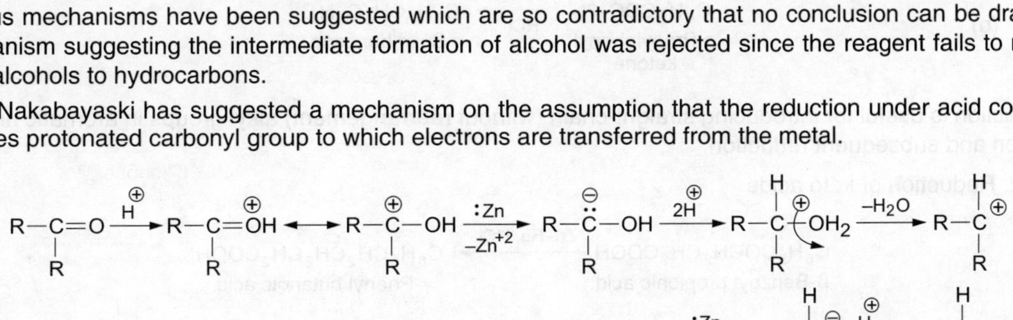

Certain types of aldehydes and ketones do not give the normal reduction products alone. Thus, α-hydroxy ketones give either ketones through hydrogenolysis* of OH group or olefins and 1, 3-diketones give exclusively monoketones with rearrangement.

$$CH_3-\overset{O}{\overset{\|}{C}}-CH_2-\overset{O}{\overset{\|}{C}}-CH_3 \xrightarrow[\text{Reduction}]{\text{Clemmensen}} CH_3-\overset{O}{\overset{\|}{C}}-\underset{CH_3}{\underset{|}{CH}}-CH_3$$

Certain cyclic 1, 3-diketones give under Clemmensen reduction a fully reduced product along with a monoketone with ring contraction.

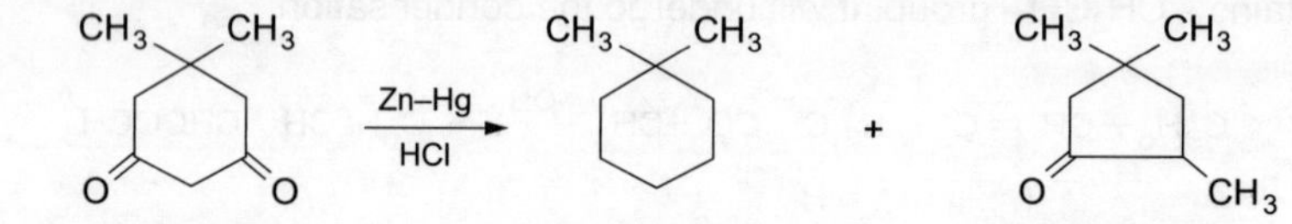

5, 5-Dimethyl cyclohexane-1, 3-dione — 1, 1-Dimethyl cyclohexane — 2, 4, 4-Trimethyl cyclopentanone

The latter probably is formed through a diradical with subsequent intramolecular C—C bond formation and pinacol-type rearrangement.

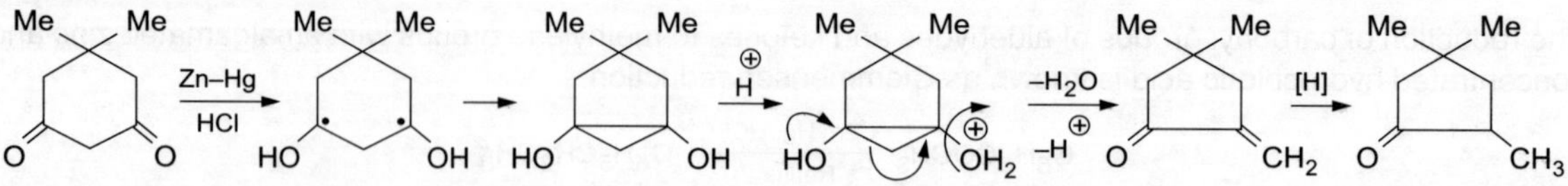

Applications

The reduction has important synthetic applications.

1. Reduction of aliphatic and mixed aliphatic–aromatic carbonyl compounds.

(a)
$$\underset{n\text{-Heptaldehyde}}{CH_3-(CH_2)_5-CHO} \xrightarrow[\text{HCl}]{\text{Zn–Hg}} \underset{n\text{-Heptane}}{CH_3-(CH_2)_5-CH_3}$$

(b)
$$\underset{n\text{-Propylphenyl ketone}}{C_6H_5COC_3H_7} \xrightarrow[\text{HCl}]{\text{Zn–Hg}} \underset{n\text{-Butyl benzene}}{C_6H_5CH_2C_3H_7}$$

The reaction is useful for introducing straight-chain (without rearrangement) alkyl groups in aromatic rings by acylation and subsequent reduction.

2. Reduction of keto acids

$$\underset{\beta\text{-Benzoyl propionic acid}}{C_6H_5COCH_2CH_2COOH} \xrightarrow{\text{Zn–Hg, HCl}} \underset{\gamma\text{-Phenyl butanoic acid}}{C_6H_5CH_2CH_2CH_2COOH}$$

α- and β-keto acids are generally not reduced.

---

* Cleavage of carbon-hetero atom bond by catalytic hydrogenation.

3. Reduction of phenolic carbonyl compounds

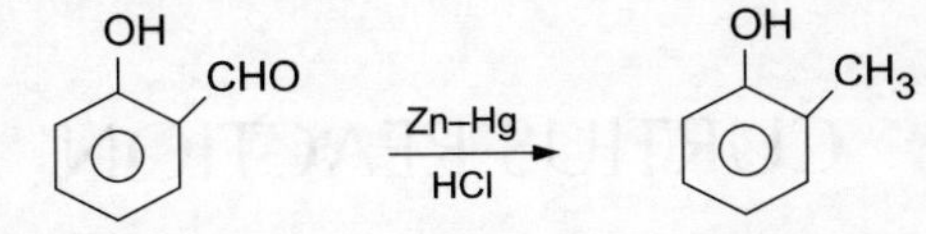

Salicylaldehyde → *o*-Cresol

4. Reduction of cyclic ketones

(a)

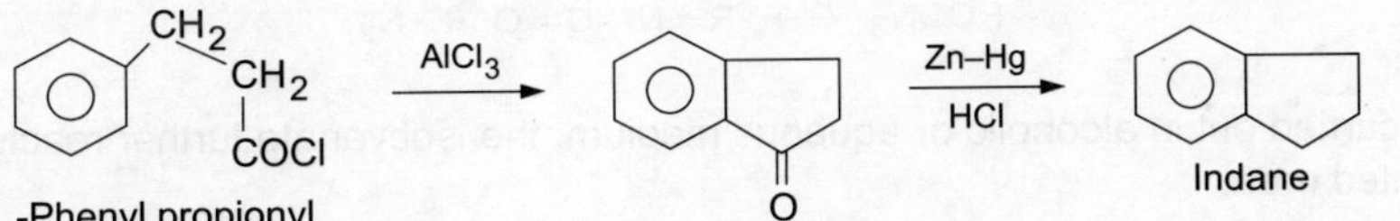

β-Phenyl propionyl chloride → α-Hydrindone → Indane

(b) In the synthesis of naphthalene

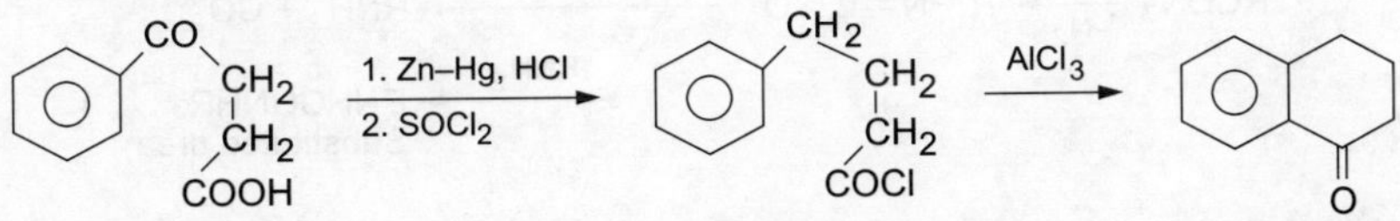

β-Benzoyl propionic acid → γ-Phenyl butanoyl chloride → α-Tetralone

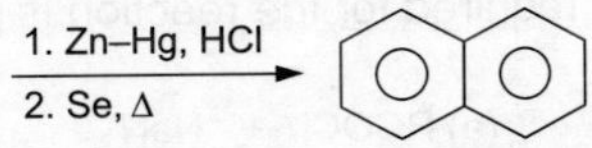

Naphthalene

5. Reduction with ring expansion

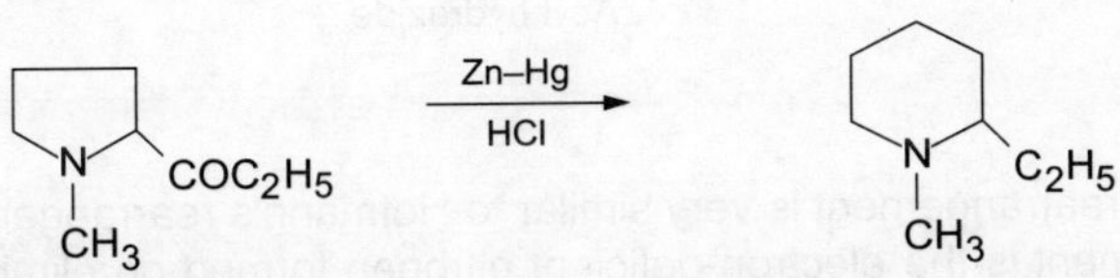

1-Methyl-2-propionyl pyrrolidine → 2-Ethyl-1-methylpiperidine

6. Reduction with ring contraction

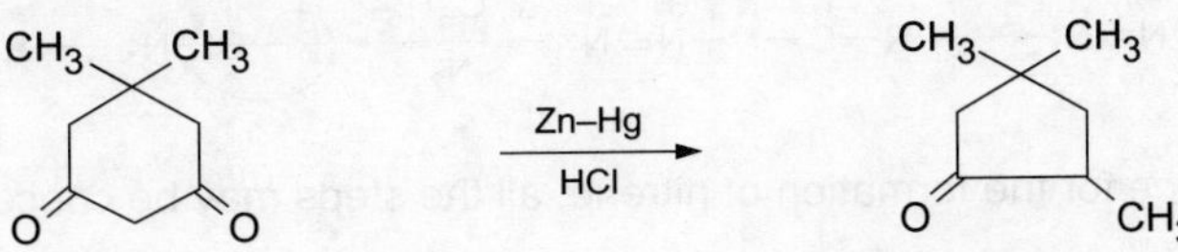

5, 5-Dimethyl cyclohexane-1, 3-dione → 2, 4, 4-Trimethyl cyclopentanone

7. Synthesis of cycloparaffins

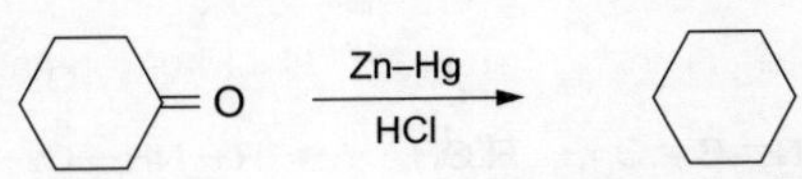

Cyclohexanone → Cyclohexane

CURTIUS REACTION

Curtius rearrangement involves the decomposition of acyl azides in an inert solvent (e.g., chloroform, benzene, etc.,) by gentle heat to isocyanate. Good yields of isocyanates have been obtained.

$$RCON_3 \xrightarrow{\Delta} R{-}N{=}C{=}O + N_2$$

If the reaction is carried out in alcoholic or aqueous medium, the isocyanate further reacts to form urethane, amine or substituted urea.

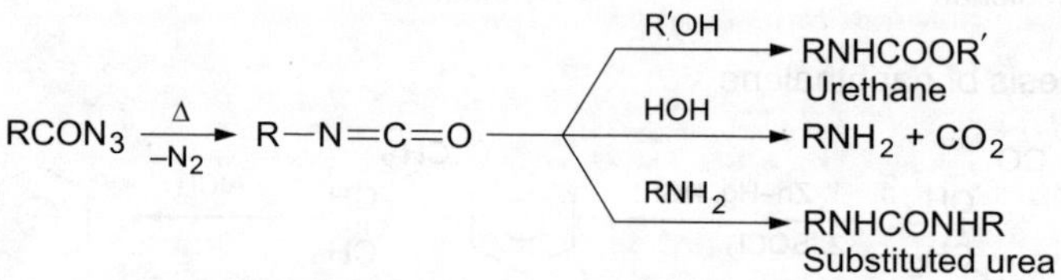

The conversion of acyl azides to isocyanates involves Curtius rearrangement while Curtius reaction involves the conversion of acids to amines, urethanes and substituted urea via Curtius rearrangement.

Acyl azide required for the reaction is prepared as below.

$$\text{(a) } \underset{\text{}}{RCOCl} + \underset{\text{Sodium azide}}{NaN_3} \longrightarrow \underset{\text{Acyl azide}}{RCON_3} + NaCl$$

$$\text{(b) } RCOOC_2H_5 \xrightarrow{NH_2NH_2} \underset{\text{Acyl hydrazide}}{RCONHNH_2} \xrightarrow{HNO_2} RCON_3 + 2H_2O$$

Mechanism

The mechanism of the rearrangement is very similar to Hofmann's rearrangement to isocyanate. The driving force of the rearrangement is the electron-deficient nitrogen formed on elimination of nitrogen molecule on heating.

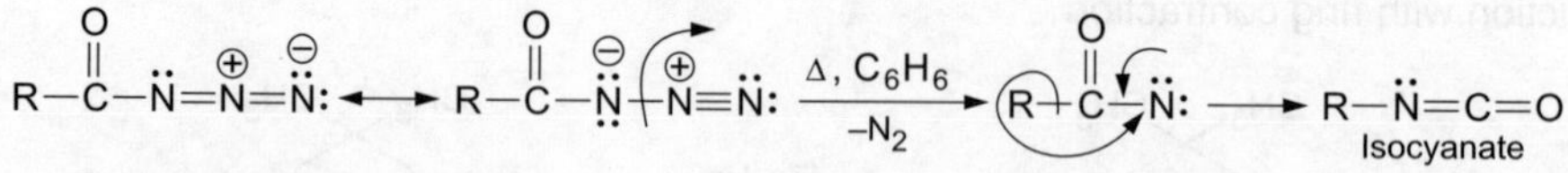

Since there is no evidence for the formation of nitrene, all the steps may be concerted.

Reactions of isocyanate

(a) With alcohols

$$R{-}N{=}C{=}O + R'OH \longrightarrow \underset{\text{Urethane}}{R{-}NH{-}\overset{O}{\overset{\|}{C}}{-}OR'}$$

(b) With water

$$R{-}N{=}C{=}O + HOH \longrightarrow R{-}NH{-}\overset{O}{\overset{\|}{C}}{-}OH \longrightarrow RNH_2 + CO_2$$

Carbamic acid

Unreacted isocyanate may further react with the amine to yield derivative of urea.

$$R{-}N{=}C{=}O + R'NH_2 \longrightarrow R{-}NH{-}\overset{O}{\overset{\|}{C}}{-}NHR'$$

Alkyl-substituted urea

The reaction is a general one and can be applied to aliphatic, aromatic, heterocyclic and unsaturated acids. These acids may contain different functional groups which remain unaffected.

Applications

This simple one-step and mild reaction affords an important and easy preparative method for primary amines, α-amino acids, aldehydes, urethanes, etc.

1. Preparation of primary amines—Primary amines, free from secondary and tertiary amines can be prepared, e.g.,

$$C_6H_5CH_2COOC_2H_5 \xrightarrow[2.\ HNO_2]{1.\ NH_2NH_2} C_6H_5CH_2CON_3 \xrightarrow[2.\ H_2O]{1.\ \Delta,\ C_6H_6} C_6H_5CH_2NH_2$$

Ethylphenyl acetate — Benzylamine

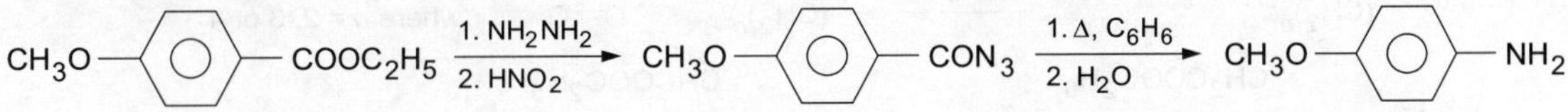

Ethyl anisate — *p*-Anisidine

Similarly, ethyl adipate gives tetramethylenediamine.

2. Preparation of α-amino acids

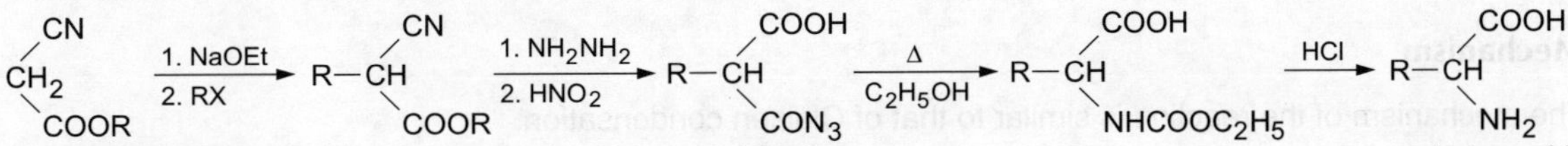

Cyanoacetic ester — Acyl azide — α-Amino acid

Many important α-amino acids may be conveniently prepared.

3. Preparation of aldehydes

$$CH_3CH(OH)COOH \xrightarrow[3.\ HNO_2]{1.\ C_2H_5OH,\ \overset{\oplus}{H}\quad 2.\ NH_2NH_2} CH_3CH(OH)CON_3 \xrightarrow[\Delta]{C_2H_5OH} CH_3CH(OH){-}NHCOOC_2H_5 \xrightarrow[(H_2O)]{NaOH}$$

Lactic acid

$$\left[CH_3{-}\overset{OH}{\overset{|}{C}H}{-}NH_2\right] \longrightarrow CH_3CHO + NH_3$$

Similarly, benzylmalonic acid gives phenylacetaldehyde.

$$\underset{\text{Benzylmalonic ester}}{C_6H_5CH_2CH(COOR)_2} \xrightarrow{NH_2NH_2} C_6H_5CH_2CH(CONHNH_2)_2 \xrightarrow{HNO_2} C_6H_5CH_2CH(CON_3)_2 \xrightarrow[\text{2. NaOH}]{\text{1. } C_2H_5OH}$$

$$C_6H_5CH_2CH(NH_2)_2 \xrightarrow{HNO_2} \left[C_6H_5CH_2CH(OH)_2\right] \xrightarrow{-H_2O} \underset{\text{Phenyl acetaldehyde}}{C_6H_5CH_2CHO}$$

4. Curtius reaction may be used for stepping down the acid series.

$$RCH_2COOH \xrightarrow[\overset{\oplus}{H}]{C_2H_5OH} RCH_2COOC_2H_5 \xrightarrow[\text{2. } HNO_2]{\text{1. } NH_2NH_2} RCH_2CON_3 \xrightarrow[\text{2. } H_2O]{\text{1. } \Delta,\ C_6H_6} RCH_2NH_2$$

$$\xrightarrow{HNO_2} RCH_2OH \xrightarrow{\text{oxdn.}} RCOOH$$

DIECKMANN REACTION

Intramolecular Claisen condensation in dibasicacid esters is called Dieckmann reaction. The resulting products are invariably cyclic β-ketone derivatives. The condensing bases may be sodium, sodium ethoxide, sodium hydride, potassium *t*-butoxide, etc.

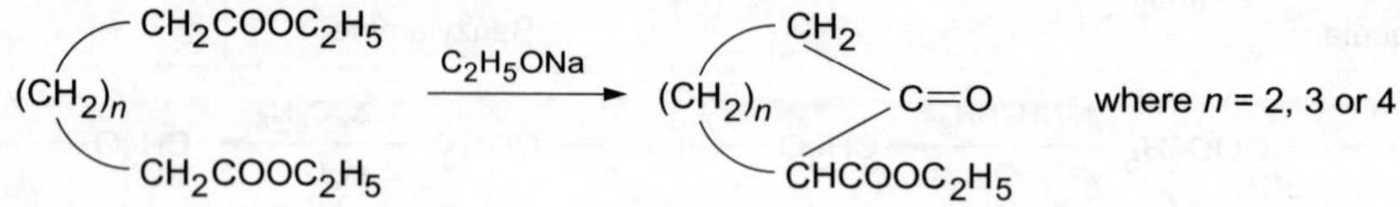

The reaction best proceeds with dibasicacid esters having 6, 7 or 8 carbon atoms which give stable rings with 5, 6, or 7 carbons. Yields for rings of 9 to 12 carbons are very low. High-dilution technique is used for the formation of large-size rings.

Mechanism

The mechanism of the reaction is similar to that of Claisen condensation.

The base abstracts a proton from one of the α-carbons. The resulting carbanion then attacks the carbonyl carbon of the other ester group. Subsequent expulsion of the alkoxide ion gives the cyclic ketone derivative.

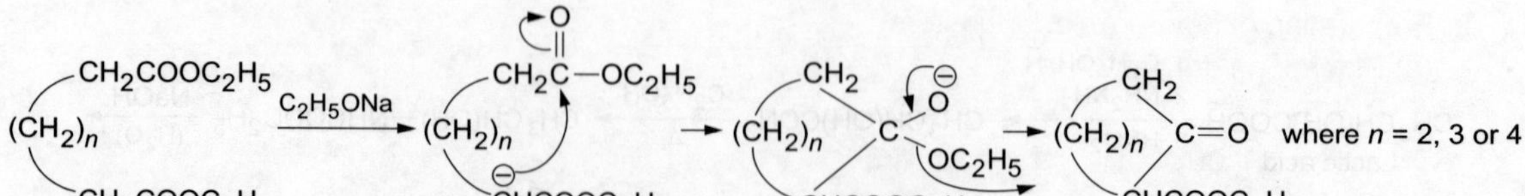

The compound on hydrolysis and decarboxylation gives cyclic ketone.

Esters of acids lower than adipic acid undergo more of intermolecular condensation with subsequent cyclisation. Thus, ethyl succinate gives cyclohexandione derivative. This may be due to reasons of stability of six-membered rings.

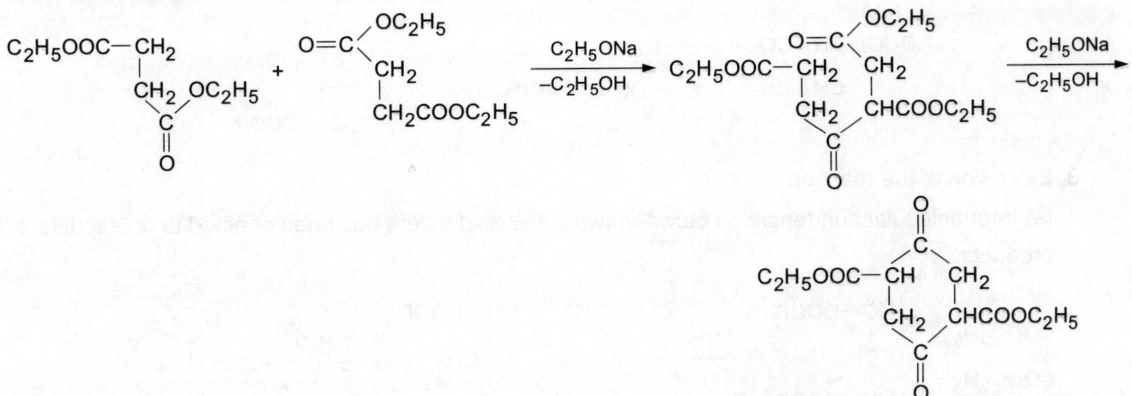

Cyclohexan-2, 5-dione-1, 4-dicarboxylic ester

Effect of experimental condition on the ring size has been observed in some compounds.

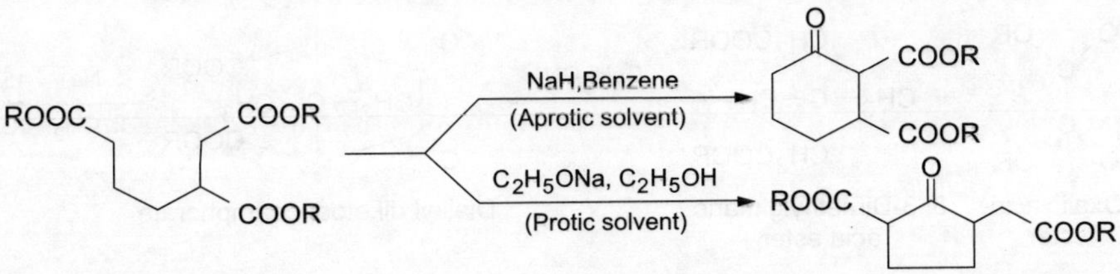

Applications and extension

The reaction affords a useful route for the synthesis of cyclopentanone and cyclohexanone derivatives. Some examples are given for illustration.

1. The reaction has been used to build up five- or six-membered rings in the synthesis of various natural products. The general process is given below.
   Synthesis of steroid

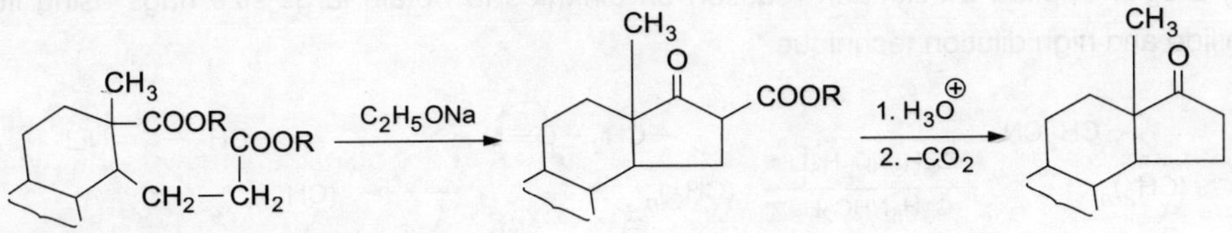

2. Preparation of heterocyclic ketoesters
   (a) Piperidone derivative

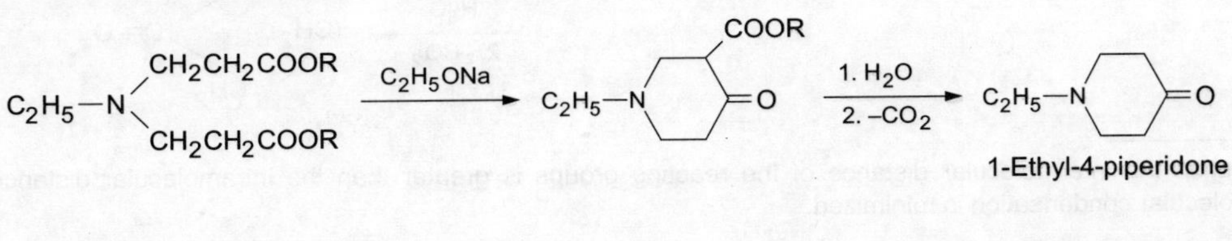

1-Ethyl-4-piperidone

(b) Thiophene derivatives—Depending on the conditions of the reaction, two isomers are obtained.

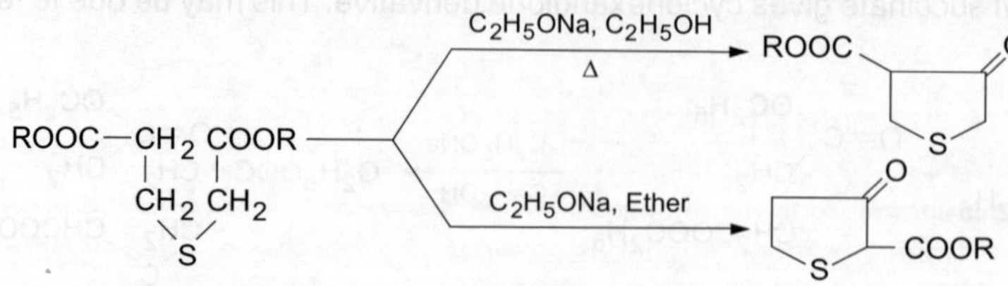

3. Extension of the reaction

(a) Intermolecular condensation between two lower acid esters has been effected to obtain different products.

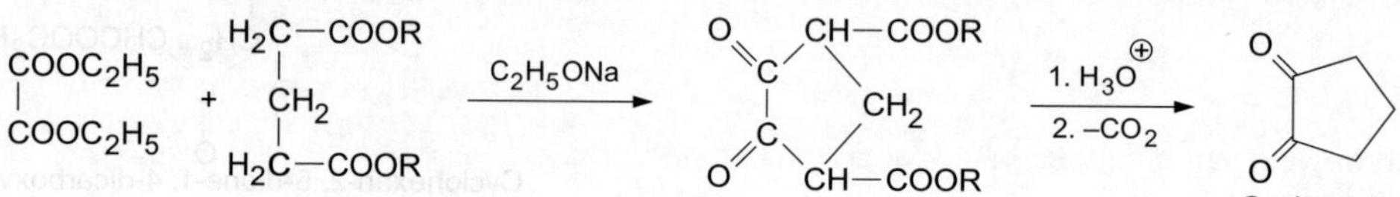

Cyclopentane-1,2-dione

Above synthesis was utilized for the synthesis of camphoric acid.

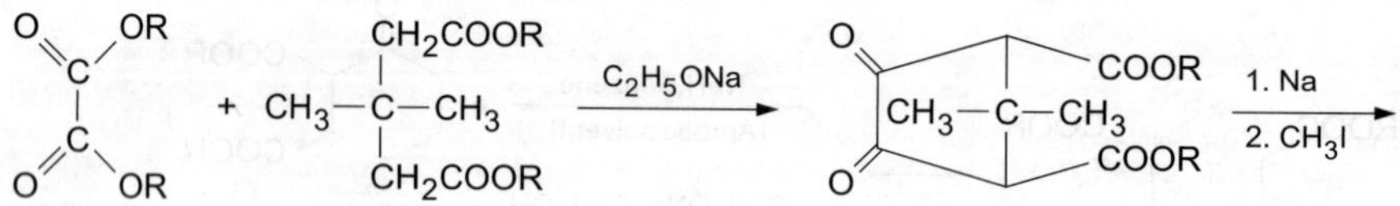

Oxalic acid ester 3, 3-Dimethylglutaric acid ester Dialkyl diketoapocamphorate

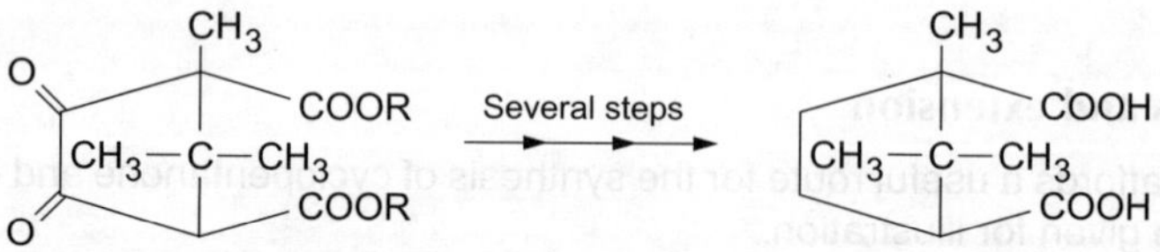

Dialkyl diketocamphorate Camphoric acid

This, incidentally, elucidates the structure of camphor.

(b) Ziegler applied Dieckmann reaction on dinitriles to obtain large-size rings using lithium ethyl anilide and high dilution technique.*

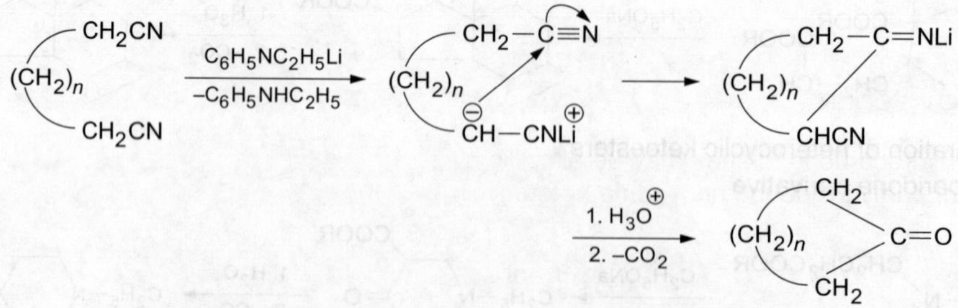

---

* On dilution the intermolecular distance of the reacting groups is greater than the intramolecular distance so that intermolecular condensation is minimized.

DIELS–ALDER REACTION

Diels–Alder reaction involves the 1, 4-addition of an alkene to a conjugated diene to form an adduct of six-membered ring. The double bond compound is called the dienophile. The reaction is initiated thermally or by Lewis acid catalyst with or without the use of solvents.

Ethylene and simple olefins give poor yields even at high temperature.

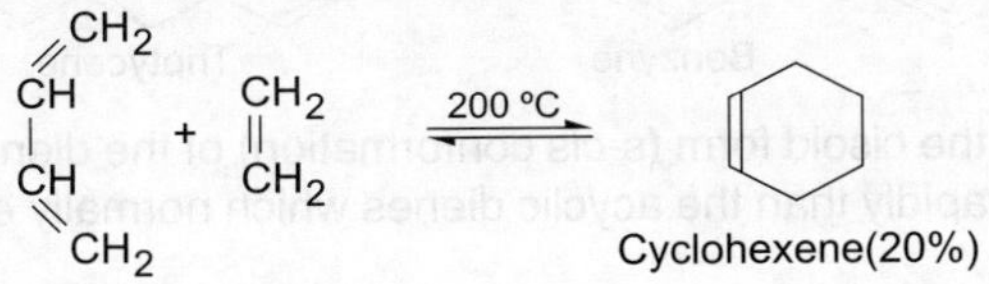

Electron-withdrawing substituents in the dienophile, such as $>C=O$, $-CHO$, $-COOR$, $-CN$, $-NO_2$, etc., promote the reaction.

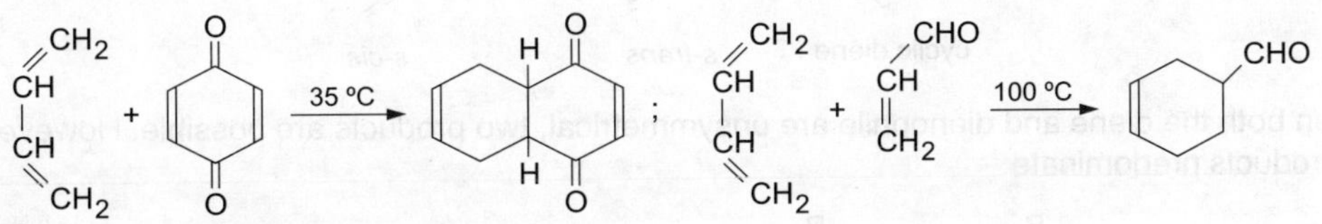

The reaction rate is also accelerated by the presence of electron-releasing groups in the dienes. Thus, the reaction between 2-methyl-1, 3-butadiene (isoprene) and acraldehyde is faster than that between 1, 3-butadiene and acraldehyde.

Triple bond compounds, allenes and benzyne may also function as dienophiles

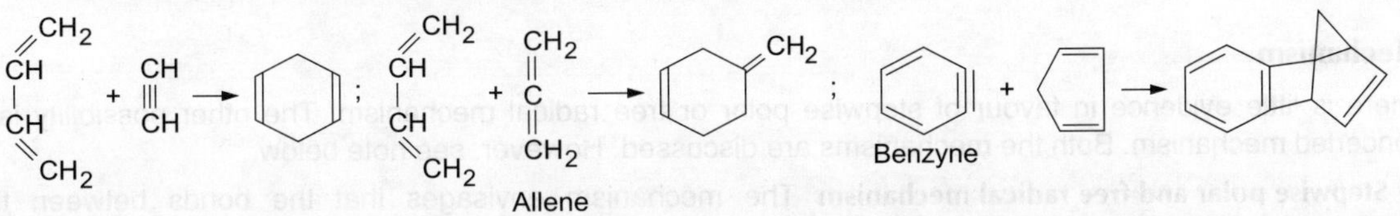

Since the reaction involves uniting of π orbitals, all carbon skeleton is not necessary in the dienophile, e.g.,

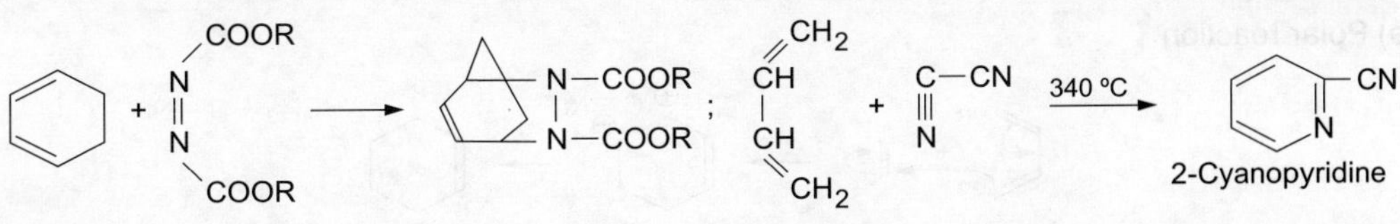

Besides acylic hydrocarbons, dienes may be alicyclic hydrocarbons, in which the conjugated double bonds may be wholly or partly inside the ring, some heterocyclic and some aromatic hydrocarbons.

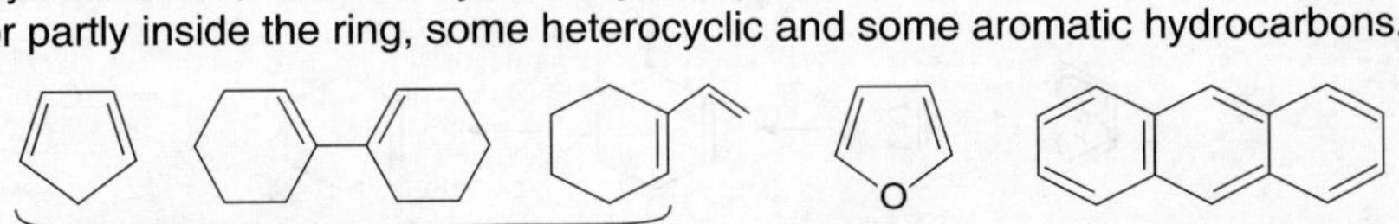

Alicyclic Heterocyclic Aromatic

Benzene, naphthalene and phenanthrene are quite unreactive but anthracene responds readily.

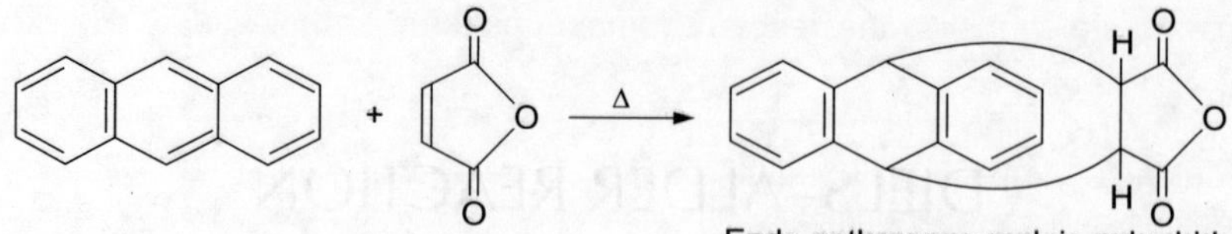

Endo anthracene maleic anhydride

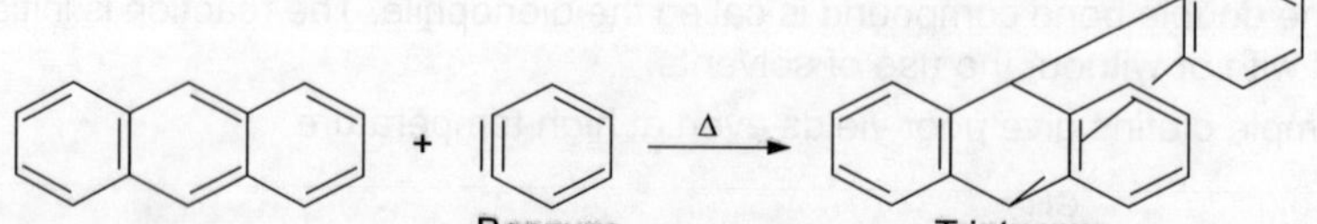

Benzyne Triptycene

The reaction occurs with the cisoid form (s-cis conformation) of the diene. Cyclic dienes are naturally in cisoid form and so react more rapidly than the acyclic dienes which normally exist in the more stable transoid forms (*s*-trans conformation).

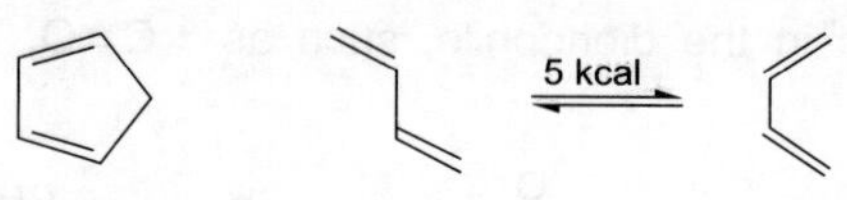

cyclic diene *s-trans* *s-cis*

When both the diene and dienophile are unsymmetrical, two products are possible. However, the 1, 2- and 1, 4-products predominate.

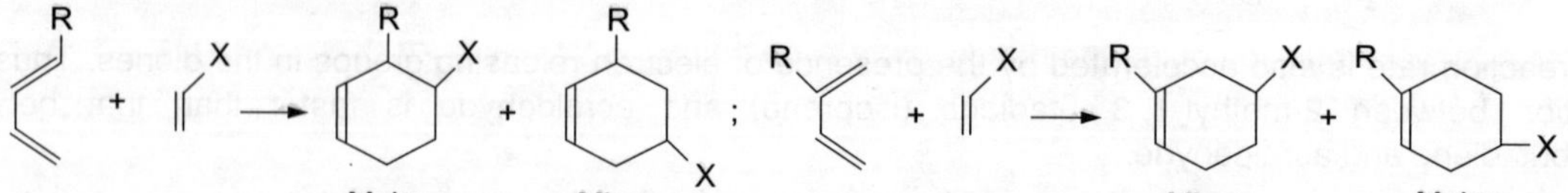

Major Minor Minor Major

Mechanism

There is little evidence in favour of stepwise polar or free radical mechanism. The other possibility is a concerted mechanism. Both the mechanisms are discussed. However, see note below.

(i) Stepwise polar and free radical mechanism The mechanism envisages that the bonds between the reactants are formed consecutively, i.e., one bond is formed followed by the other. The first bond gives a diion (a) or a diradical (b) which then forms the second bond.

(a) Polar reaction

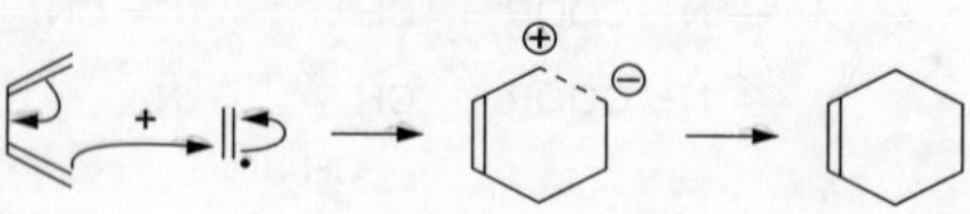

(b) Free radical reaction

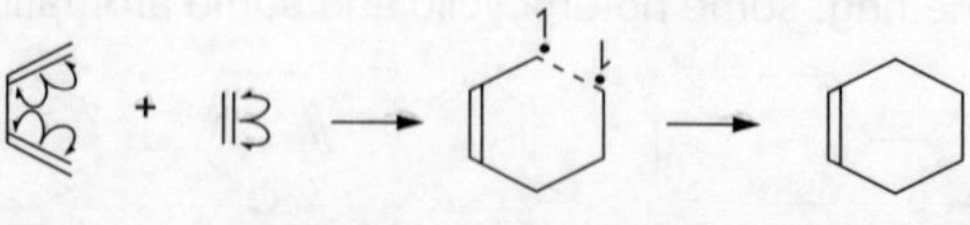

The mechanism assumes that the second bond is formed more rapidly than the rotation about the C – C bond, as otherwise a mixture of *cis* and *trans* products (nonstereospecific) would be obtained with substituted reactants, which is contrary to observation. The reaction is strictly stereospecific. The orientation of the groups (i.e., *cis* or *trans*) in the reactant remain unaltered in the product. Hence the mechanism is not favourable.

(ii) Concerted mechanism The mechanism visualises a process in which there is simultaneous (not consecutive) breaking and making of bonds through a six-centred transition state with no intermediate. It is a $4\pi + 2\pi$ cycloaddition and stereospecifically cis with respect to both reactants.

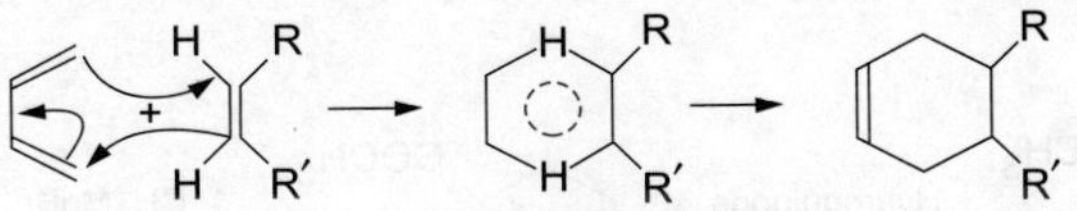

Transition state

The addition of the dienophile is always cis so that the groups cis in the olefin remain cis in the adduct. The addition is therefore stereospecific.

There are two possible modes of addition, (a) exo and (b) endo. When the greater part of the dienophile is under the diene ring in the adduct, it is called endo and in the reverse case, it is called exo. The endo adduct is more stable.

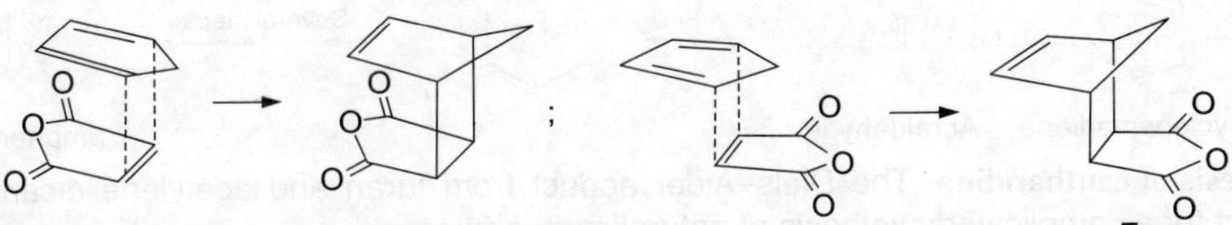
Endo ; Exo

This is because the cyclic transition state has further stabilization through secondary π-orbital overlaps for greater accumulation of double bonds in the endo adduct.

Applications

The reaction has proved of great value. Due to its high stereospecific nature, the reaction has been used to synthesize many natural products which otherwise would be difficult to prepare. The reaction can be used as a diagnostic test for conjugation in a system. Since the reaction is stereospecific, the configurations of the reactants can be determined by studying the adduct. The reaction has also been used to trap benzyne intermediate. Some reactions are given to illustrate its use.

1. Determination of configuration Maleic and fumaric acids can be identified from the products.

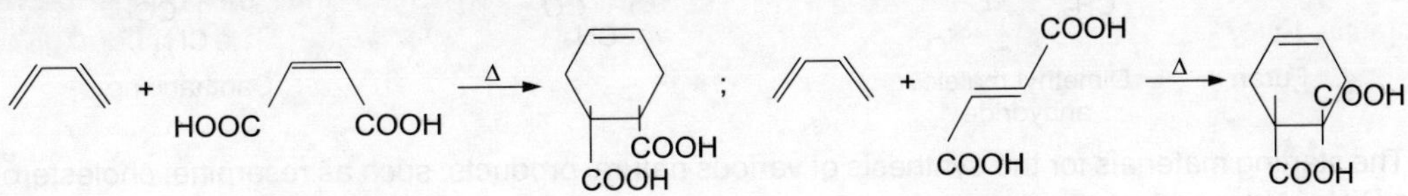

Maleic acid; *Cis*; Fumaric acid; *Trans*

2. Synthesis of quinones and polynuclear hydrocarbons

(i)

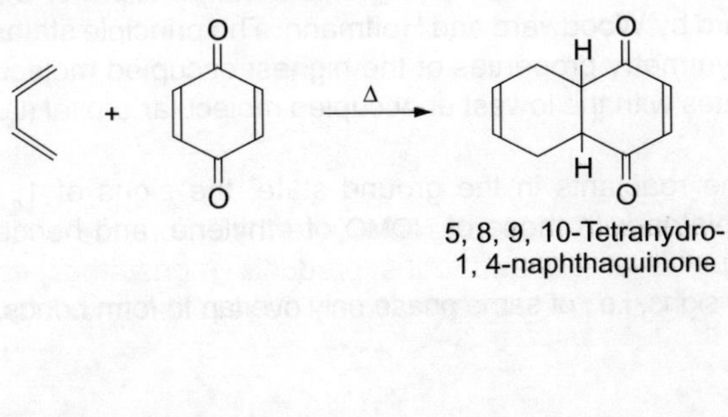

5, 8, 9, 10-Tetrahydro-1, 4-naphthaquinone

(ii) 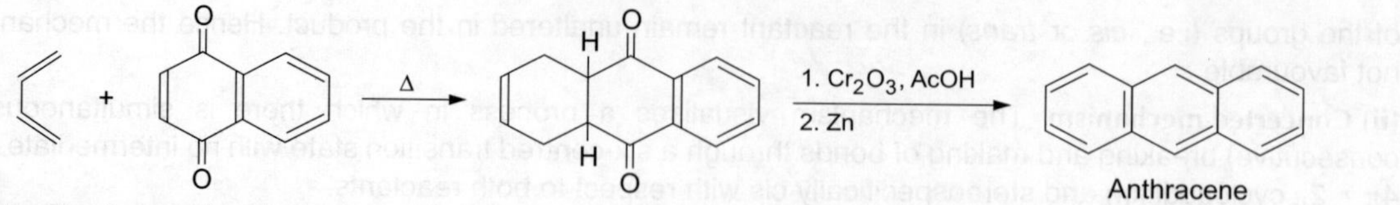

3. Synthesis of α-terpineol

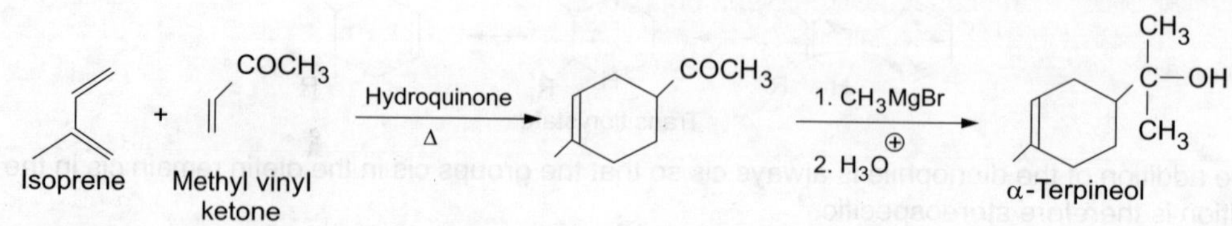

4. In the synthesis of camphene The intermediate required in the synthesis of camphene is prepared by Diels–Alder reaction.

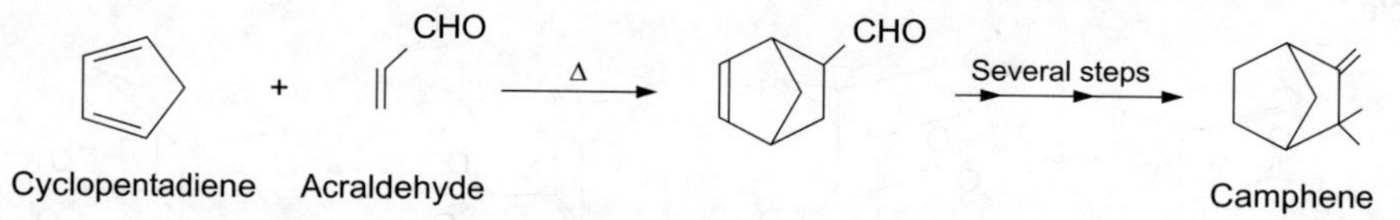

5. In the synthesis of cantharidine The Diels–Alder adduct from furan and acetylene dicarboxylate is the starting product for a complicated synthesis of natural cantharidine.

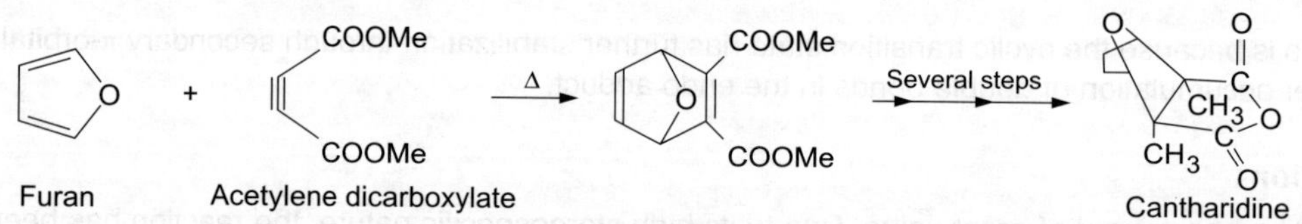

The Diels–Alder adduct obtained from furan and dimethylmaleic anhydride on hydrogenation gives cantharidine which is not the same as the natural product.

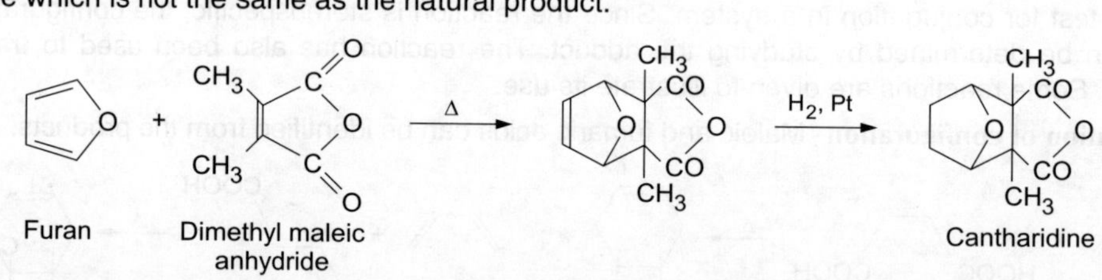

The starting materials for the synthesis of various natural products, such as reserpine, cholesterol, etc., are the Diels–Alder adducts.

Note The concerted cycloaddition is best explained from the principle of *Conservation of Orbital Symmetry* put forward by Woodward and Hoffmann. The principle states that cycloaddition is allowed when the symmetry properties of the highest occupied molecular orbital (HOMO) of one reactant correlates with the lowest unoccupied molecular orbital (LUMO) of the other and vice versa.

It is seen that in the reactants in the ground state, the signs of 1, 4-lobes of LUMO for 1, 3-butadiene correlates with those of HOMO of ethylene, and hence the addition occurs smoothly on heating.

(Orbitals of the same signs, i.e., of same phase only overlap to form bonds.)

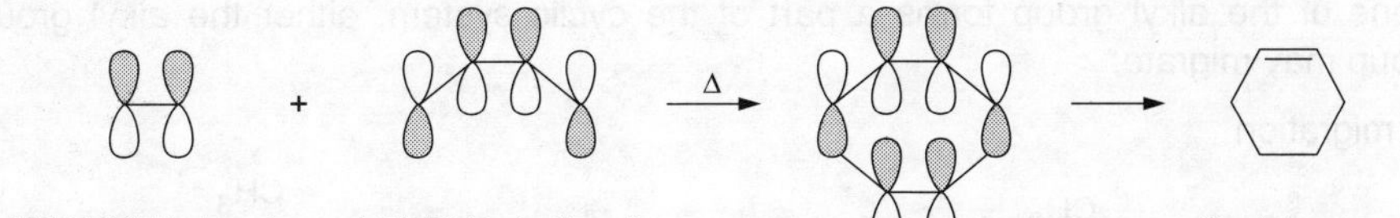

Similar correlation is observed between butadiene HOMO and ethylene LUMO.

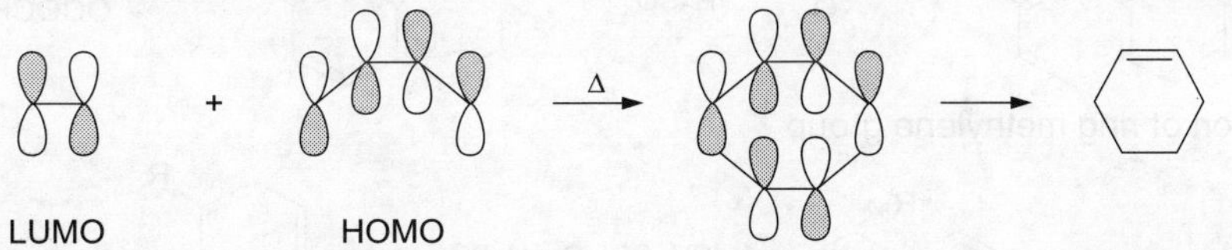

The stereospecificity (i.e., cis-addition) is thus explained.

DIENONE–PHENOL REARRANGEMENT

When 4, 4-dialkyl cyclohexadienone is treated with acid, it is converted to phenol with migration of one of the alkyl groups to the adjacent carbon. This is known as dienone–phenol rearrangement. The dienone is dissolved in acetic anhydride and treated with catalytic amount of sulphuric acid. The product on hydrolysis gives the phenol.

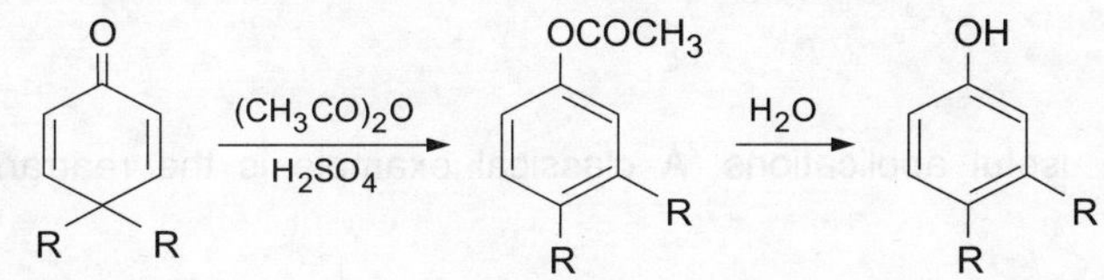

Mechanism

On protonation of the oxygen, a carbocation is generated which is stabilised by delocalization of the positive charge.

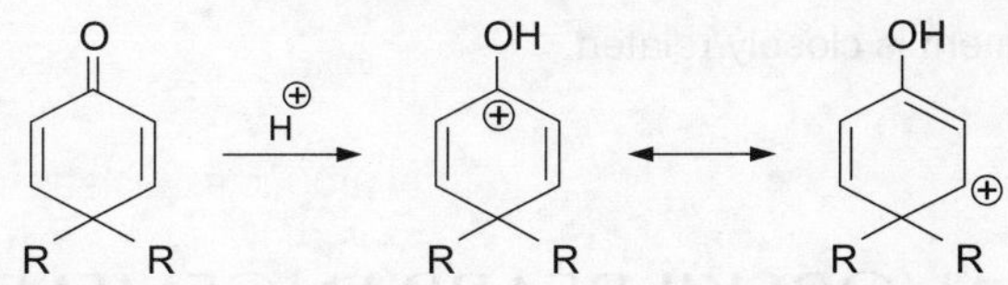

In one of the canonical structures, the positive charge is on a carbon adjacent to a highly substituted carbon. Hence, a carbocation rearrangement occurs. Subsequent loss of a proton gives the 3, 4-disubstituted phenol.

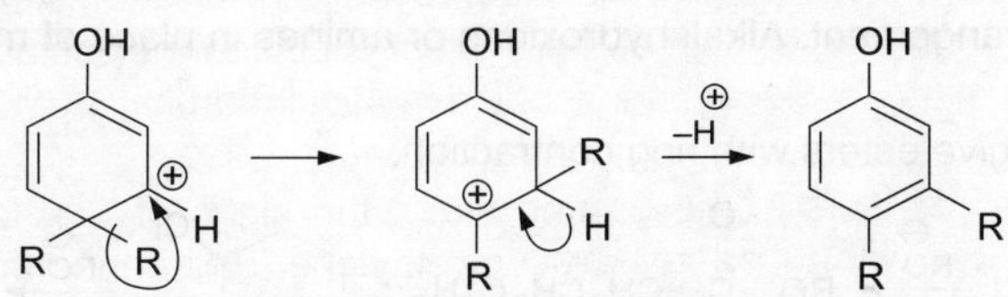

The ease of dienone-phenol rearrangement is due to the creation of a stable aromatic system.

When one of the alkyl group forms a part of the cyclic system, either the alkyl group or the ring methylene group may migrate.

(i) Alkyl migration

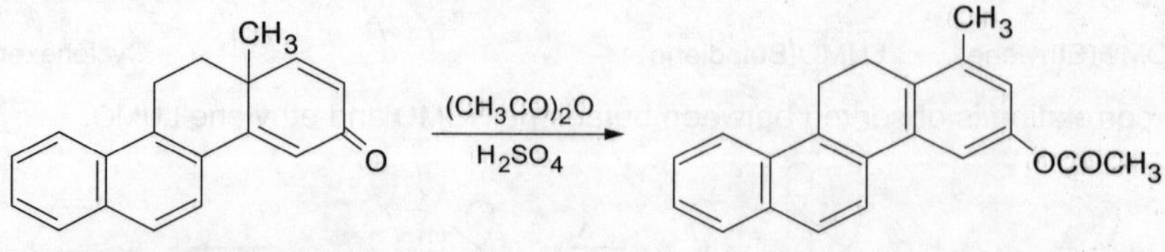

(ii) Migration of ring methylene group

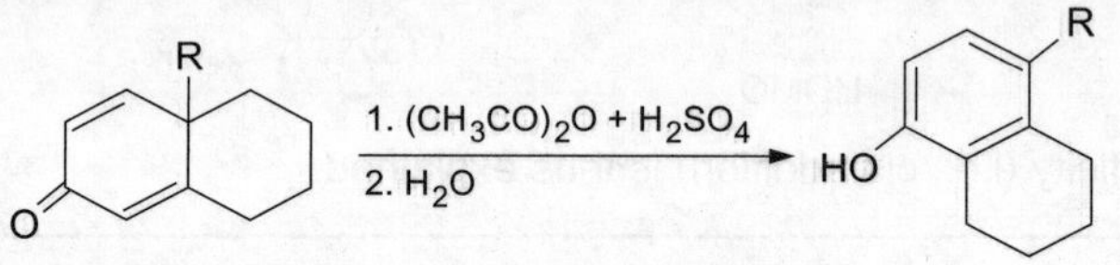

The course of the reaction depends on the structural or electronic factors and on the conditions of reaction.

A reverse rearrangement, i.e., phenol–dienone rearrangement has been observed during the electrophilic substitution in phenols in some cases.

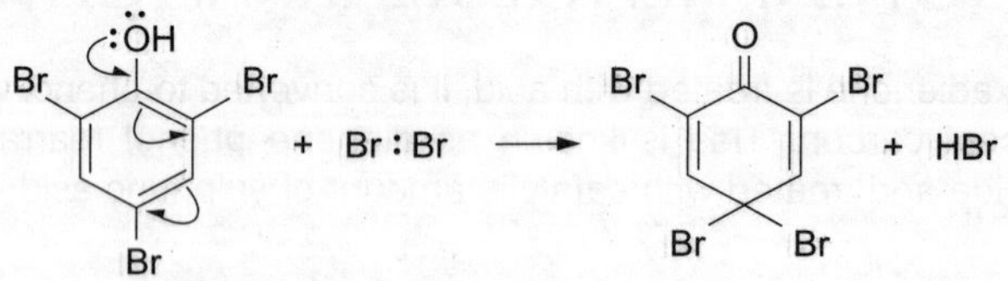

Applications

The rearrangement has useful applications. A classical example is the rearrangement of santonin to desmotropo santonin.

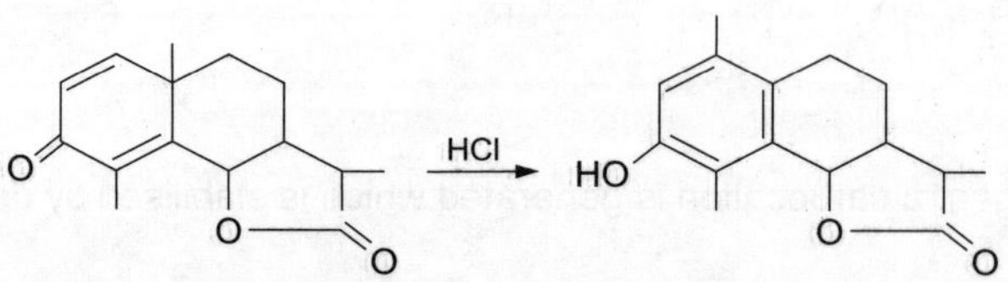

The anthrasteroid rearrangement is closely related.

FAVORSKII REARRANGEMENT

The transformation of α-haloketones to esters with rearranged carbon skeleton by the treatment with alkoxide ions is called Favorskii rearrangement. Alkali hydroxides or amines in place of metal alkoxides give acids or amides respectively.

Cyclic α-haloketones give esters with ring contraction.

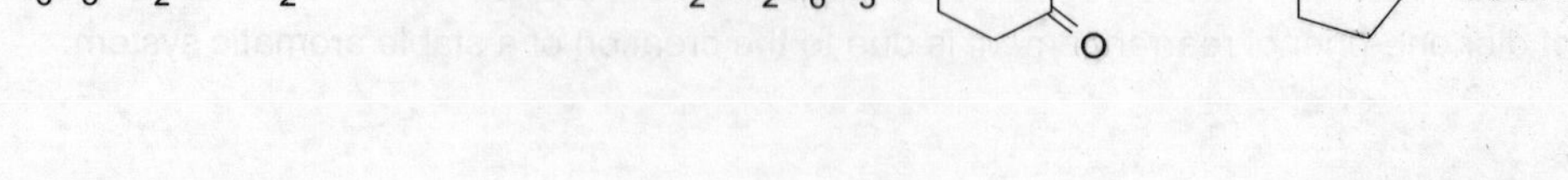

Mechanism

The mechanism of the rearrangement has been the subject of much investigation.

It was observed that both the isomeric ketones, (I) and (II) gave β-phenylpropionic acid on treatment with hydroxide ions.

$$\underset{\text{(I)}}{C_6H_5CH_2-\overset{\overset{\displaystyle O}{\|}}{C}-CH_2Cl} \xrightarrow{\overset{\ominus}{O}H} C_6H_5CH_2CH_2COOH \xleftarrow{\overset{\ominus}{O}H} \underset{\text{(II)}}{C_6H_5CH(Cl)-\overset{\overset{\displaystyle O}{\|}}{C}-CH_3}$$

This observation indicates that the chlorine is not being directly replaced by the incoming group from the other side of the carbonyl group, as otherwise (II) would give $C_6H_5CH(CH_3)COOH$ which is not obtained. Further, it was observed that a cyclic ketone (2-chlorocyclohexanone) with labelled carbon bearing the chlorine atom, on treatment with alkoxide ion gave a product in which equal amounts of ^{14}C were present at the α-carbon and at the β-carbon. This suggests a symmetrical cyclopropanone intermediate which opens up with equal ease on either side of the carbonyl group.

On the basis of the above observations, the following mechanism has been suggested.

The base abstracts an α-hydrogen to produce a carbanion. Intramolecular nucleophilic attack on the carbon bearing the chlorine displaces the chlorine atom with the formation of a transient symmetrical cyclopropanone ring. Subsequent attack of the alkoxide ion on the carbonyl carbon opens the ring with equal ease on either side of the carbonyl carbon so that the product contains 50% of ^{14}C at the α-position and 50% at the β-position.

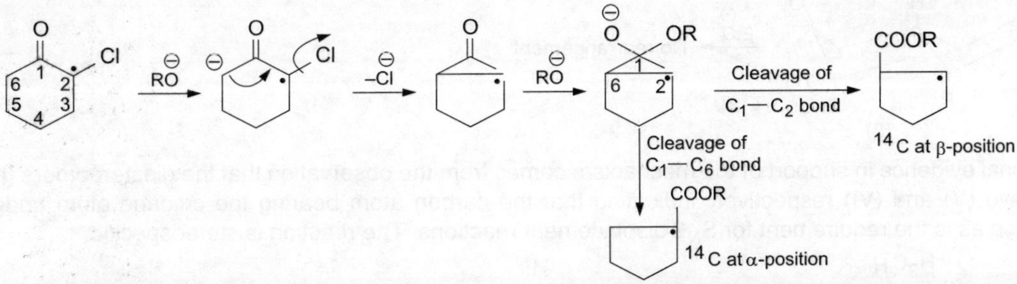

In case of unsymmetrical ketones, the unsymmetrical cyclopropanone ring which is formed, opens up to give the most stable carbanion. Thus, the two isomeric ketones (I) and (II) give the same cyclic intermediate (III) which may open on either side of the carbonyl group to give two carbanions (IV) and (V).

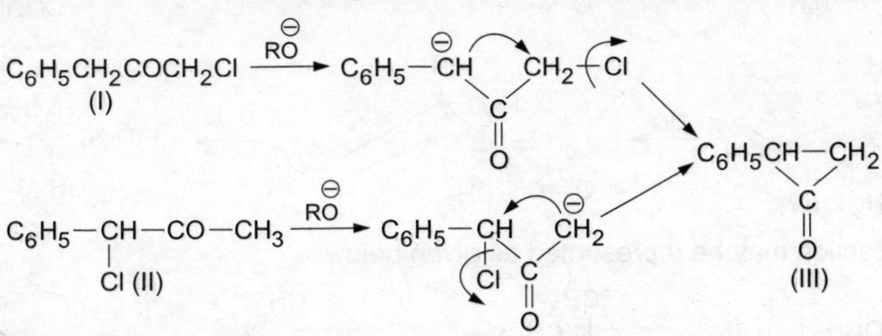

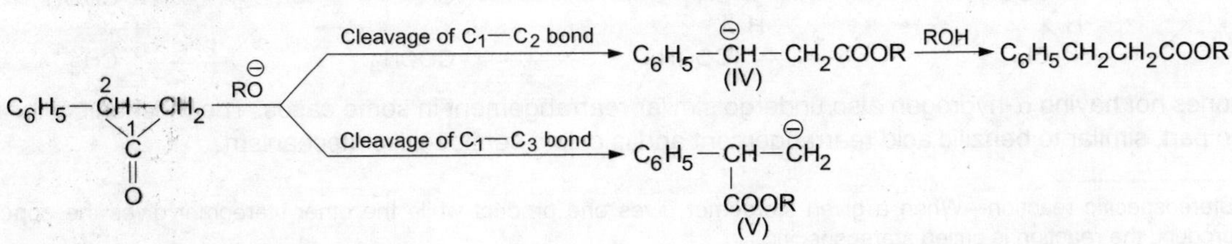

The carbanion (IV) being reasonance-stabilized is preferentially formed so that the product is $C_6H_5CH_2CH_2COOR$. Hence, both (I) and (II) give the same product.

Although the cyclopropanone intermediate has not been isolated, it has been trapped to give an adduct with furan in one case at least.

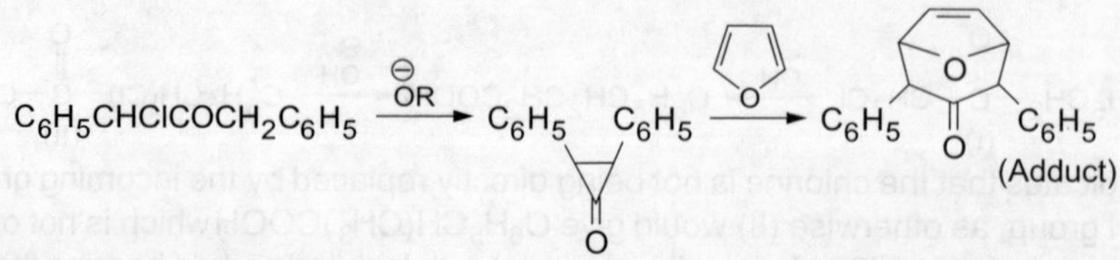

The formation of cyclopropanone intermediate probably proceeds via an intramolecular 1,3-elimination involving a backside attack of the carbanion. Thus, in nonpolar media the cyclic α-haloketone (I) with equatorial halogen underwent rearrangement but (II) with axial halogen did not, since the backside attack is restricted. (Stork and Borowitz)

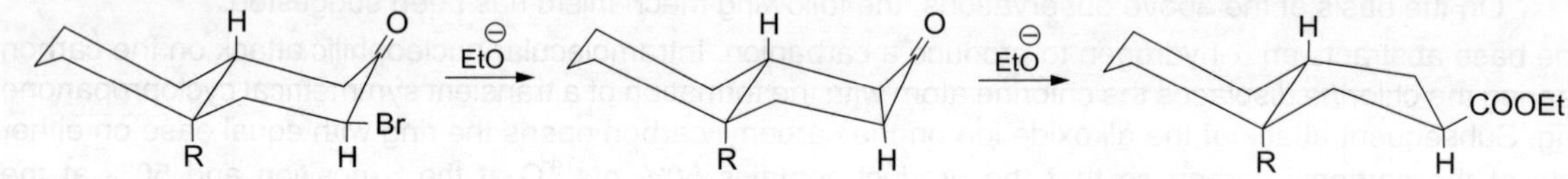

(I)

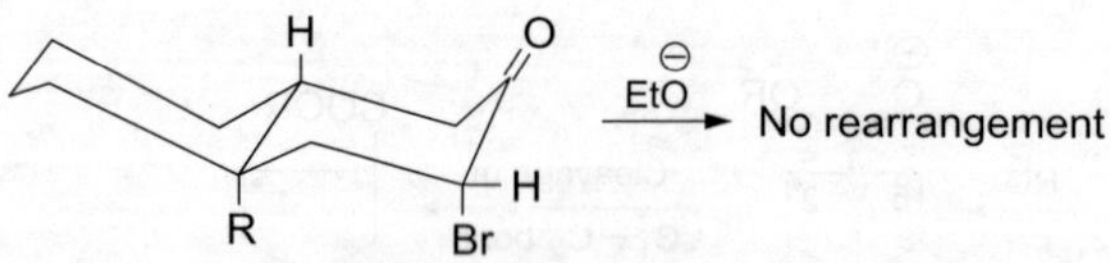

(II)

Additional evidence in support of the mechanism comes from the observation that the diastereomers (III) and (IV) gave (V) and (VI) respectively indicating that the carbon atom bearing the chlorine atom underwent inversion as is the requirement for S_N2 displacement reactions. The reaction is stereospecific.*

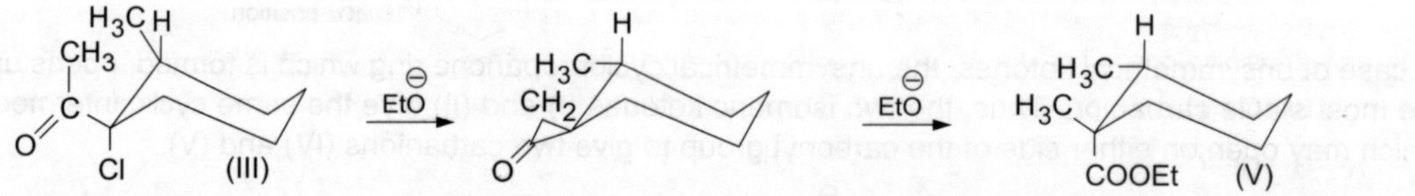

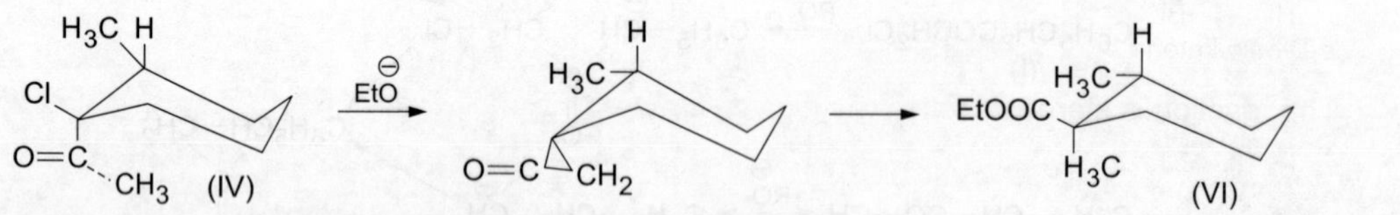

For simplicity, this reaction may be represented as given below

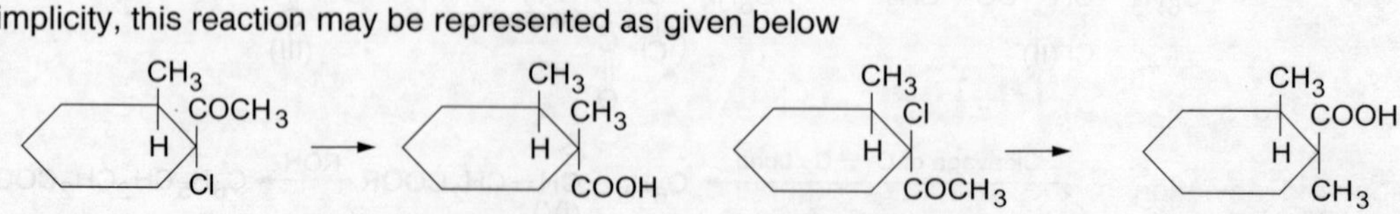

Ketones not having α-hydrogen also undergo similar rearrangement in some cases. The mechanism for this is, in part, similar to benzilic acid rearrangement and is called semibenzilic mechanism.

---

* Stereospecific reaction—When a given stereomer gives one product while the other stereomer gives the opposite product, the reaction is called stereospecific.

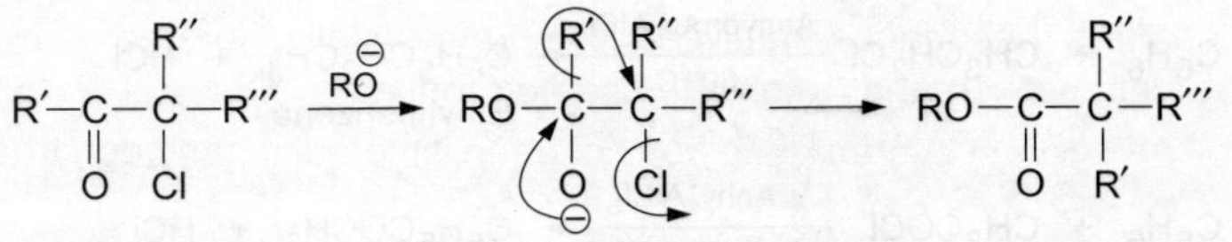

Even when there is a suitably placed α-hydrogen, the rearrangements may follow semibenzilic pattern in some compounds.

Thus, 2-bromocyclobutanone undergoes Favorskii rearrangement when treated with water as the base. When treated with D_2O, no deuterium is incorporated in the ring.

Cyclopropanone intermediate mechanism suggests incorporation of deuterium in the ring.

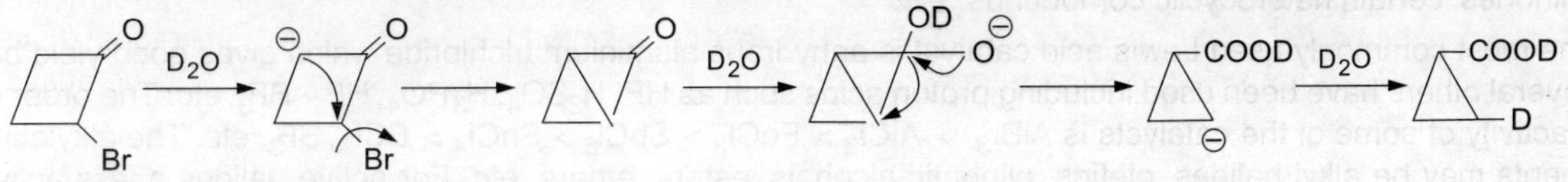

However, semibenzilic mechanism can explain the formation of the actual product without deuterium in the ring.

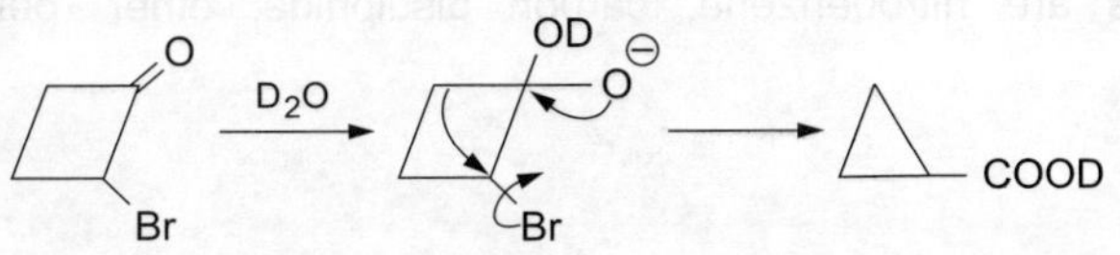

Probably, the strain in the bicyclobutanone ring restricts the operation of cyclopropanone mechanism.

Favorskii rearrangement of $\alpha_1\alpha$ (gem) and $\alpha\alpha'$ (vic) dihaloketones produce α,β-unsaturated esters.

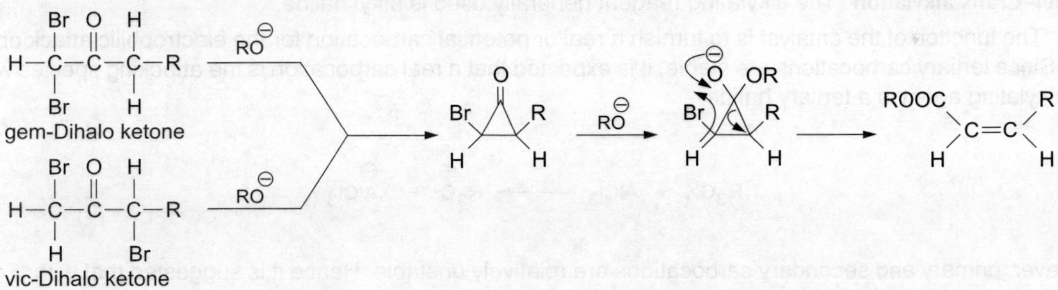

The reaction is stereoselective* as it gives *cis* olefin.

FRIEDEL–CRAFTS REACTION

Alkylation and acylation of the aromatic compounds with alkyl halides and acid halides or anhydrides respectively in the presence of a metal halide (Lewis acid) catalyst, usually aluminium chloride, is known as Friedel–Crafts reaction.

---

* Stereoselective reaction—Any reaction in which one of the stereomers is formed completely or predominantly is called a stereoselective.

Conclusion—A reaction on an optically inactive compound can be stereoselective but cannot be stereospecific.

$$C_6H_6 + CH_3CH_2Cl \xrightarrow[80\,°C]{\text{Anhydrous } AlCl_3} \underset{\text{Ethyl benzene}}{C_6H_5CH_2CH_3} + HCl$$

$$C_6H_6 + CH_3COCl \xrightarrow[C_6H_5NO_2]{\text{Anhy. } AlCl_3} \underset{\text{Acetophenone}}{C_6H_5COCH_3} + HCl$$

$$C_6H_6 + (CH_3CO)_2O \xrightarrow{\text{Anhy. } AlCl_3} C_6H_5COCH_3 + CH_3COOH$$

The aromatic compounds may be hydrocarbons, aryl halides, polyhydric phenols, amines, aldehydes, quinones, certain heterocyclic compounds, etc.

The most commonly used Lewis acid catalyst is anhydrous aluminium trichloride which gives good yield but several others have been used including proton acids such as HF, H_2SO_4, H_3PO_4, HF – BF_3, etc. The order of reactivity of some of the catalysts is $AlBr_3 > AlCl_3 > FeCl_3 > SbCl_5 > SnCl_4 > BCl_3, BF_3$, etc. The alkylating agents may be alkyl halides, olefins, aliphatic alcohols, esters, ethers, etc. For active halides a less active catalyst (e.g., $ZnCl_2$) and for unreactive halides a strong catalyst (e.g., $AlCl_3$) are used. The acylating agents employed are acid chlorides and acid anhydrides (open or cyclic).

Commonly used solvents are nitrobenzene, carbon disulphide, ether, petroleum ether, methylene chloride, etc.

Mechanism

The mechanism of the reaction is not clearly understood. The mechanisms of alkylation and acylation will be separately discussed.

Friedel–Crafts alkylation The alkylating reagent generally used is alkyl halide.

The function of the catalyst is to furnish a real or potential carbocation for the electrophilic attack on the ring. Since tertiary carbocations are stable, it is expected that a real carbocation is the attacking species when the alkylating agent is a tertiary halide.

$$R_3CX + AlCl_3 \longrightarrow R_3\overset{\oplus}{C} + X\overset{\ominus}{Al}Cl_3$$

However, primary and secondary carbocations are relatively unstable. Hence it is suggested that with 1° or 2° halides, a polarized complex with a potential carbocation is the attacking species.

$$CH_3Cl + AlCl_3 \longrightarrow \overset{\delta+}{CH_3}\cdots Cl \cdots \overset{\delta-}{AlCl_3} \text{ (Polarized complex)}$$

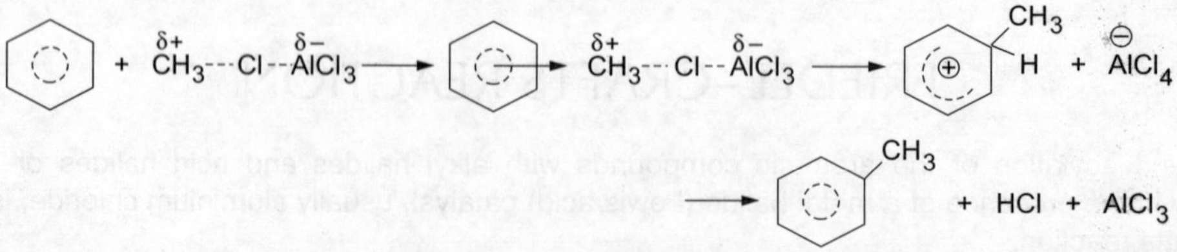

It is, however, not certain whether a polarized complex or a free carbocation attacks. For example, *n*-propyl chloride reacts with benzene to form both *n*-propyl benzene and isopropyl benzene. This indicates that an *n*-propyl carbocation is first formed which may then either attack the benzene ring or rearrange by 1, 2-hydride shift to form a greater stable isopropyl carbocation (2°) before attack. Thus,

$$CH_3CH_2CH_2Cl \xrightleftharpoons{AlCl_3} CH_3CH_2\overset{\oplus}{C}H_2\overset{\ominus}{AlCl_4}$$

$$CH_3CH_2\overset{\oplus}{C}H_2\overset{\ominus}{AlCl_4} \xrightarrow{C_6H_6} C_6H_5CH_2CH_2CH_3 + HCl + AlCl_3$$

$$CH_3CH_2\overset{\oplus}{C}H_2\overset{\ominus}{AlCl_4} \longrightarrow CH_3-\overset{\oplus}{C}H-CH_3 \xrightarrow{C_6H_6} C_6H_5CH(CH_3)_2 + HCl + AlCl_3$$

Besides alkyl halides, the alkylating agents may be aliphatic alcohols, alkenes, ethers and esters also. These in the presence of acidic catalysts, such as H_2SO_4, H_3PO_4, HF, HF – BF_3, etc., afford carbocations for the electrophilic attack on the ring.

$$\text{(i)}\ CH_3-CH{=}CH_2 \xrightarrow[\overset{\oplus}{(H)}]{H_3PO_4} CH_3-\overset{\oplus}{C}H-CH_3 \xrightarrow{C_6H_6} \underset{\text{Cumene}}{C_6H_5CH(CH_3)_2}$$

$$\text{(ii)}\ CH_3CH(OH)CH_3 \xrightarrow[-H_2O]{H_2SO_4} CH_3-\overset{\oplus}{C}H-CH_3 \xrightarrow{C_6H_6} \underset{\text{Cumene}}{C_6H_5-CH(CH_3)_2}$$

$$\text{(iii)}\ CH_2{=}CH_2 \xrightarrow[\overset{\oplus}{(H)}]{H_3PO_4} \overset{\oplus}{C}H_2-CH_3 \xrightarrow{C_6H_6} \underset{\text{Ethyl benzene}}{C_6H_5CH_2CH_3}$$

For alkyl halides the reactivity order is F > Cl > Br > I. Hence, $FCH_2CH_2CH_2Cl$ reacts with benzene to give $C_6H_5CH_2CH_2CH_2Cl$ in the presence of BF_3. Benzene rings with substituted haloalkyl groups have important synthetic applications (see applications).

Limitations

(a) Polyalkylation Since the alkyl groups are activating, di- and poly-alkylations are generally observed. To minimize polyalkylation, a large excess of the aromatic compound may be used.

(b) Rearrangement Alkylation is frequently accompanied by rearrangement of the entering group.

(c) Isomerization In the presence of excess catalyst and at high temperature, isomerization and disproportionation result.

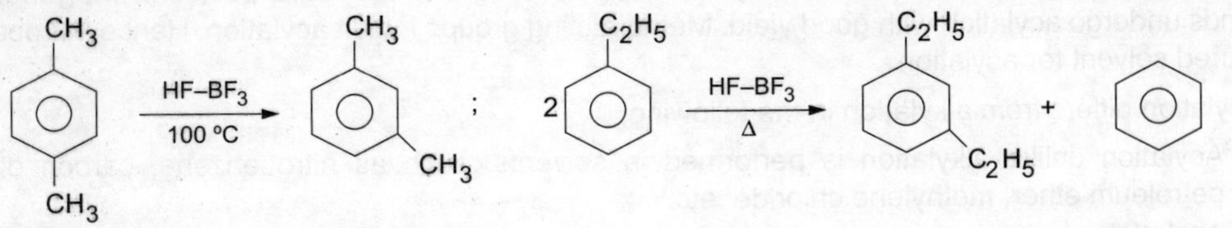

p-Xylene *m*-Xylene

(d) Effect on the reactivity of the substrates Electron-withdrawing groups inhibit the reaction while activating groups, such as OH, OR, NH_2, etc., react with the catalyst to retard the reaction. Naphthalene and heterocyclic compounds are very reactive and react with the catalyst. Naphthalene gives poor yield and heterocyclic compounds are not alkylated.

Friedel–Crafts acylation

The acylating reagents are acid chlorides or acid anhydrides. Depending on conditions probably two mechanisms operate.

(i) Generation of the attacking species which may be a free acyl cation or an ion pair

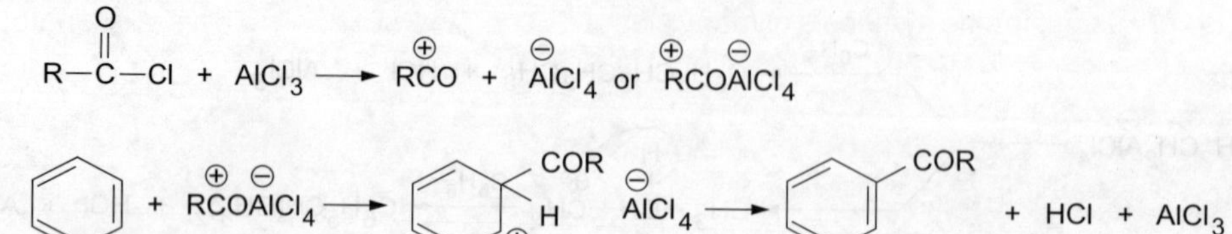

With sterically hindered acyl halides the attacking species may be the acyl cation.

(ii) Generation of 1 : 1 complex for the electrophilic attack

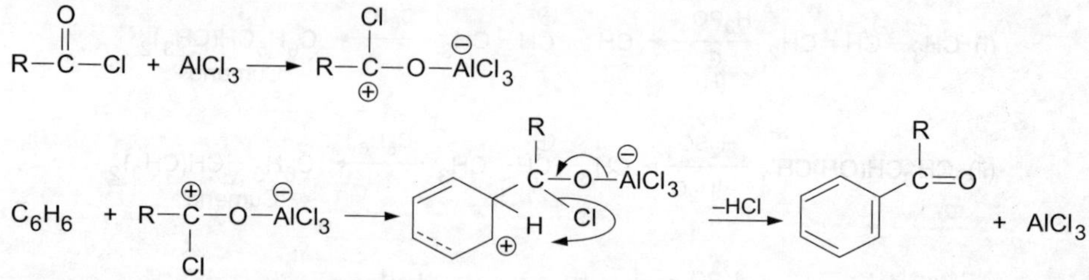

In either case, one mole of the catalyst remains complexed with the carbonyl oxygen of the ketone formed. Hence, a little more than one mole of the catalyst is required per mole of the reagent for acylation with acyl halides. When acid anhydride is the reagent, slightly more than two moles of the catalyst is required. This is because one mole of the catalyst is used up in liberating acyl halide and another mole for complexing with the product, ketone.

$$(RCO)_2O + AlCl_3 \longrightarrow RCOCl + RCOOAlCl_2$$

$$C_6H_6 + RCOCl \xrightarrow{AlCl_3} C_6H_5-\overset{\oplus}{\underset{R}{C}}-O-\overset{\ominus}{A}lCl_3$$

The product, ketone is liberated with ice-cold dilute acid.

Aromatic rings having activating groups, such as alkyl, alkoxy, halogen, acetamido, etc., are easily acylated. For reasons of steric factors, acylation mainly occurs at the para position. Many heterocyclic compounds undergo acylation with good yield. Metadirecting groups inhibit acylation. Hence, nitrobenzene is the favoured solvent for acylation.

Acylation differs from alkylation in the following;

(i) Acylation unlike alkylation is performed in solvents, such as nitrobenzene, carbon disulphide, petroleum ether, methylene chloride, etc.

(ii) Acylation requires more catalyst than alkylation for complexing with the carbonyl oxygen of the reagent.

(iii) Since acyl group is deactivating unlike alkyl group, a monosubstituted product is always obtained.

(iv) In acylation rearrangement in the substituent is not observed.

This fact has been utilized for preparing long-chain substituted arenes without rearrangement.

$$C_6H_6 + CH_3CH_2COCl \xrightarrow{AlCl_3} C_6H_5COCH_2CH_3 \xrightarrow[HCl]{Na-Hg} C_6H_5CH_2CH_2CH_3$$

n-Propyl benzene

Applications

The reaction is very useful for the synthesis of many classes of organic compounds. This is illustrated below.

(a) Hydrocarbons

(i) $C_6H_6 + C_6H_5CH_2Cl \xrightarrow{AlCl_3} C_6H_5CH_2C_6H_5$

Diphenyl methane

(ii) $3C_6H_6 + CHCl_3 \xrightarrow{AlCl_3} (C_6H_5)_3CH + 3HCl$

Triphenyl methane

(iii) 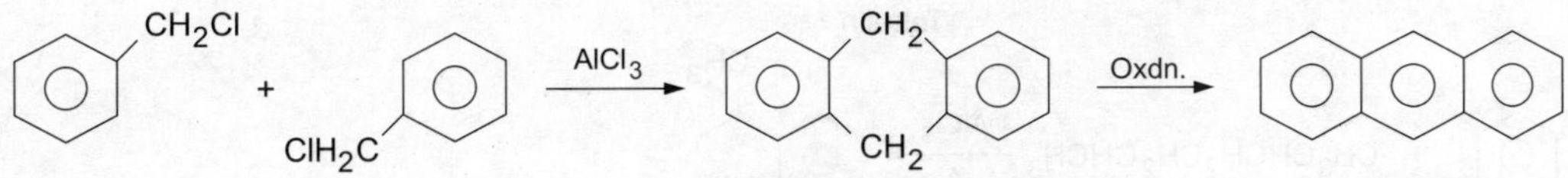

9, 10-Dihydro anthracene — Anthracene

(iv) 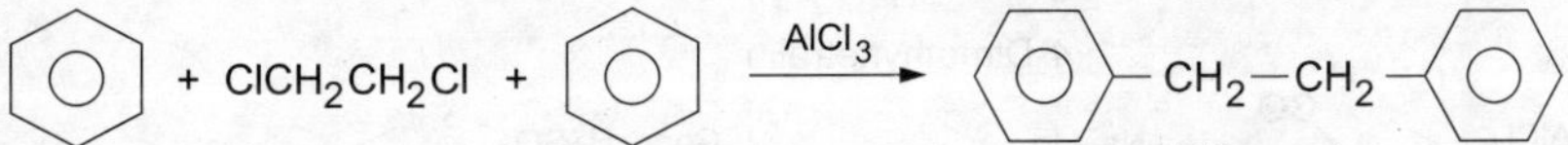

Dibenzyl

(v) 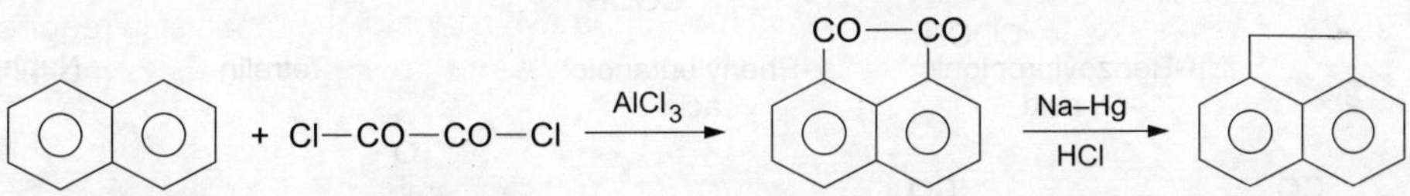

Naphthalene — Oxalyl chloride — 7, 8-Acenaphthaquinone — Acenaphthene

(b) Ketones

(i) $C_6H_6 + RCOCl \xrightarrow[PhNO_2]{AlCl_3} C_6H_5COR + HCl$

(ii) $C_6H_6 + C_6H_5CH_2COCl \xrightarrow[CS_2]{AlCl_3} C_6H_5COCH_2C_6H_5$

Benzyl phenyl ketone

(iii) 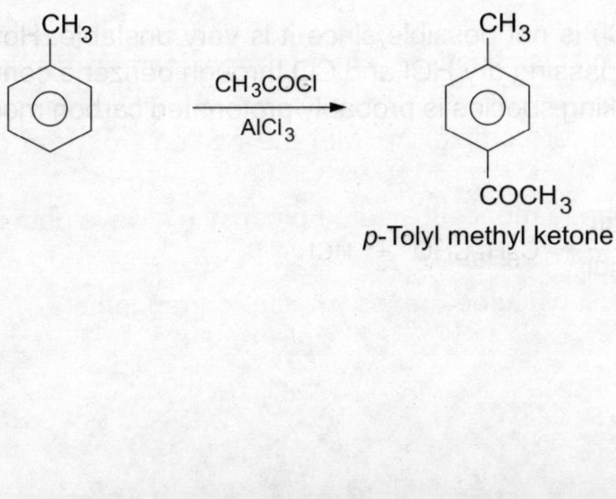

p-Tolyl methyl ketone

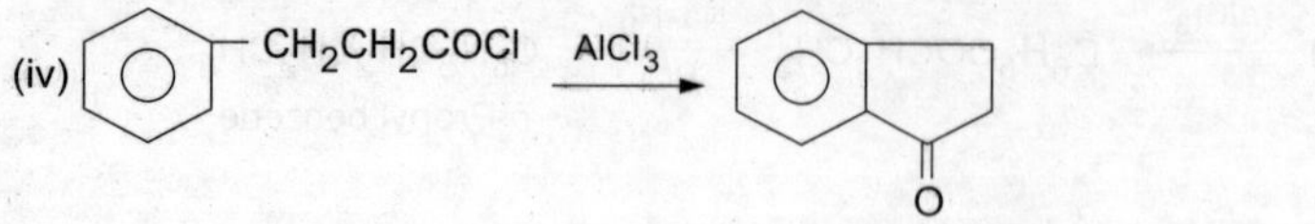

1-Hydrindone

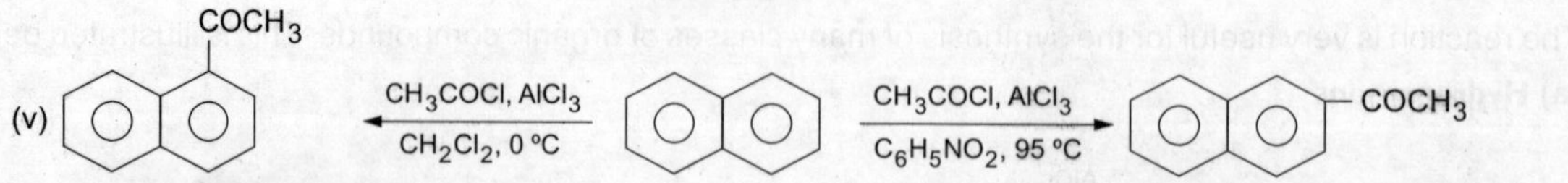

1-Naphthyl methyl ketone 2-Naphthyl methyl ketone

(c) Polynuclear hydrocarbons (cyclisation reactions) Friedel–Crafts alkylation and acylation with cyclic anhydrides have been employed to effect ring closure.

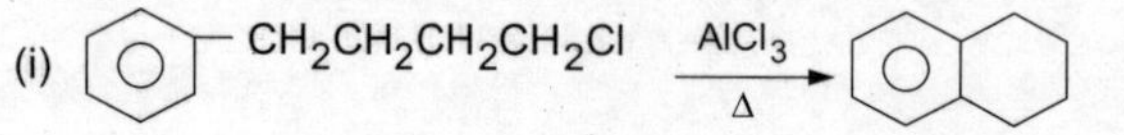

Tetralin

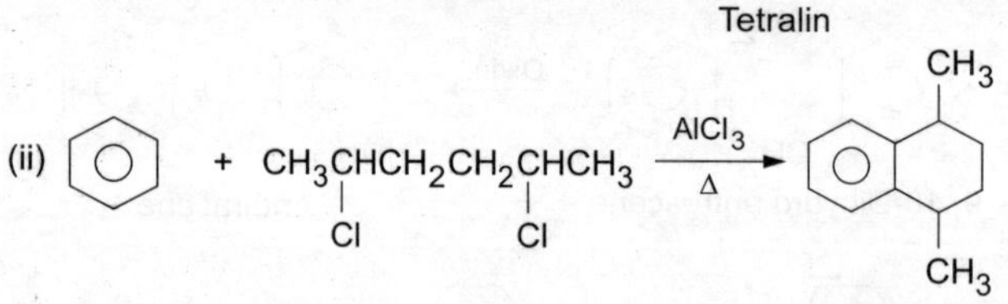

1, 4-Dimethyltetralin

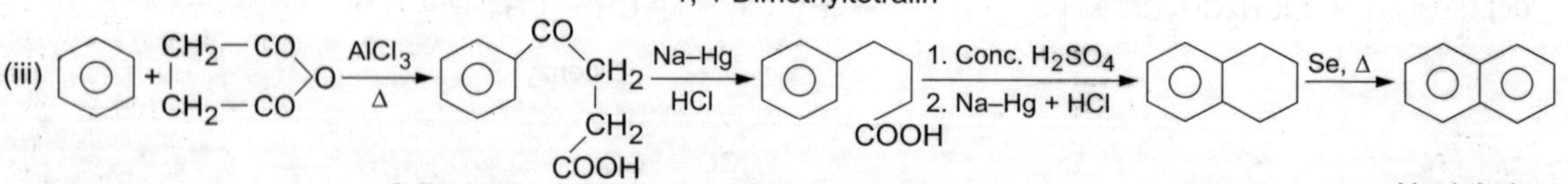

β-Benzoylpropionic acid γ-Phenylbutanoic acid Tetralin Naphthalene

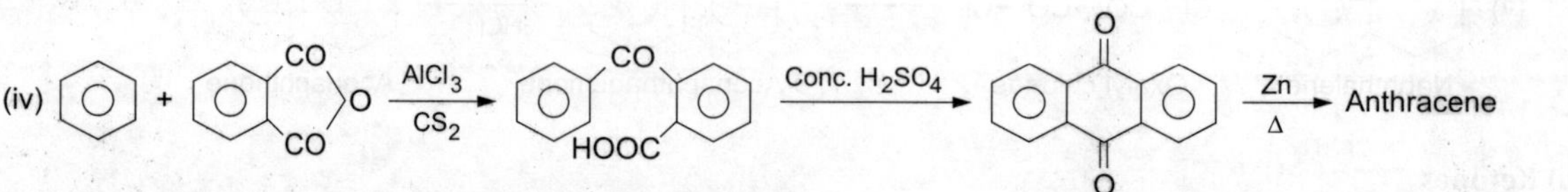

Phthalic anhydride *o*-Benzoylbenzoic acid Anthraquinone

(d) Acid chlorides

$$C_6H_6 + \underset{\text{Phosgene}}{COCl_2} \xrightarrow[Cu_2Cl_2]{AlCl_3} C_6H_5COCl + HCl$$

(e) Formylation Formylation with formyl chloride (HOCl) is not possible since it is very unstable. However, formylation has been achieved (Gattermann–Koch) by passing dry HCl and CO through benzene containing anhydrous $AlCl_3$ and a little cuprous chloride. The attacking species is probably protonated carbon monoxide ($H-\overset{\oplus}{C}=O$).

$$C_6H_6 + CO + HCl \xrightarrow[Cu_2Cl_2]{AlCl_3} C_6H_5CHO + HCl$$

FRIES REARRANGEMENT

Phenolic esters on heating with aluminium trichloride (Lewis acid) give *o*- and *p*- acyl phenol. This is known as Fries rearrangement.

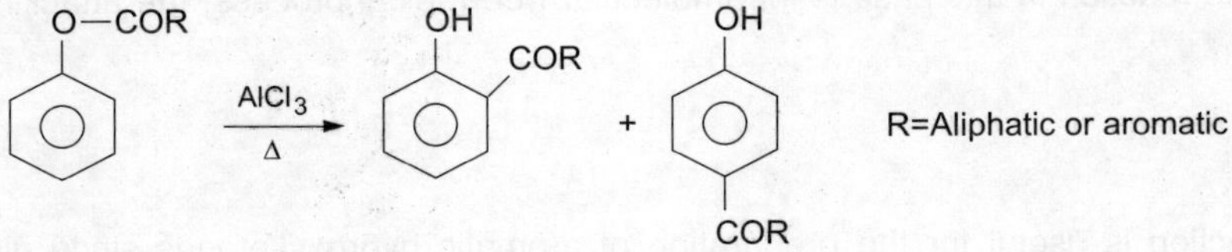

A mixture of ortho- and para-isomers is obtained. Electron-withdrawing groups in the substrate retard the reaction as in the case of Friedel–Crafts reaction. In general, low temperature favours the para-product and high temperature favours the ortho-product.

Mechanism

Exact mechanism is still not clearly understood. There is evidence for both intermolecular and intramolecular reaction mechanisms. It is, therefore, suggested that both mechanisms are operating simultaneously.

Two-step mechanism It may be taken to be Friedel–Crafts acylation in which the acylium ion, (Me$\overset{\oplus}{C}$O) is supplied by the substrate, i.e., it is self-acylation.

At first, $AlCl_3$ complexes with the oxygen of the phenoxy group from which the acylium ion is generated. The acylium ion then attacks the benzene ring as in the case of Friedel–Crafts reaction.

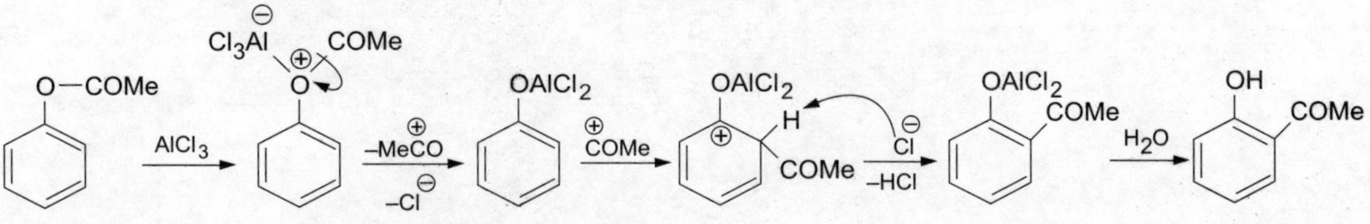

Similar attack at *p*-position gives the para-isomer.

Concerted or single-step mechanism

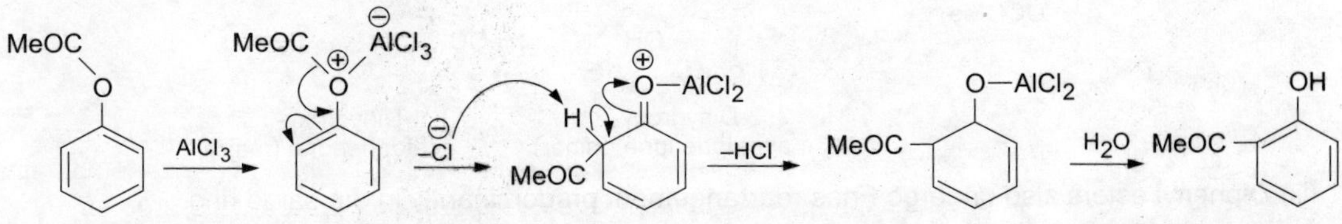

In practice, both *o*- and *p*-isomers are obtained. The amount of each isomer depends on temperature, solvent, amount of catalyst and on the structure of the substrate.

At low temperature (< 100 °C) para-isomer is the major product while at high temperature (> 100 °C) ortho-isomer is the major product. This is because the intermediate of ortho-isomer is stabilized by chelation and is hence thermodynamically more stable.

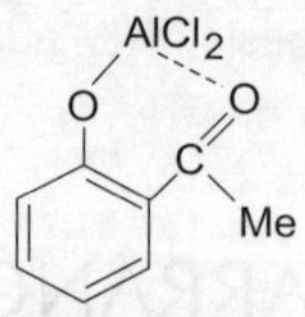

Solvent is generally not required for the reaction. Nitrobenzene may be used which reduces the reaction temperature.

Fries rearrangement has also been observed to be catalysed by light (photo Fries rearrangement). It is suggested that the reaction in this case is intramolecular free radical process, the attacking species being $R\dot{C}O\dot{O}$.

Applications

(i) This reaction is useful for the preparation of aromatic hydroxyketones since direct acylation of phenols gives very poor yield. The effect of this rearrangement on substrates bearing methyl groups at ortho, meta and para positions shows that when the para position is occupied, the acyl group substitutes exclusively to the ortho position.

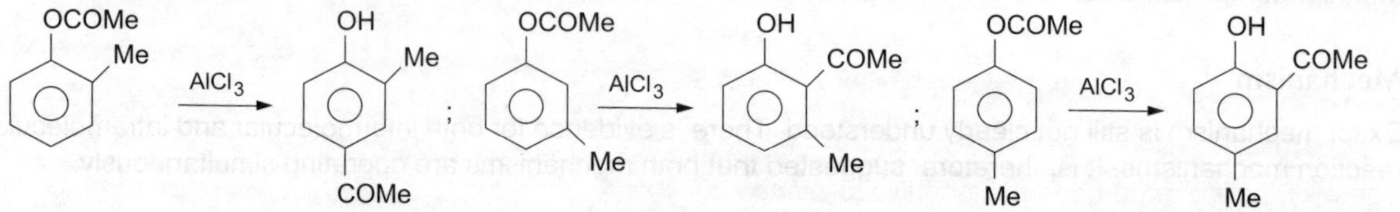

Major product; Major product; 100 %

The proportions of *o*- and *p*-isomers can be varied by controlling the conditions of reaction, viz., temperature, solvent and the amount of catalyst. The reaction is useful because it gives both the isomers which can be easily separated by steam distillation. The ortho-isomer having lower boiling point due to H-bonding distills over first, followed by the para-isomer.

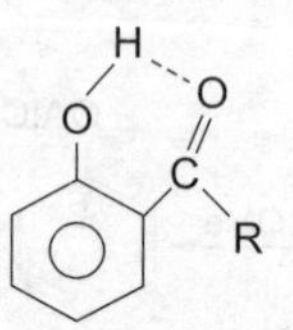

(ii) Esters of catechol give acyl catechols.

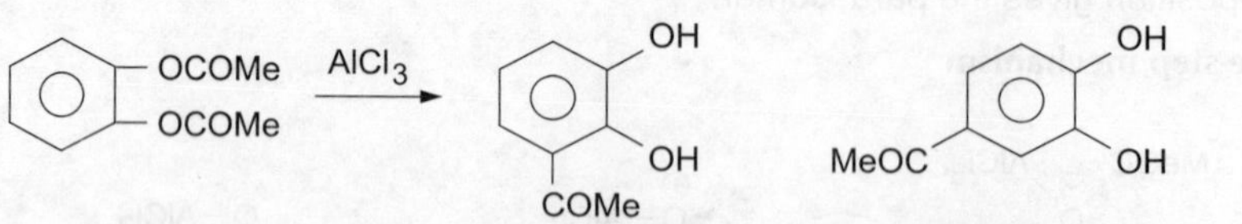

2, 3-Dihydroxy-acetophenone (minor) 3, 4-Dihydroxy-acetophenone (major)

(iii) Diphenyl esters also undergo Fries rearrangement predominantly in the same ring.

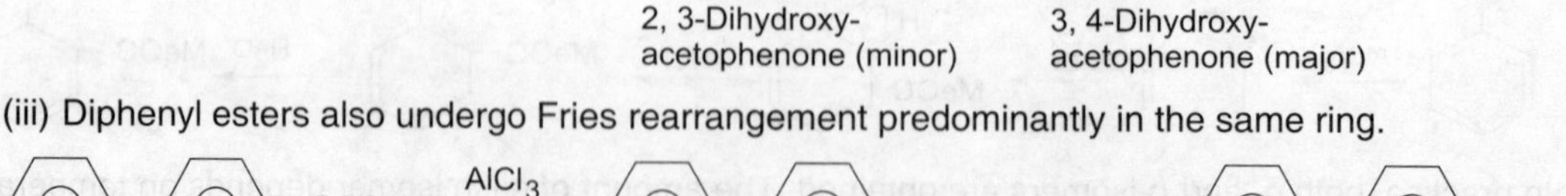

(Major) 4-Hydroxy-3-methoxybiphenyl (Minor) 4-Hydroxy-4′-methoxybiphenyl

(iv) A very useful application is in the synthesis of (±) adrenaline which is a heart stimulant.

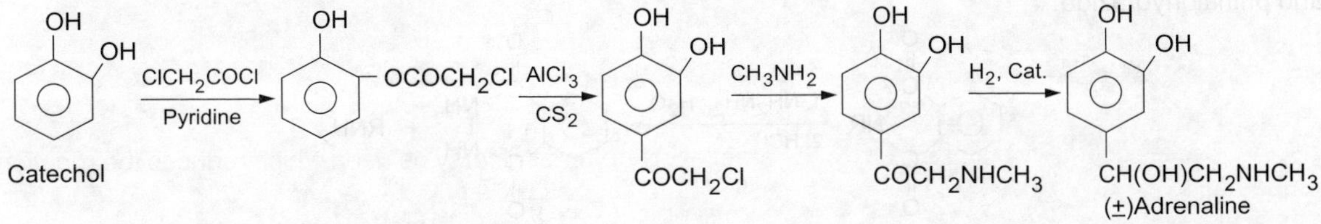

GABRIEL SYNTHESIS

The reaction involves the preparation of primary amines free from secondary or tertiary amines by reacting alkyl halides with alkali phthalimide and subsequent hydrolysis.

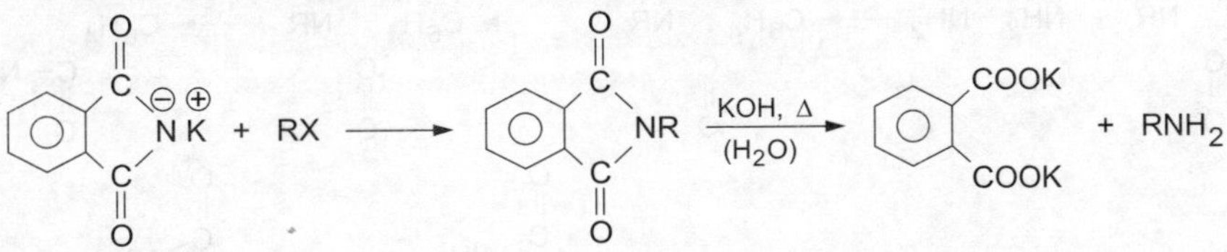

Mechanism

The alkyl halide undergoes nucleophilic displacement by the phthalimide anion (S_N2 displacement) to form *N*-substituted phthalimide. The latter is then hydrolysed either with acid or alkali. Usually a prolonged heating is required in both the mediums. The mechanism of hydrolysis is similar to amide hydrolysis.

(a) Base-catalysed hydrolysis

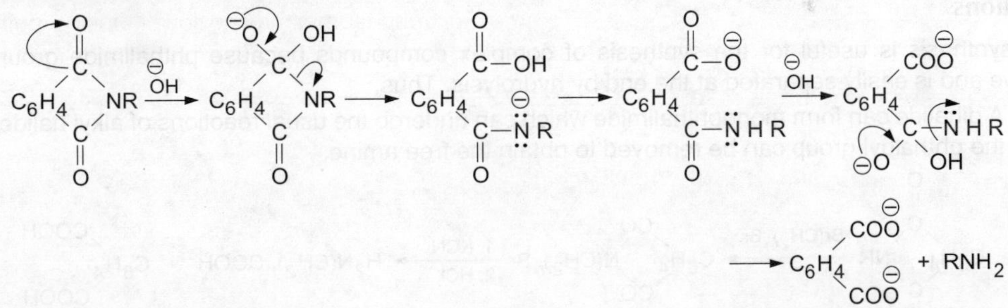

(b) Acid-catalysed hydrolysis

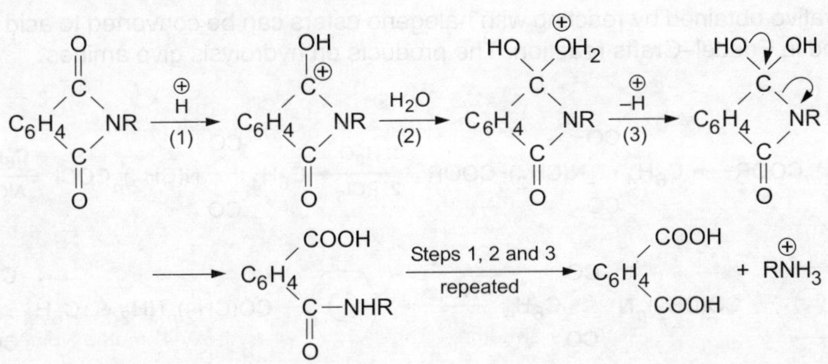

When substituted phthalimide is difficult to hydrolyse, hydrazine hydrate may be used to obtain free amine and phthalohydrazide.

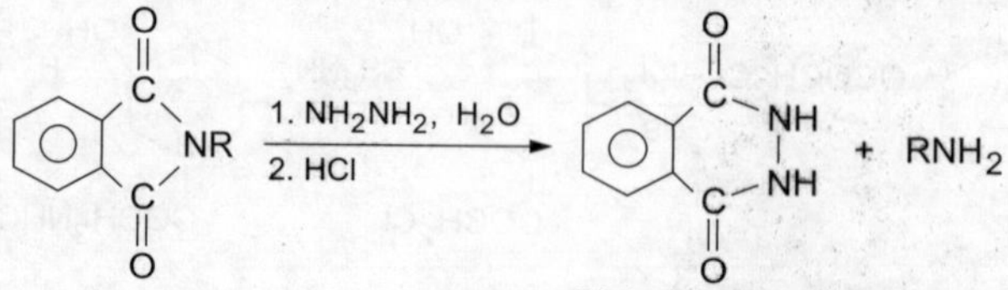

Phthalohydrazide

The reaction, called *hydrazinolysis,* proceeds under milder conditions than alkaline hydrolysis.

Probable mechanism for hydrazinolysis

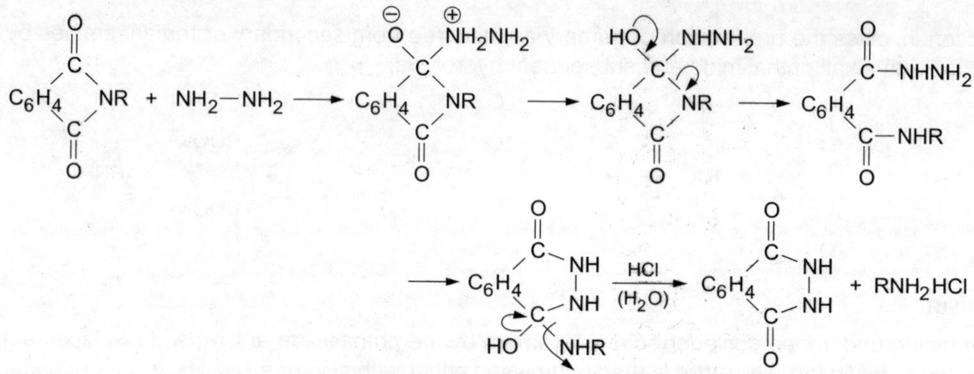

A better solvent for Gabriel synthesis is dimethylformamide.

Applications

Gabriel synthesis is useful for the synthesis of complex compounds because phthalimide group is fairly unreactive and is easily separated at the end by hydrolysis. Thus,

(a) A dihalide can form monophthalimide which can undergo the usual reactions of alkyl halides. Finally the phthaloyl group can be removed to obtain the free amine.

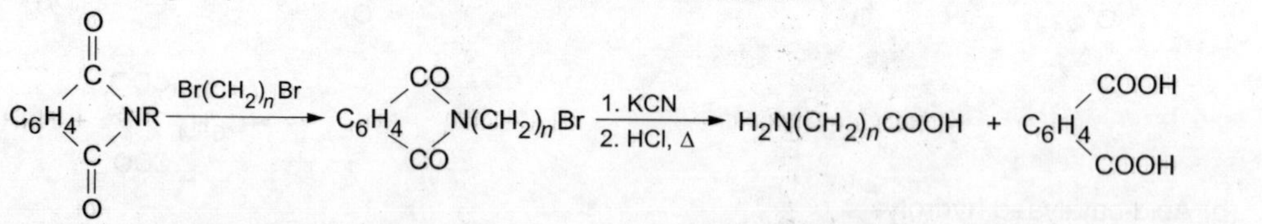

(b) Phthalimide derivative obtained by reacting with halogeno esters can be converted to acid chlorides which can be used in Friedel–Crafts reaction. The products on hydrolysis give amines.

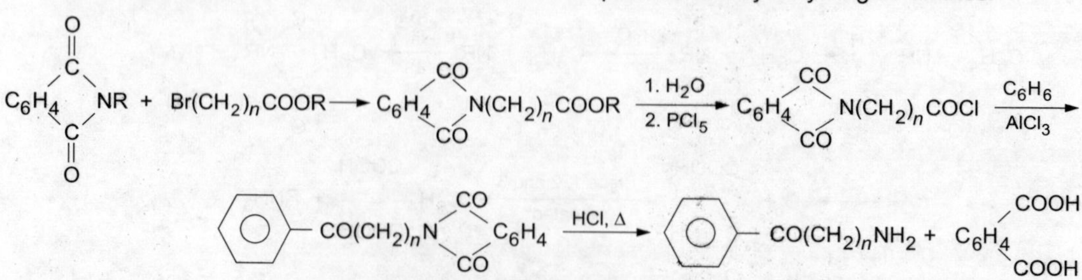

(c) Various amino acids can be prepared by using derivatives of malonic esters

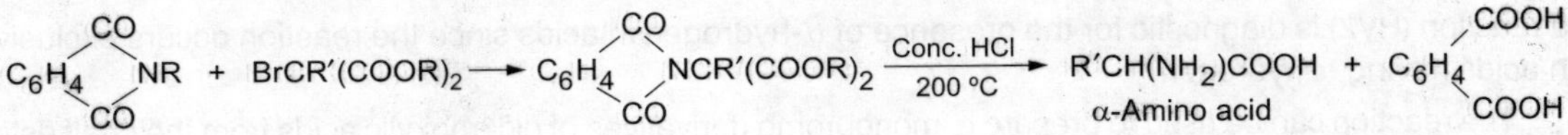

HELL–VOLHARD–ZELINSKY REACTION

Aliphatic carboxylic acids react with bromine or chlorine (but not iodine and fluorine) in the presence of small amount of red phosphorus to give exclusively mono α-halogenated acids. This is known as Hell–Volhard–Zelinsky (HVZ) reaction. The reaction is given only by aliphatic acids having α-hydrogen. Bromine reacts smoothly.

$$CH_3CH_2COOH + Br_2 \xrightarrow{\text{Red P}} CH_3CHBrCOOH + HBr$$

Chlorine reacts similarly but the reaction is less specific due to some free radical chlorination.

$$\underset{}{CH_3CH_2COOH} + Cl_2 \xrightarrow{h\nu} \underset{\alpha\text{-Chloropropionic acid}}{CH_3CH(Cl)COOH} + \underset{\beta\text{-Chloropropionic acid}}{CH_2(Cl)CH_2COOH}$$

Halogen from the catalyst does not enter the α-position of the acid, e.g.,

$$RCH_2COOH + Cl_2 \xrightarrow{PBr_3} RCH(Cl)COOH$$

Mechanism

Since acylhalides undergo halogenation without a catalyst, it is considered that red phosphorus and halogen first form phosphorus trihalide

$$2P + 3Br_2 \longrightarrow 2PBr_3$$

which reacts with the acid to give acid bromide.

$$RCH_2COOH + PBr_3 \longrightarrow RCH_2COBr + POBr + HBr$$

The acid bromide then undergoes α-halogenation through its enol form as in the case of acid-catalysed halogenation of ketones.

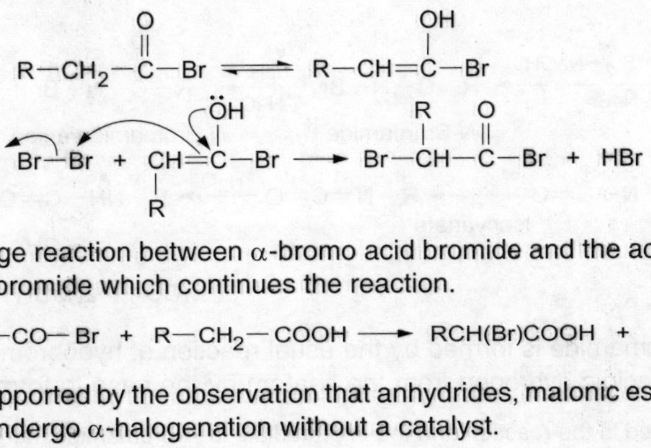

Finally, the interchange reaction between α-bromo acid bromide and the acid molecule gives α-bromo acid and regenerates acid bromide which continues the reaction.

$$R{-}CH(Br){-}CO{-}Br + R{-}CH_2{-}COOH \longrightarrow RCH(Br)COOH + RCH_2COBr$$

The mechanism is supported by the observation that anhydrides, malonic esters, nitro compounds, etc., which can enolise, easily undergo α-halogenation without a catalyst.

Applications

The reaction (HVZ) is diagnostic for the presence of α-hydrogen in acids since the reaction occurs exclusively with acids having α-hydrogen.

The reaction can be used to prepare α-monobromo derivatives of dicarboxylic acids from their half esters.

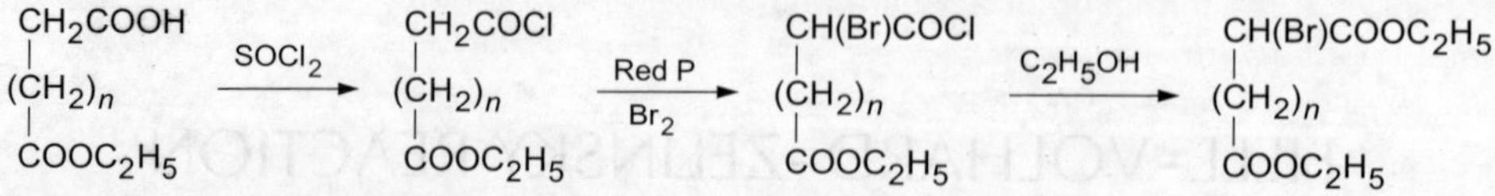

The yield is generally very high.

The α-halogen can be easily replaced by nucleophilic reagents to give various useful substituted products, e.g., α-amino and α-hydroxyacids which are of biochemical significance.

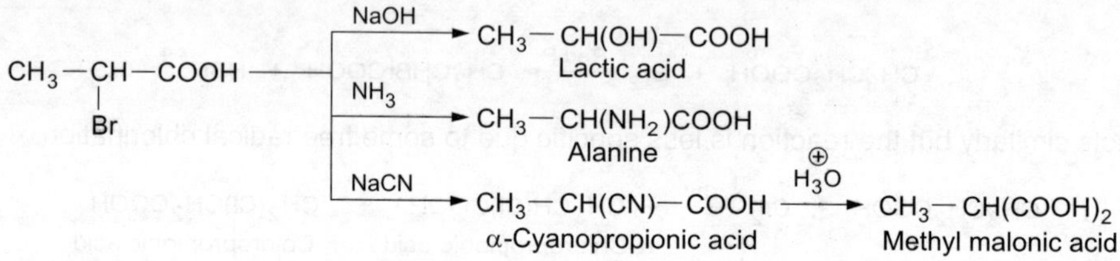

HOFMANN REARRANGEMENT OR HOFMANN BROMAMIDE* REACTION

The reaction involves the conversion of an amide into a primary amine with one carbon less, by the action of alkaline hypohalite (NaOH solution + Br_2 or Cl_2). The overall reaction is

$$RCONH_2 + Br_2 + 4NaOH \longrightarrow RNH_2 + 2NaBr + Na_2CO_3 + 2H_2O$$

where R may be aliphatic, aromatic or heterocyclic.

Mechanism

The mechanism has been suggested on the basis of the intermediates isolated during the course of reaction.

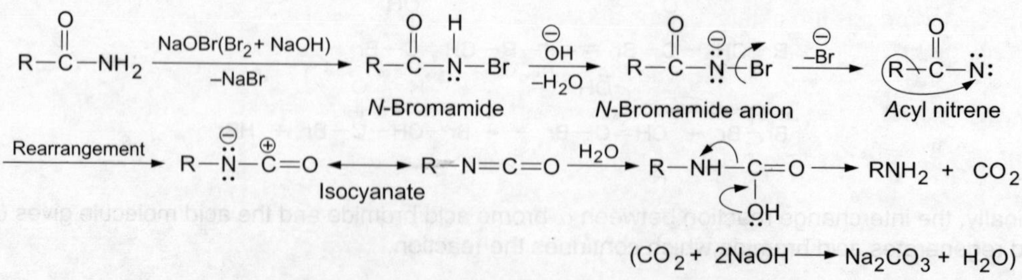

In the first step *N*-bromamide is formed by the usual reaction of hypobromite on primary amines. This follows the removal of the acidic hydrogen from the N-atom by the base to form *N*-bromamide anion in the

* Since bromine is mostly used in the reaction and the intermediate is *N*-bromamide, hence the name.

second step. In the third step loss of bromine results in the formation of the highly reactive acylnitrene. In the fourth step, migration of R to the electron-deficient nitrogen gives the isocyanate. The latter reacts with water to give carbamic acid which spontaneously eliminates carbon dioxide to yield the amine.

By careful control of experimental conditions the intermediates, *N*-bromamide, its anion and isocyanate (in aprotic solvent) have been isolated. This confirms the mechanism.

The possibility of the formation of acylnitrene, however, has been rejected, for if it is formed it would react with water to give hydroxamic acid,

$$R-\overset{O}{\overset{\|}{C}}-\ddot{N}: + H_2O \longrightarrow R-\overset{O}{\overset{\|}{C}}-NHOH \text{ (Hydroxamic acid)}$$

which has not been detected.

Hence, the loss of Br and the migration of R in *N*-bromamide anion is suggested to be concerted.

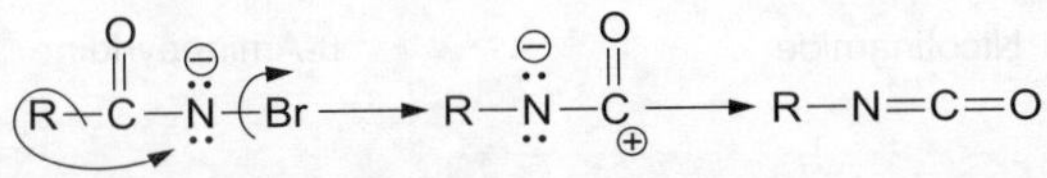

Since no cross-over products are obtained when two different amides are rearranged, it is assumed that the rearrangement is intramolecular and the migrating group never completely separates during the migration.

This is further confirmed by the fact that if R is chiral (asymmetric), it migrates with unchanged configuration. Thus, camphoramidic acid (I) having the COOH and $CONH_2$ groups in cis position undergoes Hofmann rearrangement to give the amino acid (II) in which the COOH and NH_2 groups are also in cis position, since it readily forms lactam.

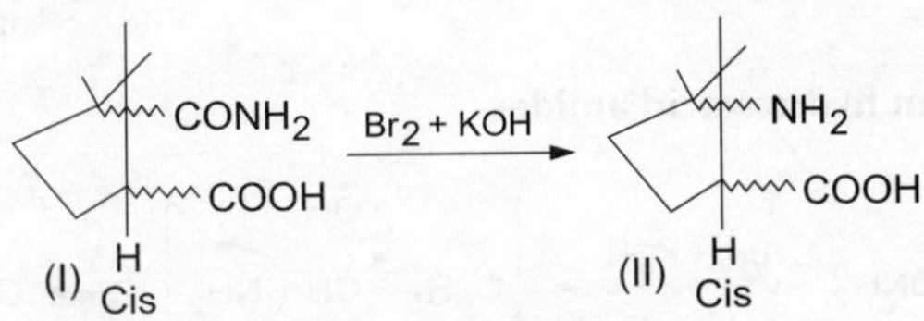

Similarly, D-α-phenylpropionamide gives D-α-phenylethylamine on subjecting to Hofmann rearrangement.

$$CH_3\overset{*}{C}H(C_6H_5)CONH_2 \longrightarrow CH_3\overset{*}{C}H(C_6H_5)NH_2$$

The rate of reaction increases when the migrating group is more electron-donating and decreases when electron-withdrawing. If R is an alkyl group with more than eight carbons, low yields are obtained.

Some side products are obtained, e.g., addition of $RCONH_2$ to RNCO gives RCONHCONHR and when R is a primary group nitriles are obtained.

Applications

1. Formation of amines It is a very useful method for the preparation of amines.

(a) Acids and amides to amines.

(i) $$RCOOH \xrightarrow[2.\ \Delta]{1.\ NH_4OH} RCONH_2 \xrightarrow{Br_2 + KOH} RNH_2$$

(ii) $$\underset{\beta,\ \beta\text{-Dimethyl butyramide}}{Me_3CCH_2CONH_2} \xrightarrow{NaOBr} \underset{\text{Neopentyl amine}}{Me_3CCH_2NH_2}$$

(b) Higher amides (with more than eight carbons) give nitriles which can be reduced to amines.

$$RCH_2CONH_2 \xrightarrow{Br_2 + KOH} RCH_2CN \xrightarrow{Na + Alcohol} RCH_2CH_2NH_2$$

(c) Urea gives the valuable reagent hydrazine.

$$\underset{\text{Urea}}{H_2NCONH_2} \xrightarrow{Br_2 + KOH} NH_2NH_2$$

The yield of amines is poor with β, γ-unsaturated acids.

2. Preparation of β-amino pyridine from nicotinamide

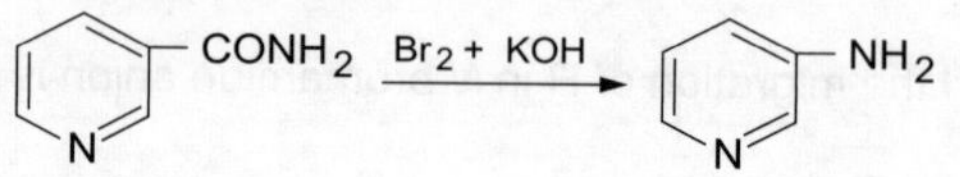

Nicotinamide β-Aminopyridine

3. Synthesis of amino acids

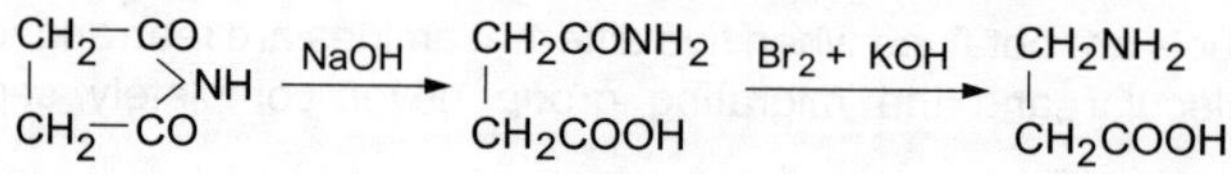

Succinimide β-Alanine

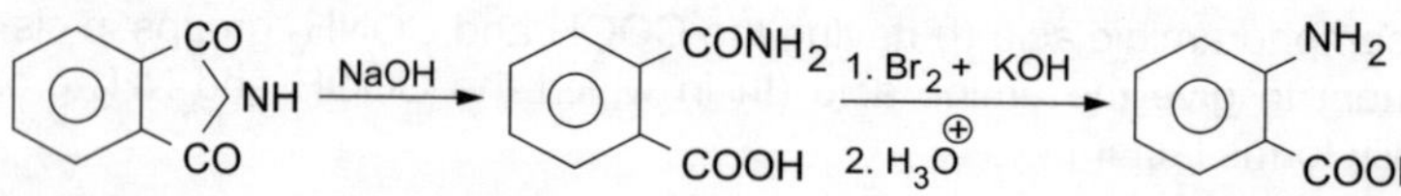

Phthalimide Anthranilic acid

4. Preparation of aldehydes from hydroxyacid amides

(i) $$\underset{\text{Mandelic acid amide}}{C_6H_5-CH(OH)-CONH_2} \xrightarrow{Br_2 + KOH} \left[C_6H_5-\overset{\ddot{O}H}{\overset{|}{C}H}-\ddot{N}H_2 \right] \longrightarrow C_6H_5-\overset{O}{\overset{||}{C}}-H + NH_3$$

(ii) Methanolic α, β-unsaturated acid amides on treatment with NaOCl give urethane which on hydrolysis with HCl gives a good yield of aldehyde.

$$R-CH{=}CH-CO-NH_2 \xrightarrow[CH_3OH]{NaOCl} R-CH{=}CH-NHCOOCH_3 \xrightarrow[(H_2O)]{HCl} R-CHO$$

N.B. This reaction is generally confused with Hofmann elimination which relates to the cleavage of quaternary ammonium hydroxides.

HOUBEN–HOESCH REACTION

Polyhydroxy phenols, phenolic ethers and some reactive heterocyclic compounds (e.g., pyrrole) undergo acylation with nitrile and hydrochloric acid in the presence of a Lewis acid, the most common being zinc chloride and aluminium trichloride. This particular Friedel–Crafts acylation with nitriles is called Houben–Hoesch reaction.

The reaction is carried out by passing dry HCl gas through an equimolecular mixture of nitrile and phenol in dry ether containing $ZnCl_2$. The resulting ketimine chloride on hydrolysis gives the aromatic hydroxy ketone. Thus, resorcinol gives 2, 4-dihydroxyacetophenone.

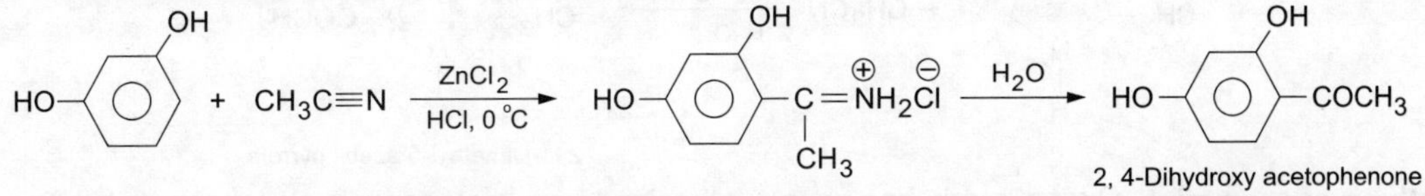

2, 4-Dihydroxy acetophenone

The reaction is very successful with polyhydroxy phenols especially the *m*-polyhydroxy phenols. The reaction, however, is not successful with phenol due to the formation of imino-ether hydrochloride as almost the exclusive product resulting from the attack on the hydroxy oxygen.

$$C_6H_5OH + RCN \xrightarrow[HCl]{ZnCl_2} C_6H_5O-\underset{}{\overset{R}{C}}=\overset{\oplus}{N}H_2\overset{\ominus}{Cl}$$

Hydrolysis gives phenyl ester.

Besides a variety of aliphatic nitriles (e.g., acetonitrile, mono- and trichloro-aceto nitriles), aromatic nitriles have also been found to give good yield. Ether, chloroform, ethyl acetate, etc., may be used as solvent.

Mechanism

The mechanism of the reaction is complex and not fully understood. The attacking species is supposed to be the imine hydrochloride (I). The resulting imine salt (II) on hydrolysis gives the product.

$$R-C\equiv N + 2HCl + ZnCl_2 \longrightarrow \underset{(I)}{R-\overset{\oplus}{C}=NH\ HCl} + [ZnCl_3]^{\ominus}$$

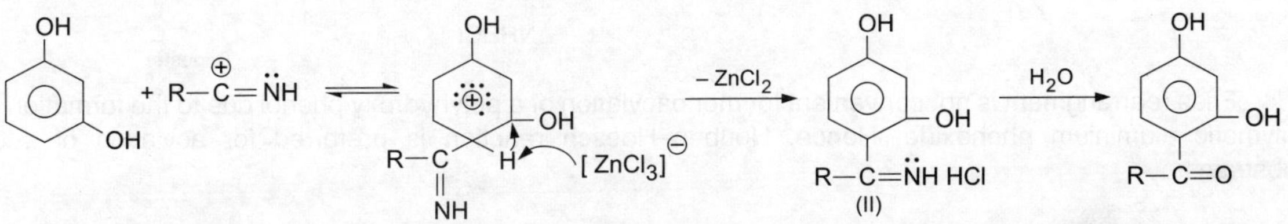

When hydrogen cyanide is employed in place of nitrile, aromatic aldehyde may be obtained. This modification is called Gattermann synthesis of aromatic aldehydes. By this method aldehydes of various aromatic compounds have been prepared.

Applications

The reaction provides a convenient method for the synthesis of polyhydroxy acetophenones and polyhydroxy benzophenones. Many natural products of medicinal value have been synthesized by this reaction.

1. Synthesis of ω-substituted acetophenones When benzyl cyanide is used, ω-phenylaceto phenones are obtained.

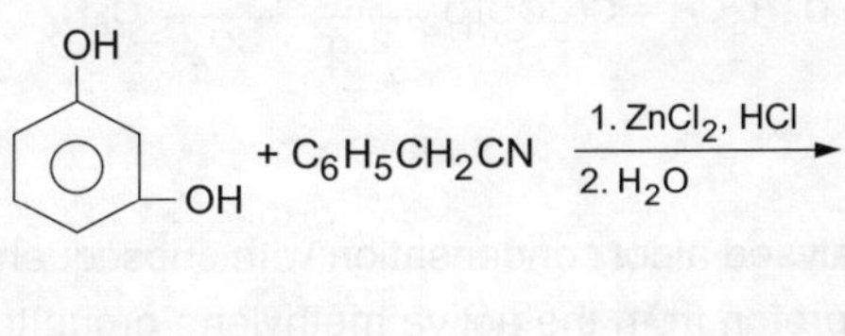

2, 4-Dihydroxy-ω-phenyl acetophenone

Similarly, on reacting with chloromethyl cyanide ($ClCH_2CN$), 2, 4-dihydroxy-ω-chloroacetophenone is obtained.

2. Synthesis of heterocyclic ketones A few pyrryl ketones have been synthesized.

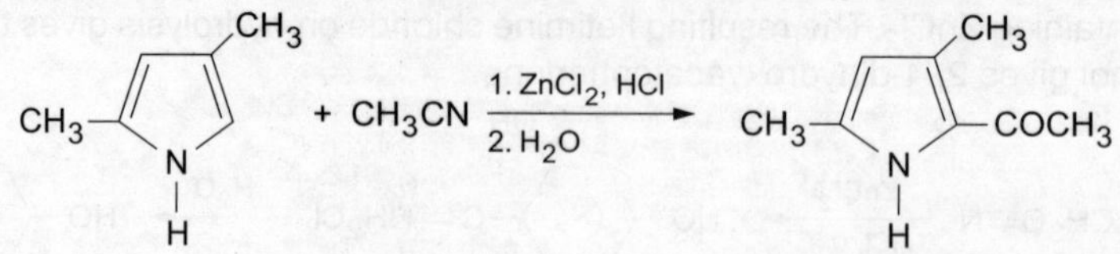

2, 4-Dimethyl-5 acetyl pyrrole

3. Synthesis of coumarins Oxocoumarin has been synthesized from malononitrile and resorcinol.

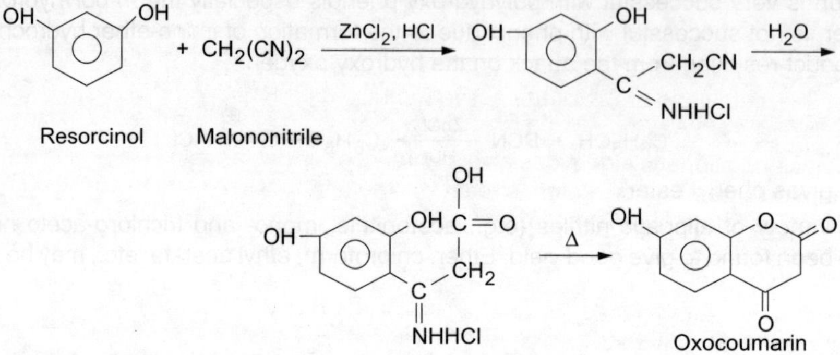

Resorcinol Malononitrile

Oxocoumarin

4. Synthesis of thioesters Thioester may be prepared by using thiocyanate (RSCN).

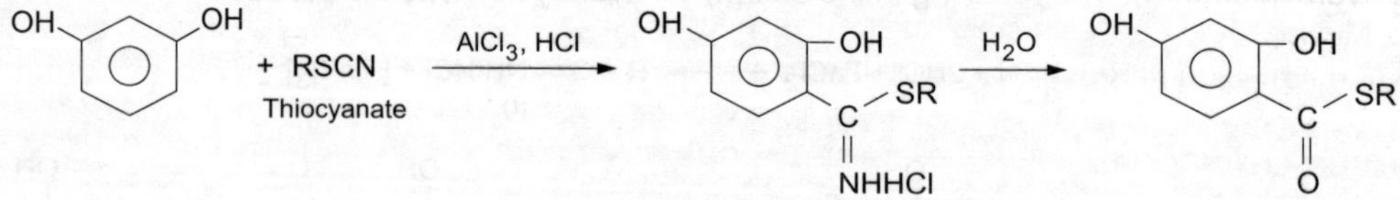

Thiocyanate Thioester

Fries rearrangment is not convenient for monoacylation of a polyhydroxy phenol due to the formation of polymeric aluminium phenoxide. Hence, Houben–Hoesch reaction is preferred for acylation of such substrates.

KNOEVENAGEL REACTION

Condensations of aldehydes and ketones with compounds having active methylene group in the presence of basic catalyst to form α,β-unsaturated compounds is called Knoevenagel reaction. The basic catalysts may be ammonia or its derivatives. Thus, primary, secondary or tertiary amines, e.g., aniline, di- or tri-alkyl amines, pyridine, piperidine, etc., are used.

$$\underset{}{C_6H_5CHO} + \underset{\text{Malonic ester}}{H_2C(COOR)_2} \xrightarrow[\text{piperidine}]{\text{Pyridine-}} C_6H_5CH{=}C(COOR)_2 \xrightarrow[2.\ \Delta,\ -CO_2]{1.\ H_2O} \underset{\text{Cinnamic acid}}{C_6H_5{-}CH{=}CH{-}COOH}$$

Mechanism

The initial stage of the reaction is base-catalysed aldol condensation with subsequent dehydration.

In the first step the base removes a proton from the active methylene group to generate a carbanion. The carbanion then attacks the carbonyl carbon of the substrate to form an alkoxide ion which abstracts the proton from the protonated catalyst to form a hydroxy compound. Subsequent dehydration gives the α, β-unsaturated compound which is hydrolysed and decarboxylated to obtain α, β-unsaturated acid. The reaction with a malonic ester is as shown:

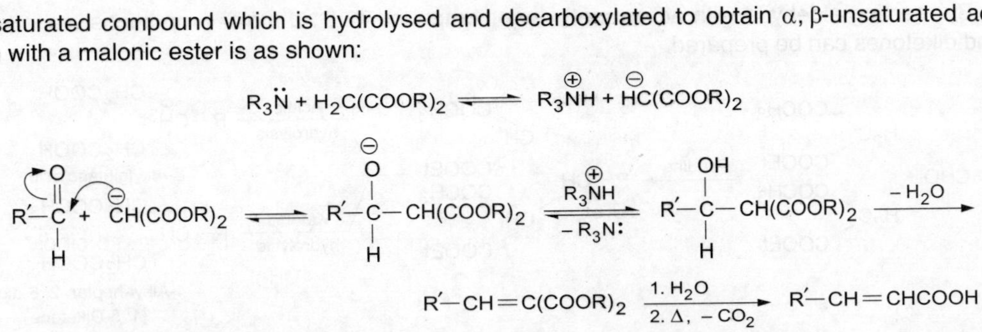

High reactivity of the methylene group of the active methylene compound prevents self-condensation of the aldehyde.

Both aromatic and aliphatic aldehydes give this reaction. For steric and electronic reasons ketones are less reactive than aldehydes. Hence, ketones react with compounds having powerful active methylene group only, e.g., ethyl acetoacetate, cyanoacetic acid and its ester but not usually with malonic ester for which stronger bases have to be used.

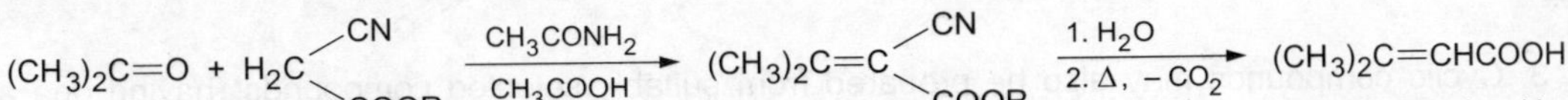

3-Methylcrotonic acid

The intermediate unsaturated product formed during the course of reaction with aldehydes tends further to undergo Michael reaction especially in the presence of excess of the active methylene compound. The Michael condensation product may be hydrolysed and decarboxylated to obtain dibasic acid.

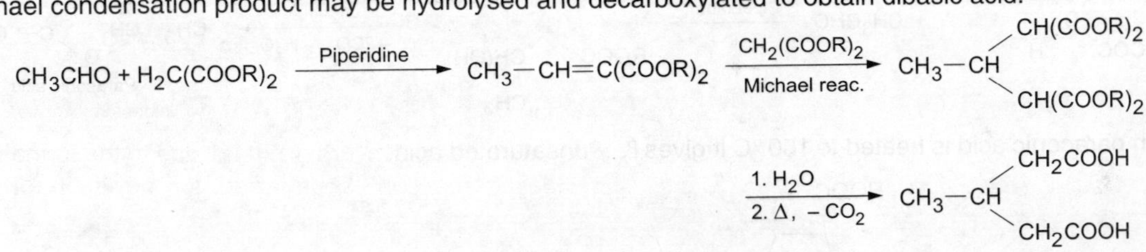

3-Methylglutaric acid

Hence, Knoevenagel reaction best proceeds with aromatic aldehydes.

Applications

1. Various α, β-unsaturated acids such as crotonic, cinnamic, fumaric and β-piperonyl acrylic acids can be prepared.

(a) $CH_3CHO + H_2C(COOR)_2 \xrightarrow{\text{Pip}} CH_3{-}CH{=}C(COOR)_2 \xrightarrow[2.\ \Delta,\ -CO_2]{1.\ H_2O} CH_3{-}CH{=}CH{-}COOH$

Crotonic acid

(b) $C_6H_5CHO + H_2C(COOR)_2 \xrightarrow{\text{Pip}} C_6H_5{-}CH{=}C(COOR)_2 \xrightarrow[2.\ \Delta,\ -CO_2]{1.\ H_2O} C_6H_5{-}CH{=}CH{-}COOH$

Cinnamic acid

(c) $HOOC{-}CHO + H_2C(COOR)_2 \xrightarrow{\text{Pip}} HOOC{-}CH{=}C(COOR)_2 \xrightarrow[2.\ \Delta,\ -CO_2]{1.\ H_2O} HOOC{-}CH{=}CH{-}COOH$

Glyoxalic acid — Maleic acid

(d) 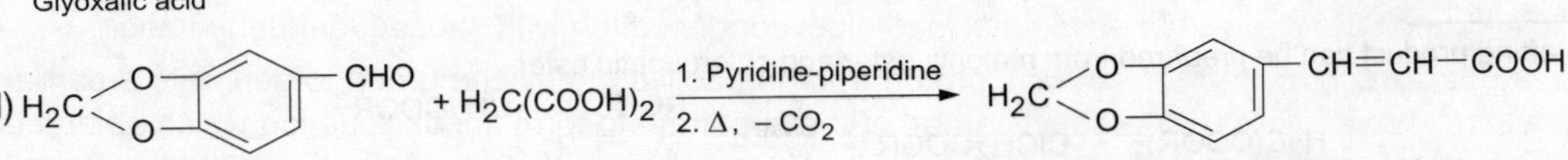

Piperonal — β-Piperonyl acrylic acid

2. By reacting aldehyde with active methylene compound in 1 : 2 molar proportions, various dibasic acids and diketones can be prepared.

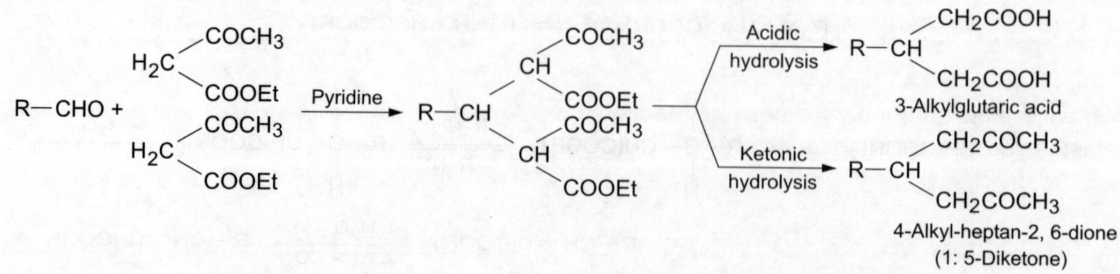

The 1 : 5-diketones may be cyclised by the treatment with alcoholic alkali to obtain cyclohexene derivatives.

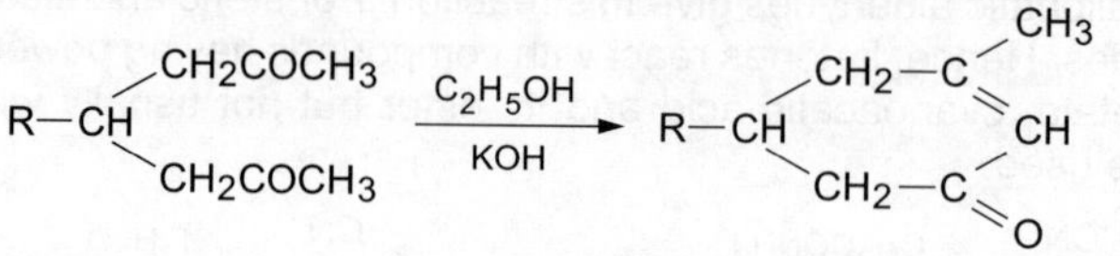

3. Cyclic compounds may also be prepared from suitably selected compounds* having one active hydrogen. The reaction proceeds up to aldol stage and then the aldol is cyclised to paraconic acid.

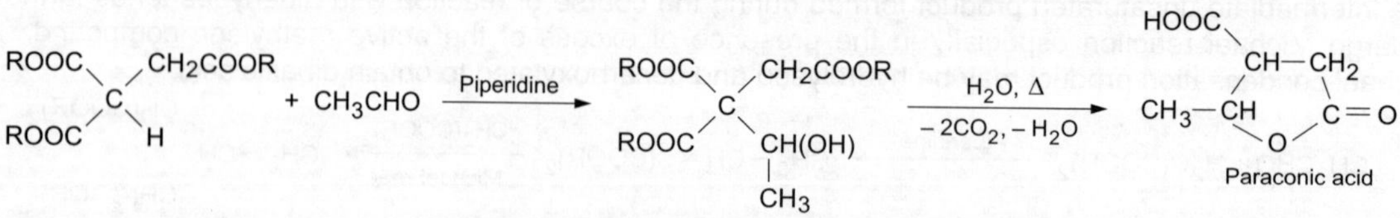

When paraconic acid is heated to 150 °C it gives β, γ-unsaturated acid.

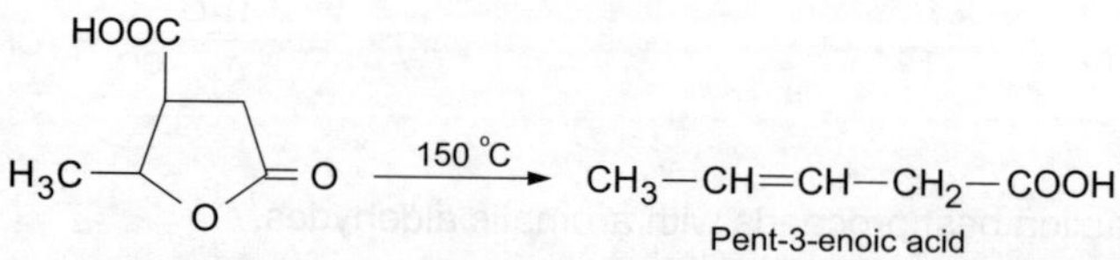

MANNICH REACTION

The condensation of a compound containing active hydrogen with formaldehyde and ammonia or 1° or 2° amines usually as their hydrochlorides (HCl being used as catalyst) to form aminomethyl or substituted aminomethyl derivatives is known as Mannich reaction. The base, called Mannich base, is usually isolated as its hydrochloride. Aryl amines do not normally respond to this reaction.

$$C_6H_5COCH_3 + HCHO + (CH_3)_2NH{\cdot}HCl \longrightarrow C_6H_5COCH_2CH_2N(CH_3)_2{\cdot}HCl + H_2O$$

---

* The starting product can be prepared from malonic ester and chloroacetic ester.

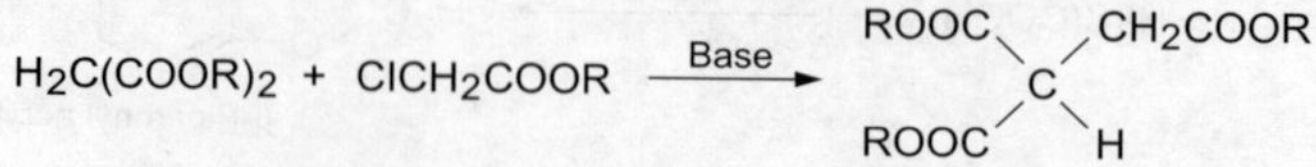

Thus, the overall reaction is (active hydrogens underlined):

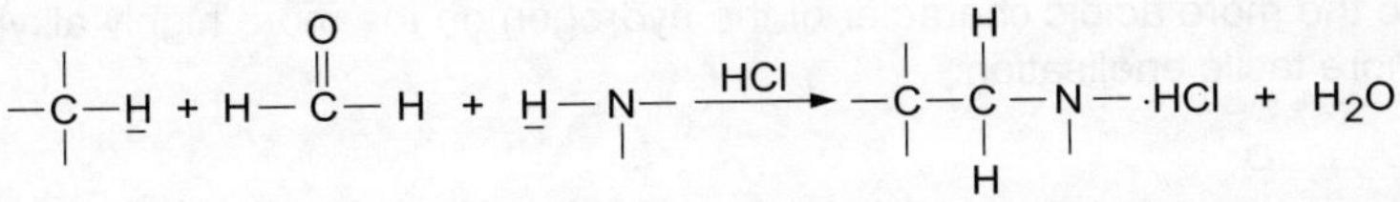

With ammonia or primary amines, the reaction may proceed further since the first formed Mannich base still contains hydrogen on the nitogen atom, i.e., active hydrogen.

$$CH_3COCH_3 + HCHO + CH_3NH_2HCl \longrightarrow CH_3COCH_2CH_2NH(CH_3){\cdot}HCl + H_2O$$

$$CH_3COCH_3 + CH_3COCH_2CH_2NH(CH_3){\cdot}HCl \xrightarrow{HCHO} (CH_3COCH_2CH_2)_2\,NCH_3{\cdot}HCl + H_2O$$

Hence, 2° amine is preferred for the reaction.

Similarly, three successive reactions with ammonia give a 3° amine.

$$3CH_3COCH_3 + 3HCHO + NH_3{\cdot}HCl \longrightarrow (CH_3COCH_2CH_2)_3\,N{\cdot}HCl + 3H_2O$$

Thus, with a 1° or 2° amine, the reaction may proceed further to give a 3° amine.

The compounds containing active hydrogens which react include aldehydes, ketones, esters, phenols, nitroalkanes, α- and γ- methyl pyridines, α- and γ- methyl quinolines, acetylenes, etc.

Ketones with active hydrogen are more commonly used. If the compound contains more than one active hydrogen, all of them may be substituted by amino methyl groups.

(a) $CH_3COCH_3 \xrightarrow[HCHO]{R_2NH} CH_3COCH_2CH_2NR_2 \xrightarrow[HCHO]{R_2NH} CH_3COCH(CH_2NR_2)_2 \xrightarrow[HCHO]{R_2NH} CH_3COC(CH_2NR_2)_3$

(b)

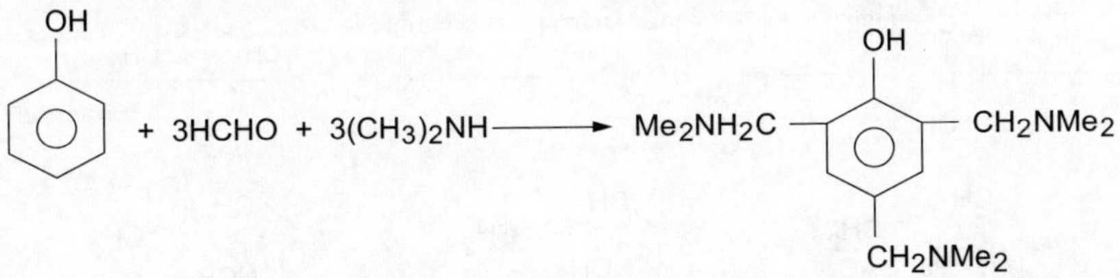

Mechanism

It is suggested that in the first step, the amine and HCHO in the presence of ($\overset{\oplus}{H}$) condense to form imminium cation.

(i)

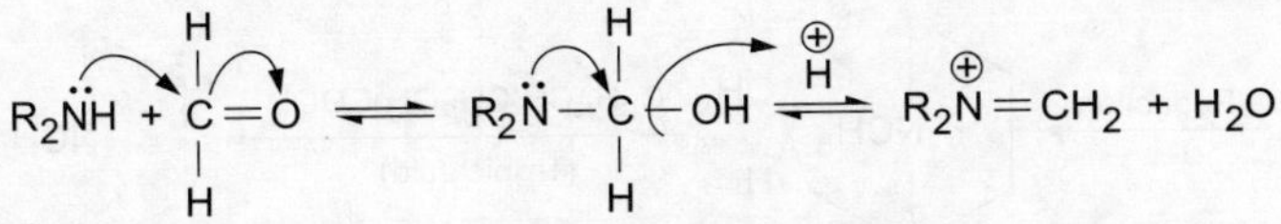

It is then attacked by the enolate anion of the active hydrogen compound in the second step to form the Mannich base.

(ii)

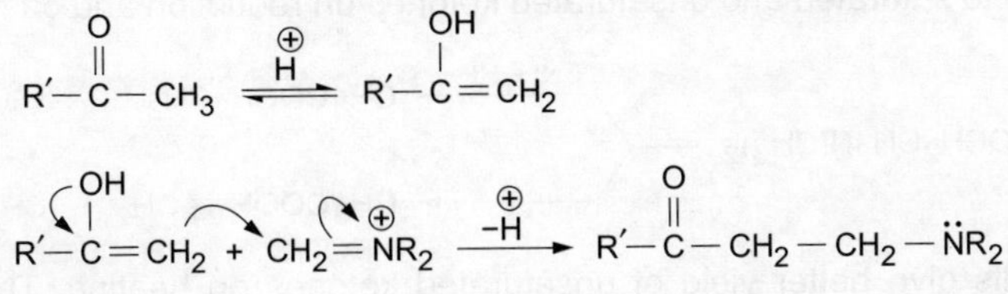

Base has also been used as catalyst.

With unsymmetrical ketones the more highly alkylated α-carbon is substituted by the aminomethyl group. This is due to the more acidic character of the hydrogen on the more highly alkylated carbon and for that matter due to more facile enolisation.

$$CH_3-\overset{O}{\overset{\|}{C}}-CH(CH_3)_2 + HCHO + R_2NH \longrightarrow CH_3COC(CH_3)_2CH_2NR_2$$

Applications

1. Many important natural products, especially alkaloids, have been synthesized by this reaction. A classical example is Robinson's synthesis of tropinone by a double Mannich condensation and subsequent synthesis of atropine.

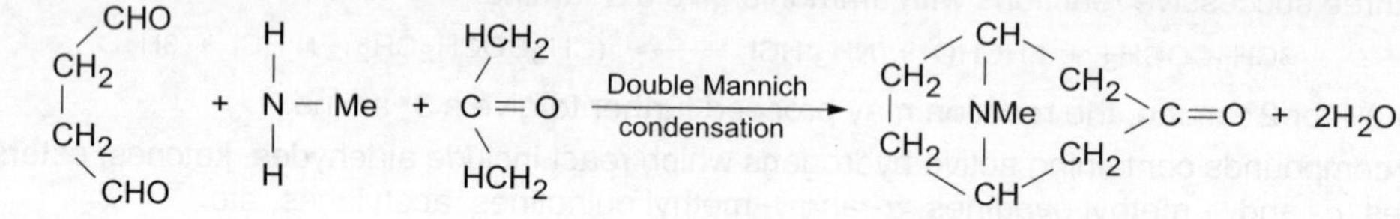

Succinaldehyde Tropinone

Mechanism

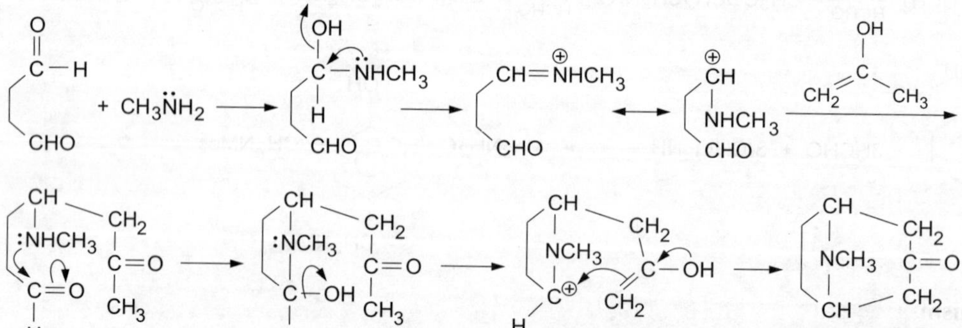

Tropinone

Better yield of tropinone is obtained by the use of calcium acetone dicarboxylate in place of acetone.

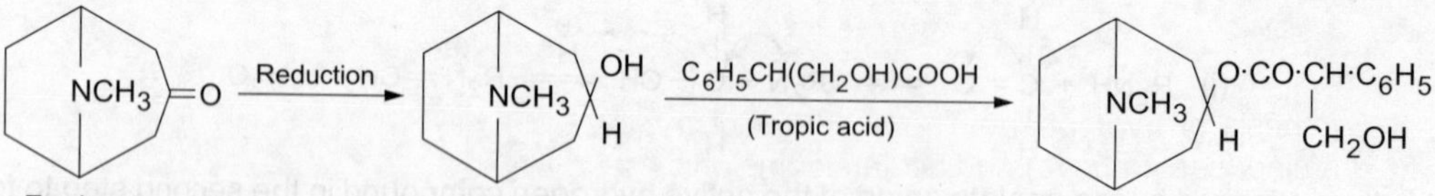

Tropinone Atropine

2. Decomposition to saturated and unsaturated ketones on reduction and on heating respectively.

$$CH_3COCH_2CH_2N(CH_3)_2 \xrightarrow{Ni + HI} CH_3COCH_2CH_3$$

$$CH_3COCH_2CH_2N(CH_3)_2 \xrightarrow{\Delta} CH_3COOH=CH_2 + (CH_3)_2NH$$

Quaternary salts give better yield of unsaturated ketones on heating. The reaction is useful for introducing vinyl group.

3. Building up of ring system—The easy elimination of R_2NH from Mannich base has synthetic applications. Thus, the unsaturated ketones obtained by heating the quaternary salts may be used for building ring systems.

(i) $$CH_3COCH_3 + HCHO + (CH_3)_2NH \longrightarrow CH_3COCH_2CH_2N(CH_3)_2 \xrightarrow[\Delta]{CH_3I}$$

$$\underset{\text{Quaternary salt}}{CH_3COCH_2CH_2\overset{\oplus}{N}(CH_3)_3\overset{\ominus}{I}} \xrightarrow{\Delta} CH_3COCH{=}CH_2 + (CH_3)_3NHI$$

(ii)

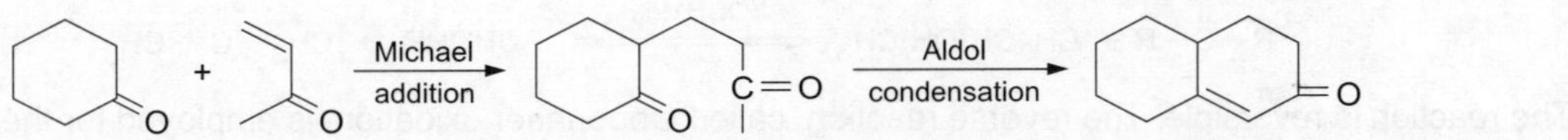

4. The imminium salt, being a strong electrophile, replaces the active hydrogens of indole, phenol, nitroalkane, etc., e.g.,

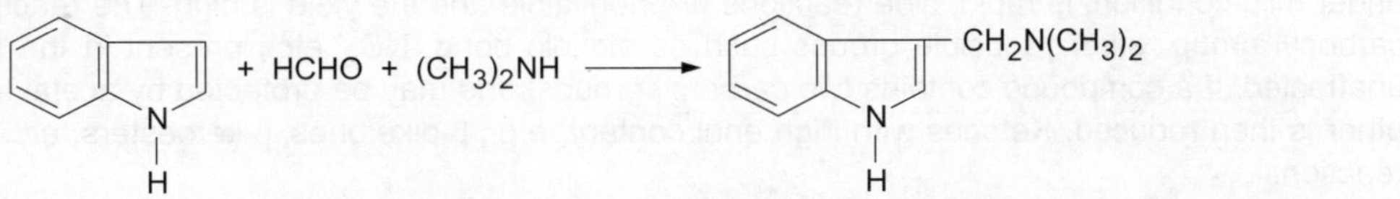

Gramine

The product may be quaternised and the amino group may be substituted by other groups.

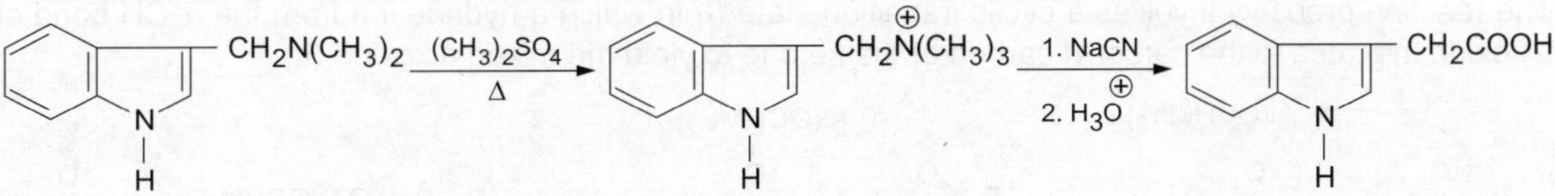

β-Indole acetic acid (Heteroauxin)

5. Tutocaine, a commercially useful anaesthetic, is prepared as below.

$$CH_3COCH_2CH_3 + HCHO + (CH_3)_2NHHCl \longrightarrow CH_3\cdot COCH(CH_3)\cdot CH_2N(CH_3)_2HCl \xrightarrow{\text{Redn.}}$$

$$CH_3-CH(OH)-CH\cdot(CH_3)\cdot CH_2\cdot N(CH_3)_2\cdot HCl \xrightarrow{p\text{-}H_2NC_6H_4COOH} \underset{\text{Tutocaine}}{CH_3-CH(O-COC_6H_4NH_2(p))-CH(CH_3)-CH_2-N(CH_3)_2\cdot HCl}$$

6. Synthesis of tryptophan—The amino acid, tryptophan is synthesized from the quaternary salt of gramine (see 4 above) and acetamidomalonic ester.

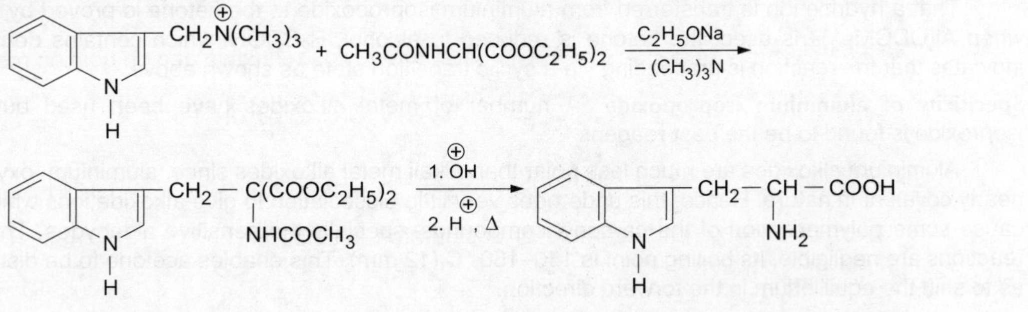

MEERWEIN–PONNDORF–VERLEY REDUCTION

The reaction involves the reduction of aldehydes or ketones to alcohols by treatment with aluminium isopropoxide in excess of isopropyl alcohol.

$$R-\overset{\overset{\displaystyle O}{\|}}{C}-R' + CH_3CH(OH)CH_3 \underset{}{\overset{Al(OCHMe_2)_3}{\rightleftharpoons}} RCHOHR' + CH_3-\overset{\overset{\displaystyle O}{\|}}{C}-CH_3$$

The reaction is reversible. The reverse reaction, called Oppenauer oxidation, is employed for the oxidation of alcohols, using aluminium *t*-butoxide as catalyst in the presence of excess acetone.

The reaction shifts in the forward direction by the removal of acetone by distillation. The reaction occurs under mild condition, is rapid, side reactions are negligible and the yield is high. The reaction is specific for carbonyl group, other reducible groups such as olefinic bond, NO_2, etc., present in the substrate remain unaffected. If a compound contains two carbonyl groups, one may be protected by acetal formation and the other is then reduced. Ketones with high enol content, e.g., β-diketones, β-ketoesters, etc., do not give this reaction.

Mechanism

The reaction probably involves a cyclic transition state (I) in which a hydride ion from the α-CH bond of the alkoxide migrates to the carbonyl carbon of the ketone to yield the mixed alkoxide (II).

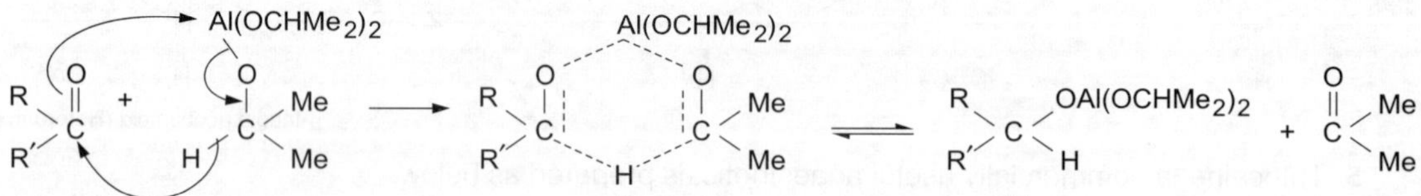

(I) (II)

An excess of isopropyl alcohol is used so that it exchanges with the mixed alkoxide (II) to liberate the reduced ketone (III), i.e., the desired alcohol.

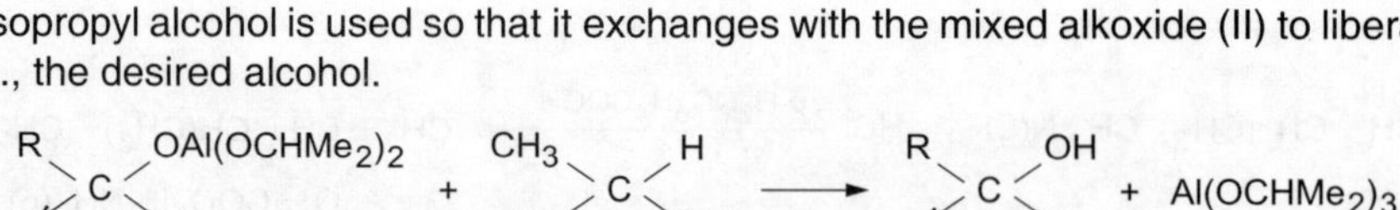

(III)

Thus, for the reduction one hydrogen is supplied by the catalyst and the other hydrogen by the solvent.

That a hydride ion is transferred from aluminium isopropoxide to the ketone is proved by the fact that when $Al(ODCMe_2)_3$ is used, the ketone is reduced to alcohol, R_2CDOH, which contains deuterium. This indicates that the reaction is proceeding via a cyclic transition state as shown above.

Specificity of aluminium isopropoxide A number of metal alkoxides have been used but aluminium isoproxide is found to be the best reagent.

Aluminium alkoxides are much less polar than alkali metal alkoxides since, aluminium–oxygen bond is nearly covalent in nature. Hence, this undergoes very little dissociation to give alkoxide ions which generally cause some polymerization of the carbonyl compounds, specially the sensitive aldehydes. Thus, the side reactions are negligible. Its boiling point is 140–150 °C (12 mm). This enables acetone to be distilled over so as to shift the equillibrium in the forward direction.

Applications

The reduction has many useful applications.

1. The reaction has been employed to reduce α,β-unsaturated aldehydes to α,β-unsaturated alcohols.

$$\underset{\text{Acraldehyde}}{CH_2{=}CH{-}CHO} \xrightarrow[(CH_3)_2CHOH]{Al(OCHMe_2)_3} \underset{\text{Allyl alcohol}}{CH_2{=}CH{-}CH_2OH}$$

$$\underset{\text{Crotonaldehyde}}{CH_3{-}CH{=}CH{-}CHO} \xrightarrow[(CH_3)_2CHOH]{Al(OCHMe_2)_3} \underset{\text{Crotyl alcohol}}{CH_3{-}CH{=}CH{-}CH_2OH}$$

2. Reduction of aromatic ketones

$$\underset{\text{Acetophenone}}{C_6H_5COCH_3} \xrightarrow[Me_2CHOH]{Al(OCHMe_2)_3} \underset{\alpha\text{-Methyl benzylalcohol}}{C_6H_5CHOHCH_3}$$

3. Reduction of alicyclic ketones

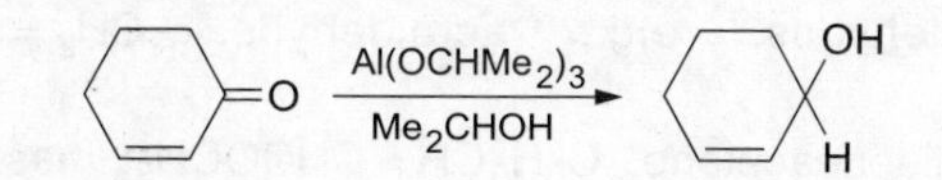

2-Cyclohexene-1-one → 2-Cyclohexene-1-ol

4. Reduction of α-halogenated ketones

$$\underset{\text{Trichloroacetone}}{CH_3COCCl_3} \xrightarrow[Me_2CHOH]{Al(OCHMe_2)_3} \underset{\text{Trichloropropanol-2}}{CH_3CHOHCCl_3}$$

5. Reduction of ketoesters

$$\underset{\text{Ethyl trimethylpyruvate}}{Me_3C{\cdot}CO{\cdot}COOC_2H_5} \xrightarrow[Me_2CHOH]{Al(OCHMe_2)_3} \underset{\text{Ethyl trimethylacetate}}{Me_3C{\cdot}CH(OH){\cdot}COOC_2H_5}$$

6. The reduction has been helpful during the course of synthesis of chloromycetin and oestradiol.

(a)

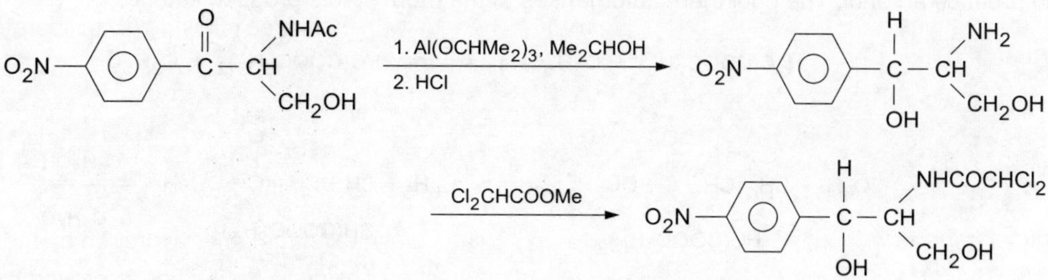

Chloromycetin

(b)

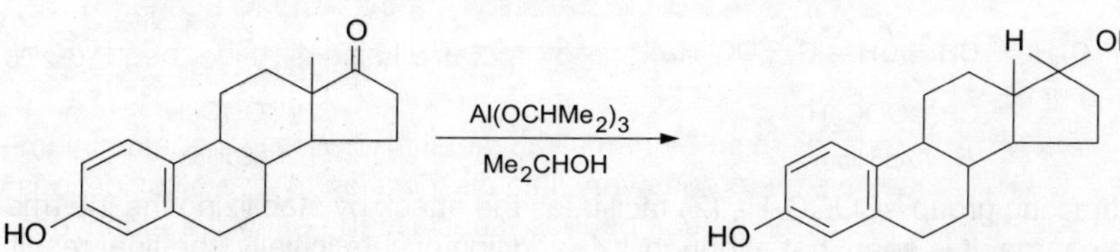

Oestrone → Oestradiol

MICHAEL REACTION

The base-catalysed addition of compounds having active methylene group (or relatively acidic hydrogens) to an activated olefinic bond of the type $-\overset{|}{C}=\overset{|}{C}-Z$ (Z = electron-withdrawing) is classified as Michael reaction.

$$\underset{\text{Ethyl cinnamate}}{C_6H_5-CH=CH-COOC_2H_5} + \underset{\text{Malonic ester}}{H_2C(COOC_2H_5)_2} \xrightarrow{C_2H_5ONa} C_6H_5-\underset{\underset{CH(COOC_2H_5)_2}{|}}{CH}-CH_2-COOC_2H_5$$

The compounds having an active methylene group or having relatively acidic hydrogens are called *donors* and the compounds having an activated olefinic bond are called *acceptors.* A large variety of donors and acceptors are employed in Michael reaction.

The donors include malonic ester, cyanoacetic ester, acetoacetic ester, phenylacetic acid ester, cyanoacetamide, aliphatic nitro compounds, benzyl cyanide, sulphones, cyclopentadienes, indenes, fluorenes, etc.

The acceptors include (a) aldehydes, e.g., acraldehyde, $CH_2=CH-CHO$; cinnamaldehyde, $C_6H_5CH=CHCHO$.

(b) ketones, e.g., benzylideneacetone, $C_6H_5CH=CHCOCH_3$; mesityloxide, $(CH_3)_2C=CHCOCH_3$; quinones, etc.

(c) nitriles, e.g., acrylonitrile, $CH_2=CH-CN$.

(d) esters of α,β-unsaturated acids, e.g., $C_6H_5-CH=CH-COOC_2H_5$.

Various types of basic catalysts are used. Most commonly used are alkali metal alkoxides, such as sodium or potassium ethoxides, potassium tertiary butoxide, potassium isopropoxide, etc. Mild basic catalysts such as 2° amines, 3° amines, piperidine and pyridine have been used with success.

Mechanism

The base generates a carbanion from the donor, malonic ester. The carbanion then adds to the β-carbon of the α,β-unsaturated ester acceptor, ethyl cinnamate to yield the anion (I) which takes up a proton from alcohol to produce an enol. The enol then tautomerises to the more stable product, ketone.

$$H_2C(COOC_2H_5) + C_2H_5ONa \rightleftharpoons \overset{\ominus}{H C}(COOC_2H_5)_2 + C_2H_5OH$$

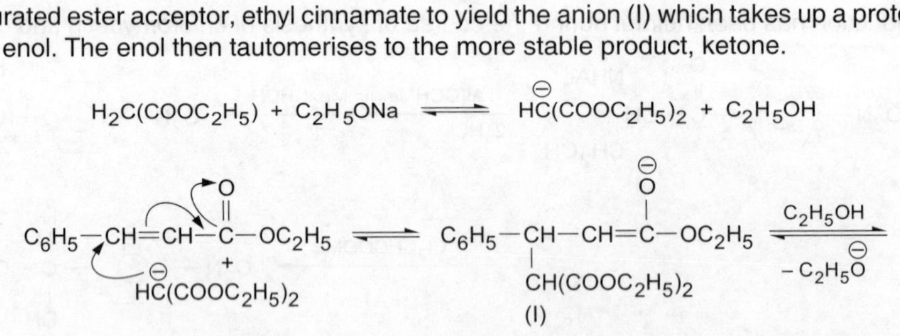

(1, 4-Addition) (α, β-Addition)

The electron-attracting group $-COOC_2H_5$ (Z) facilitates the attack by stabilizing the intermediate anion (I) by dispersal of the charge. It is seen that although 1,4- addition occurs initially, the final result is addition to the α,β-unsaturated carbons. This is because the enol reverts to the more stable ketone (recall that vinyl alcohol is unknown). In the presence of strong base, the product may undergo cyclisation. No cyclisation occurs with mild bases such as 2° or 3° amines and piperidine.

Compounds with two double bonds in conjugation with the electron-withdrawing group may undergo nucleophilic attack at β-carbon or δ-carbon to give three products. Thus:

(a) On attack at β-carbon

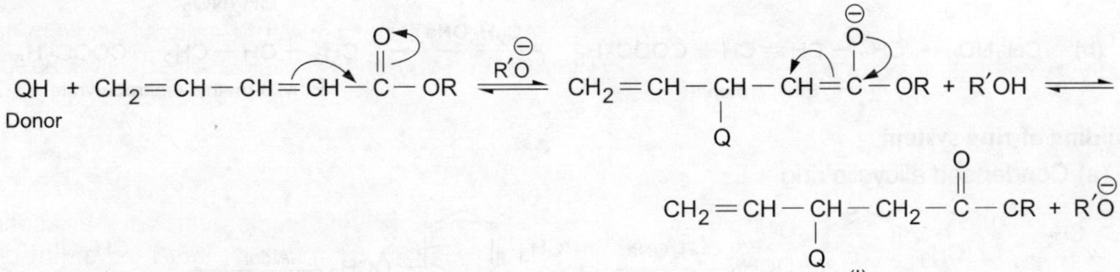

(I)

(b) On attack at δ-carbon

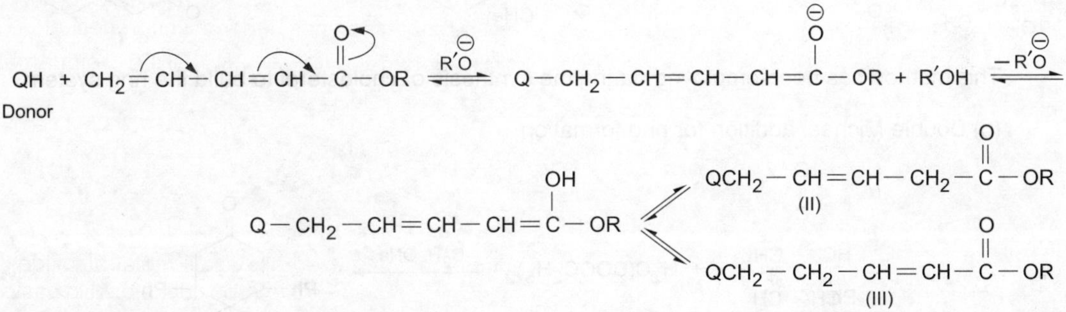

Since the double bond is conjugated in (III), it is the most stable of the three products. Hence it is the predominant product.

Applications

The reaction is of great synthetic importance since a variety of organic compounds can be synthesized with the help of this reaction.

1. Synthesis of polybasic acids

(a) Tricarballylic acids

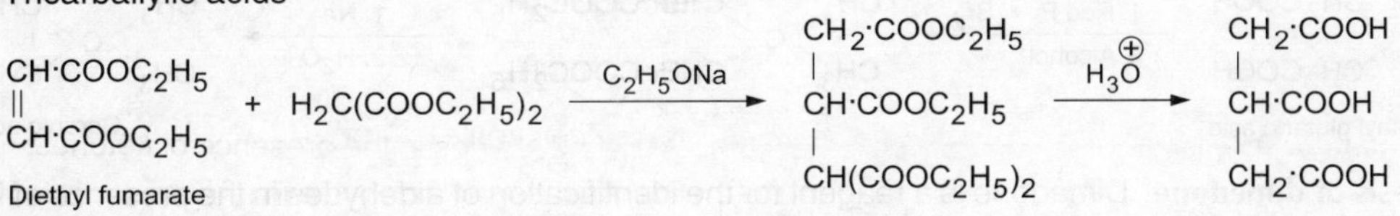

Diethyl fumarate

Propan-1, 2, 3-tricarboxylic acid

Esters of tricarballylic acid are used as plasticisers.

(b) Aconitic acid

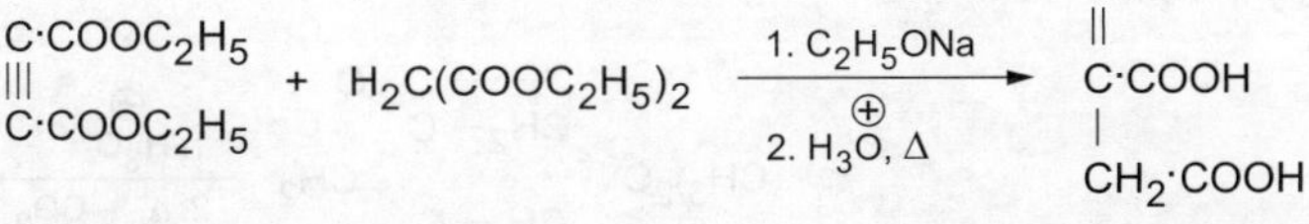

Aconitic acid

Aconitic acid is used in the preparation of medicines for releaving pain (analgesic) and reducing fever (febrifuge). Its esters are used as plasticisers.

2. Preparation of cyano– and nitro– compounds

(a)

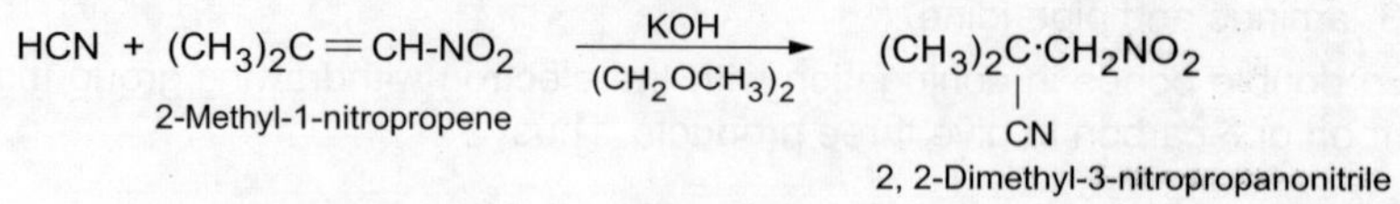

(b)

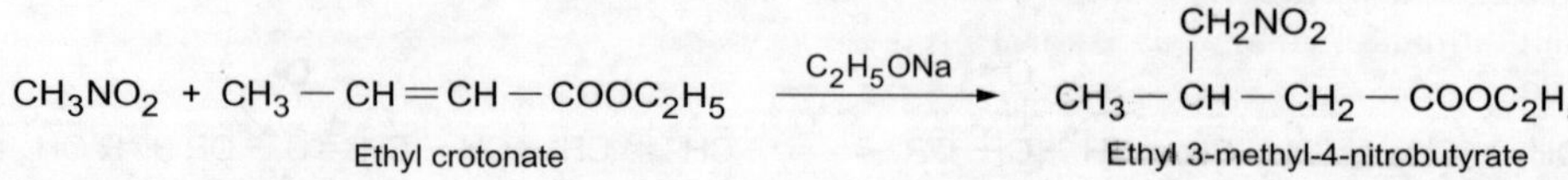

3. Building of ring system

(a) Condensed alicyclic ring

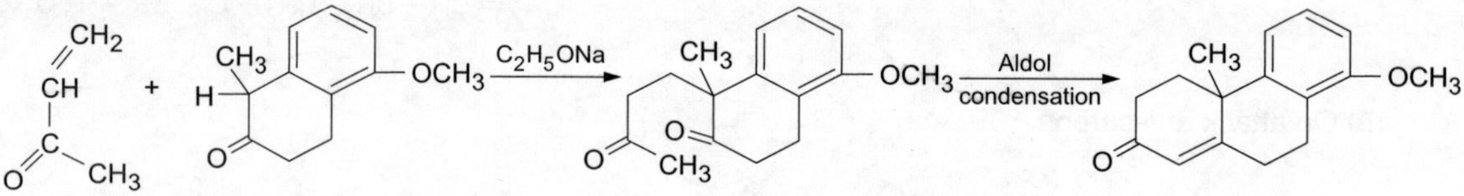

This method has been employed during the synthesis of cholesterol to build the ring system.

(b) Double Michael addition for ring formation

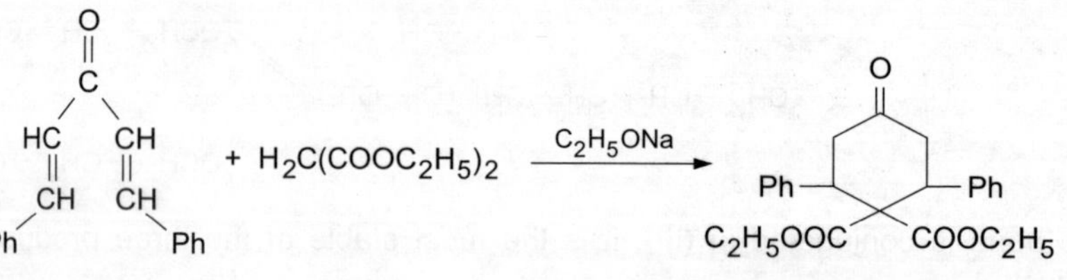

(c) Cyclopropane derivative—Caronic acid

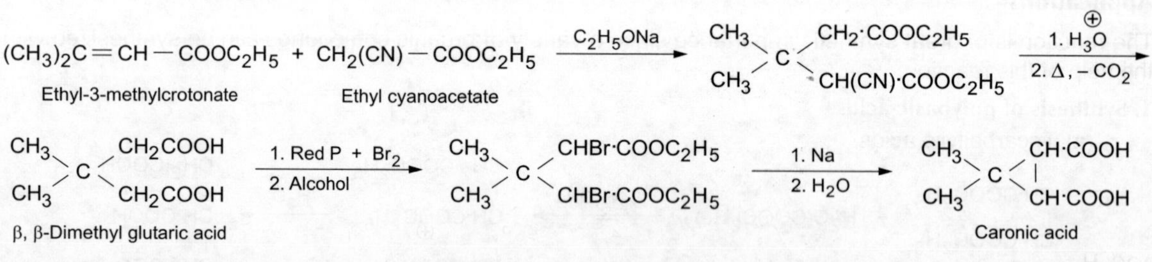

4. Synthesis of dimedone Dimedone is a reagent for the identification of aldehydes in the presence of ketones.

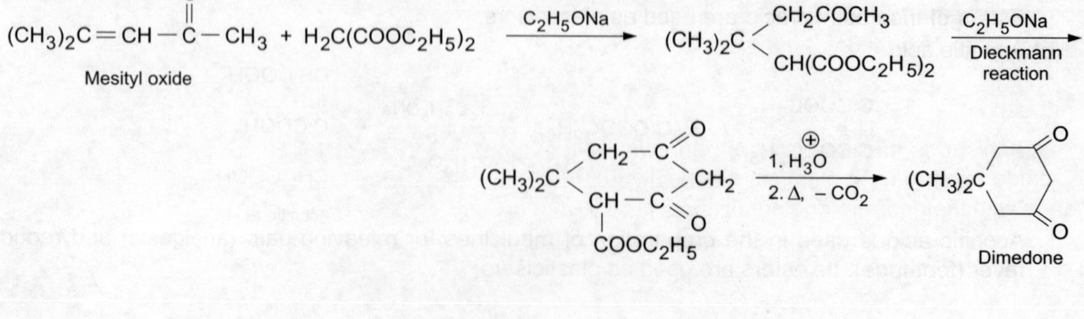

Dimedone is also employed for the separation of aldehydes from ketones because it reacts only with aldehydes.

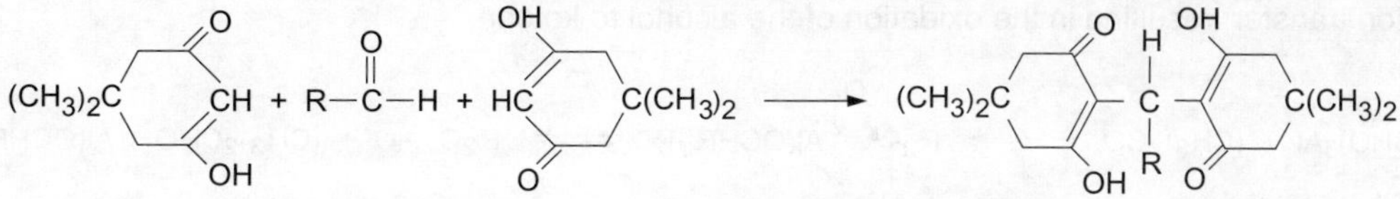

Reaction with formaldehyde is quantitative and hence, the reagent is used for the quantitative estimation of formaldehyde.

5. Synthesis of amino acids

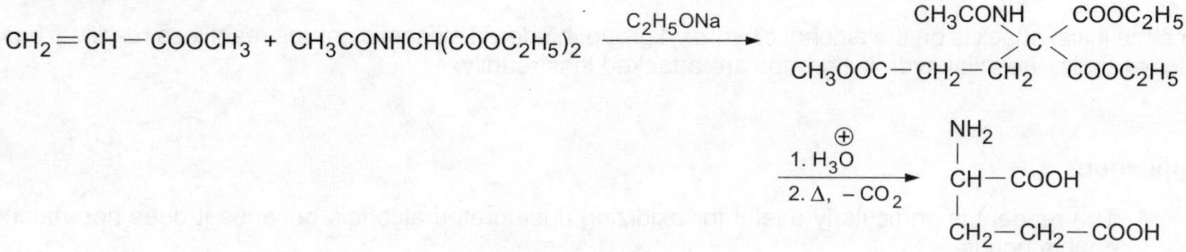

(DL) Glutamic acid

Michael reaction has been employed to synthesize anthracene from naphthalene.

OPPENAUER OXIDATION

The reaction is the reverse of Meerwein–Ponndorf–Verley reduction. The reaction involves the oxidation of a secondary alcohol with a ketone and a base to the corresponding ketone of the alcohol.

Commonly used ketones are acetone, methyl ethyl ketone and cyclohexanone. Commonly used bases are aluminium *tert*-butoxide, aluminium isoporpoxide, potassium *tert*-butoxide, etc.

Thus, when a secondary alcohol in acetone or cyclohexanone is refluxed with aluminium *tert*-butoxide in benzene or toluene solution, the secondary alcohol is dehydrogenated to a ketone and the hydrogens are transferred to acetone or cyclohexanone converting them to alcohols.

$$\underset{2^\circ\text{ Alcohol}}{R_2CHOH} + \underset{\text{Acetone}}{(CH_3)_2CO} \xrightleftharpoons{Al(OCMe_3)_3} \underset{\text{Ketone}}{R_2CO} + \underset{2^\circ\text{ Alcohol}}{CH_3CHOHCH_3}$$

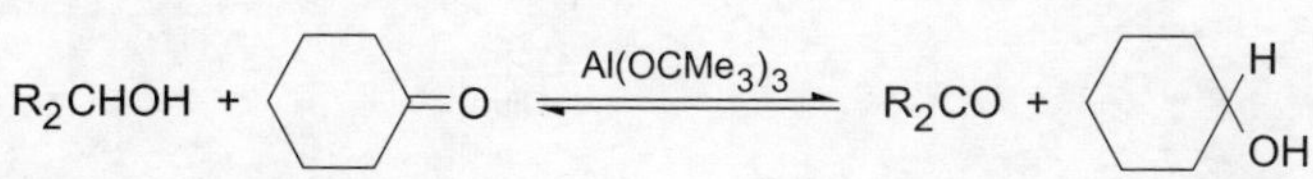

Cyclohexanone Cyclohexanol

Primary alcohols may also be oxidized to aldehydes if acetone is replaced by a better hydrogen acceptor, e.g., *p*-benzoquinone. The equillibrium can be controlled by the amount of acetone, an excess of which favours the oxidation of the alcohol.

Mechanism

The mechanism is the reverse of Meerwein–Ponndorf–Verley reaction. The alcohol and aluminium *tert*-butoxide react to form aluminium derivative of the 2° alcohol. [Metal alkoxides undergo rapid acid–base exchange with their corresponding alcohols.]

$$3R_2CHOH + Al(OCMe_3)_3 \rightleftharpoons (R_2CHO)_3Al + 3Me_3C(OH)$$

The aluminium derivative then forms with acetone a cyclic transition state which undergoes internal hydride ion transfer, resulting in the oxidation of the alcohol to ketone.

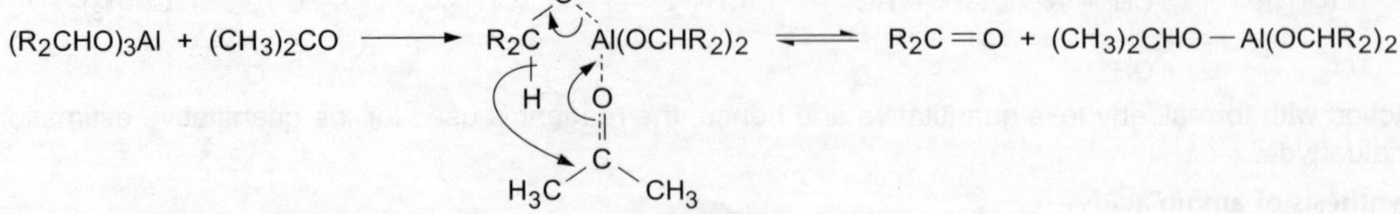

Since the initial attack is on the alcoholic hydroxyl group, hindered alcoholic groups react less readily. Thus, in cyclohexanols, the axial hydroxyl groups are attacked less readily.

Applications

1. The reagent is particularly useful for oxidizing unsaturated alcohols because it does not affect the double bonds.

(a)
$$CH_3-\underset{OH}{CH}-CH{=}CH-CH{=}\underset{CH_3}{C}-CH{=}CH_2 \xrightarrow[\text{Acetone–benzene}]{Al(OCMe_3)_3} CH_3-\overset{O}{\overset{\|}{C}}-CH{=}CH-CH{=}\underset{CH_3}{C}-CH{=}CH_2$$

6-Methyl-3, 5, 7-octatriene-2-ol → 6-Methyl-3, 5, 7-octatriene-2-one

(b)
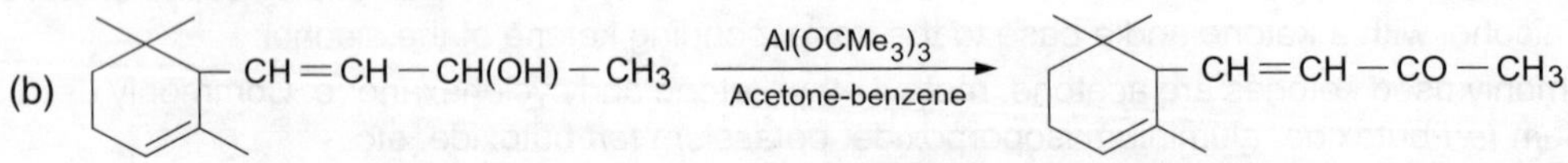

α-Ionol → α-Ionone

2. Primary unsaturated alcohols have been oxidized to aldehydes in the presence of good hydrogen acceptors, e.g., *p*-benzoquinone. In some cases acetaldehyde or cinnamaldehyde have been used.

(a)
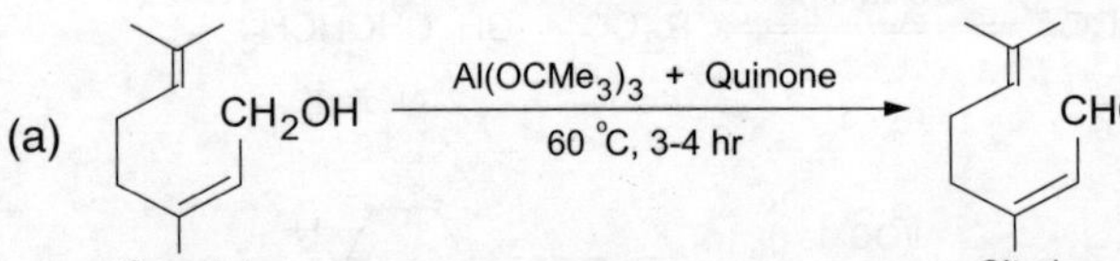

Geraniol → Citral

(b)
$$(CH_3)_2C{=}CH-CH_2-CH_2-CH_2OH + C_6H_5-CH{=}CH-CHO$$

5-Methyl-4-hexene-1-ol + Cinnamaldehyde

$$\xrightarrow{Al(OCMe_3)_3} (CH_3)_2C{=}CH-CH_2-CH_2-CHO + C_6H_5-CH{=}CH-CH_2OH$$

5-Methyl-4-hexenal + Cinnamyl alcohol

The reaction is successful with low-boiling aldehydes which can be distilled off as it is formed.

(c) The terminal CH_2OH group of the unsaturated side chain in Vit A_1 is oxidized to aldehyde group by using aluminium isopropoxide in the presence of acetaldehyde and benzene and prolonged heating at 70 °C.

3. The β,γ-unsaturated alcohols undergo oxidation with migration of double bond to form α,β-unsaturated ketones.

$$R-CH=CH-CH_2-CH(OH)-R \xrightarrow[p\text{-Benzoquinone}]{Al(OCMe_3)_3} R-CH_2-CH=CH-CO-R$$

This reaction finds numerous applications in steroid chemistry.

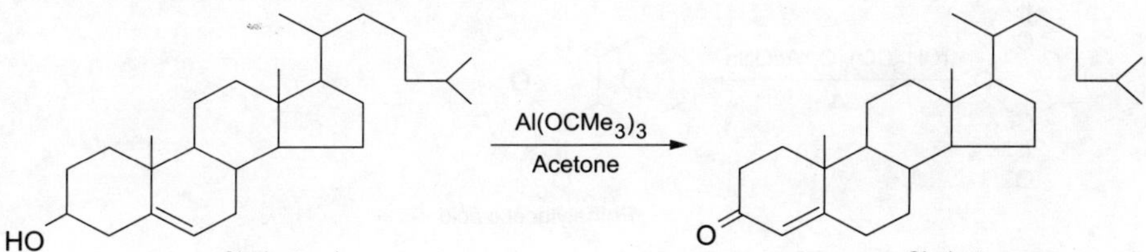

Cholesterol Cholestenone

4. Formates (but not acetates or benzoates) have been oxidized to ketones.

$$R_2CH-O-\overset{O}{\overset{\|}{C}}-H \xrightarrow{[O]} R_2CH-O-\overset{O}{\overset{\|}{C}}-OH \xrightarrow{-CO_2} R_2CH-OH \xrightarrow[\text{Acetone}]{Al(OCMe_3)_3} R_2C=O$$

5. Alicyclic alcohols have been oxidized to alicyclic ketones.

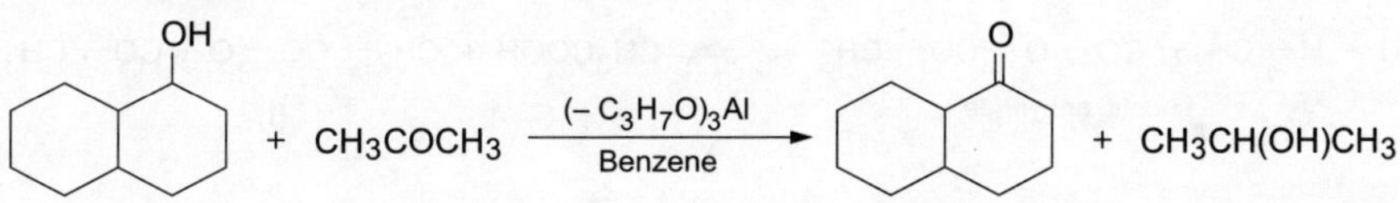

α-Decanol α-Decalone

Sensitive alcohols can be oxidized under mild conditions by using fluorenone which is a strong hydrogen acceptor.

PERKIN REACTION

In Perkin reaction, condensation has been effected between aromatic aldehydes and aliphatic acid anhydrides in the presence of sodium or potassium salt of the acid corresponding to the anhydride, to yield α,β-unsaturated aromatic acids.

The acid anhydride should have at least two α-hydrogens.

$$C_6H_5CHO + (CH_3CO)_2O \xrightarrow[170-180\,^{\circ}C,\,5\,h]{AcONa} C_6H_5-CH=CH-COOH + CH_3COOH$$

Besides simple aromatic aldehydes, their vinylogs, heterocyclic aldehydes and even phthalic anhydride (as the carbonyl component) give this reaction.

(a) $$C_6H_5-CH=CH-CHO \xrightarrow[\Delta]{(CH_3CO)_2O,\ AcONa} C_6H_5-CH=CH-CH=CH-COOH$$

5-Phenyl-pent-2,4-dienoic acid

(b) 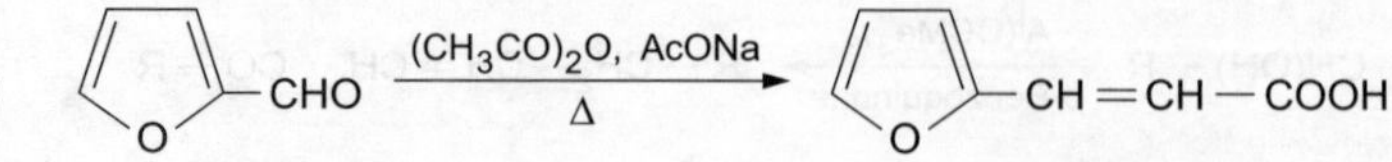

3-(α-Furyl)-acrylic acid

(c) 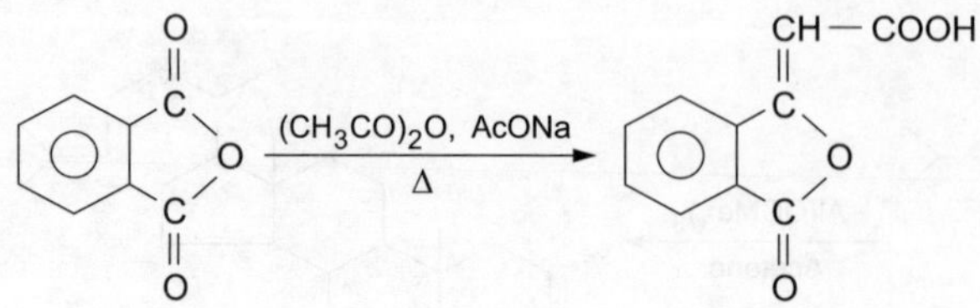

Phthalylacetic acid

Mechanism

It is suggested that the acetate ion abstracts a proton from the α-carbon of the anhydride producing a carbanion (I) which then attacks the carbonyl group of the aldehyde. The product (II) then abstracts a proton from the acid to form aldol-type compound (III). The latter then undergoes dehydration in the presence of hot (ca 140 °C) acetic anhydride.

On pouring the hot mixture in water, the mixed anhydride is hydrolysed to α, β-unsaturated acid (IV).

$$CH_3COONa \rightleftharpoons CH_3CO\overset{\ominus}{O} + \overset{\oplus}{Na}$$

$$CH_3CO\overset{\ominus}{O} + H-CH_2-CO-O-CO-CH_3 \rightleftharpoons CH_3COOH + \overset{\ominus}{C}H_2-CO-O-CO-CH_3$$

Acetic anhydride (I)

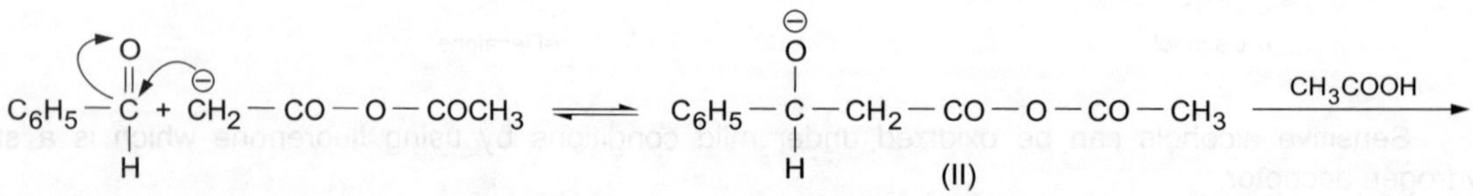

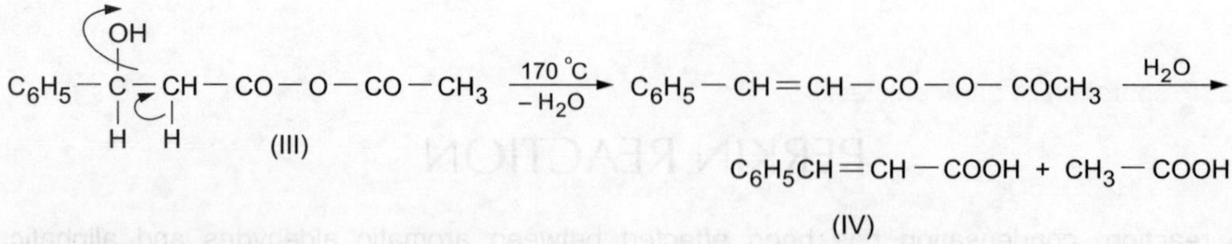

Prolonged heating (about 5 h) and high temp. is required, since a weak base (acetate ion) has to react with a weak acid (anhydride).

That the anhydride adds to the aldehyde is proved by the fact that when benzaldehyde, acetic anhydride and trimethyl amine or pyridine are heated, cinnamic acid is obtained, but when benzaldehyde, sodium acetate and pyridine are heated, it is not obtained. Thus, the alkali salt acts only as the catalyst.

Meta-directing groups in the aromatic ring promotes the reaction. When anhydride with one α-H atom is used, no dehydration is possible and an aldol-type product is isolated.

The reaction is specific for aromatic aldehydes which cannot undergo self-condensation in the presence of the basic catalyst.

Applications

Perkin reaction has many useful synthetic applications.

1. Preparation of α-substituted unsaturated acids

$$C_6H_5-CHO + (CH_3CH_2CO)_2O \xrightarrow[\Delta]{AcONa} C_6H_5-CH=C(CH_3)-COOH$$

α-Methylcinnamic acid

2. Synthesis of coumarin

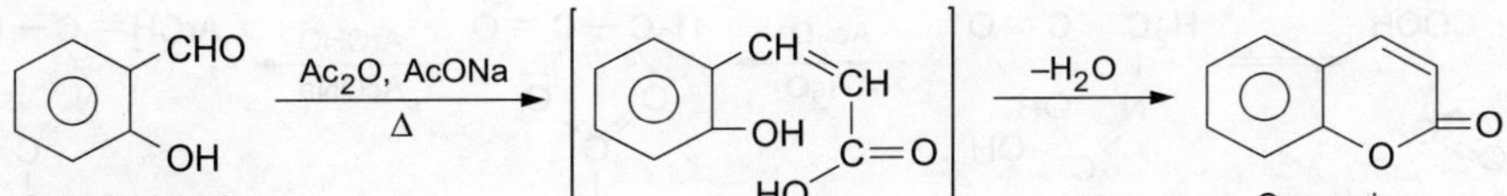

Salicylaldehyde → Coumarin

3. Synthesis of carbostyril (nitrogen analogue of coumarin)

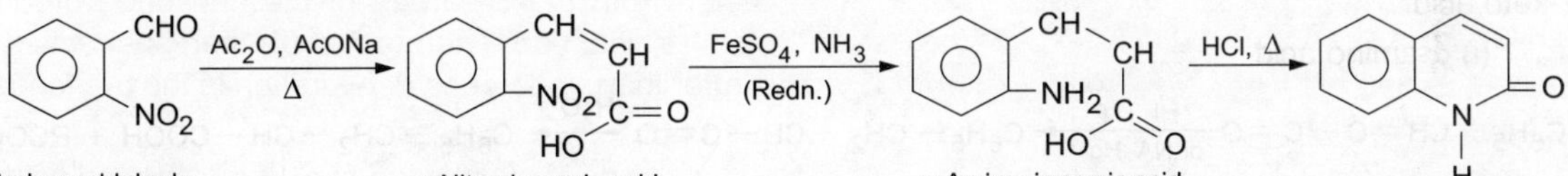

o-Nitrobenzaldehyde → *o*-Nitrocinnamic acid → *o*-Aminocinnamic acid → Carbostyril

4. Synthesis of phenanthrene

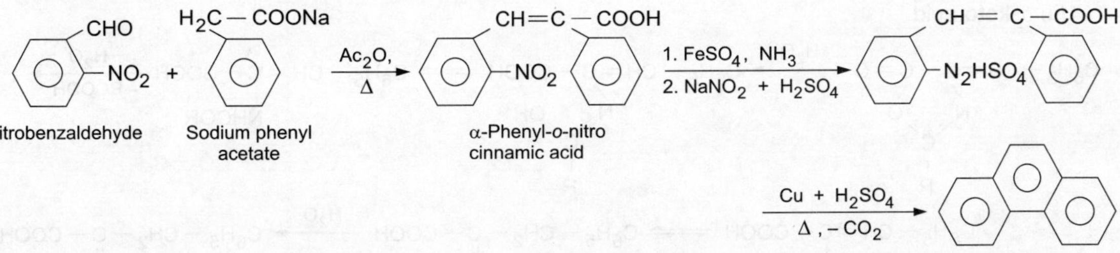

o-Nitrobenzaldehyde + Sodium phenyl acetate → α-Phenyl-*o*-nitro cinnamic acid → Phenanthrene

5. Preparation of paraconic acid

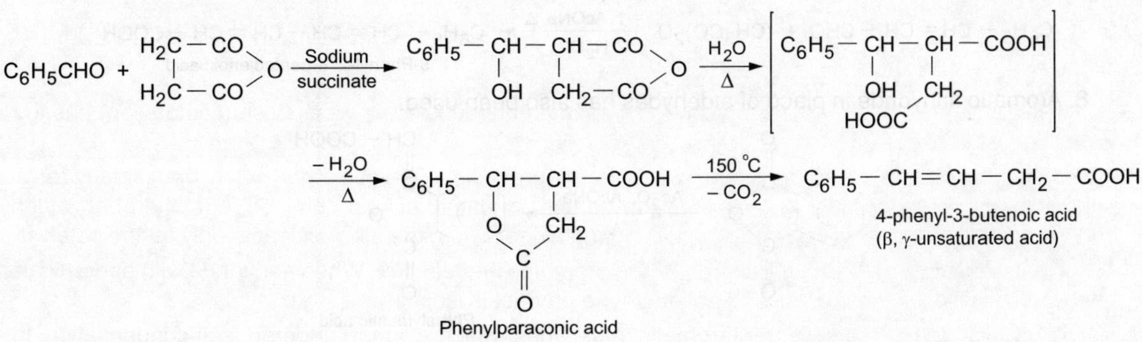

Phenylparaconic acid → 4-phenyl-3-butenoic acid (β, γ-unsaturated acid)

6. Erlenmeyer's Azlactone synthesis

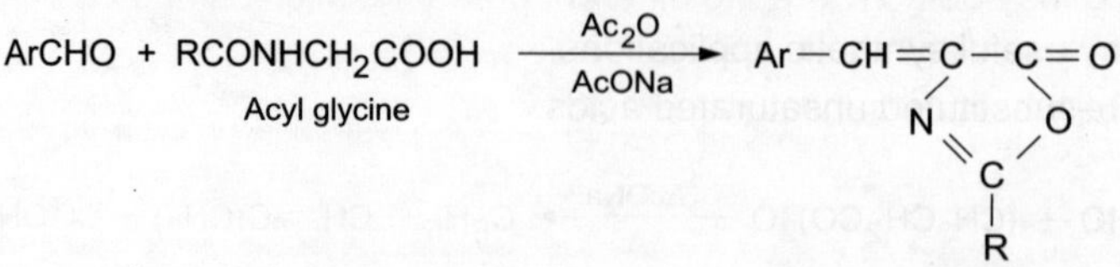

Acyl glycine — Azlactone

It is believed that benzoyl or acetyl glycine first forms a cyclic compound in hot acetic anhydride. The active methylene group of the cyclic compound then reacts with the aldehyde.

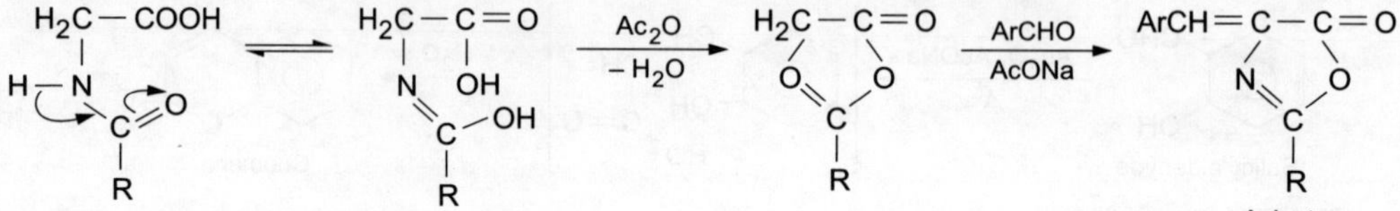

Azlactone

Azlactone on reduction followed by hydrolysis gives α-amino acid and on simple hydrolysis gives α-keto acid.

(i) α-amino acid

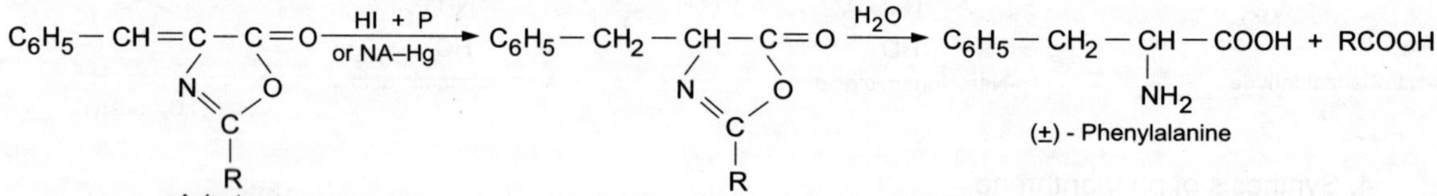

Azlactone — (±) - Phenylalanine

(ii) α-keto acid

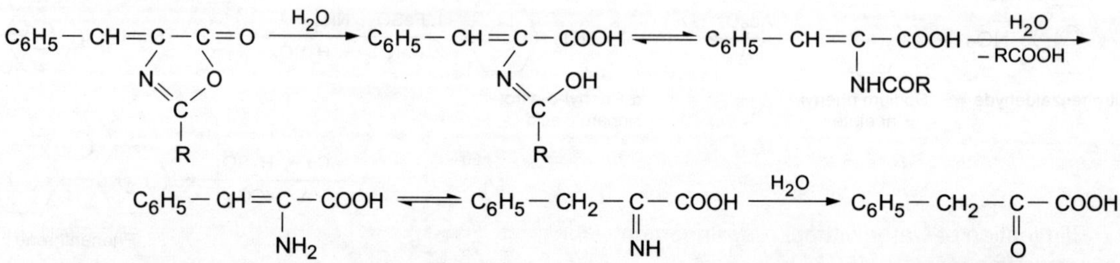

Phenylpyruvic acid

7. Preparation of vinylogs of cinnamic acid

$$C_6H_5-CH=CH-CHO + (CH_3CO)_2O \xrightarrow[2. H_2O]{1. AcONa, \Delta} C_6H_5-CH=CH-CH=CH-COOH$$

5-Phenyl-2, 4-pentadienoic acid

8. Aromatic anhydride in place of aldehydes has also been used.

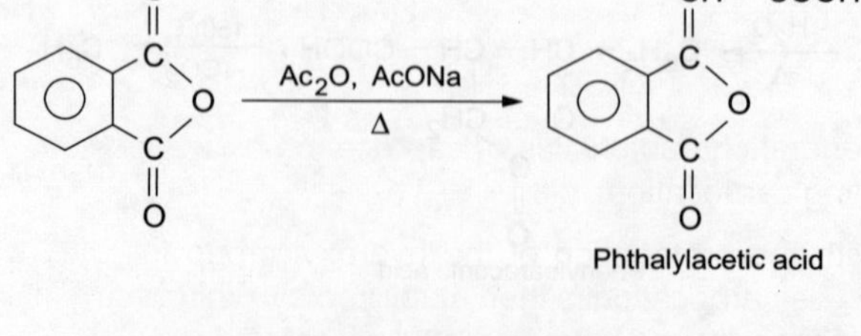

Phthalylacetic acid

Phthalylacetic acid may be converted to different products (Michael and Gabriel), thus:

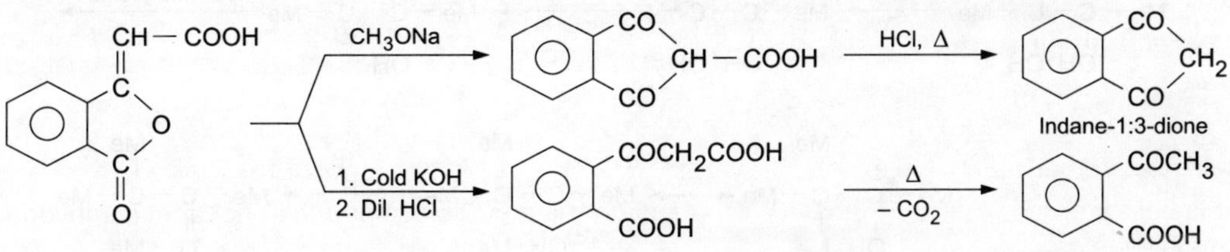

Indane-1:3-dione

o-Acetylbenzoic acid

PINACOL–PINACOLONE REARRANGEMENT

The acid-catalysed rearrangement of vic diols (1, 2-diols) to ketones or aldehydes with elimination of water is known as pinacol or pinacol–pinacolone rearrangement. The name was given from the classical example of the conversion of pinacol to pinacolone.

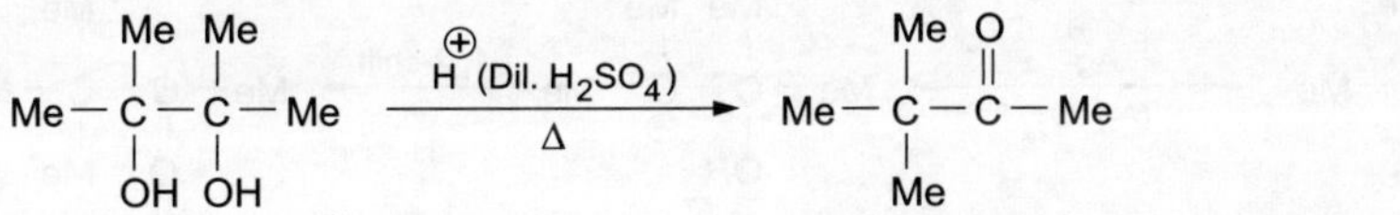

Pinacol — Pinacolone (Methyl-*t*-butyl ketone)

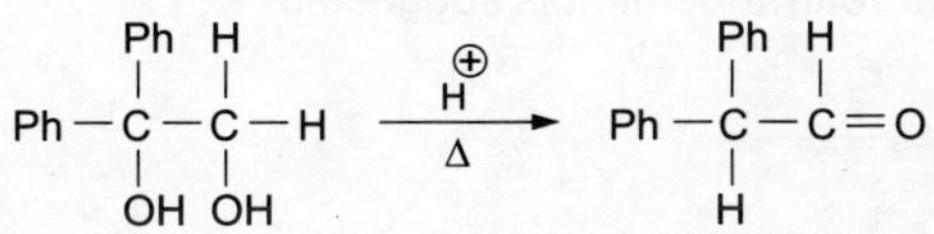

2, 2-Diphenyl-1, 2-glycol — 2, 2-Diphenyl acetaldehyde

Elimination of water without rearrangement—the normal reaction of alcohols—may be achieved under drastic conditions (Al_2O_3, 450 °C).

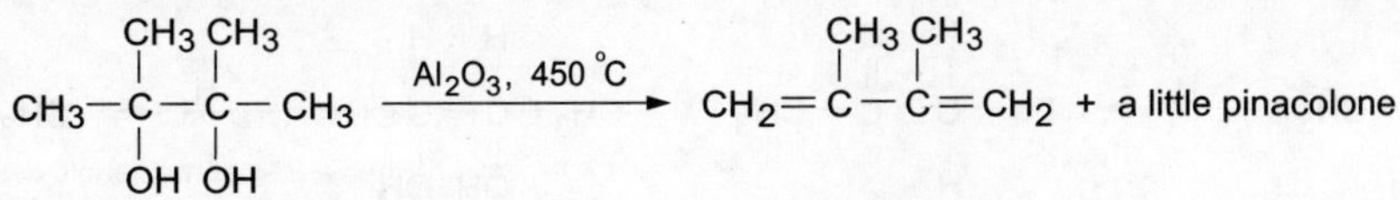

The rearrangement has been successfully carried out with various polysubstituted glycols.

Mechanism

The reaction involves the general characteristics of carbocation rearrangement in which the driving force is the stabilization of the resulting carbocation.

The reaction starts with the protonation of the hydroxyl group followed by elimination of water and formation of carbocation (I). The carbocation is then stabilized by Whitmore 1, 2-shift. Finally, elimination of a proton from the stable carbocation (II) gives the carbonyl compound.

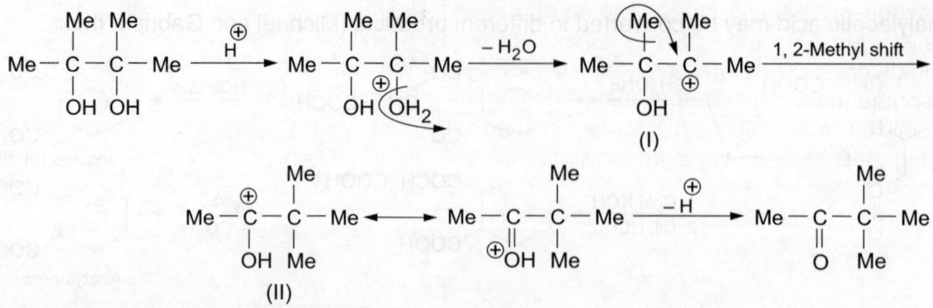

The carbocation (I), though tertiary, prefers to form (II) for its resonance stability.

The mechanism is supported by the fact that any carbocation in which the positive charge is on the carbon adjacent to the one bearing the hydroxyl group $\left(-\overset{|}{\underset{\oplus}{C}}-\overset{|}{\underset{|}{C}}-OH\right)$ also undergoes similar rearrangement. Thus,

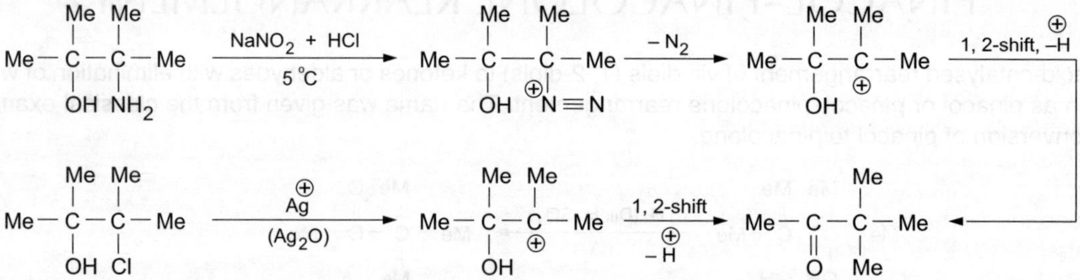

The loss of water and migration of the alkyl group may be very rapid or simultaneous. Probably the migrating group does not become completely free before it is partially bonded (III) to the adjacent positively charged carbon, i.e., a type of intramolecular rearrangement is suggested.

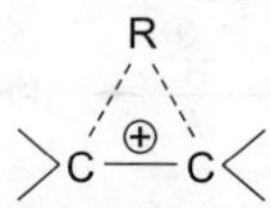

(III)

Evidence in favour of this are (a) the migrating group retains its configuration, if chiral and (b) no cross over products are obtained when a mixture of two nearly similar 1, 2-diols is treated with acid.

Migratory aptitude Migration order in general is H > aryl > alkyl.

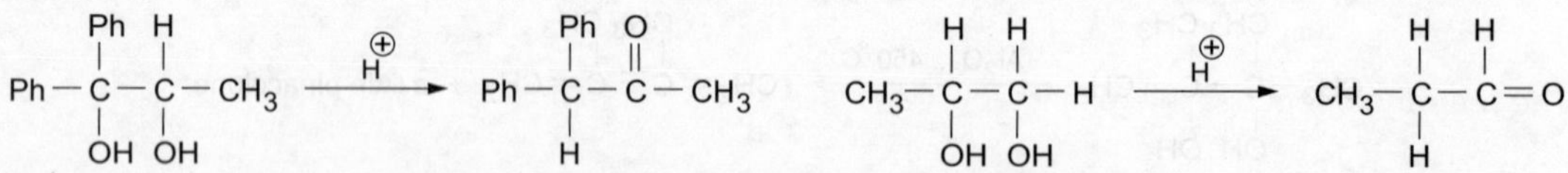

As the migrating group migrates with its electron pair, the more nucleophilic group might be expected to migrate. Thus, the order of migration amongst the aryl groups is *p*-anisyl > *p*-tolyl > phenyl > *p*-chlorophenyl, etc.

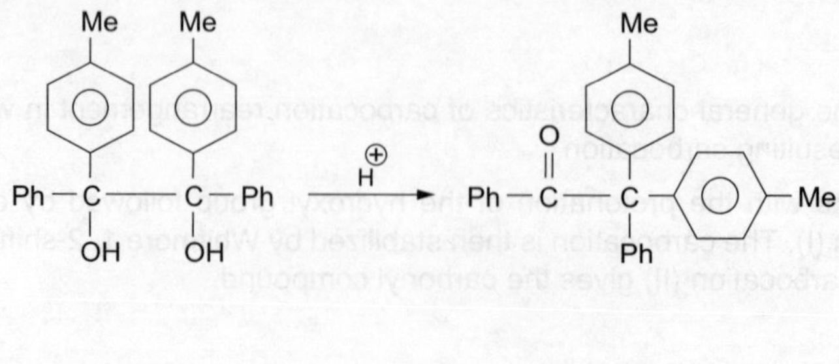

Obviously, electron-withdrawing groups will retard the migration. The migratory aptitude amongst the alkyl groups is $Me_3C > Me_2CH > Me$. However, the stability of the initially formed carbocation may offset the migratory aptitude order. The initial carbocation is formed by the loss of that hydroxyl group which results in the formation of the most stable carbocation. Thus, in the compound 1, 1-dimethyl-2, 2-diphenyl glycol, the resonance-stabilized carbocation (IV) is formed instead of (V) and so it is the methyl group and not the phenyl group which migrates, contrary to the above sequence.

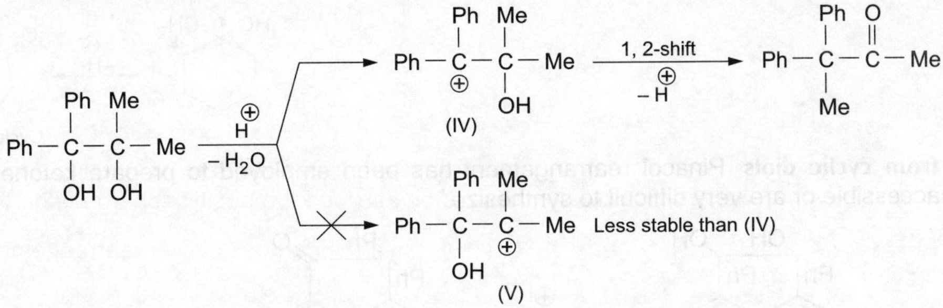

Steric hindrance may affect the rate of migration—*p*-anisyl group migrates 1000 times faster than *o*-anisyl group.

The migrating group attacks from the trans position (back side) to the leaving group. This has important effect in cyclic systems. Thus, the two isomers of 1, 2-dimethyl-cyclohexane-1, 2-diol give different products due to different orientations of the methyl and hydroxyl groups. The one (VI) in which the Me and OH groups are *trans* to each other gives 2, 2-dimethylcyclohexanone by methyl shift. The other (VII) in which the Me and OH groups are *cis* to each other undergoes ring methylene group shift instead of Me-shift with consequent ring contraction to give 1-acetyl-1-methylcyclopentane (VIII).

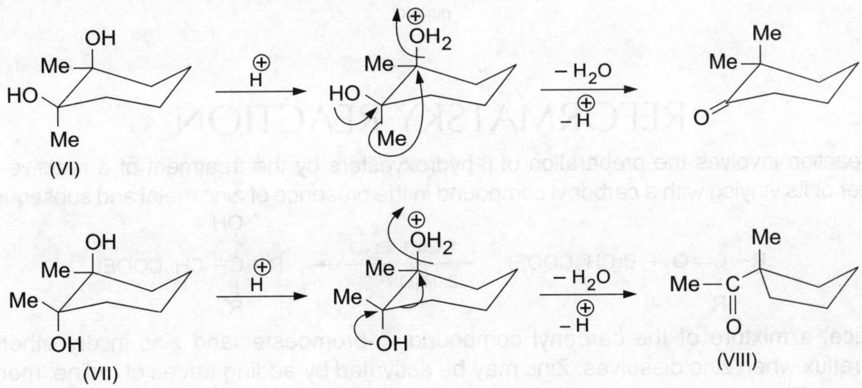

The rearrangement has interesting applications in synthesis.

Applications

1. Synthesis of carbonyl compounds from alkenes Isobutyraldehyde may be prepared on a large scale from isobutylene.

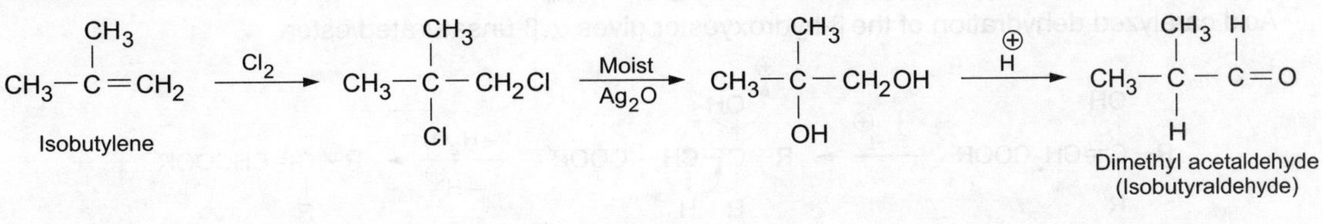

2. Ring expansion of cyclic ketones Cyclohexanone can be converted to cycloheptanone in good yield.

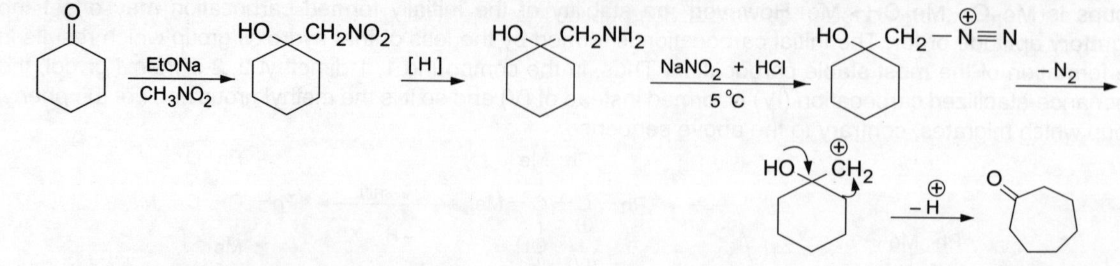

Cycloheptanone

3. Ketones from cyclic diols Pinacol rearrangement has been employed to prepare ketones which are otherwise inaccessible or are very difficult to synthesize.

(i)

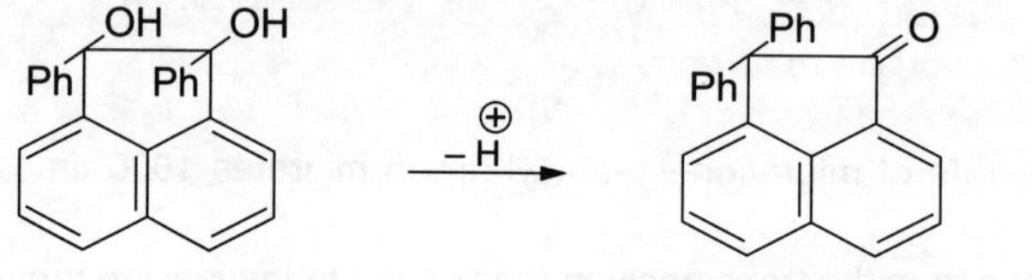

7, 8-Diphenylacenaphthene -7, 8-diol 7-Oxo-8, 8-diphenylacenaphthene

(ii)

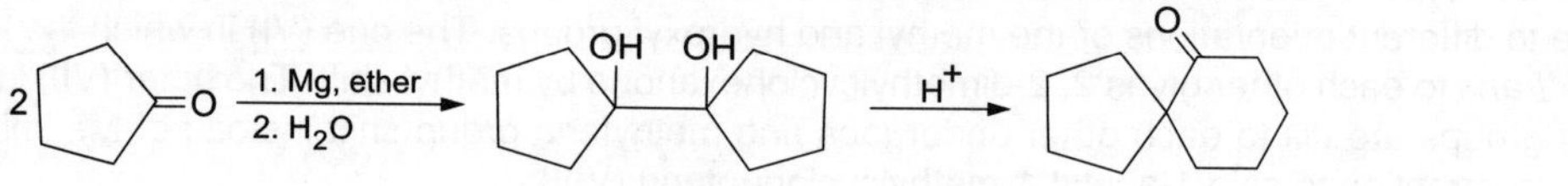

Cyclopentanone pinacol

REFORMATSKY REACTION

Reformatsky reaction involves the preparation of β-hydroxyesters by the treatment of a reactive organic halide e.g., α-haloester or its vinylog with a carbonyl compound in the presence of zinc metal and subsequent hydrolysis.

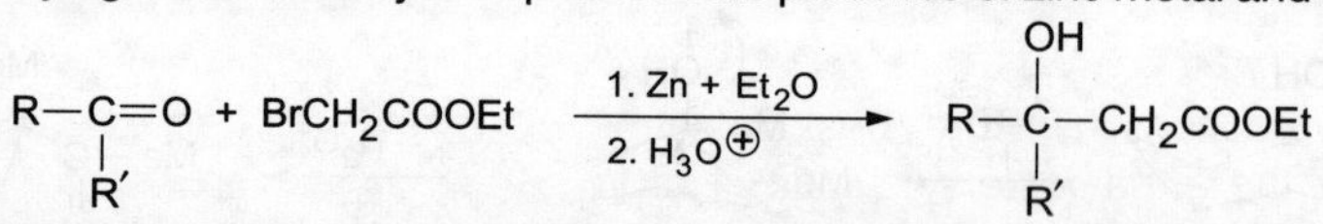

In practice, a mixture of the carbonyl compound, α-bromoester and zinc in dry ether is cautiously heated under reflux when zinc dissolves. Zinc may be activated by adding traces of iodine, mercuric bromide or copper powder. The mixture is then treated with ice-cold dilute sulphuric acid and ether layer separated. Ether is distilled off when β-hydroxyester is obtained.

Generally used solvents for this reaction are ether, benzene, toluene, THF etc. In place of zinc, activated indium, tin or zinc-copper couple have been used.

The aldehyde or ketone may be aliphatic, aromatic, or heterocyclic and may contain various functional groups which remain unaffected (difference from Grignard reagent).

Acid catalyzed dehydration of the β-hydroxyester gives α, β-unsaturated ester.

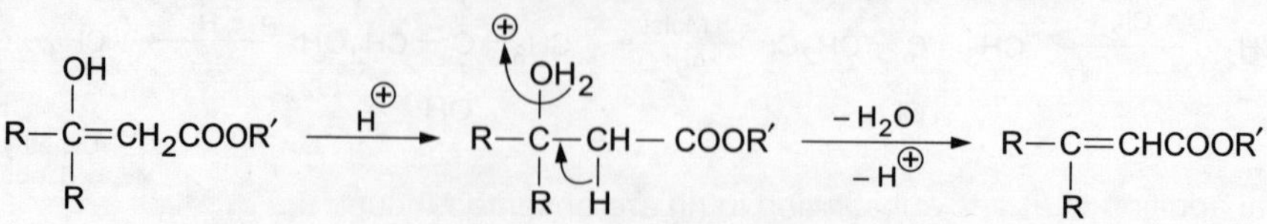

Mechanism At first zinc and the α-bromoester react to form an organo-zinc intermediate (I). The zinc salt of the enol ester then adds to the carbonyl group of the aldehyde or ketone. Subsequent hydrolysis gives β-hydroxyester.

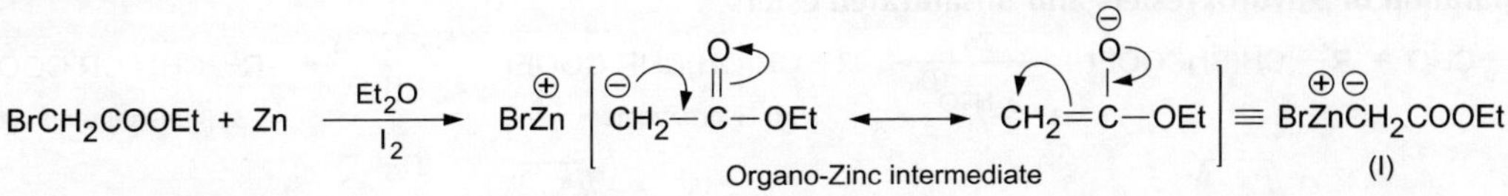

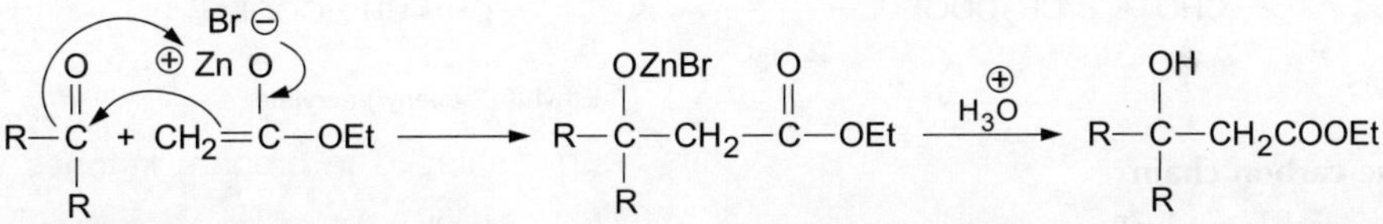

The initial formation of the oragno-zinc intermediate (I) has been substantiated. The X-ray crystallography of the solid derived on treatment of t-butyl bromoacetate with zinc indicates its structure to be (II). This structure may be seen has some characteristic resemblance to (I).

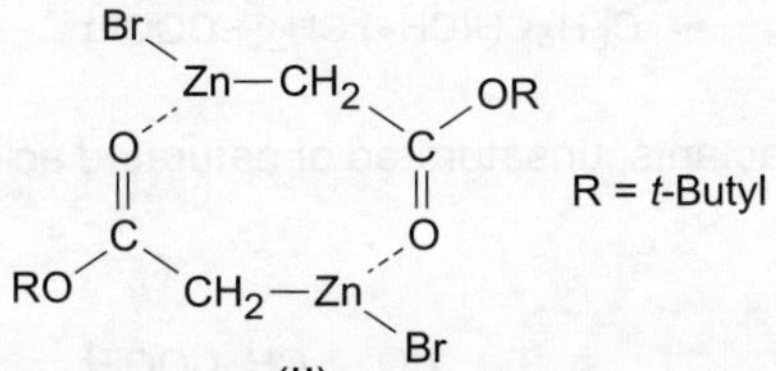

(II)

Reformatsky reaction is closely related to Grignard reaction. The initially formed intermediate, $BrZnCH_2COOEt$ is analogous to RMgX. Grignard reagent cannot be derived from α- haloesters since it reacts with active halogens. The organo-zinc compounds are less reactive than Grignard reagent and do not normally react with their own ester group. It cannot however add to sterically hindered carbonyl compounds i.e., with too highly substituted ketones. In such case it reacts perforce with its own ester group producing a β-ketoester.

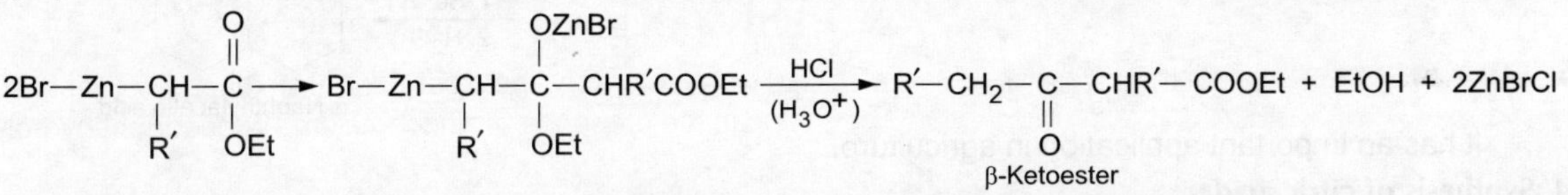

Reformatsky reaction, therefore, best proceeds with aldehydes, methyl ketones and cyclic ketones. Reactivity order of the α-haloesters is iodo > bromo > chloro. Zinc-copper couple may be used with chloroesters with advantage. The β- and γ-haloesters are much less reactive. However, γ-bromocrotonic ester being a vinylog of α- haloester is as much reactive.

Besides aldehydes and ketones, nitriles (Blaise reaciton) and carboxylic esters have been used as substrates.

(i) 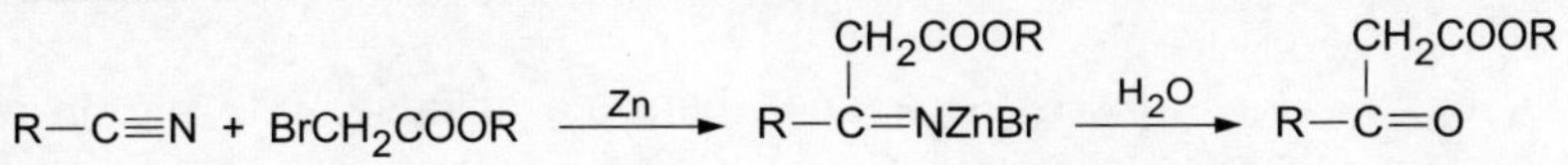

(ii) 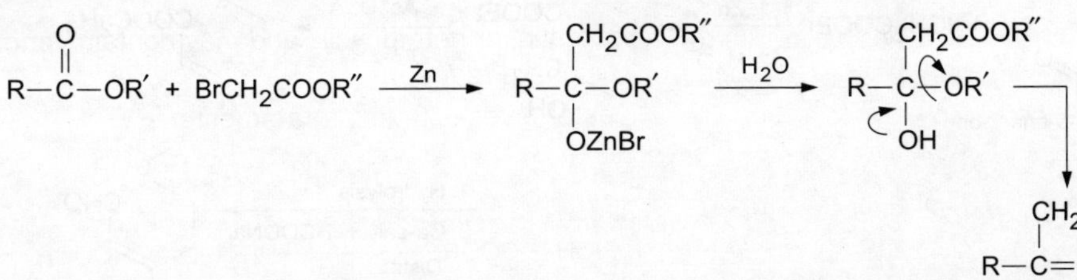

Normal addition in (i) and substitution in (ii) are observed though the products are the same.

Applications

The reaction has many valuable applications:

1. Preparation of β-hydroxyesters and unsaturated esters

$$R{-}CHO + R'{-}CH(Br)COOEt \xrightarrow[2.\ H_3O^{\oplus}]{1.\ Zn} \underset{\beta\text{-Hydroxyester}}{R{-}CH(OH)CHR'COOEt} \xrightarrow[-H_2O]{H_2SO_4,\ \Delta} \underset{\alpha,\beta\text{-unsaturated ester}}{R{-}CH{=}CR'COOEt}$$

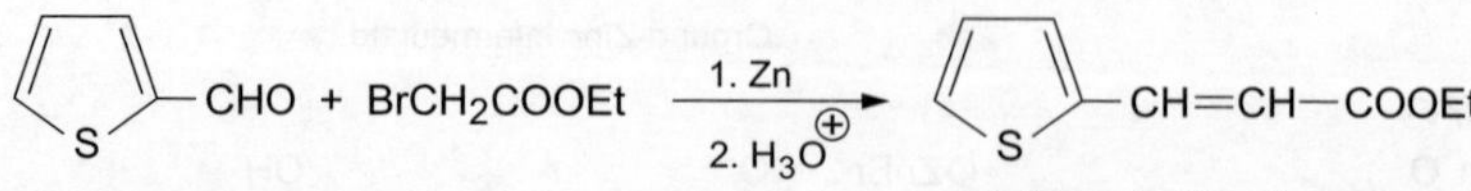

Ethyl-β-(2-thienyl)-acrylate

2. Lengthening of the carbon chain

$$C_6H_5COCH_3 + BrCH_2COOEt \xrightarrow[2.\ H_3O^{\oplus}]{1.\ Zn} C_6H_5{-}C(OH)(CH_3){-}CH_2{-}COOEt \xrightarrow[-H_2O]{H_2SO_4,\ \Delta} C_6H_5{-}C(CH_3){=}CH{-}COOEt$$

$$\xrightarrow{H_2,\ Pt} C_6H_5CH(CH_3){\cdot}CH_2{-}COOEt \xrightarrow{H_2O} \underset{\beta\text{-Phenylbutyric acid}}{C_6H_5CH(CH_3){\cdot}CH_2{-}COOH}$$

By suitable selection of the reactants, unsaturated or saturated acids or esters with branching at α- and β- carbons can be synthesized.

3. Synthesis of arylacetic acid

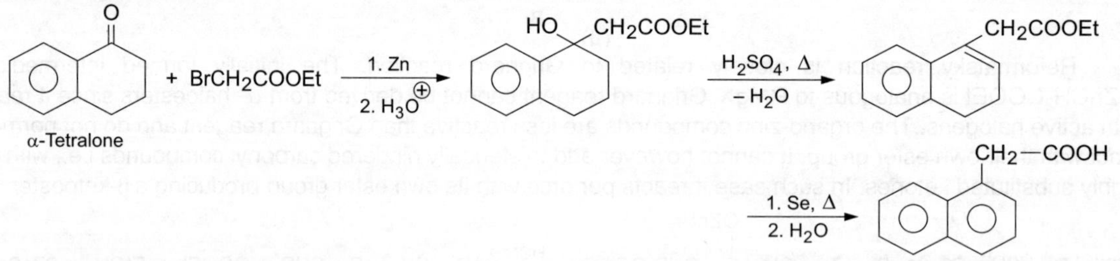

α-Tetralone

α-Naphthylacetic acid

It has an important application in agriculture.

4. Synthesis of citric acid

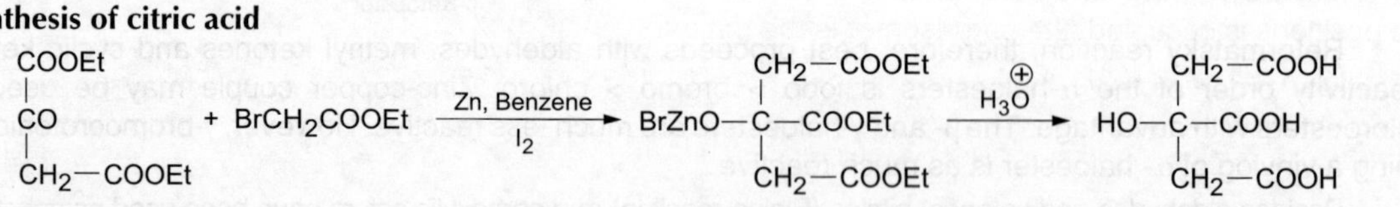

Oxalacetic ester

Citric acid

5. Synthesis of citral

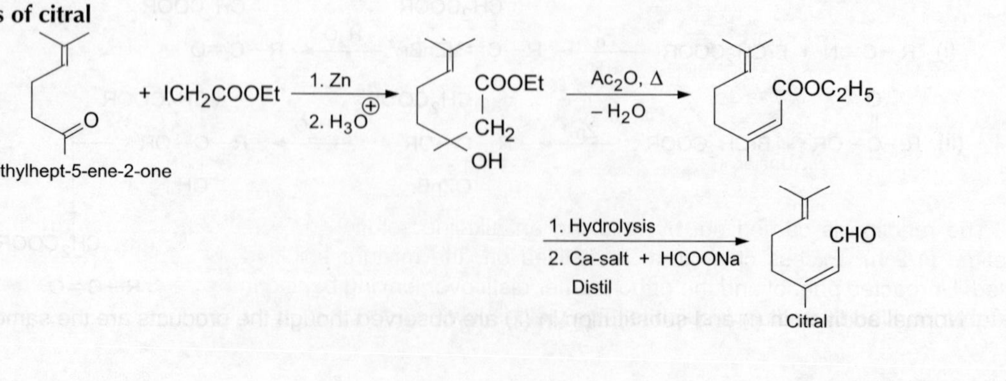

6-Methylhept-5-ene-2-one

Citral

6. Synthesis of camphoronic acid

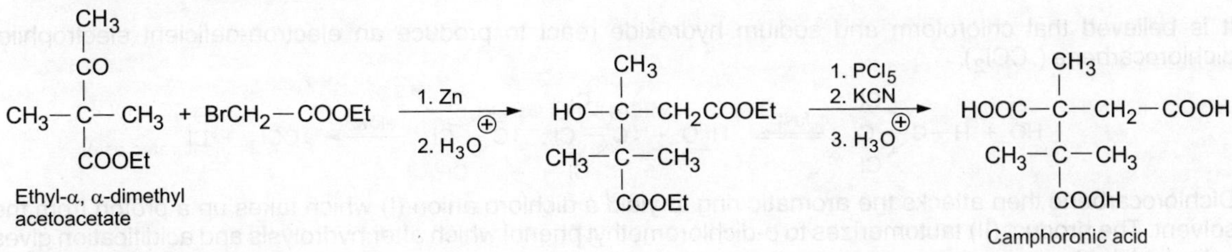

7. Synthesis of vitamin A_1

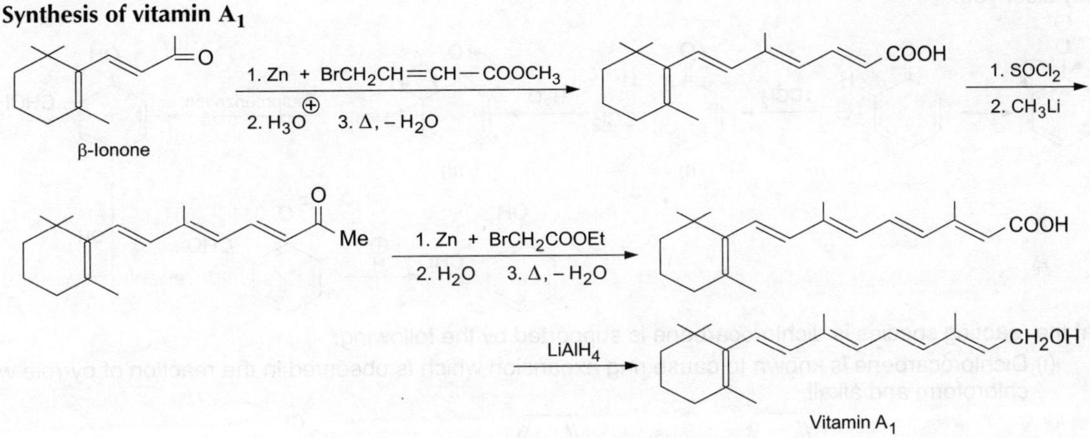

REIMER–TIEMANN REACTION

Formylation of phenols with chloroform in alkaline solution is known as Reimer–Tiemann reaction (RTR). The method is applicable to phenols and some heterocyclic compounds.

A mixture of ortho- and para-isomers is obtained in which the ortho isomer predominates. If one of the ortho positions is occupied, the para-isomer is the major product.

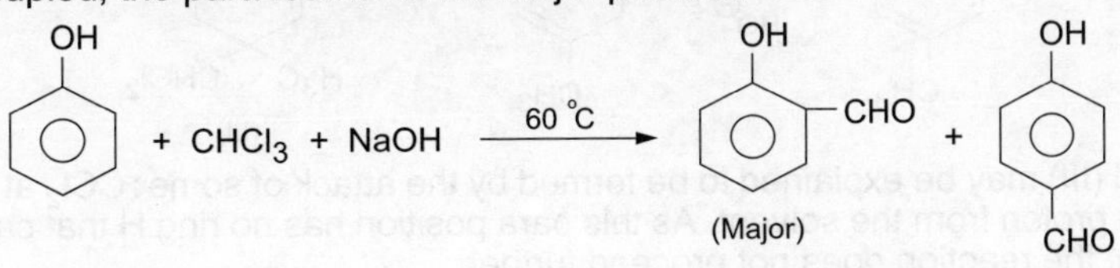

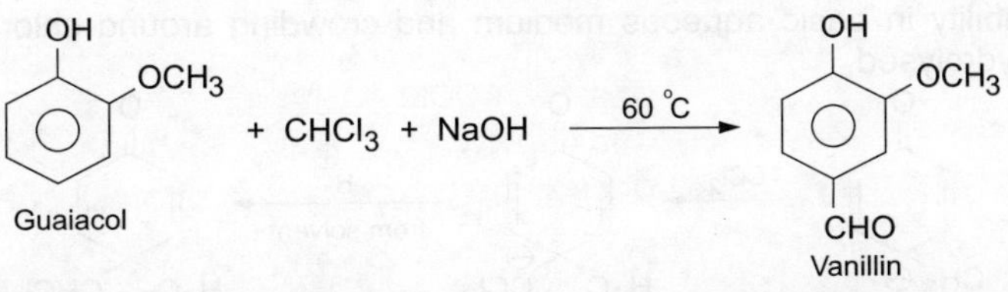

The reaction is carried out by refluxing an alkaline solution of phenol and chloroform at 60 °C for sometime (1/2 h). Excess chloroform is distilled off, the mixture acidified with sulphuric acid and steam distilled. Unreacted phenol and the ortho-isomer distil over leaving behind the para-isomer. The two isomers are further purified by sodium bisulphite. The yield is low.

Mechanism

It is believed that chloroform and sodium hydroxide react to produce an electron-deficient electrophile, dichlorocarbene (: CCl_2).

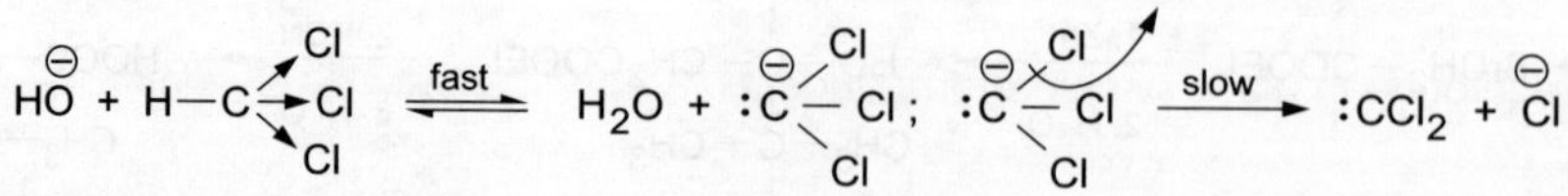

Dichlorocarbene then attacks the aromatic ring to yield a dichloro anion (I) which takes up a proton from the solvent. The product (II) tautomerizes to *o*-dichloromethyl phenol which after hydrolysis and acidification gives salicylaldehyde.

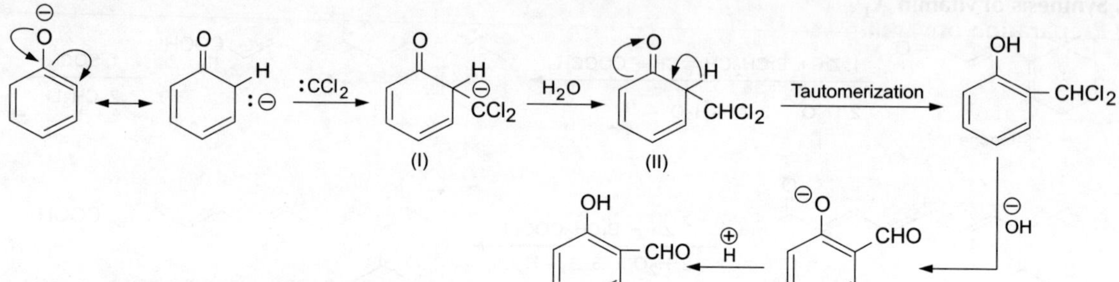

That the reacting species is dichlorocarbene is supported by the following:

(i) Dichlorocarbene is known to cause ring expansion which is observed in the reaction of pyrrole with chloroform and alkali.

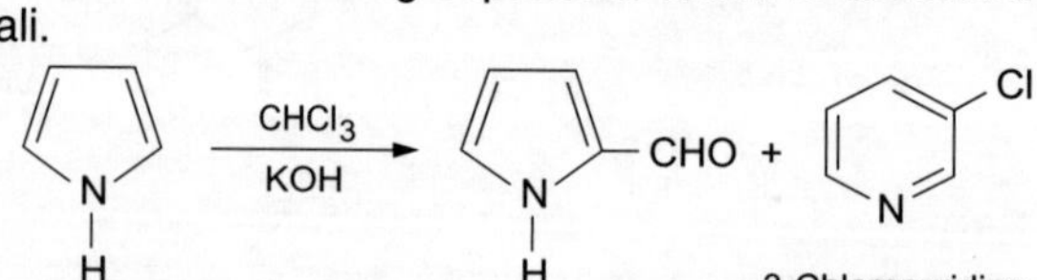

Pyrrole   3-Chloropyridine (Ring expansion)

(ii) When *p*-cresol instead of phenol is used besides the normal aldehyde, a ketone (III) with dichloromethyl group is obtained as a by-product.

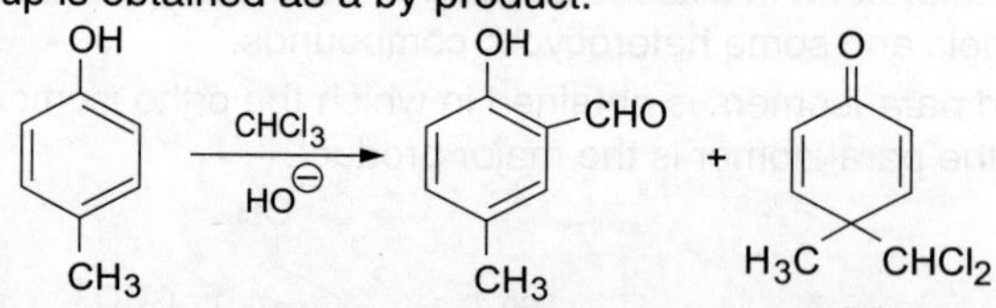

(III)

The compound (III) may be explained to be formed by the attack of some : CCl_2 at the para position and subsequent gain of a proton from the solvent. As this para position has no ring H that can be lost as proton to re-aromatise the ring, the reaction does not proceed further.

Due to its insolubility in basic aqueous medium and crowding around chlorine atoms, the dichloro compound (III) is not hydrolysed.

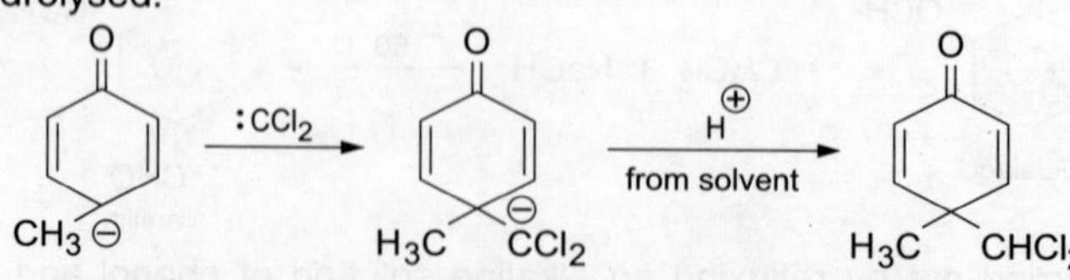

(III)

The presence of negative groups such as CN, COOH, NO_2, SO_3H, etc., decreases the yield.

The yield is nearly 50% and a large amount of phenol remains unreacted. This is probably due to the formation of diphenylacetal derivative.

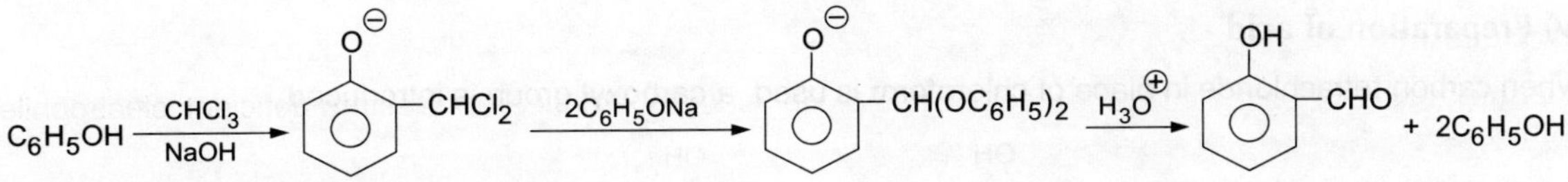

Carbon tetrachloride in place of chloroform under RTR condition gives salicylic acid.

Applications

The reaction affords a good method for introducing aldehyde or carboxyl group in phenols.

(i) Preparation of vanillin

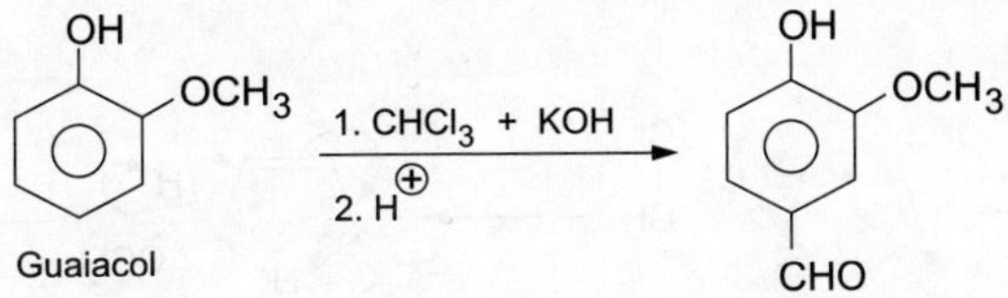

Guaiacol

Vanillin

(ii) Preparation of piperonal

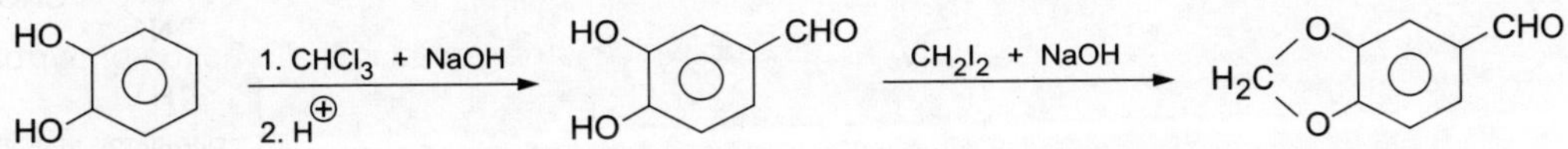

Catechol

Piperonal

(iii) Formylation of heterocyclic compounds

(a)

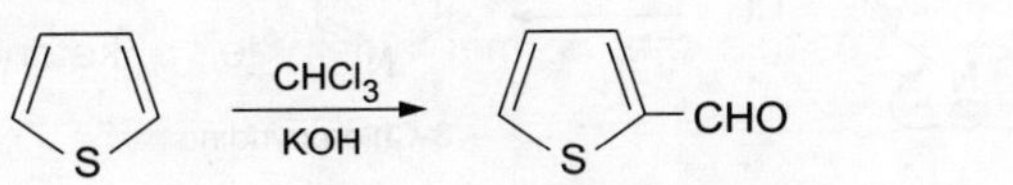

Thiophene-2-aldehyde

(b)

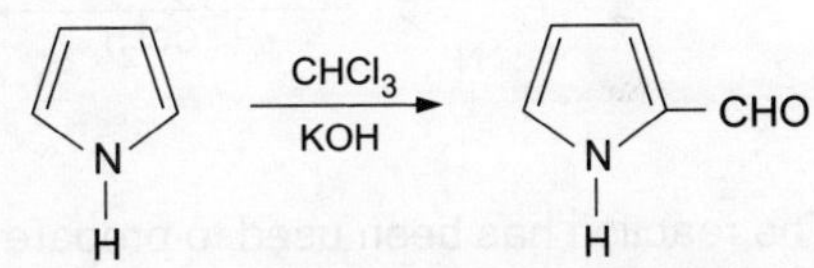

Pyrrole-2-aldehyde

(c)

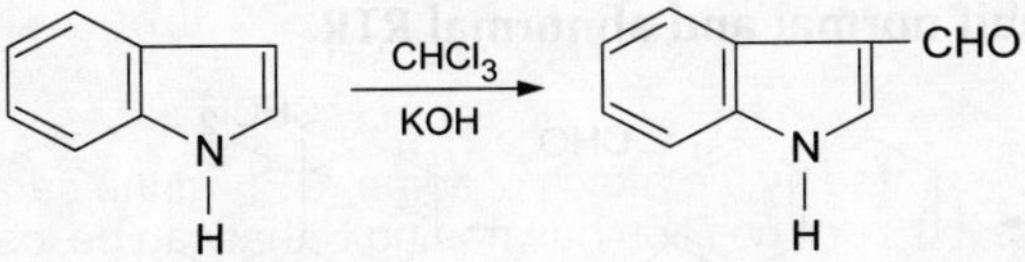

β-Indole-aldehyde

The compound has been used to synthesize the amino acid, tryptophan.

(iv) Formylation of naphthol

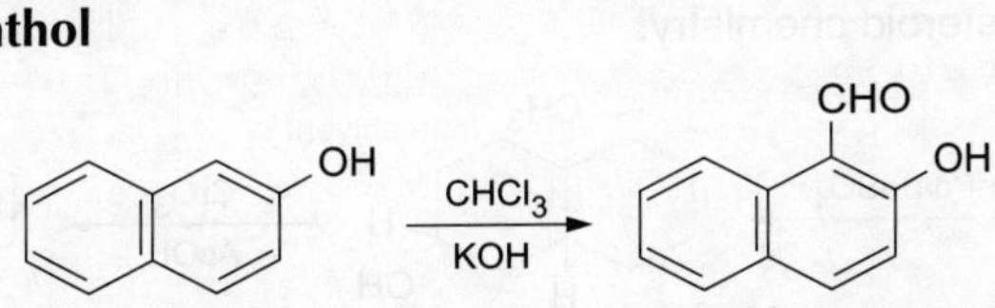

2-Naphthol

2-Hydroxy-1-naphthaldehyde

(v) Preparation of acid

When carbon tetrachloride in place of chloroform is used, a carboxyl group is introduced.

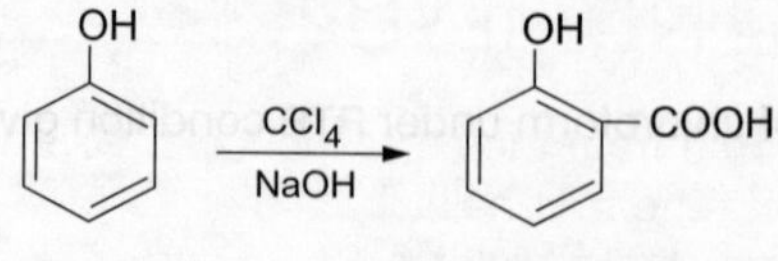

Salicylic acid

(vi) Abnormal Reimer–Tiemann reaction

Pyrrole undergoes normal and abnormal RTR

Normal reaction—

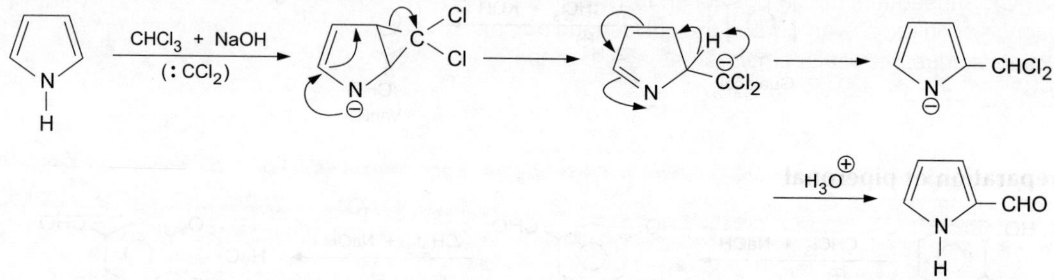

Pyrrole-2-aldehyde

Abnormal reaction (Ring expansion)—

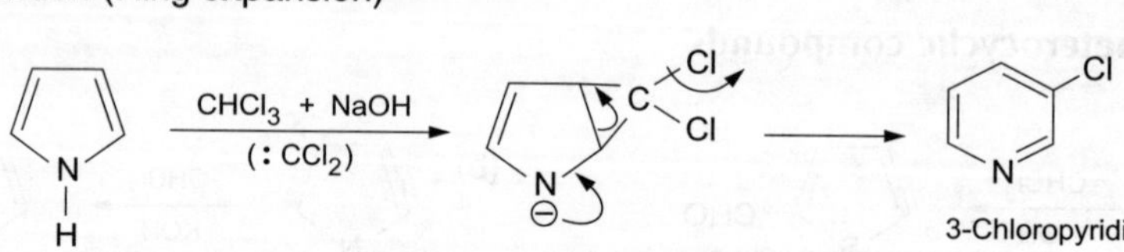

3-Chloropyridine

The reaction has been used to prepare pyridine and its derivatives.

(vii) Certain phenolic compounds also exhibit normal and abnormal RTR

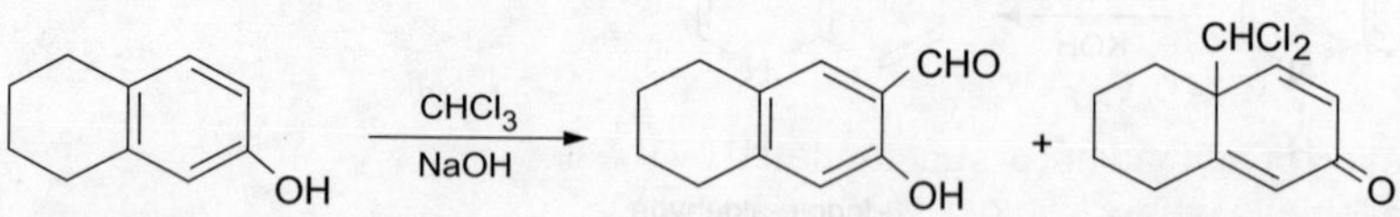

ar-2-Tetralol (Normal product) (Abnormal product)

The abnormal product may be reduced and then oxidized to give a product with angular methyl group. The process has been utilized in steroid chemistry.

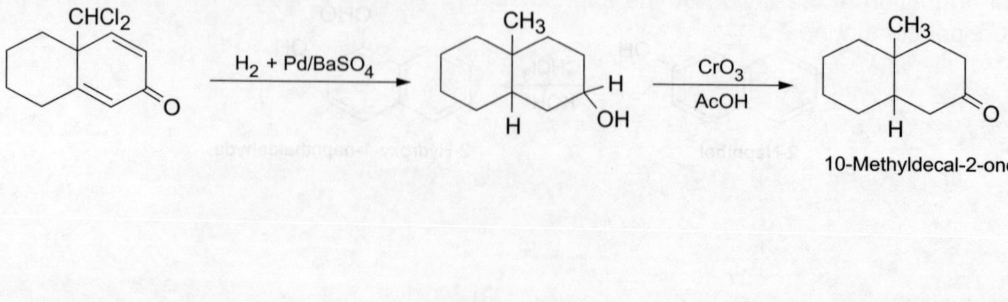

10-Methyldecal-2-one

SANDMEYER REACTION

Alkyl halides are more often prepared from the corresponding alcohols by reacting the alcohols with PCl_3, $SOCl_2$ or concentrated HCl / $ZnCl_2$. The aryl halides cannot be prepared from phenols by these methods. Direct halogenation of aromatic compounds yields a mixture of isomers from which it is difficult to isolate the desired isomer.

Sandmeyer reaction affords a useful method for introducing a halogen substituent at the desired position of an aromatic ring.

The method involves the conversion of an aromatic primary amine into an aryl diazonium salt by treatment with nitrous acid in the presence of mineral acids (usually HCl or H_2SO_4) at low temperature (0–5 °C). Subsequent decomposition of the diazonium salt by heating with cuprous chloride or bromide in the presence of an excess amount of the corresponding halogen acid gives aryl chloride or bromide. The overall reaction is, thus, the replacement of the amino group of the aromatic amine by halogens.

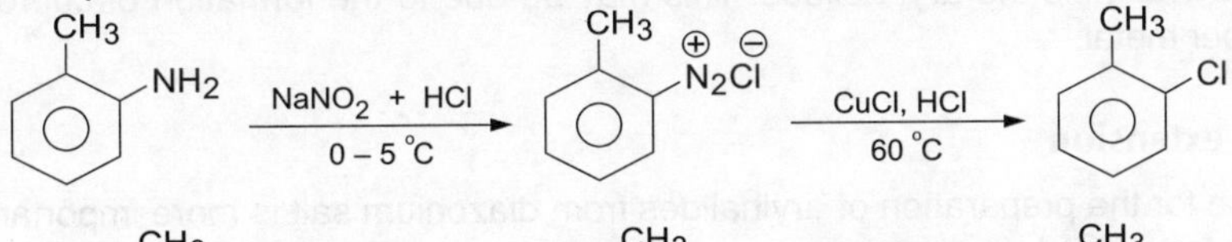

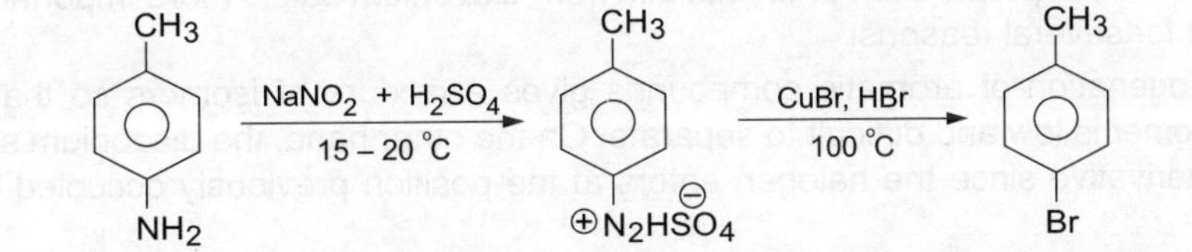

Mechanism

It seems that cuprous copper has the power to reduce diazonium ion to aryl radical by oxidation–reduction involving one-electron transfer. The copper first acts as reducing and then as oxidizing agent.

$$C_6H_5-\overset{\oplus}{N}\equiv N\overset{\ominus}{Cl} + \overset{I}{Cu}Cl \longrightarrow C_6H_5-\overset{\oplus}{N}\equiv N + \overset{I}{Cu}\overset{\ominus}{Cl_2}$$

$$C_6H_5-\overset{\oplus}{N}\equiv N + \overset{I}{Cu}\overset{\ominus}{Cl_2} \longrightarrow {}^{\bullet}C_6H_5 + N_2 + \overset{II}{Cu}Cl_2$$

$${}^{\bullet}C_6H_5 + \overset{II}{Cu}Cl_2 \longrightarrow C_6H_5Cl + \overset{I}{Cu}Cl$$

The formation of aryl radical is substantiated by the decomposition of benzene diazonium chloride in the presence of acrylonitrile when 2-chloro-3-phenylpropionitrile is obtained through free radical addition.

$${}^{\bullet}C_6H_5 + CH_2{=}CH-CN \longrightarrow C_6H_5-CH_2-{}^{\bullet}CH-CN \xrightarrow{CuCl_2} C_6H_5-CH_2-\underset{Cl}{CH}-CN + \overset{I}{Cu}Cl$$

The formation of the halide by the cupric copper may also involve a carbocation intermediate or an organo-copper compound.

$${}^{\bullet}C_6H_5 + \overset{II}{Cu} \longrightarrow \overset{\oplus}{C_6H_5} + \overset{I}{Cu} \xrightarrow{\overset{\ominus}{Cl}} C_6H_5Cl + \overset{I}{Cu}$$

$$\text{or} \quad {}^{\bullet}C_6H_5 + \overset{II}{Cu} + \overset{\ominus}{Cl} \longrightarrow C_6H_5-Cu-Cl \longrightarrow C_6H_5Cl + \overset{I}{Cu}$$

For the preparation of aryl iodide, the aryl diazonium salt is treated with potassium iodide solution. The cuprous catalyst is unnecessary because iodide ion is sufficient to decompose the diazonium salt. However, in this case also oxidation–reduction is probably involved since enough iodine is liberated in the reaction.

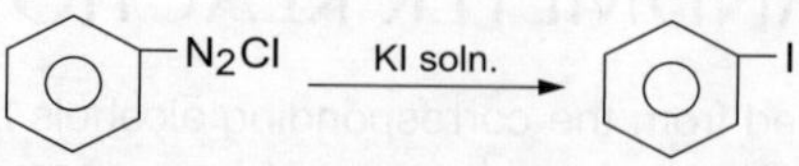

Aryl fluoride is prepared by treating the diazonium salt with fluoboric acid or fluoborate. Sparingly soluble diazonium fluoborate which separates is washed and dried. The dry salt is then decomposed by heating.

$$C_6H_5\overset{\oplus}{N_2}\overset{\ominus}{Cl} \xrightarrow{HBF_4} C_6H_5\overset{\oplus}{N_2}\overset{\ominus}{BF_4} \xrightarrow{150-160\,^{\circ}C} C_6H_5F + N_2 + BF_3$$

This reaction is known as Schiemann reaction.

Gattermann modification It has been found that copper powder or copper bronze in place of cuprous chloride acts similarly to yield the aryl halides. This may be due to the formation of cuprous copper on the surface of the copper metal.

Applications and extension

Sandmeyer reaction for the preparation of arylhalides from diazonium salt is more important and useful than direct halogenation for several reasons.

(i) Direct halogenation of aromatic compounds gives a mixture of isomers so that the yield of the desired isomer is low and difficult to separate. On the other hand, the diazonium salts give only one halogen derivative since the halogen enters at the position previously occupied by the diazonium group.

(ii) Aryl iodides and fluorides which are seldom prepared by direct halogenation can be prepared by Sandmeyer reaction and Schiemann reaction respectively.

(iii) In some cases direct halogenation at a particular position is not possible for reasons of electronic factors but this has been possible through Sandmeyer reaction, e.g.,

(a) Preparation of *m*-dichlorobenzene

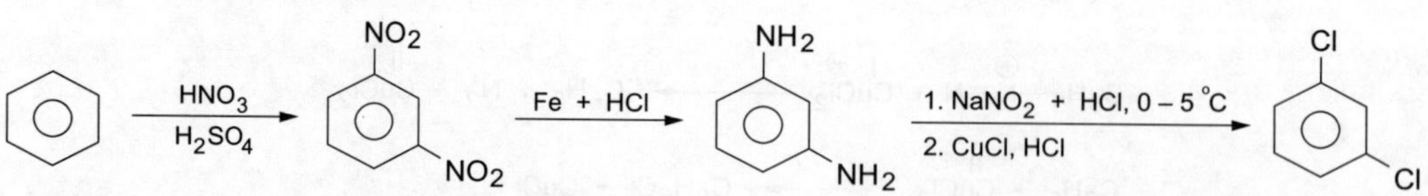

(b) Preparation of 2-chloronaphthalene

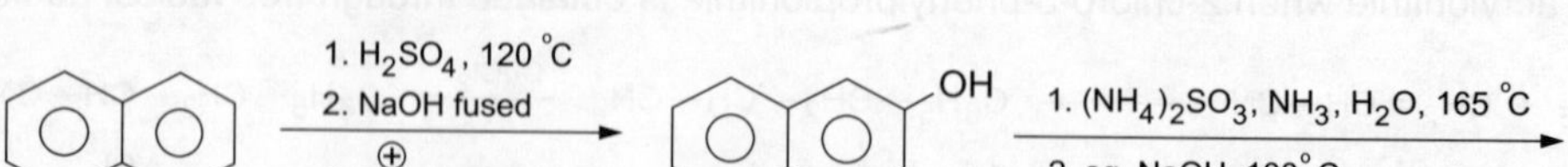

β-Naphthol

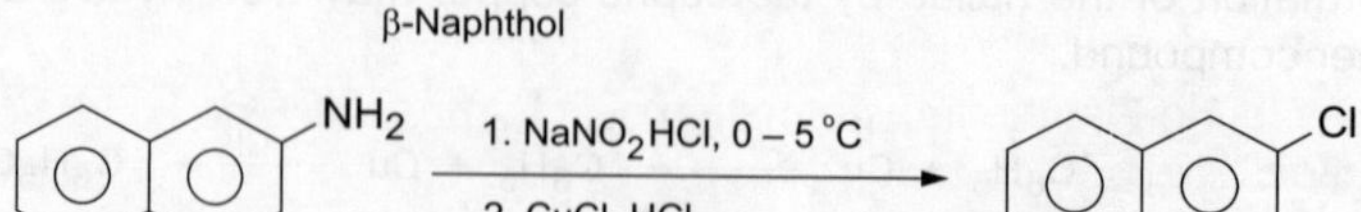

β-Naphthylamine 2-Chloronaphthalene

(c) Preparation of acids— Diazonium salts on treatment with cuprous cyanide and potassium cyanide give nitriles which on hydrolysis give acids.

$$C_6H_6 \xrightarrow[H_2SO_4]{HNO_3} C_6H_5NO_2 \xrightarrow{H} C_6H_5NH_2 \xrightarrow[0-5\,^\circ C]{NaNO_2\ +\ HCl} C_6H_5\overset{\oplus}{N_2}\overset{\ominus}{Cl} \xrightarrow[KCN]{CuCN}$$

$$C_6H_5CN \xrightarrow{H_3\overset{\oplus}{O}} C_6H_5COOH$$

(d) Removal of amino group from aromatic rings—Amino groups of aromatic amines after conversion to the corresponding diazonium salt and treatment with hypophosphorous acid are removed from the aromatic rings. The reaction has been successfully used to prepare compounds which cannot be prepared by direct substitution. Thus, *m*-nitrotoluene may be prepared form toluene. Toluene on nitration gives *o*- and *p*-nitrotoluenes. The para-isomer after separation is processed as below.

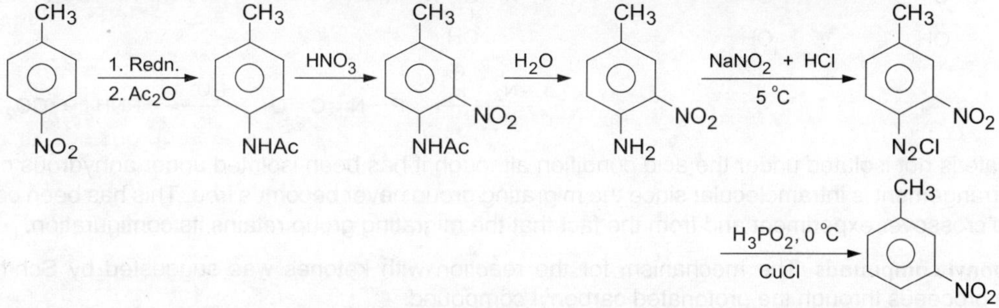

SCHMIDT REACTION

Carboxylic acids and hydrazoic acid react in the presence of sulphuric acid to give amines. This reaction is known as Schmidt reaction.

$$RCOOH + N_3H \xrightarrow{H_2SO_4} RNH_2 + CO_2 + N_2$$

Free hydrazoic acid is highly toxic and hence sodium azide is slowly added to the solution of the carboxylic acid in sulphuric acid when hydrazoic acid is liberated.

The reaction is closely related to Hofmann and Curtius reactions, all of which involve the formation of isocyanate intermediate through the migration of a group from carbon to nitrogen.

Schmidt reaction also occurs between ketones or aldehydes and hydrazoic acid when ketones give substituted amides and aldehydes give a mixture of nitriles and *N*-formyl derivatives.

$$R_2CO + N_3H \xrightarrow{H_2SO_4} RCONHR + N_2$$

$$RCHO + N_3H \xrightarrow{H_2SO_4} \underset{\substack{\text{Nitrile}\\ \text{(Major)}}}{RCN} \text{ and } \underset{\substack{N\text{-Formyl derivative}\\ \text{(Minor)}}}{RNHCHO}$$

The rearrangements in these cases closely resemble the Beckmann rearrangement. Dialkyl and cyclic ketones react more readily than alkyl aryl ketones. With alkyl aryl ketones, it is the aryl group which migrates.

Mechanism

(a) Acids (i) It was found that the transformation occurs most rapidly without heating with sterically hindered acids (e.g., mesitoic acid) which readily form acyl cations in sulphuric acid. This clue led to suggest the formation of protonated acyl azide (I), in the first step, which eliminates nitrogen to form the intermediate (II). The intermediate (II) then undergoes rearrangement to form isocyanate which is hydrolysed under the reaction conditions to amine and carbon dioxide.

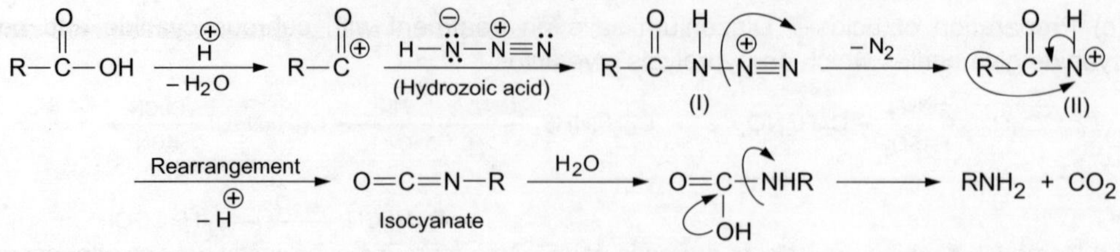

(ii) Acids which do not form acyl cation react through the protonated acid on heating as below.

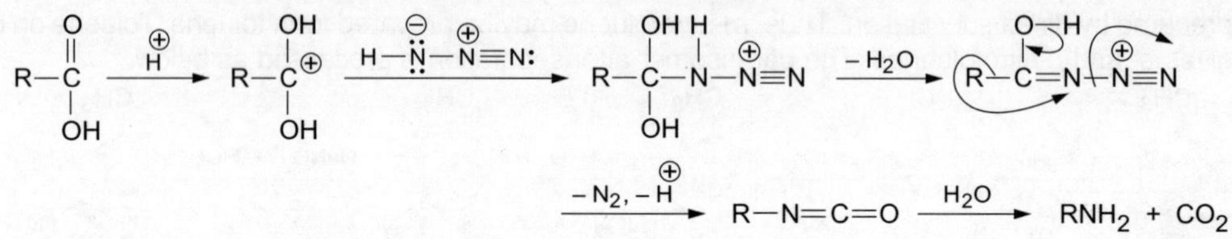

Isocyanate is not isolated under the acid condition although it has been isolated under anhydrous condition. The rearrangement is intramolecular since the migrating group never becomes free. This has been concluded from the crossover experiment and from the fact that the migrating group retains its configuration.

(b) Carbonyl compounds The mechanism for the reaction with ketones was suggested by Schmidt. The reaction proceeds through the protonated carbonyl compound.

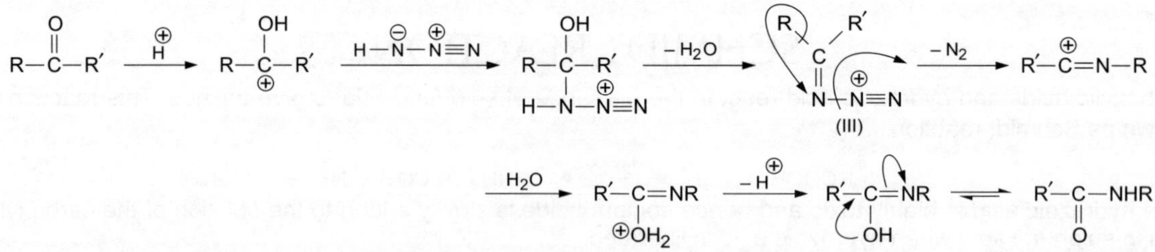

Steps from (III) onwards resemble Beckmann rearrangement.

In the case of aldehyde the intermediate (III) will have the structure (IV) in which migration of H will give nitrile and migration of R will give formyl derivative.

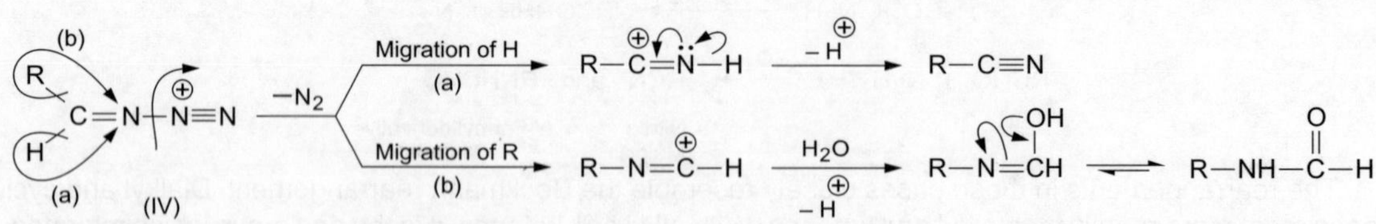

Sulphuric acid is the most common catalyst for Schmidt reaction but Lewis acids have also been used.

Applications

1. Preparation of amines Primary amines in good yield are obtained directly from the acids, provided the acids do not contain groups sensitive to concentrated sulphuric acid. The reagent, however, is dangerous to handle due to its poisonous and explosive nature.

(a) $$C_6H_5CH_2COOH + N_3H \xrightarrow[CHCl_3]{H_2SO_4} C_6H_5CH_2NH_2 + N_2 + CO_2$$

Phenylacetic acid — Benzyl amine

(b) 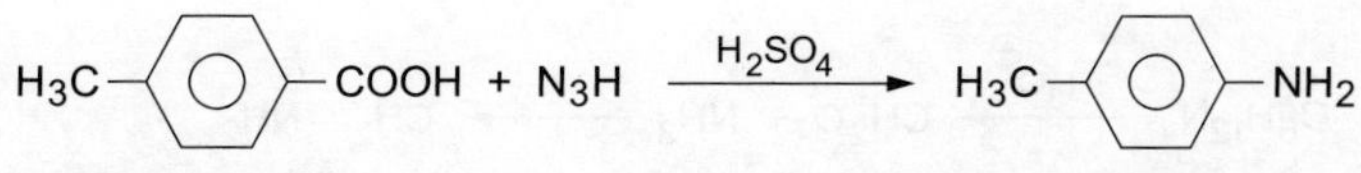

p-Toluic acid — *p*-Toluidine

2. Preparation of α-amino acids Ethyl acetoacetate and hydrazoic acid react in the presence of sulphuric acid to give α-amino acid.

$$CH_3 \cdot CO \cdot CHR \cdot COOC_2H_5 \xrightarrow[H_2SO_4]{N_3H} CH_3CONHCHR \cdot COOC_2H_5 \xrightarrow[H^{\oplus}]{H_2O} R \cdot CH(NH_2) \cdot COOH$$

Note that the reaction with ketones is virtually the insertion of NH group between the carbonyl group and the alkyl group of the ketone.

3. Preparation of lactams Cyclic ketones react to give lactams. Cyclohexanone gives ∈-caprolactam.

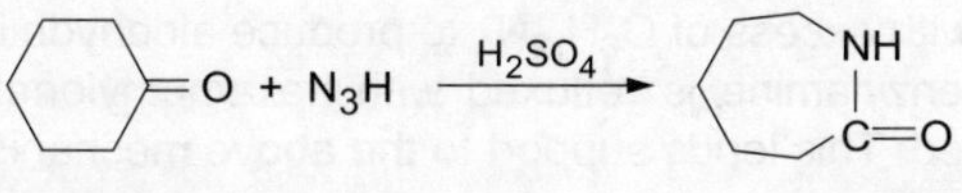

With excess of N_3H substituted tetrazoles are obtained from ketones. Cardiazole, a heart stimulant has been prepared from cyclohexanone and N_3H.

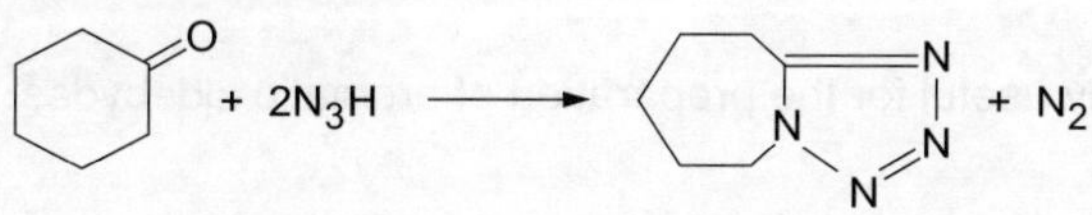

SOMMELET REACTION

Sommelet reaction involves the oxidation of chloromethyl group ($-CH_2Cl$) to an aldehyde group by the use of hexamethylenetetramine ($C_6H_{12}N_4$) and subsequent hydrolysis in acidic medium (pH 3–6.5). The reaction is successful with benzylic halide ($ArCH_2Cl$).

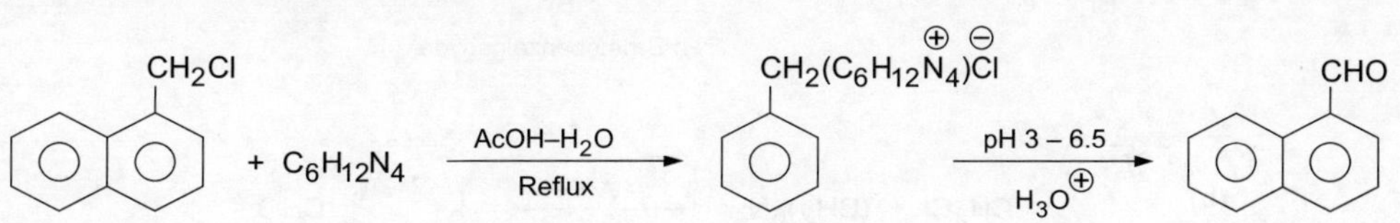

Quaternary salt — 1-Naphthaldehyde

Mechanism

The mechanism of the reaction is not clearly understood. According to Angyal and co-workers, the halide reacts with hexamethylenetetramine to form a quaternary salt (I) which is hydrolysed to amine (II). Hexamethylene tetramine is also hydrolysed to formaldehyde and ammonia which subsequently form methylene amine (III). The amine (II) then transfers a hydride ion to methylene amine (III) to form an imine (IV), which is finally hydrolysed to aldehyde.

(i) $$C_6H_5CH_2Cl + C_6H_{12}N_4 \longrightarrow \underset{(I)}{C_6H_5CH_2(C_6H_{12}\overset{\oplus}{N_4})\overset{\ominus}{Cl}} \xrightarrow{H_2O} \underset{(II)}{C_6H_5CH_2NH_2}$$

(ii) $$C_6H_{12}N_4 \xrightarrow{H_3O^{\oplus}} CH_2O + NH_3 \longrightarrow \underset{(III)}{CH_2{=}\overset{\oplus}{N}H_2}$$

(iii) $$\underset{(II)}{C_6H_5{-}\underset{H}{C}H{-}\ddot{N}H_2} + \underset{(III)}{CH_2{=}\overset{\oplus}{N}H_2} \longrightarrow \underset{(IV)}{C_6H_5{-}CH{=}\overset{\oplus}{N}H_2} + CH_3NH_2$$

(iv) $$C_6H_5{-}CH{=}\overset{\oplus}{N}H_2 \xrightarrow{H_3O^{\oplus}} C_6H_5CHO + NH_3$$

Reaction of benzylamine with excess of $C_6H_{12}N_4$ to produce aldehyde is the actual Sommelet reaction (the last three steps). When benzylamine is refluxed with hexamethylenetetramine (hexamine) in acidic medium benzaldehyde is obtained. This lends support to the above mechanism.

Strong deactivating groups as also *o*-substituents decrease the yield. When both the *o*-positions are substituted, as in 2, 4-dinitrobenzylchloride, the reaction completely fails. The yield is also very poor with phenolic compounds.

The reaction is generally useful for the preparation of aromatic aldehydes.

Applications

The reaction has proved useful for the preparation of aldehydes from amines and halides. Various types of aromatic, heterocyclic, some aliphatic aldehydes and amines have been prepared.

(a)

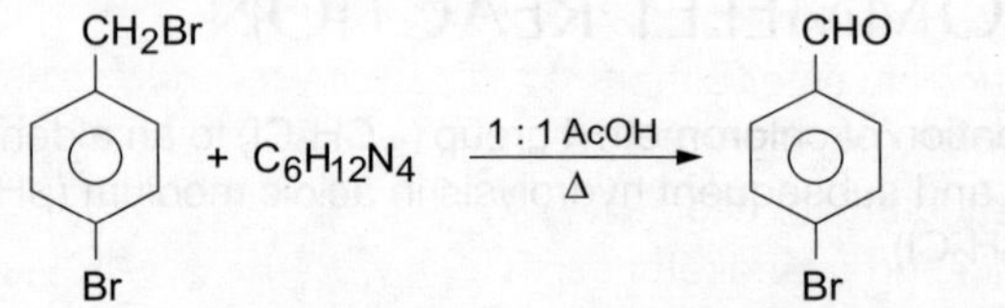

p-Bromobenzaldehyde

(b)

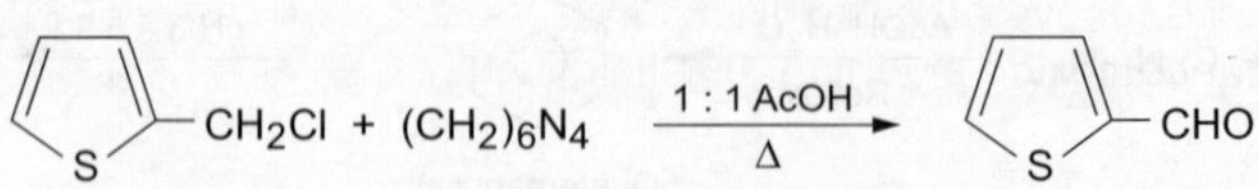

Thiophene-2-aldehyde

(c)

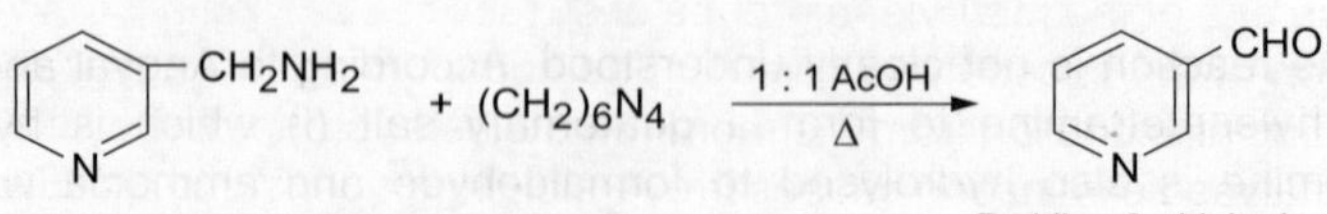

Pyridine-3-aldehyde

$$\text{(d)}\quad CH_3-(CH_2)_4-CH_2NH_2 + (CH_2)_6N_4 \xrightarrow[\Delta]{HCl} \underset{n\text{-Hexanal}}{CH_3-(CH_2)_4-CHO}$$

$$\text{(e)}\quad C_6H_5CH_2Cl + (CH_2)_6N_4 \xrightarrow[\Delta]{\text{Excess } NH_3} \underset{\text{Benzylamine}}{C_6H_5CH_2NH_2}$$

The reaction (e) has been utilized for the preparation of an aminoketone intermediate required in the synthesis of chloromycetin.

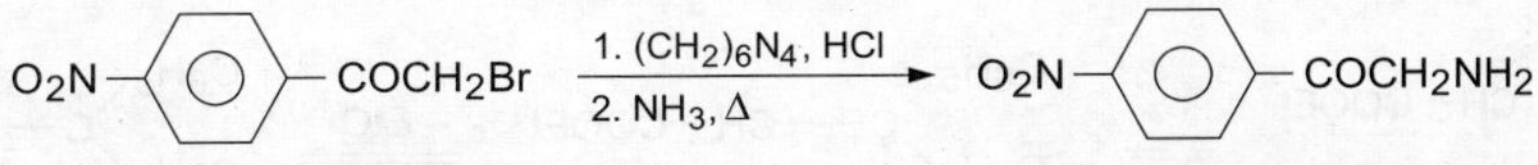

p-Nitro-ω-bromoacetophenone — Intermediate for chloromycetin

Another way to oxidize benzilic halides to aldehydes is the Kröhnke reaction. The reaction consists of treatment with pyridine followed by *p*-nitrosodimethylaniline and subsequent hydrolysis.

$$C_6H_5CH_2Cl + C_5H_5N \longrightarrow [C_6H_5CH_2\overset{\oplus}{N}C_5H_5]\overset{\ominus}{Cl} \xrightarrow[2.\ H_3O^{\oplus}]{1.\ p\text{-}ONC_6H_4\text{-}N(CH_3)_2,\ \overset{\ominus}{O}H} C_6H_5CHO$$

STOBBE CONDENSATION

Aldehydes and ketones condense with the esters of succinic acid in the presence of bases such as C_2H_5ONa, Me_3COK or NaH to give the salts of α, β-unsaturated half esters but not the alcohol. This is known as Stobbe condensation.

$$R_2C{=}O + H_2\overset{\overset{\displaystyle COOC_2H_5}{|}}{C}-CH_2COOC_2H_5 \xrightarrow[Me_3COH]{Me_3COK} R_2C{=}\overset{\overset{\displaystyle COOC_2H_5}{|}}{C}-CH_2COOK$$

The reaction is specific for succinic ester although the carbonyl compound may be varied over a wide range. The carbonyl compounds which may be used are:

(a) Aliphatic and α,β-unsaturated aldehydes

(b) Aliphatic, aromatic, alicyclic and cyanoketones as also ketoesters.

However, ketones are more often used than aldehydes. In practice, the reaction mixture—ketone, diethyl succinate and ether solution of sodium ethoxide—is allowed to stand at room temperature for several days and then the product is recovered by acidification. The yield is improved and the reaction time is reduced on using potassium tertiary butoxide in tertiary butyl alcohol as base.

Mechanism

The mechanism of Stobbe condensation is not very clear. According to the accepted mechanism, the base accepts a proton from one of the methylene groups of succinic ester. The succinic ester carbanion then adds to the carbonyl carbon of the substrate to give (I). The adduct (I) then undergoes cyclization (ester–lactone interchange) generating alkoxide ion from the more remote ester group. The cyclized product (II) is a lactone. Subsequent base-catalysed elimination causes irreversible ring opening to produce a salt of unsaturated half ester (III).

Lactones have been isolated from the reaction mixture in some cases, which support the mechanism.

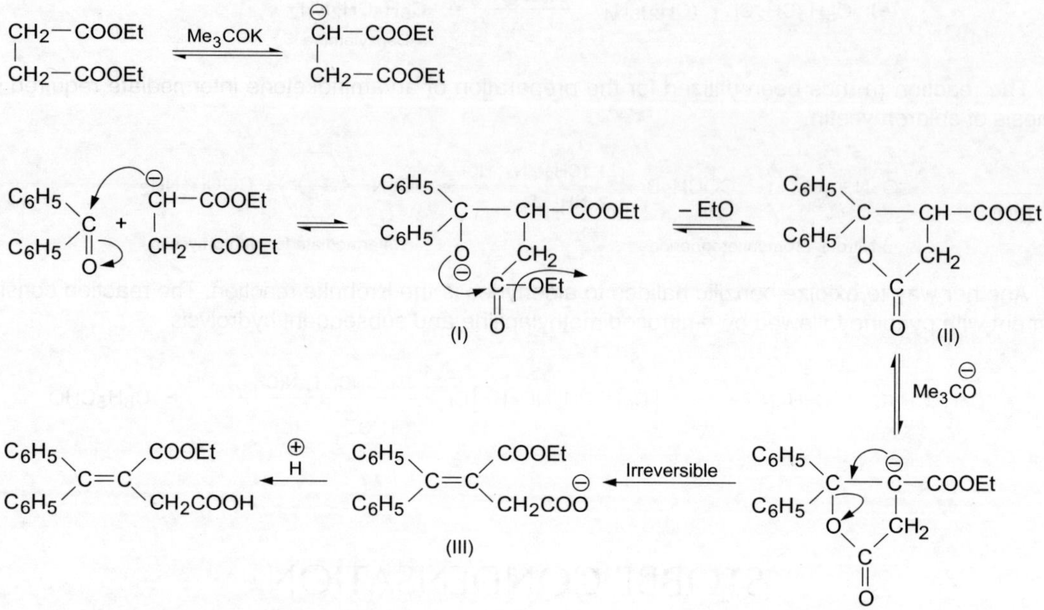

Applications

Stobbe condensation has been used to prepare a large number of varieties of unsaturated and saturated acids. The condensation has also been useful for the synthesis of many types of polycyclic ring systems. It has also been used during the synthesis of estrone. Some of its synthetic applications are given below.

1. Synthesis of acids

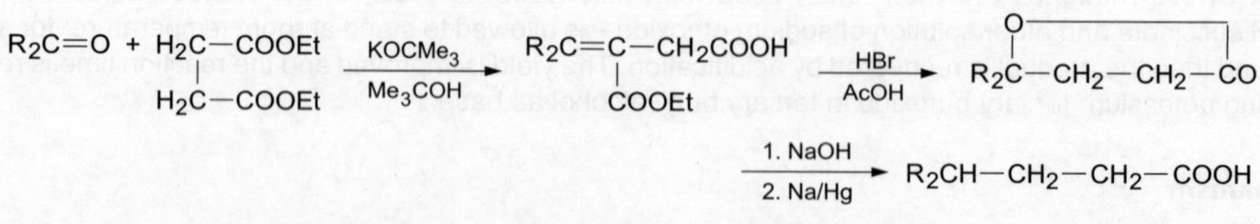

2. Synthesis of polycyclic rings (a) Naphthol and indenone derivatives—Stobbe condensation product with aryl ketones on cyclodehydration gives polycyclic rings. Since Stobbe condensation product is a substituted olefin, the aryl group may be *cis* to CH_2COOH group or to COOH group so that two products may be obtained on cyclodehydration.

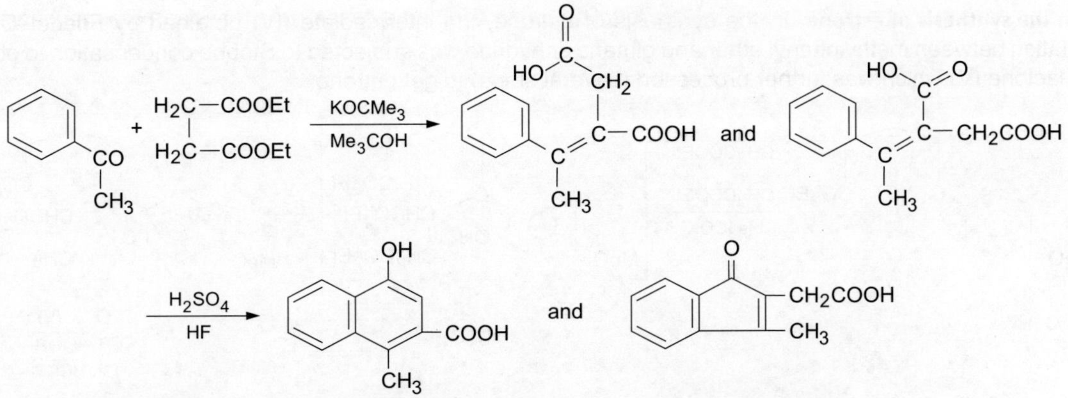

Naphthol derivative

Indenone derivative

(b) Tetralone derivative—

(i)

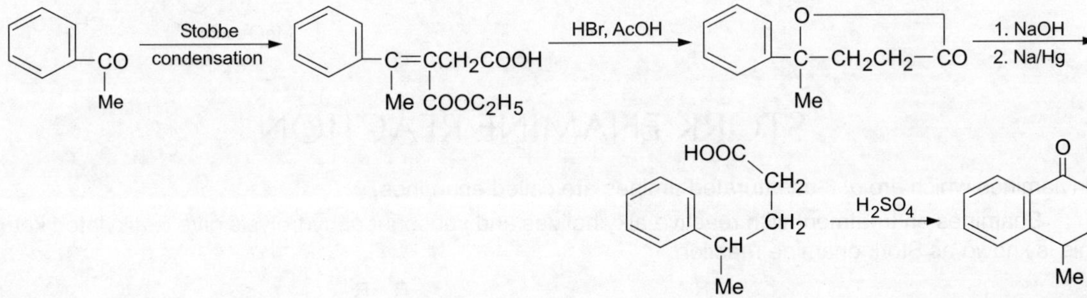

4-Methyl tetralone

(ii)

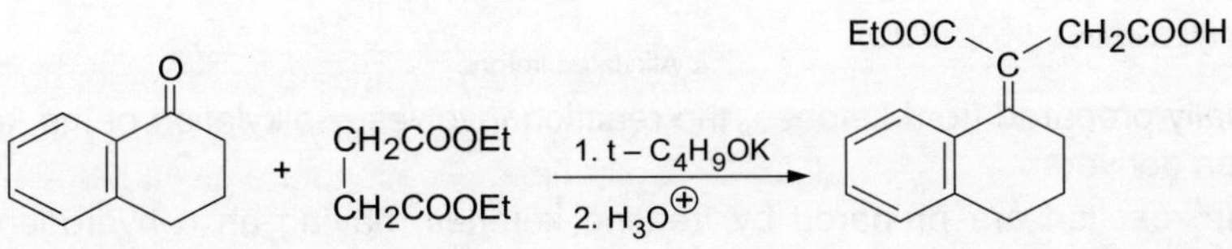

(c) Phenanthrene derivative—

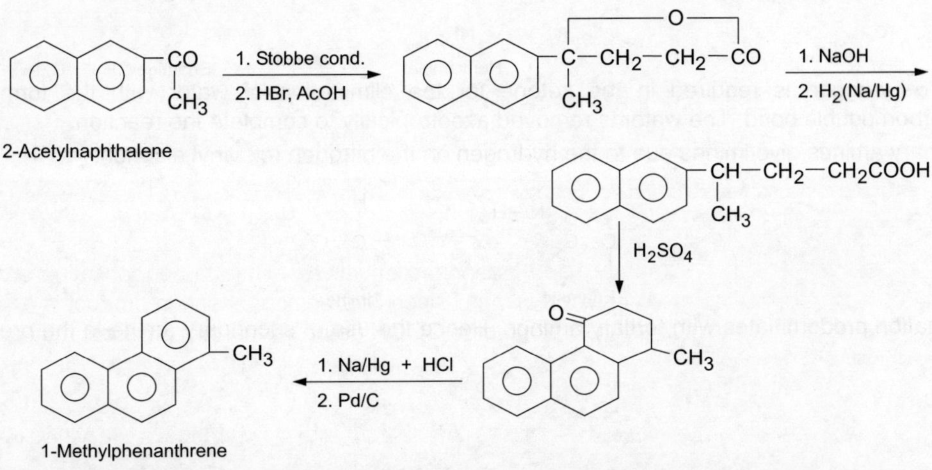

2-Acetylnaphthalene

1-Methylphenanthrene

3. In the synthesis of estrone In the synthesis of estrone, the intermediate (IV) obtained by Friedel–Crafts acylation between methylphenyl ether and glutaric anhydride was subjected to Stobbe condensation to obtain the lactone (V) which was further processed (several steps) to get estrone.

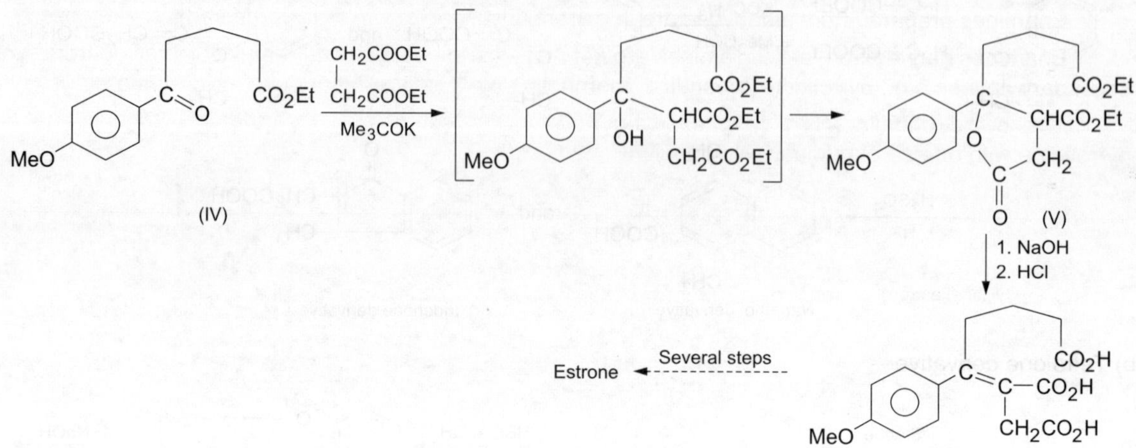

STORK ENAMINE REACTION

Vinylamines which are α, β-unsaturated amines are called enamines.

Enamines on treatment with reactive alkylhalides and subsequent hydrolysis give α-alkylated ketones. This is known as Stork enamine reaction.

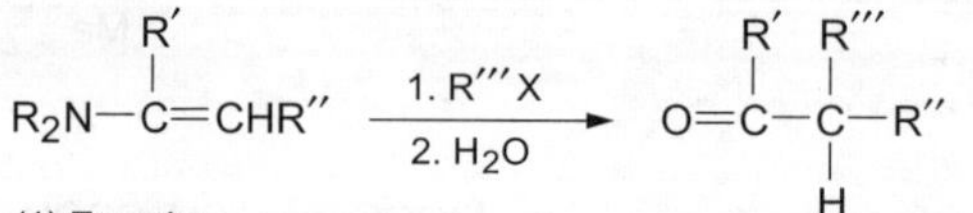

(1) Enamine α-Alkylated ketone

Since enamines are normally prepared from ketones, the reaction involves α-alkylation of the ketone from which the enamine has been derived.

Enamines required for the reaction are prepared by treating ketones, having an α-hydrogen with secondary amines.

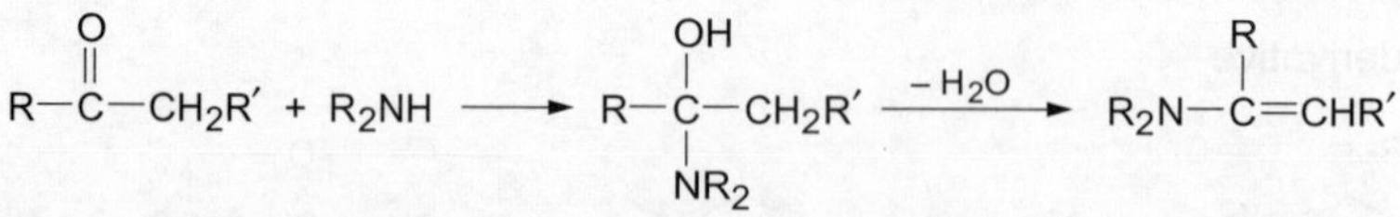

Hemiaminal Enamine

An α-hydrogen is required in the ketone for the elimination of water with the formation of a carbon-carbon double bond. The water is removed azeotropically to complete the reaction.

Primary amines give imines due to the hydrogen on the nitrogen (cf. vinyl alcohol).

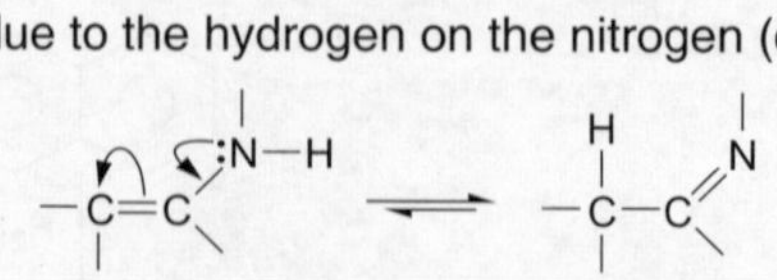

Enamine Imine

and elimination predominates with tertiary amines. Hence the use of secondary amine in the preparation of enamines.

The reaction is not successful with ordinary primary or secondary halides due to *N*-alkylation. With tertiary halides elimination is significant. The reaction is succesful with active alkyl halides e.g., allyl, benzyl, propergyl halides etc. Alkyl group is attached to the less substituted side of the ketone.

Enamines prepared from aldehydes are in general less stable than those prepared from ketones.

Enamines derived from acyclic amines are not resistant to heat or acid. Enamines obtained from cyclic secondary amines e.g., pyrrolidine, piperidine, morpholine etc. react faster and are more stable.

The cyclic enamine, N-1-cyclohexenyl-pyrrolidine (I) is prepared by boiling cyclohexanone and pyrrotidine with a trace of *p*-toluene-sulphonic acid as catalyst.

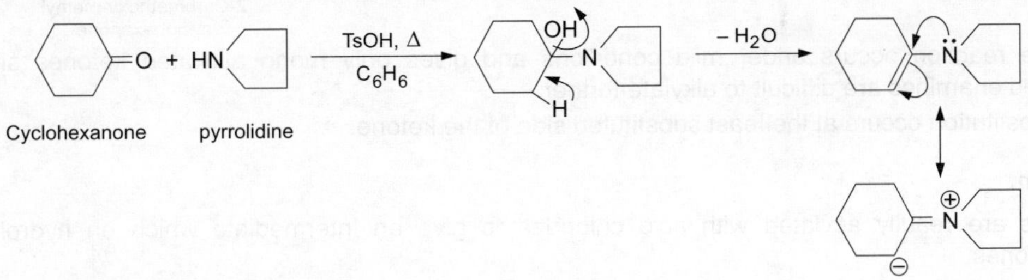

(I)

The water is removed azeotropically.

It is seen that enamines are resonance hybrides (I) and the β-carbon is the nucleophilic centre. Hence, enamines are useful intermediates for organic synthesis.

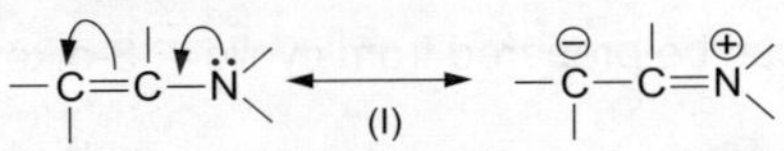

From the resonance structure it is seen that the β-carbon is suseptible to electrophilic attack. Enamines are easily hydrolysed to regenerate ketones. Hence substitution followed by hydrolysis gives varidly substituted ketones.

Applications

The nucleophilic behaviour of enamines has been utilized in various important synthesis. Stork and coworkers have widely investigated the properties of enamines.

On reacting with alkyl halides nucleophilic displacement in the alkyl halide results in the formulation of imine salt (II) which after hydrolysis gives α-alkylated ketone (III).

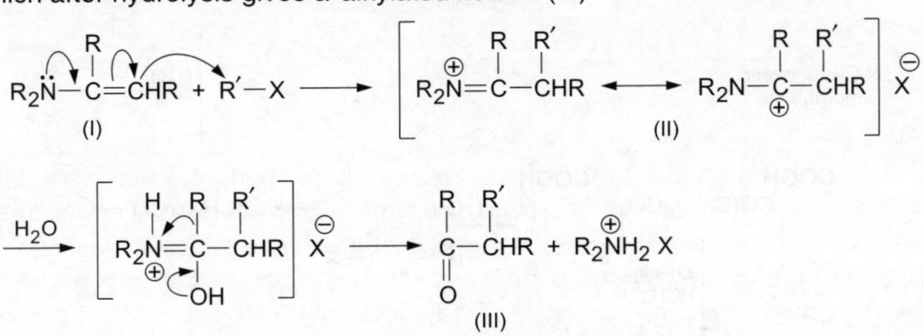

Alkylation

Enamines undergo alkylation at the β-carbon by reactive alkyl halides. With α-bromoacetic esters, the β-carbon is substituted by carbmethoxy methyl group.

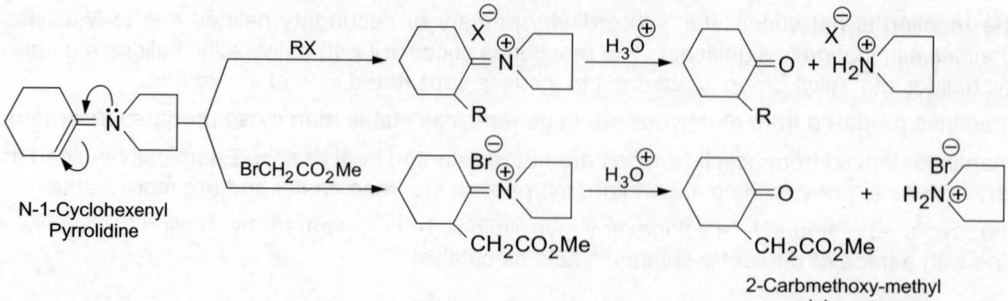

N-1-Cyclohexenyl Pyrrolidine

2-Carbmethoxy-methyl cyclohexanone

The reaction occurs under mild conditions and gives only mono alkylated ketones since mono substituted enamines are difficult to alkylate further.

Substitution occurs at the least substituted side of the ketone.

Acylation

Enamines are readily acylated with acid chlorides to give an intermediate which on hydrolysis gives 1, 3-diketones.

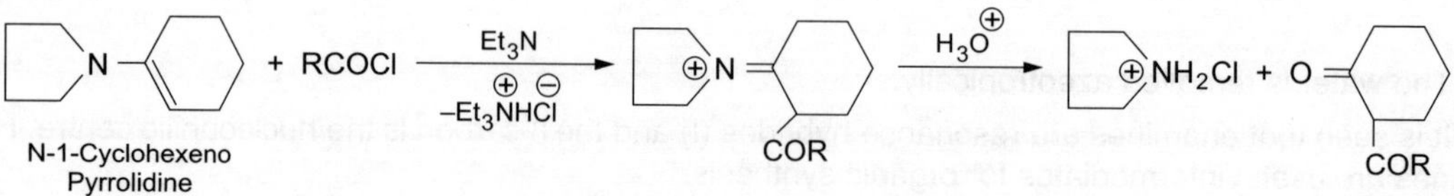

N-1-Cyclohexeno Pyrrolidine

1, 3-Diketone

Long chain carboxylic acids can be prepared from cyclic 1, 3-diketones.

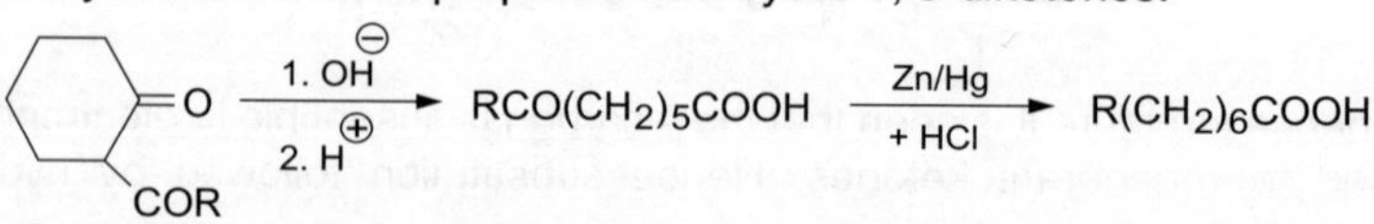

The length of the carboxylic acid chain depends upon the size of the cyclic ketone used in the preparation of enamine.

By using dicarboxylic acid chlorides, the carbon chain of the dicarboxylic acid may be extended still further.

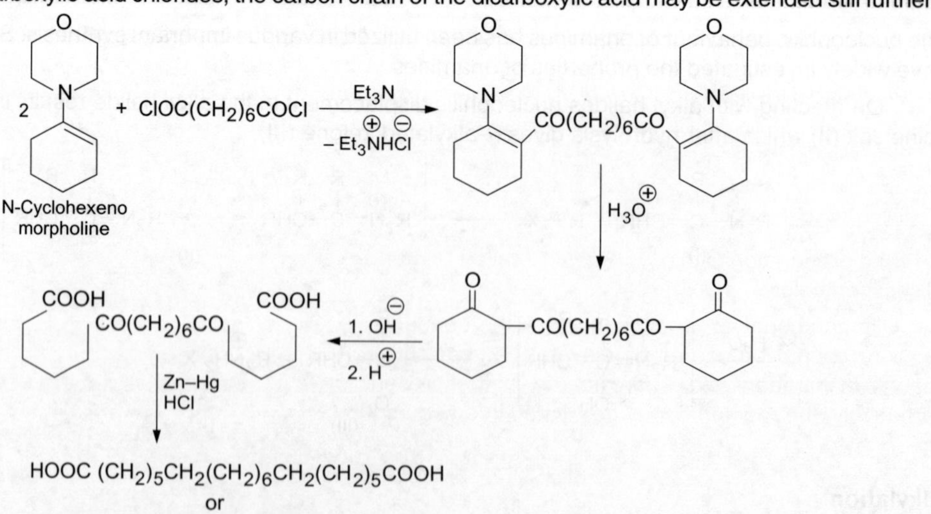

N-Cyclohexeno morpholine

$$HOOC\,(CH_2)_5CH_2(CH_2)_6CH_2(CH_2)_5COOH$$

or

$$HOOC\,(CH_2)_{18}COOH$$

Since acylated enamines are weak bases, Et_3N is used to absorb the acid produced in the reaction.

Michael type condensation

Enamines react with activated aryl halides e.g., 2, 4-dinitrochlorobenzene and with α, β-unsaturated ketones, esters, cyanides etc. The reaction is a Michael type of reaction in which the enamine acts as addend.

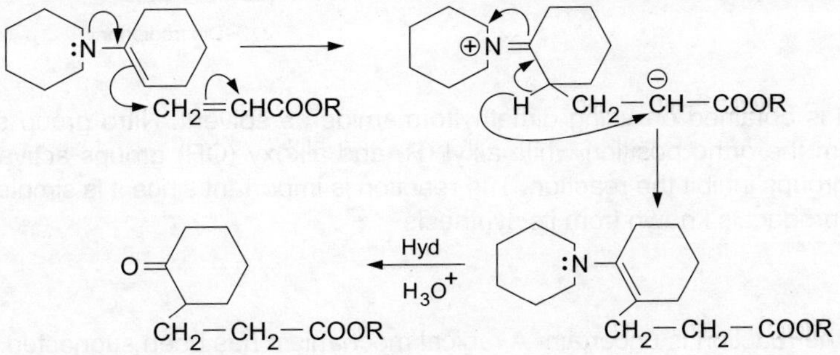

Two molecules of acetylene add together in the presence of cuprous chloride and ammonium chloride to give vinyl acetylene.

$$2HC\equiv CH \xrightarrow[CuCl]{NH_4Cl} HC\equiv C-CH=CH_2$$

In the same way terminal alkynes add to the double bond of enamines.

$$RC\equiv CH + \;\rangle C=\overset{|}{C}-NR_2 \xrightarrow[NH_4Cl]{CuCl} RC\equiv C-\underset{|}{\overset{|}{C}}-CH-NR_2$$

Enamines derived from aldehydes only add to Michael type olfins and also to ketenes to form stable four membered rings.

Enamines derived from ketones add to isocyanates to give β-lactams.

ULLMANN REACTION

Ullmann reaction encompasses the synthesis of diphenyl amines, diphenyl ethers and diphenyls.

(i) $C_6H_5NHCOCH_3 + C_6H_5Br + K_2CO_3 \xrightarrow[Reflux]{Cu} (C_6H_5)_2NH + CO_2 + CH_3COOK + KBr$

(ii) $C_6H_5OH + C_6H_5Br + KOH \xrightarrow[Reflux]{Cu} (C_6H_5)_2O + KBr + H_2O$

(iii) $2C_6H_5I + Cu \xrightarrow[\Delta]{C_6H_5NO_2} C_6H_5-C_6H_5 + CuI_2$

The preparation of diaryls [Eq. (iii)], called Ullmann coupling reaction, is the most important reaction and is discussed below.

Ullmann coupling reaction involves the condensation of aryl halides in the presence of finely divided copper or copper bronze at an elevated temperature (100–350 °C) to yield diaryl derivatives. Thus, iodobenzene in nitrobenzene when heated in the presence of copper powder gives diphenyl in 80% yield. Alternatively, the reactants may be heated in a sealed tube.

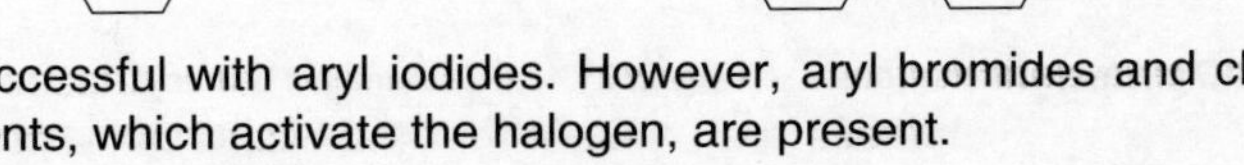

The reaction is successful with aryl iodides. However, aryl bromides and chlorides also react when electronegative substituents, which activate the halogen, are present.

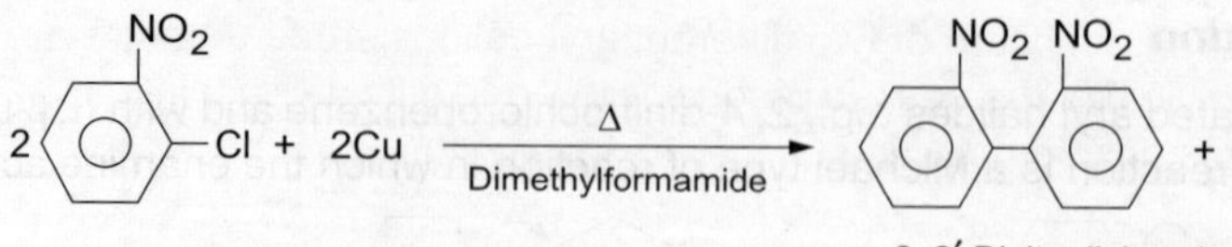

2, 2′-Dinitrodiphenyl

A better yield is obtained on using dimethylformamide as solvent. Nitro group strongly activates the halides but only from the ortho position while alkyl (R) and alkoxy (OR) groups activate from all positions. Electron-releasing groups inhibit the reaction. The reaction is important since it is simple, straightforward and the structure of the product is known from its synthesis.

Mechanism

The mechanism of the reaction is uncertain. A radical mechanism has been suggested.

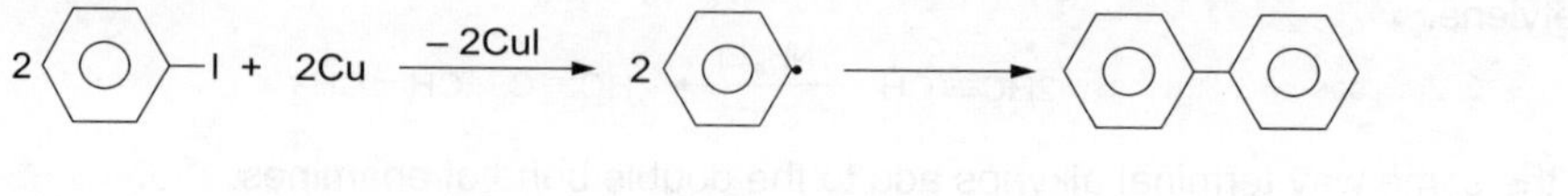

There are evidence against the radical mechanism and hence a mechanism similar to that of Wurtz reaction has been suggested.

$$C_6H_5I + Cu \longrightarrow C_6H_5CuI \quad \ldots (1)$$

$$C_6H_5CuI + C_6H_5I \longrightarrow C_6H_5-C_6H_5 + CuI_2 \quad \ldots (2)$$

The fact that iodides give good results suggests that iodides undergo step (I) more readily.

Applications

The reaction provides methods for the preparation of compounds which cannot be readily prepared by other methods. The yields of the products are high in most cases.

(A) A large number of biaryls and polyaryls have been synthesized by the Ullmann coupling reaction.

1. Symmetrical biaryls

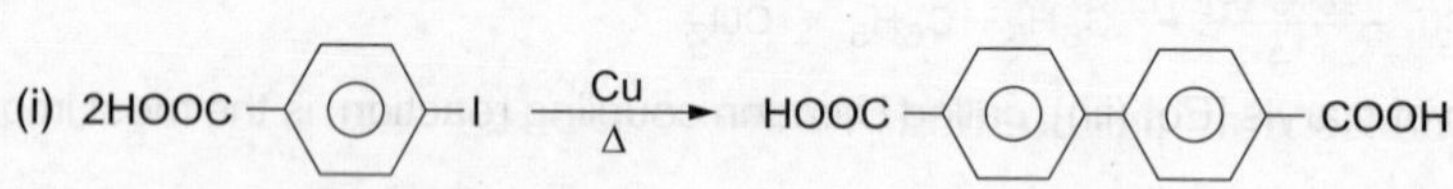

p-Iodobenzoic acid 4, 4′-Diphenic acid

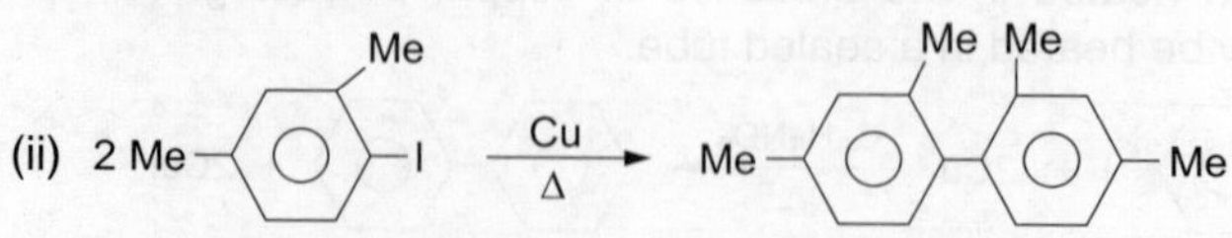

2,4-Dimethyl iodobenzene 2, 2′, 4, 4′-Tetramethyl biphenyl

2. Unsymmetrical diaryls With a mixture of two different aryl halides, three products are obtained which has poor synthetic value for the yield of the desired product is low and difficult to isolate. In some cases, however, the unsymmetrical product is only formed, e.g.,

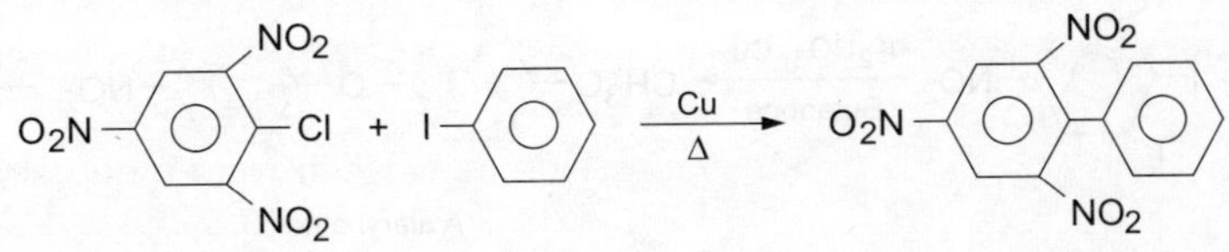

Picryl chloride → 2, 4, 6-Trinitro biphenyl

3. Polyaryl hydrocarbons

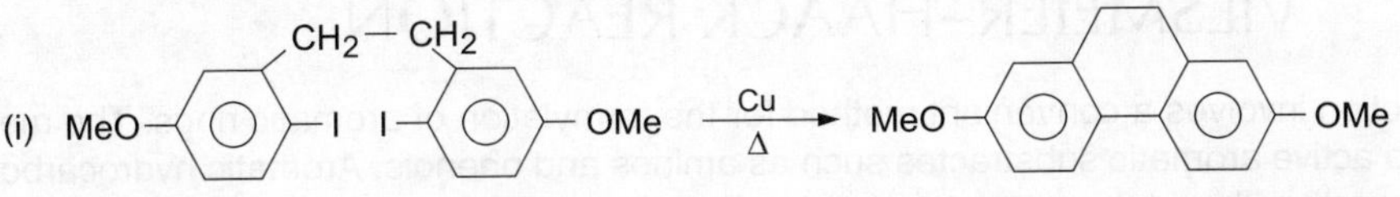

2, 2′-Diiodo-5,5′-dimethoxy dibenzyl → 2, 7-Dimethoxy-9,10-dihydrophenanthrene

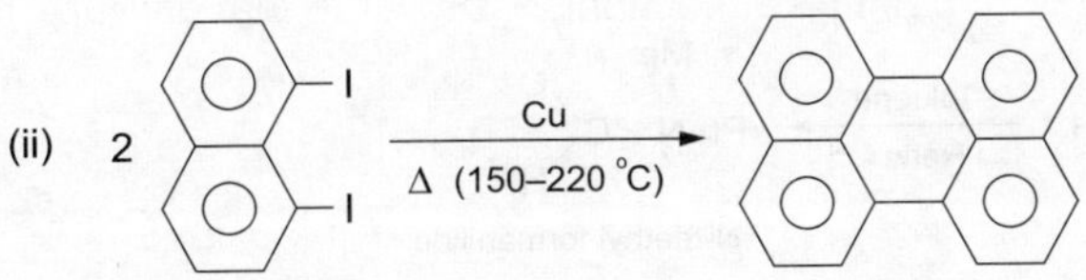

1, 8-Diiodonaphthalene → Perylene

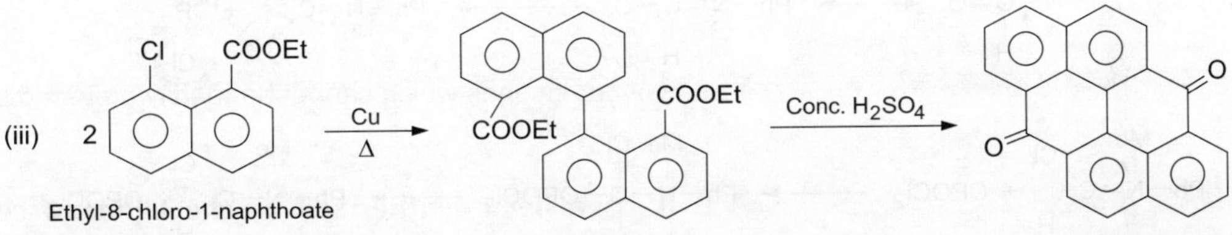

Ethyl-8-chloro-1-naphthoate → Anthanthrone

Anthanthrone and its halogen derivatives are used as dye.

(B) Ullmann reaction also provides methods for the preparations of diarylamines and diaryl ethers

1. Diarylamines An arylamine and an arylhalide are refluxed in the presence of anhydrous potassium carbonate and copper powder.

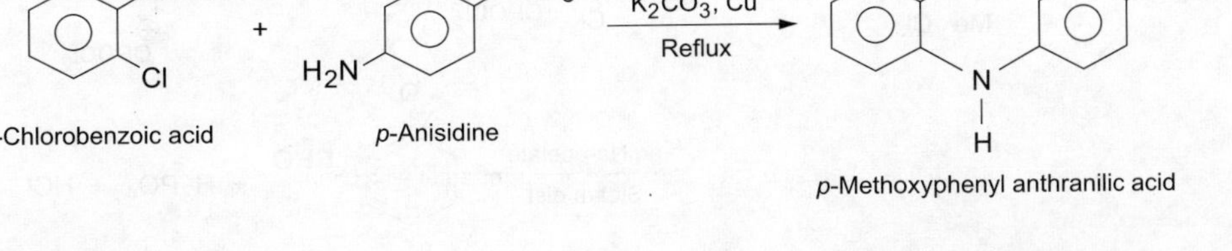

o-Chlorobenzoic acid + *p*-Anisidine → *p*-Methoxyphenyl anthranilic acid

2. Diaryl ethers A phenolic compound and an aryl halide are refluxed in the presence of potassium hydroxide or K_2CO_3 and copper. The reaction has been employed in the synthesis of thyroxine.

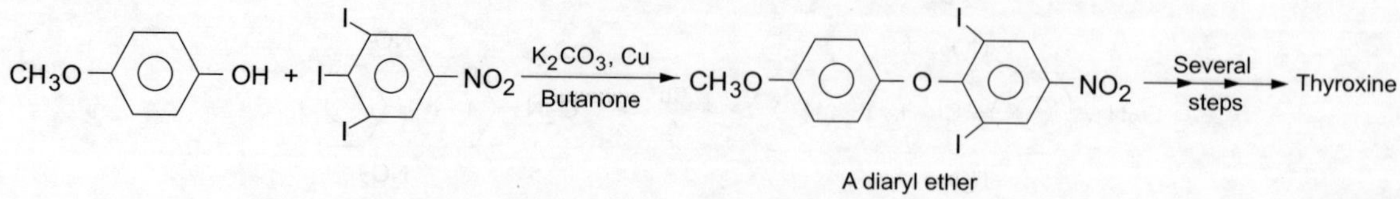

VILSMEIER–HAACK REACTION

Vilsmeier–Haack reaction involves a convenient method for the formylation of aromatic rings. The method is however applicable to active aromatic substractes such as amines and phenols. Aromatic hydrocarbons and haterocyclics more reactive than benzene can also be formylated. The reagent used for formylation is N-phenyl-N-methyl formanilide which is prepared from N-methyl aniline, formic acid and phosphorous oxychloride. Cobalt chloride may be substituted for phosphorous oxychloride.

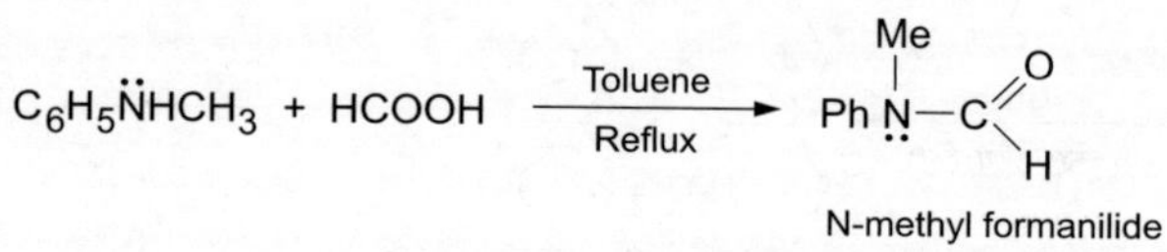

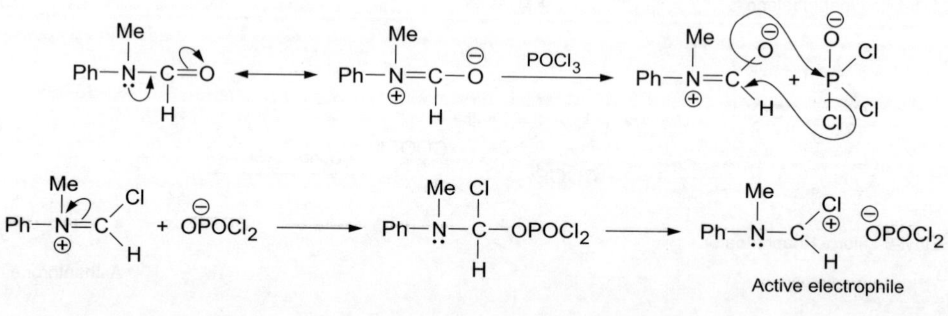

Nuclear Magnetic Resonance and other evidence support the formation of the active electrophile.

The formylation of aromatic compounds with N-methyl formanilide probably proceeds as given below:

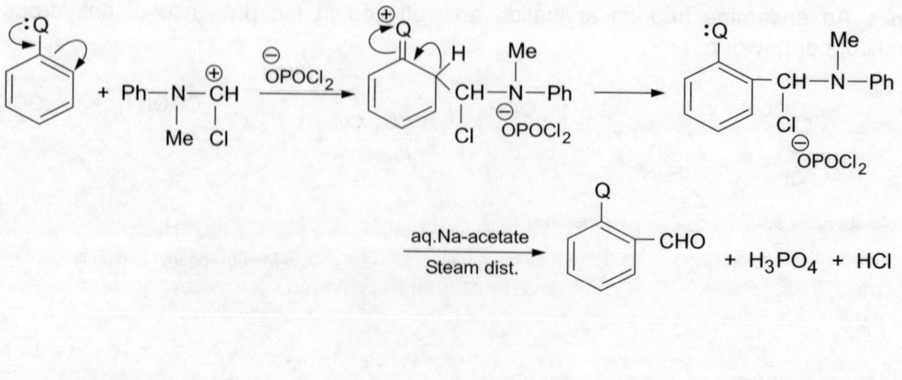

Phenolic ethers and dialkyl anilines are smoothly formylated at ortho and para positions.

Amongst hydrocarbons only anthracene is formylated at position-9.

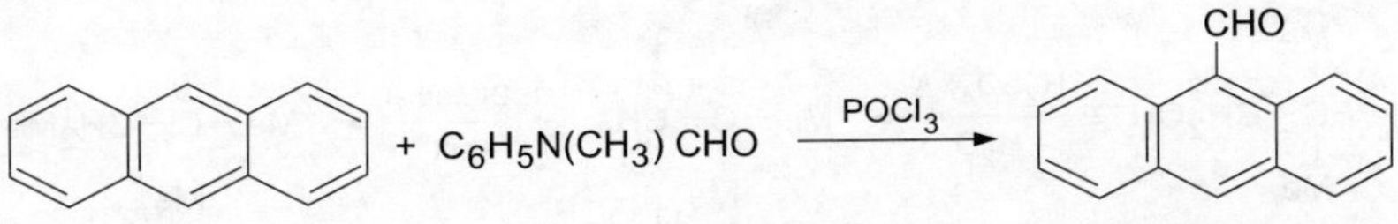

9-Anthraldehyde

Synthesis of aromatic aldehydes has considerable importance, for the aldehydes are used as intermediates in the synthesis of other valuable compounds.

WAGNER–MEERWEIN REARRANGEMENT

Reactions involving the change in the carbon skeleton through the rearrangement of the carbocation intermediate are collectively known as Wagner–Meerwein rearrangement.

When neopentyl bromide is hydrolysed under S_N1 condition it is found that instead of the expected neopentyl alcohol (Me_3CCH_2OH), 2-methyl-butan-2-ol and 2-methyl but-2-ene are formed.

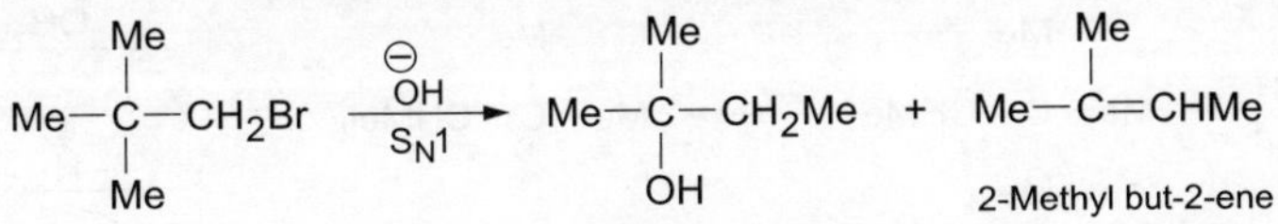 ...(i)

2-Methyl butan-2-ol 2-Methyl but-2-ene

Similarly, neopentyl alcohol on dehydration gives 2-methyl-but-2-ene and 2-methyl-but-1-ene.

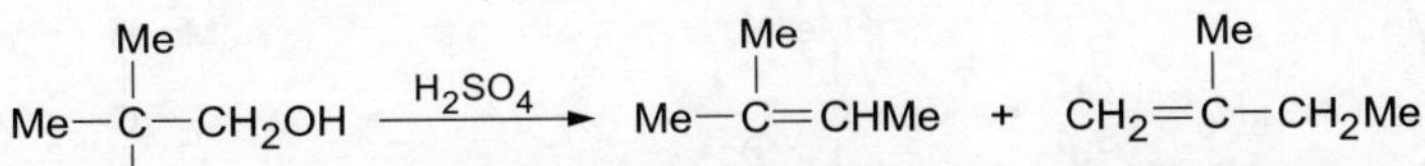 ... (ii)

2-Methyl but-2-ene 2-Methyl but-1-ene

In both cases, changes in the carbon skeleton are observed. Such rearrangement was first observed in bicyclic terpenes.

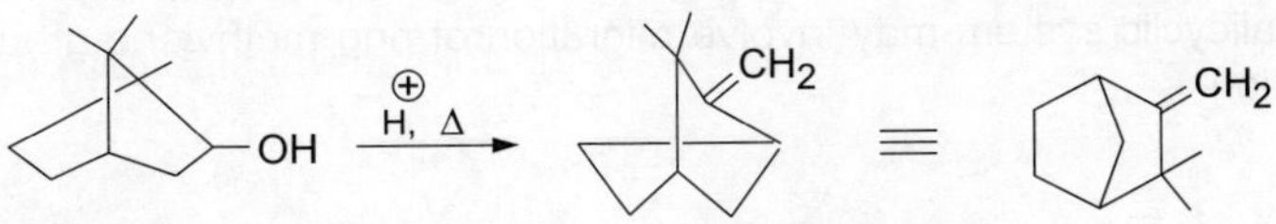 ... (iii)

Isoborneol Camphene

Mechanism of the dehydration of alcohol is discussed below.

Mechanism

Protonation of the hydroxyl group of the alcohol followed by the loss of water molecule affords a 1° carbocation. The 1° carbocation then rearranges to the relatively more stable 3° carbocation by 1, 2-methyl shift before the product is formed. The greater stability of the 3° carbocation provides the necessary force for the migration of the methyl group from the adjacent carbon. The rearranged carbocation then stabilizes itself by the loss of a β-hydrogen to form olefin. Zaitsev's rule governs as to which of the two β-hydrogens will be eliminated.

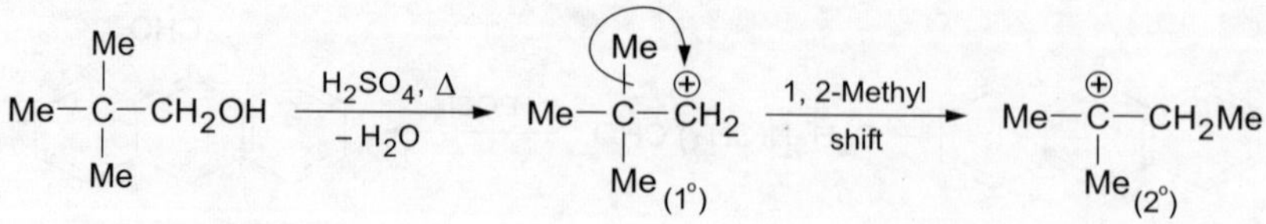

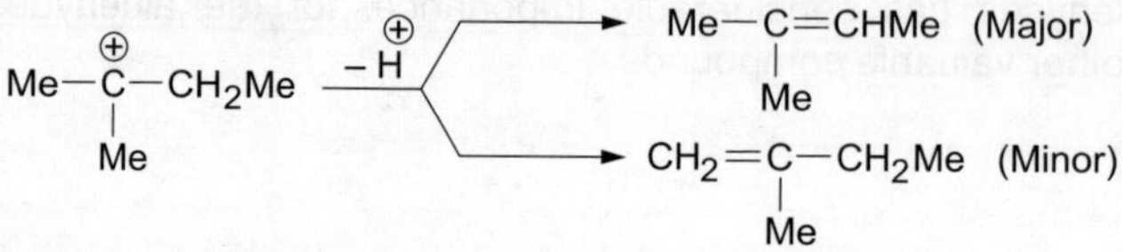

... (1)

[Hydrolysis of neopentyl halide similarly gives first a rearranged 3° carbocation which can either accept a nucleophile from the solvent to give alcohol or eliminate a proton to give olefin; see Eq. (1)]

Rearrangement does not occur if the initially formed carbocation can stabilize by other factors. Thus, 3, 3-dimethyl-2-bromo butane (neopentyl type) undergoes S_N1 hydrolysis with rearrangement,

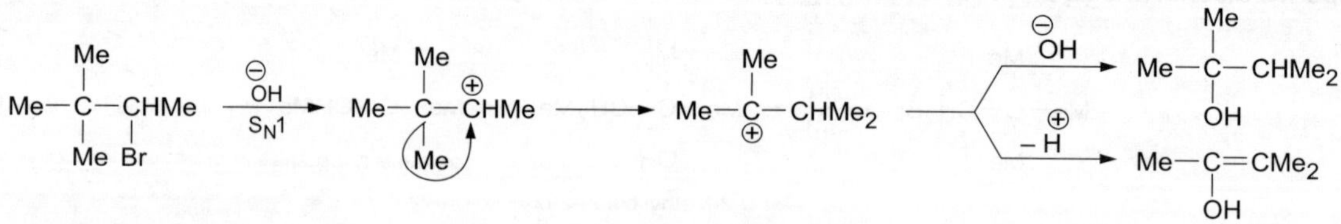

while its phenyl analogue gives product without rearrangement.

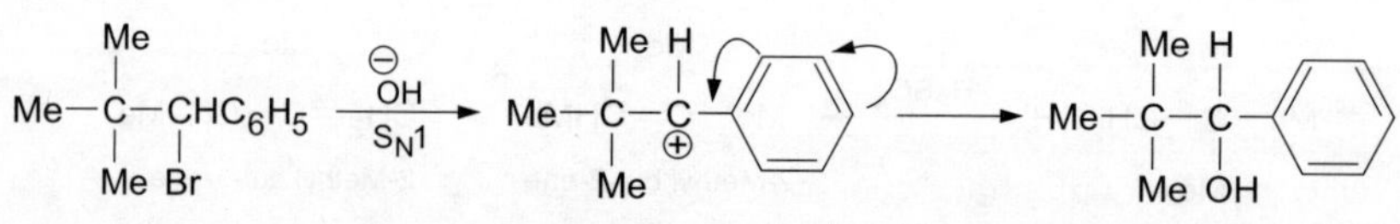

Benzilic cation
(stable)

The benzilic cation is stabilised by the phenyl group through delocalization and so does not rearrange. Rearrangement in the alicyclic system may involve migration of ring methylene group resulting in the ring expansion and contraction.

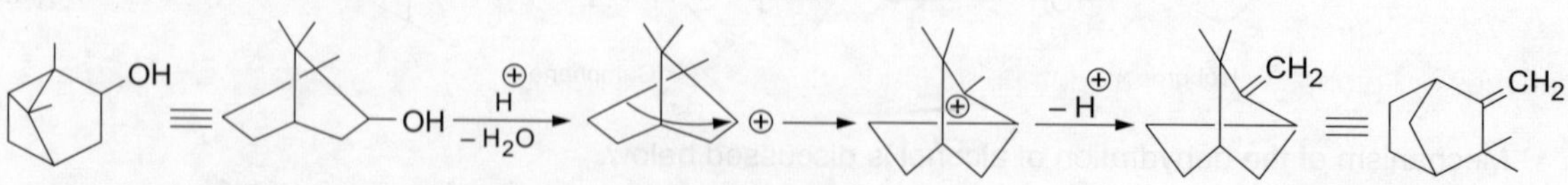

Isoborneol Camphene

Other examples are the conversions of camphene hydrochloride to isobornyl chloride, bornyl chloride to camphene, pinene hydrochloride to bornyl chloride, etc.

Some simpler examples are:

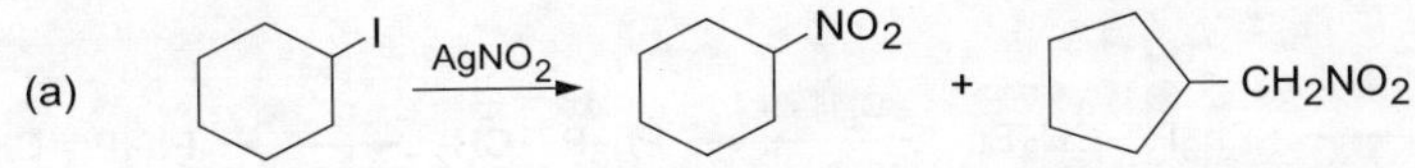

Iodocyclohexane Nitrocyclohexane Cyclopentylnitromethane

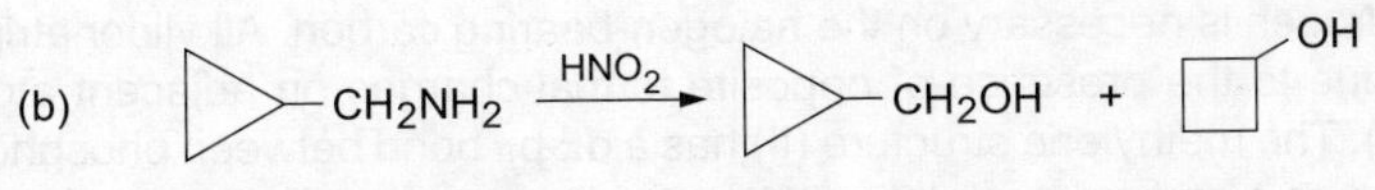

Cyclopropylcarbinylamine Cyclopropylcarbinol Cyclobutanol

The migrating group besides being alkyl and ring methylene groups may be hydride ion or aryl group.

$$CH_3-CH_2-CH_2-Br + AlBr_3 \xrightarrow{\Delta} CH_3-CH(H)-\overset{\oplus}{C}H_2 + \overset{\ominus}{Al}Br_4 \longrightarrow CH_3-\overset{\oplus}{C}H-CH_3 + \overset{\ominus}{Al}Br_4$$

$$\longrightarrow CH_3-CHBr-CH_3 + AlBr_3$$

The aryl group migrates faster than alkyl group. Electron-releasing group in the aryl group increases the rate of migration while electron-withdrawing group decreases the rate of migration. Thus, elimination is many times faster in neophyl bromide than in neopentyl bromide. This is because the rearranged phenonium ion is relatively more stable due to delocalization than the rearranged carbocation from neopentyl bromide. Hence the former has lower energy and more easily formed than the latter.

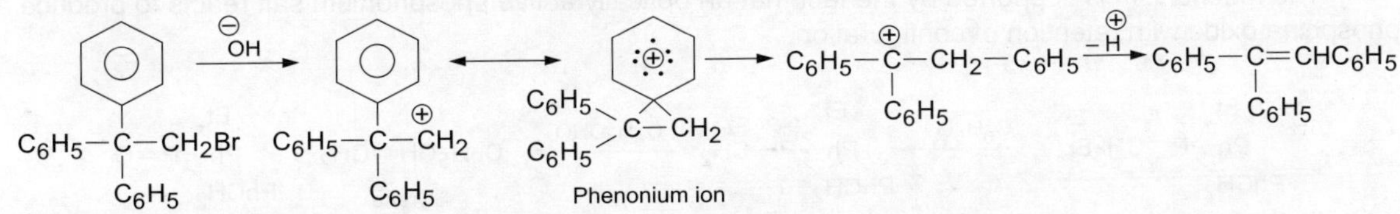

Pinacol and benzilic acid rearrangements are also examples of this carbon to carbon migration of H, R and aryl groups with consequent change in the carbon skeleton. This rearrangement has important applications especially in steroid chemistry.

WITTIG REACTION

Wittig reacton affords an important and useful method for the synthesis of alkenes by the treatment of aldehydes or ketones with alkylidenetriphenylphosphorane ($Ph_3P = CR_2$) or simply known as phosphorane.

$$Ph_3P{=}CH_2 + Ph_2C{=}O \longrightarrow Ph_2C{=}CH_2 + Ph_3P{=}O$$

1, 1-Diphenyl ethylene   Triphenyl phosphonium oxide

The Wittig reagent, alkylidenetriphenylphosphorane, is prepared by treating trialkyl or triarylphosphine usually the latter with an alkyl halide in ether solution. The resulting phosphonium salt is treated with a strong base (such as C_6H_5Li, BuLi, $NaNH_2$, NaH, C_2H_5ONa, etc.) which removes a halacid to give the reagent, methylenetriphenyl phosphorane (II).

$$Ph_3P + CH_3Br \longrightarrow Ph_3\overset{\oplus}{P}-CH_3\overset{\ominus}{Br} \xrightarrow{C_6H_5Li} \underset{(I)}{Ph_3\overset{\oplus}{P}-\overset{\ominus}{C}H_2} \longleftrightarrow \underset{(II)}{Ph_3P{=}CH_2} + C_6H_6 + LiBr$$

In the alkyl halide a hydrogen is necessary on the halogen-bearing carbon. Alkylidenetriphenylphosphoranes are also called ylides due to the presence of opposite formal charges on adjacent atoms as in one of the resonance structures (I). The methylene structure (II) has a $d\pi$-$p\pi$ bond between phosphorus and carbon. The ylide may be considered as a carbanion stabilized by the adjacent phosphonium cation.

The carbonyl compound is directly treated with the ethereal solution of the reagent.

Mechanism

The reaction probably proceeds by the nucleophilic attack of the ylide on the carbonyl carbon. The dipolar complex (betain) so formed decomposes to olefine and triphenylphosphine oxide via a four-centred transition state.

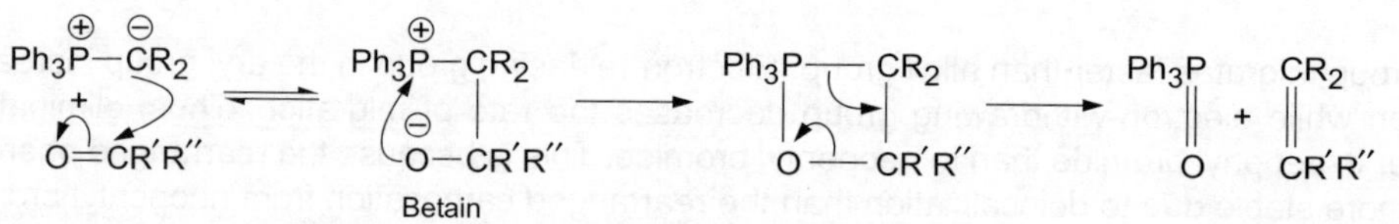

The mechanism is supported by the fact that an optically active phosphonium salt reacts to produce a phosphine oxide with retention of configuration.

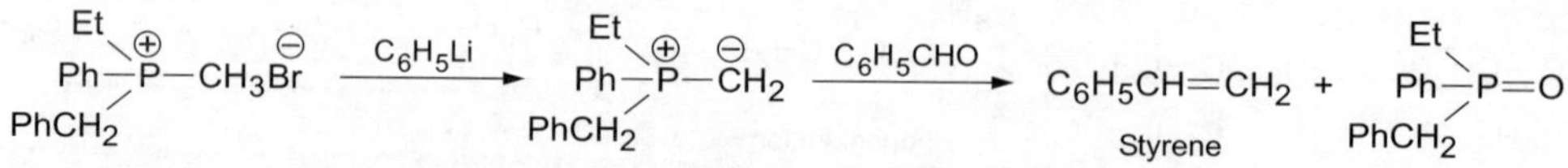

Since desired alkyl groups can be introduced in the alkyl halide and the carbonyl compound, it is extremely useful for the synthesis of desired substituted alkenes. Double or triple bonds even when conjugated with the carbonyl group ($>C{=}O$) does not interfere. The reaction with the carbonyl group of esters is very slow and does not interfere.

Phosphorous ylides react in the same manner with the C=O groups of ketenes and isocyanates as also with the N=O and C=N groups of nitroso and imine compounds respectively.

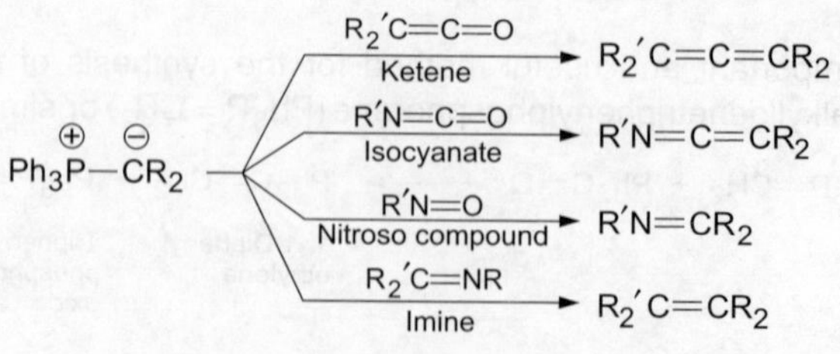

Applications

The reaction has many useful synthetic applications. Many natural products which are otherwise difficult to prepare can be synthesized by Wittig reaction.

1. Formation of exocyclic methylene group

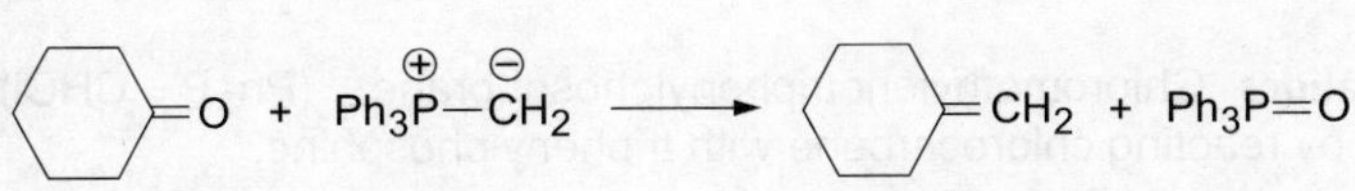

Cyclohexanone → Methylene cyclohexane

This method of introducing exocyclic methylene group is extremely valuable and has been widely used in the preparation of methylene steroids.

2. Preparation of β, γ-unsaturated acids

$$R_2C{=}O + Ph_3\overset{\oplus}{P}-\overset{\ominus}{C}H-CH_2CO\overset{\ominus}{O} \longrightarrow R_2C{=}CHCH_2CO\overset{\ominus}{O} + Ph_3P{=}O$$

In all other methods isomerization to α, β-unsaturated acids results.

3. Preparation of natural products

(i) β-carotene (pro vitamin A)

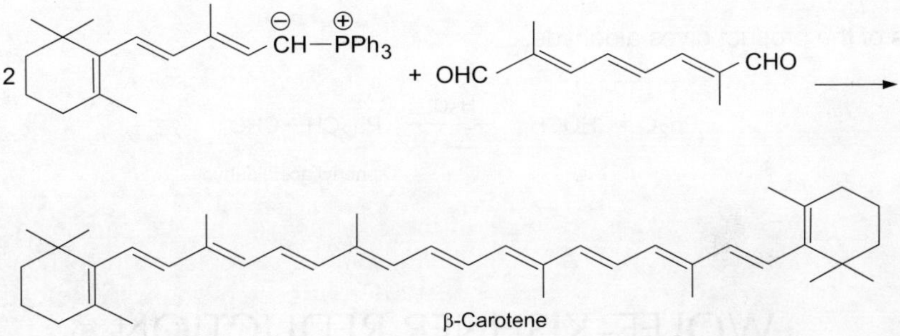

β-Carotene

(ii) Vitamin A

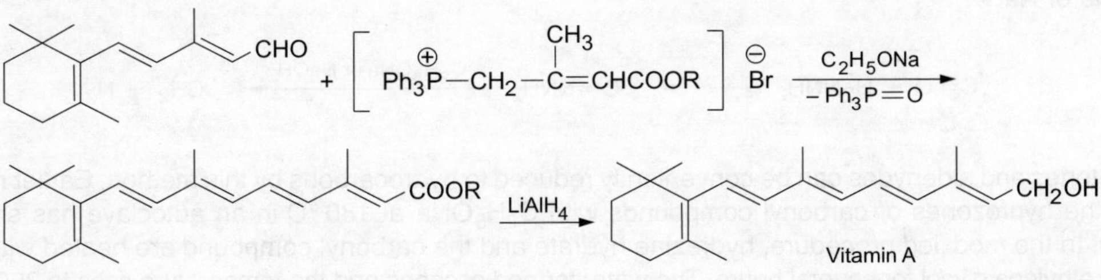

Vitamin A

4. Formation of large rings containing 5 to 16 carbons

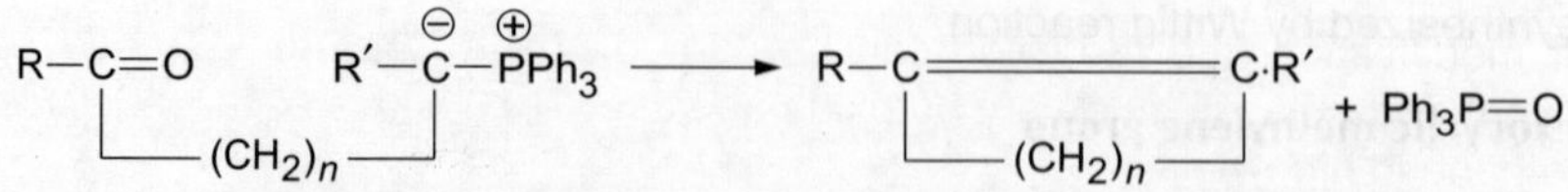

5. Synthesis of vinyl halides Chloromethylenetriphenylphosphorane ($Ph_3P = CHCl$) required for this synthesis is prepared by reacting chlorocarbene with triphenylphosphine.

$$:CHCl + Ph_3P \longrightarrow Ph_3\overset{\oplus}{P}-\overset{\ominus}{\ddot{C}}HCl \quad \text{or} \quad (Ph_3P{=}CHCl)$$

$$\text{(i)} \quad C_6H_5CHO + Ph_3\overset{\oplus}{P}-\overset{\ominus}{C}HCl \longrightarrow C_6H_5CH{=}CHCl + Ph_3P{=}O$$

(ii) 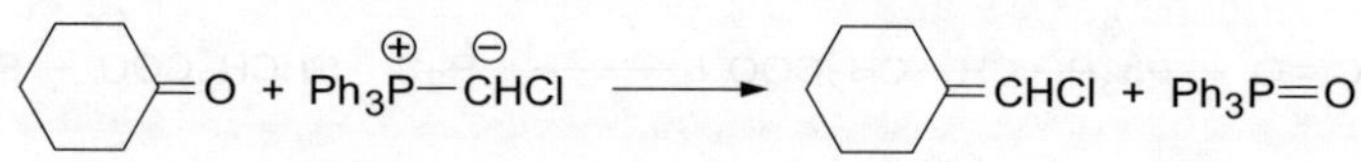

6. Synthesis of ethers Methoxymethylenetriphenylphosphorane reacts with carbonyl compounds to give diphenyl substituted vinyl methyl ethers.

$$Ph_2C{=}O + Ph_3P{=}CHOCH_3 \longrightarrow Ph_2C{=}CHOCH_3$$

Hydrolysis of the product gives aldehyde.

$$Ph_2C{=}CHOCH_3 \xrightarrow{H_2O} \underset{\text{Diphenyl acetaldehyde}}{Ph_2CH-CHO}$$

WOLFF–KISHNER REDUCTION

Wolff–Kishner reduction involves the conversion of carbonyl groups of aldehydes and ketones to methylene groups by heating their hydrozones, semicarbazones or azines in the presence of strong base such as C_2H_5ONa or NaOH.

$$>C{=}O + H_2NNH_2 \longrightarrow >C{=}NNH_2 \xrightarrow[\Delta]{C_2H_5ONa \text{ or } NaOH} >CH_2 + N_2$$

Thus, ketones and aldehydes can be conveniently reduced to hydrocarbons by this method. Earlier method of heating the hydrozones of carbonyl compounds with C_2H_5ONa at 180 °C in an autoclave has since been modified. In the modified procedure, hydrazine hydrate and the carbonyl compound are heated with KOH or NaOH in ethylene glycol for several hours. The water formed escapes and the temperature rises to 200 °C when the hydrazone decomposes with the formation of hydrocarbon with evolution of nitrogen.

$$R_2C{=}O + H_2NNH_2 \longrightarrow R_2C{=}N{\cdot}NH_2 \xrightarrow[\Delta]{C_2H_5ONa\text{ , Glycol}} R_2CH_2 + N_2$$

In a further modification, the reduction can be carried out at room temperature by using dimethyl sulphoxide as solvent and potassium tertiary butoxide as base. The yield is excellent. Thus, benzophenone gives diphenyl methane in high yield.

$$(C_6H_5)_2C{=}O \xrightarrow{H_2N{\cdot}NH_2} (C_6H_5)_2C{=}N{\cdot}NH_2 \xrightarrow[Me_2SO,\ 30\,^{\circ}C]{Me_3COK,} \underset{\text{Diphenyl methane}}{C_6H_5{\cdot}CH_2{-}C_6H_5} + N_2$$

Unlike Clemmensen reduction, the reaction does not fail with acid-sensitive or high molecular weight substrates.

Mechanism

First step involves the formation of the anion of the hydrazone (I) which is protonated at the carbonyl carbon to form a substituted diimine (II). This is followed by simultaneous loss of nitrogen and formation of hydrocarbon. (Compounds of the type (II) are unstable and decompose to hydrocarbon and nitrogen probably through carbanion or free radical mechanism.)

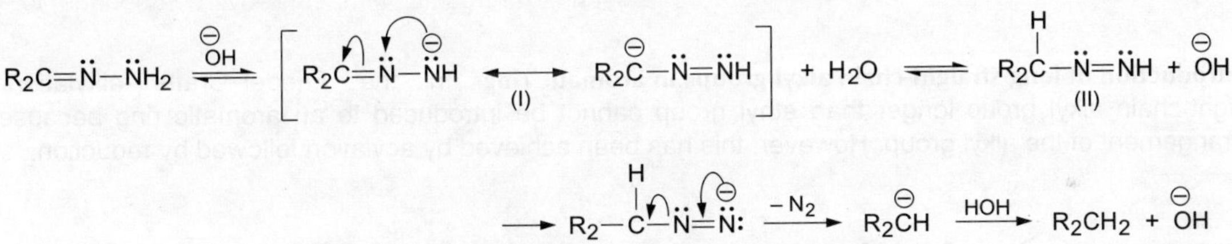

During the course of reduction, semicarbazones and azines are first converted to hydrazones before reduction.

$$\underset{\text{Semicarbazone}}{R_2C{=}N{\cdot}NH{\cdot}CO{\cdot}NH_2} + H_2O \longrightarrow R_2C{=}N{\cdot}NH_2$$

$$\underset{\text{Azine}}{R_2C{=}N{-}N{=}CR_2} + 2NH_2{\cdot}NH_2 \longrightarrow 2R_2C{=}N{\cdot}NH_2$$

The method is specific for the reduction of carbonyl groups only, for other functional groups in the substrate remain unaffected. The method is, however, not suitable for α,β-unsaturated ketones.

Applications

Wolff–Kishner reduction has been frequently used for the reduction of carbonyl groups to methylene groups in various types of syntheses.

The method unlike Clemmensen reduction is applicable for the reduction of high molecular weight and acid-sensitive compounds.

1. Reduction of high molecular weight compounds High molecular weight compound, e.g., 24-keto-cholesterol, has been successfully reduced.

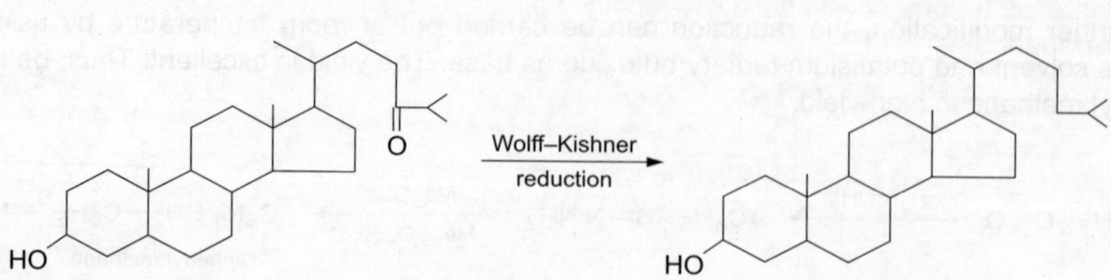

24-Ketocholesterol Cholesterol

2. Reduction of camphor to camphane

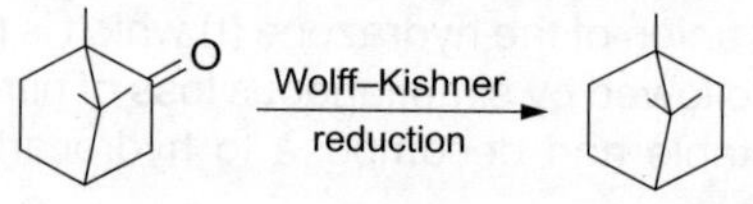

Camphor Camphane

3. Introduction of long straight-chain alkyl groups in aromatic rings In the Friedel–Crafts alkylation a straight-chain alkyl group longer than ethyl group cannot be introduced to an aromatic ring because of rearrangement of the alkyl group. However, this has been achieved by acylation followed by reduction.

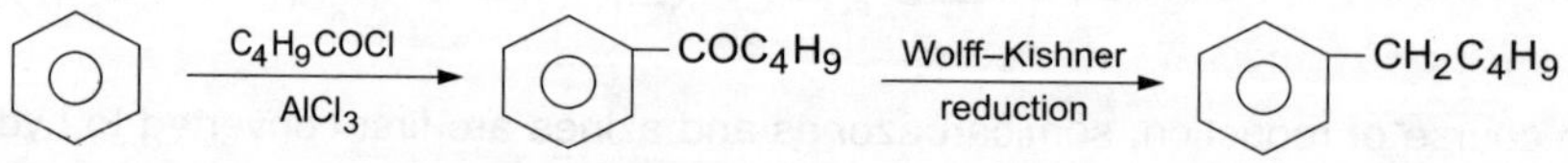

n-Butyl phenyl ketone *n*-Pentyl benzene

4. In the structure determination of oestrone The formation of 7-methoxy-1 : 2-cyclopenteno-phenanthrene, a compound of known structure, by the reduction of oestrone methyl ether followed by dehydrogenation with selenium indicates the carbon skeleton of oestrone as also the position of the methoxy group.

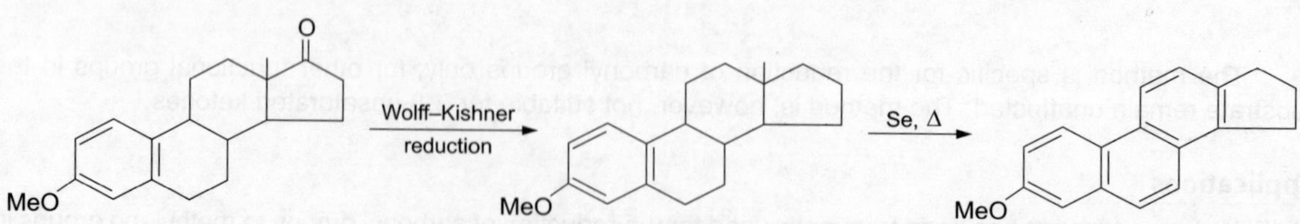

Oestrone methyl ether

7-Methoxy-1:2-cyclopenteno phenanthrene

WOLFF REARRANGEMENT

α-Diazoketones on treatment with solid silver oxide split off nitrogen and rearrange to ketene. This is known as Wolff rearrangement.

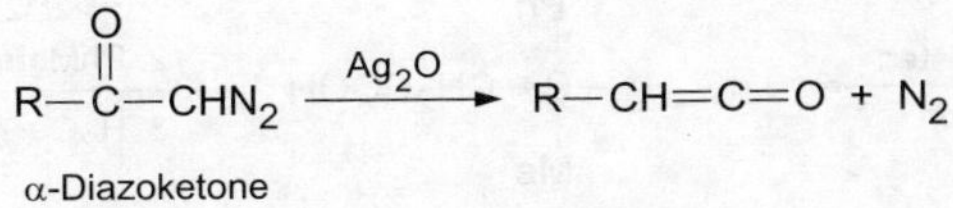

The rearrangement may also occur on irradiation or on heating. When the reaction is carried out in the presence of water, alcohol, ammonia or amine, the highly reactive ketene readily reacts with the nucleophiles present, e.g., H_2O, ROH, etc., to give respectively acids, esters, amides or substituted amides of the next higher homologue of the acid from which the α-diazoketone is prepared.

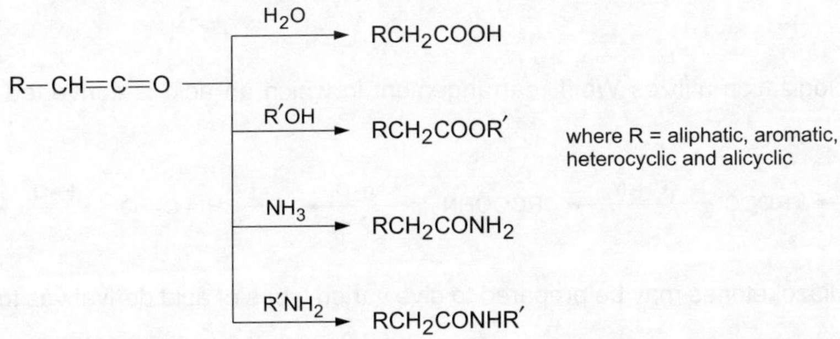

Mechanism

It has been shown (Huggett *et al.*) with isotopically labelled carbon (^{13}C) in a series of transformations* that the carbonyl carbon of α-diazoketone is present in the resulting acid as the carboxyl carbon when the reaction is carried out in the presence of water. Obviously, migration must have occurred during the rearrangement. On the basis of this, the following mechanism has been suggested:

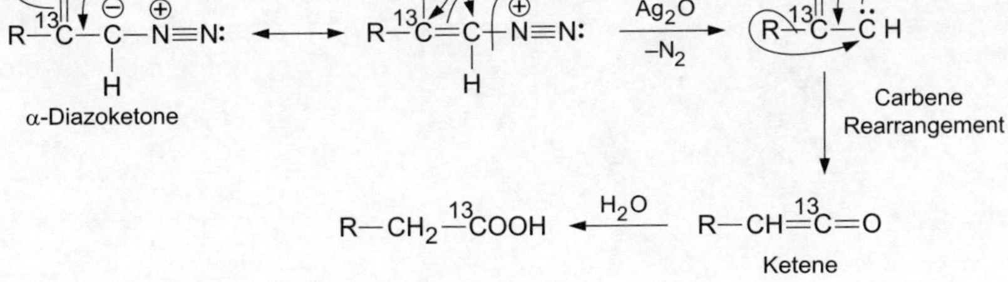

---

* $$^{13}CO_2 + PhMgBr \longrightarrow Ph^{13}COOH \xrightarrow[2.\ CH_2N_2]{1.\ SOCl_2} Ph^{13}COCHN_2 \xrightarrow[H_2O]{Ag_2O} PhCH_2{}^{13}COOH$$

$$\xrightarrow[\text{Quinoline}]{CuO.\ Cr_2O_3} {}^{13}CO_2 + PhCOOH$$

Splitting of nitrogen and migration of R group may be concerted. In some cases ketenes have been isolated. The group R migrates with retention of configuration. This has been confirmed by the following observation.

A higher homologue of an optically active acid (I) obtained by Arndt–Eistert–Wolff rearrangement on degradation by Barbier–Weiland method gave the original acid with the same configuration (Lane and Wallis).

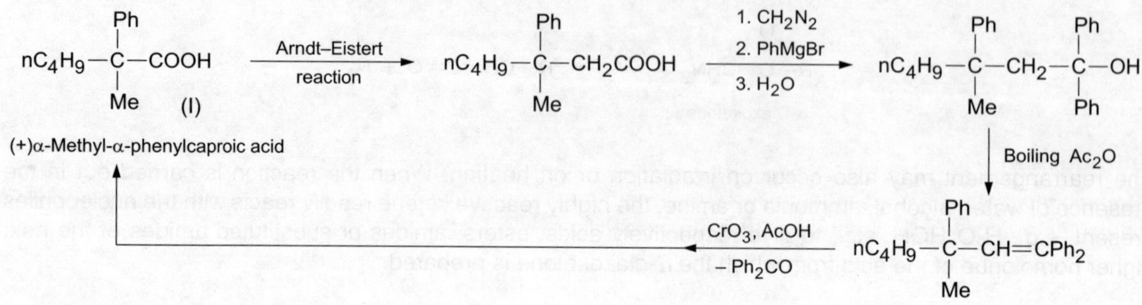

Application

Arndt–Eistert homologization utilizes Wolff rearrangement in which an acid is converted to its next higher homologue.

$$\mathrm{RCOOH} \xrightarrow{\mathrm{SOCl_2}} \mathrm{RCOCl} \xrightarrow{\mathrm{CH_2N_2}} \mathrm{RCOCHN_2} \xrightarrow[-\mathrm{N_2}]{\mathrm{Ag_2O}} \mathrm{R{-}CH{=}C{=}O} \xrightarrow{\mathrm{H_2O}} \mathrm{R{-}CH_2COOH}$$

Various classes of diazoketones may be prepared to give varied types of acid derivatives for further synthetic applications.

❑

Chapter 3
Important Reagents

Introduction

Organic reactions involve reagents and substrates. A group of organic compounds serves as substrates for a particular type of reaction when treated with a specific reagent.

Chemical reagents bring about various types of changes in organic molecules to yield products of immense value. Reagents have been found that can degrade complex molecules to simple known molecules which enabled us to elucidate the structures of complex compounds. A suitable choice of reagent and reaction conditions are essential for the success of a reaction for the desired product.

A few of the most important and widely used reagents along with a few novel catalysts for the synthesis of a large varieties of natural products, commercially useful chemicals of medicinal and industrial importance have been included in this section. Their preparations, mode of applications and mechanistic aspects along with their uses have been briefly described. The reagents have been described in alphabetic order for convenience.

ANHYDROUS ALUMINIUM CHLORIDE

This important catalyst is prepared by either of the two methods.

1. Reductive chlorination of bauxite ore Bauxite ore is mixed with coke asphalt and heated strongly to remove water. The mixture is placed into a kiln and rapidly heated to a high temperature and then a stream of chlorine gas is passed. Aluminium trichloride is formed and sublimes out of the kiln. It is cooled and the white crystals are collected in well-stoppered bottles.

$$Al_2O_3 + 3C \xrightarrow{\Delta} 2Al + 3CO \; ; \; 2Al + 3Cl_2 \longrightarrow 2AlCl_3$$

2. Direct chlorination Small pieces of clean aluminium metal or its scrap are placed in a hard glass tube which is heated strongly while passing a stream of chlorine through the tube. Aluminium trichloride sublimes out of the tube and is collected.

$$2Al + 3Cl_2 \xrightarrow{\Delta} 2AlCl_3$$

The second method is suited for laboratory purpose.

Uses

Aluminium trichloride has an electron-deficient atom and functions as Lewis acid. It initiates the reaction by accepting an electron pair and furnishing a real or potential carbocation.

$$RX + AlCl_3 \longrightarrow \overset{\delta+}{R}\text{----}X\text{----}\overset{\delta-}{AlCl_3} \longrightarrow \overset{\oplus}{R} + \overset{\ominus}{XAlCl_3}$$

It is a versatile catalyst and has been used in a large number of reactions. A few of them are mentioned below.

1. Friedel–Crafts alkylation and acylation

Aluminium trichloride is found to be the best catalyst for these reactions.

(i) $C_6H_6 + RX \xrightarrow{AlCl_3} C_6H_5R + HX$

(ii) $C_6H_6 + RCOCl \xrightarrow{AlCl_3} C_6H_5COR + HCl$

(iii) $2C_6H_6 + COCl_2 \xrightarrow{AlCl_3} C_6H_5COC_6H_5 + 2HCl$

The reactions may be employed to prepare hydrocarbons, polynuclear hydrocarbons, cyclic ketones, etc. Thus,

(iv) $C_6H_6 + RCOCl \xrightarrow{AlCl_3} C_6H_5COR \xrightarrow[HCl]{Na-Hg} C_6H_5CH_2R$

(v) $3C_6H_6 + CHCl_3 \xrightarrow{AlCl_3} \underset{\text{Triphenylmethane}}{(C_6H_5)_3CH}$

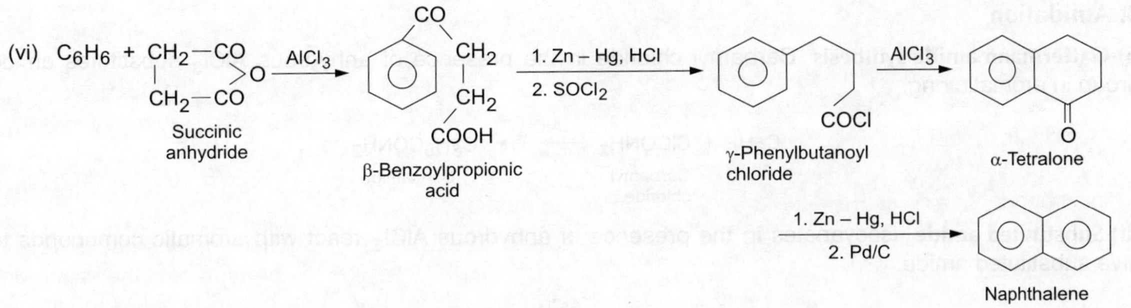

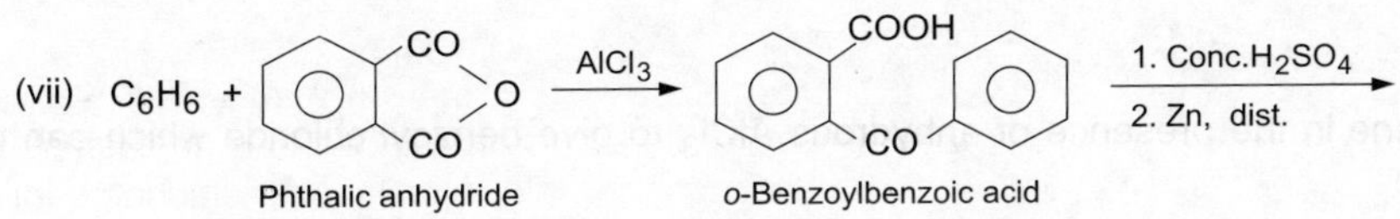

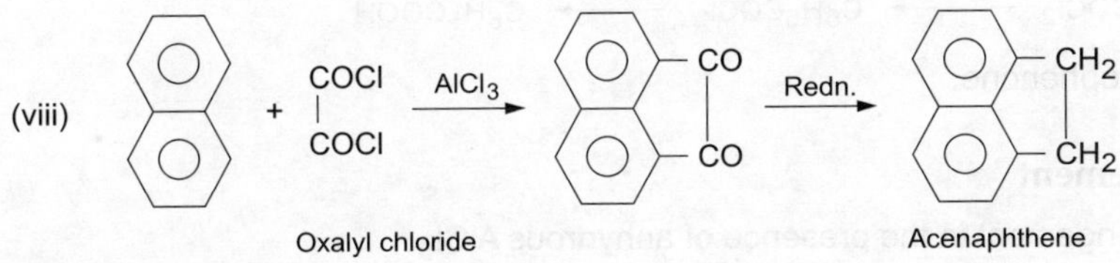

2. Fries reaction

Phenyl esters on treatment with anhydrous aluminium trichloride are converted to *o*- or *p*-hydroxy ketones. The reaction involves rearrangement through migration of a group from oxygen to carbon.

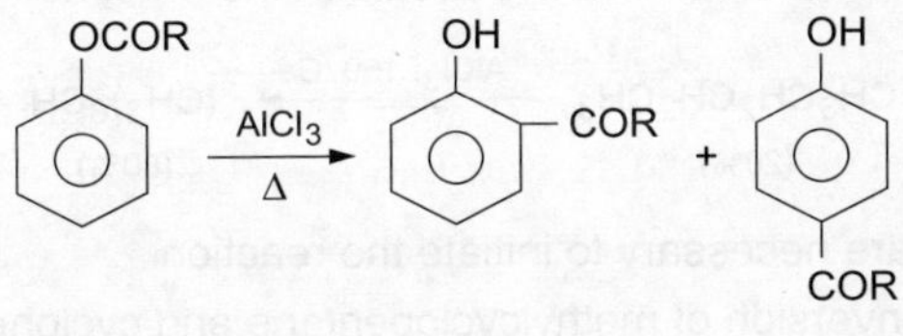

3. Gattermann–Koch aldehyde synthesis

A mixture of dry carbon monoxide and hydrochloric acid gas is passed through a solution of benzene in ether or nitrobenzene containing anhydrous aluminium trichloride and a little cuprous chloride. The mixture of carbon monoxide and hydrochloric acid behaves as formyl chloride. Cuprous chloride is necessary to perform the reaction at atmospheric pressure otherwise 100–250 atmospheric pressure is required for the reaction.

$$\text{ArH} + \text{CO} + \text{HCl} \xrightarrow[\text{Cu}_2\text{Cl}_2]{\text{AlCl}_3} \text{ArCHO}$$

Formylation has also been effected by dichloromethyl methyl ether in the presence of anhydrous aluminium trichloride.

$$\text{ArH} + \text{Cl}_2\text{CHOCH}_3 \xrightarrow{\text{AlCl}_3} \text{ArCHO}$$

4. Amidation

(i) Gattermann amide synthesis Carbamyl chloride in the presence of anhydrous $AlCl_3$ substitutes amide group in aromatic ring.

$$\underset{}{C_6H_6} + \underset{\text{Carbamyl chloride}}{ClCONH_2} \xrightarrow{AlCl_3} \underset{\text{Benzamide}}{C_6H_5CONH_2}$$

(ii) Substituted amide Isocyanates in the presence of anhydrous $AlCl_3$ react with aromatic compounds to give substituted amide.

$$C_6H_6 + RNCO \xrightarrow{AlCl_3} C_6H_5CONHR$$

5. Carboxylation

Phosgene reacts with benzene in the presence of anhydrous $AlCl_3$ to give benzoyl chloride which can be hydrolysed to acid.

$$C_6H_6 + COCl_2 \xrightarrow{AlCl_3} C_6H_5COCl \xrightarrow{H_3O^{\oplus}} C_6H_5COOH$$

Excess of benzene may give benzophenone.

6. Wagner–Meerwein rearrangement

Long-chain halides undergo rearrangement in the presence of anhydrous $AlCl_3$.

$$CH_3CH_2CH_2Br \xrightarrow[\Delta]{AlCl_3} CH_3CHBrCH_3$$

7. Isomerization

Reforming of gasoline fraction to increase branching occurs in the presence of $AlCl_3$, e.g.,

$$\underset{(20\%)}{CH_3CH_2CH_2CH_3} \xrightleftharpoons{AlCl_3,\ 150\,^{\circ}C} \underset{(80\%)}{(CH_3)_3CH}$$

Traces of alkyl halide or alcohol are necessary to initiate the reaction.

Another example is interconversion of methylcyclopentane and cyclohexane.

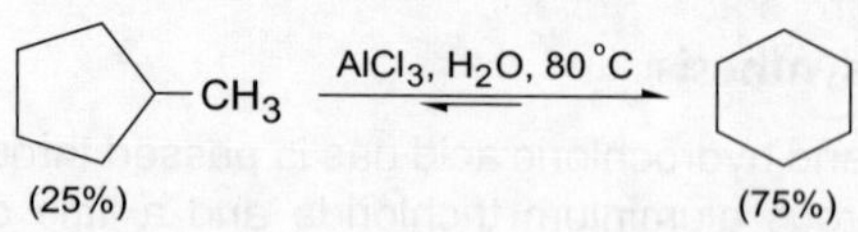

8. Dealkylation

Tertiary alkyl groups are lost more easily.

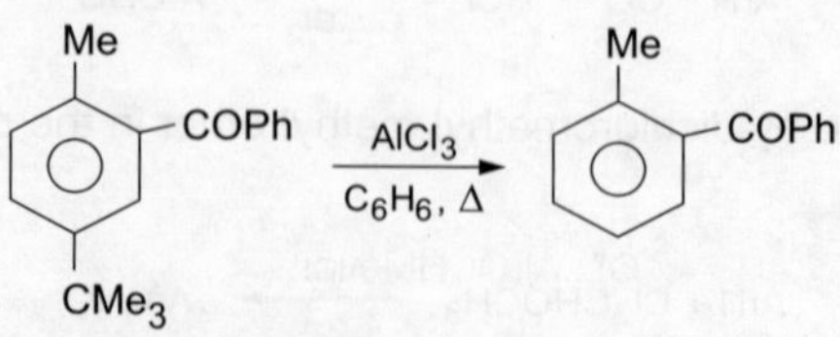

9. Addition to olefines

Alkyl halides add to olefins in the presence of anhydrous $AlCl_3$.

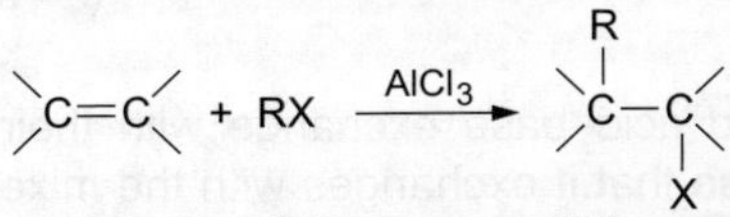

Certain Diels–Alder reactions are accelerated by $AlCl_3$ under milder conditions.

ALUMINIUM ISOPROPOXIDE, $(Me_2CHO)_3Al$

Aluminium isopropoxide is a good reducing agent. It reduces by transfer of hydride ions.

Preparation

The reagent is prepared by refluxing anhydrous isopropyl alcohol with aluminium amalgam in the presence of a small amount of carbon tetrachloride as catalyst. After the evolution of hydrogen ceases, the mixture is distilled under reduced pressure when aluminium isopropoxide distils over at 140–150 °C (12 mm) as a colourless liquid.

Uses

It is a specific reducing agent for the reduction of carbonyl compounds to alcohols without affecting other sensitive reducible groups. With excess of the reagent at elevated temperature, diaryl ketones may be reduced to hydrocarbons.

The reduction is carried out by heating the carbonyl compound with the reagent in isopropyl alcohol and distilling off the acetone as it is formed.

$$R_2C{=}O + (Me_2CHO)_3Al \rightleftharpoons Me_2CO + R_2CHO-Al(OCHMe_2)_2$$

$$R_2CHO-Al(OCHMe_2)_2 \xrightarrow{Me_2CHOH} R_2CHOH + (Me_2CHO)_3Al$$

Since the reaction is reversible, the reagent can also be employed for the oxidation of alcohols. The reverse reaction is known as Oppenauer oxidation. The position of equilibrium can be controlled by the amount of acetone present. The equilibrium shifts forward on distilling out the acetone as it is formed. An excess of acetone favours oxidation (reverse reaction).

The reagent is better than other metallic alkoxides because it is relatively less polar. The aluminium–oxygen bond is almost covalent and does not give alkoxide ions which generally cause much condensation of carbonyl compounds.

Mechanism

The reaction proceeds by complexing the carbonyl oxygen of the substrate with aluminium and then transfer of hydride ion to the carbonyl carbon of the substrate in the cyclic transition state (I), resulting in the formation of a mixed alkoxide (II).

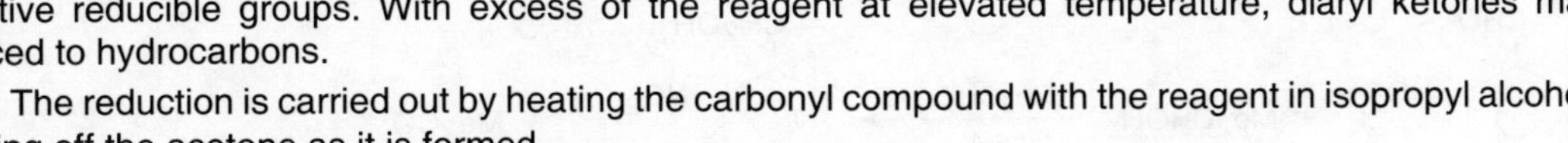

(I) (II)

$$RCH_2O{-}Al(OCHMe_2)_2 \xrightarrow{Me_2CHOH} \underset{(III)}{RCH_2OH} + Al(OCHMe_2)_3$$

(R = Saturated or unsaturated)

Metal alkoxides undergo rapid acid–base exchange with their corresponding alcohols. Hence, an excess of isopropyl alcohol is used so that it exchanges with the mixed alkoxide (II) to liberate the reduced aldehyde (III), i.e., the desired alcohol. Hence, the hydrogens for the reduction are supplied one each by the catalyst and the solvent. That a hydride ion is transferred from the reagent to the carbonyl compound is proved by the fact that with $(Me_2CDO)_3Al$, the carbonyl compound gave RCHD(OH). This indicates that the reaction proceeds via the cyclic transition state.

Applications

Some of its important applications are given below.

1. Meerwein–Ponndorf reduction

(i) $$\underset{\text{Crotonaldehyde}}{CH_3{-}CH{=}CH{-}CHO} + Me_2CHOH \xrightarrow[\Delta]{(Me_2CHO)_3Al} \underset{\text{Crotyl alcohol}}{CH_3{-}CH{=}CH{-}CH_2OH} + Me_2CO\uparrow$$

(ii) $$\underset{\text{2-Pentanone}}{CH_3{-}CO{-}CH_2{-}CH_2{-}CH_3} + Me_2CHOH \xrightarrow[\Delta]{(Me_2CHO)_3Al} \underset{\text{2-Pentanol}}{CH_3{-}CH(OH){-}CH_2{-}CH_2{-}CH_3} + Me_2CO\uparrow$$

(iii) 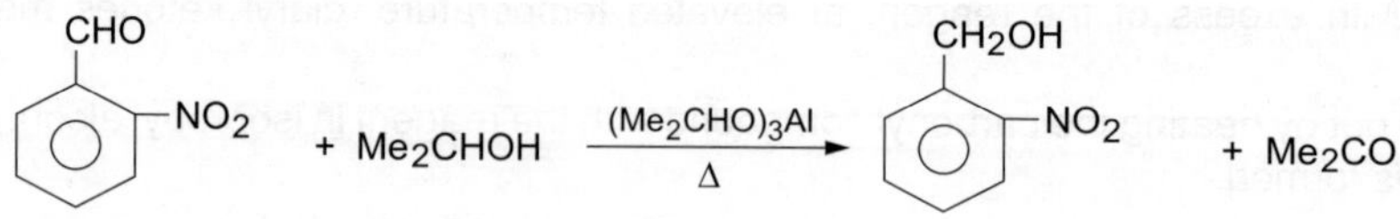

2-Nitrobenzaldehyde 2-Nitrobenzyl alcohol

(iv) $$\underset{\text{Acetophenone}}{C_6H_5{-}CO{-}CH_3} + Me_2CHOH \xrightarrow[\Delta]{(Me_2CHO)_3Al} \underset{\alpha\text{-Methyl benzyl alcohol}}{C_6H_5{-}CHOH{-}CH_3} + Me_2CO$$

(v) 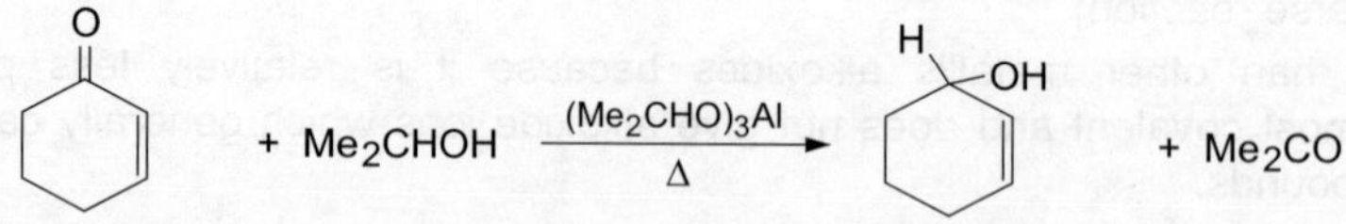

2-Cyclohexene-1-one 2-Cyclohexene-1-ol

(vi) $$\underset{\text{Trichloracetone}}{Cl_3C{-}CO{-}CH_3} + Me_2CHOH \xrightarrow[\Delta]{(Me_2CHO)_3Al} \underset{\text{1, 1, 1-Trichloropropanol-2}}{Cl_3C{-}CHOH{-}CH_3} + Me_2CO$$

(vii) $$\underset{\text{Ethyl trimethylpyruvate}}{(CH_3)_3C{-}CO{-}CO_2C_2H_5} + Me_2CHOH \xrightarrow[-Me_2CO]{(Me_2CHO)_3Al,\ \Delta} \underset{\text{Ethyl trimethylacetate}}{(CH_3)_3C{-}CHOH{-}CO_2C_2H_5}$$

2. Reduction of diaryl ketones to hydrocarbons

With excess reagent and at higher temperature complete reduction has been achieved.

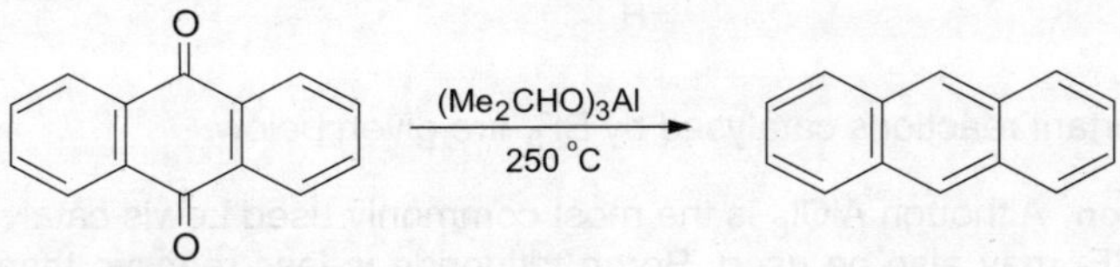

Anthraquinone Anthracene

3. In Oppenauer oxidation

Although aluminium-tertiary butoxide is the generally used catalyst for this reaction, aluminium isopropoxide has also been used for the oxidation. An excess of acetone or better hydrogen acceptors like quinones or aryl ketones are used along with the reagent.

(i) $$RCHOHR + CH_3COCH_3 \xrightarrow{(Me_2CHO)_3Al} RCOR + CH_3CHOHCH_3$$

(ii)

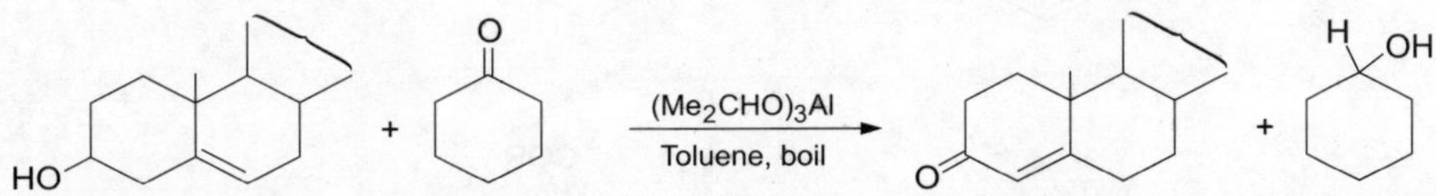

Cholesterol Cyclohexanone Cholestenone Cyclohexanol

The reagent has also been used to reduce camphor to borneol and isoborneol, carvone to carveol, oestrone to oestradiol and in the synthesis of chloromycetin.

BORON TRIFLUORIDE, BF_3

Preparation

Boron trifluoride is prepared by the following methods.

1. Ignition of boron in a current of fluorine gives boron trifluoride.

$$2B + 3F_2 \xrightarrow{\text{Ignition}} 2BF_3$$

2. By heating calcium fluoride and boron trioxide with concentrated sulphuric acid.

$$3CaF_2 + 3H_2SO_4 + B_2O_3 \xrightarrow{\Delta} 2BF_3 + 3CaSO_4 + 3H_2O$$

3. By heating borax, fluorspar and conc. H_2SO_4 (large-scale preparation).

$$Na_2B_4O_7{\cdot}10H_2O + 6CaF_2 + 8H_2SO_4 \xrightarrow{\Delta} 4BF_3 + 2NaHSO_4 + 6CaSO_4 + 17H_2O$$

It is a colourless fuming gas.

Uses

Boron trifluoride is used as a Lewis acid catalyst in organic reactions. Boron in BF_3 has a vacant orbital. Hence it has a strong tendency to coordinate with an unshared electron pair of donor elements, e.g., oxygen and nitrogen to form a relatively stable coordination complex which catalyses the reaction.

$$H_3\overset{\oplus}{N}: \rightarrow \overset{\ominus}{B}F_3, \quad R-\overset{H}{\underset{H}{\overset{|}{\underset{|}{\overset{\oplus}{N}}}}}: \rightarrow \overset{\ominus}{B}F_3, \quad R_2\overset{\oplus}{\ddot{O}}: \rightarrow \overset{\ominus}{B}F_3, \text{ etc.}$$

Some of the important reactions catalysed by BF_3 are given below.

(a) Friedel–Crafts reaction Although $AlCl_3$ is the most commonly used Lewis catalyst for this reaction, other Lewis acids including BF_3 may also be used. Boron trifluoride is less reactive than $AlCl_3$ but it has certain advantages over $AlCl_3$ such as (i) less by-products are formed, (ii) it forms a relatively stable coordination complex and (iii) a suitable catalyst for those electrophilic regents (e.g., alcohols, acids, ethers, etc.) which produce water, alcohol or acid as by-products.

(i) Alkylation

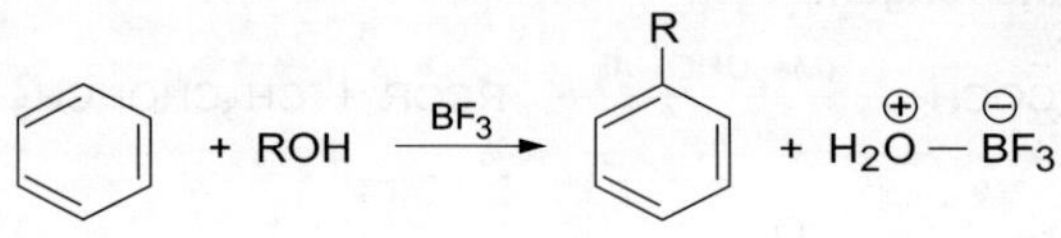

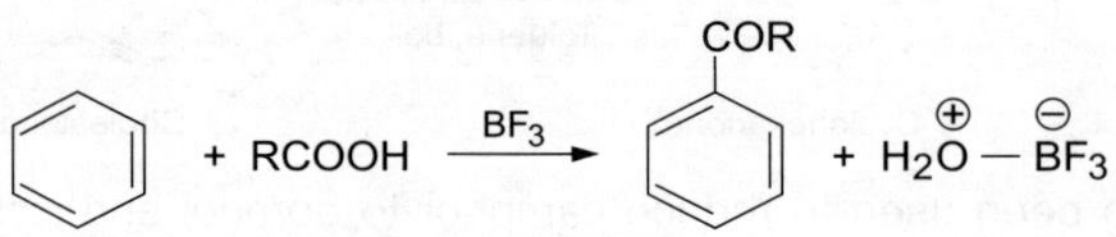

Boron trifluoride brings about alkylation with alkyl fluorides but not with other alkyl halides. This gives a method for introducing halo alkyl groups in aromatic rings.

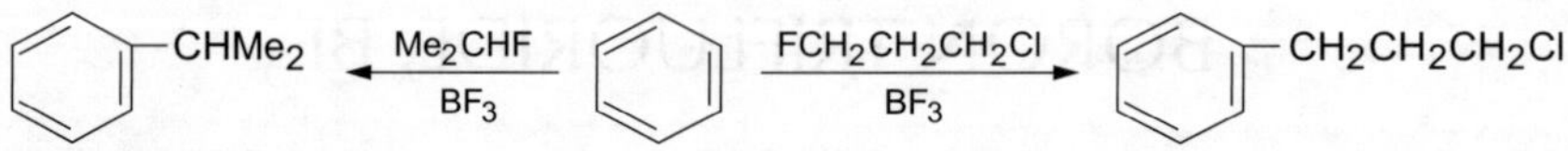

Isopropylbenzene (cumene) 3-Phenyl-*n*-propyl chloride

Alkylation may be effected with olefins in the presence of BF_3.

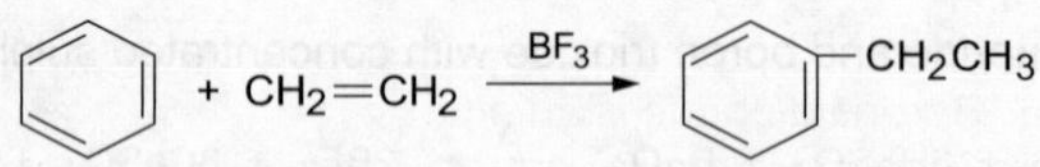

Ethylbenzene

Boron trifluoride and $AlCl_3$ catalyse alkylation in certain substrates to yield different isomers.

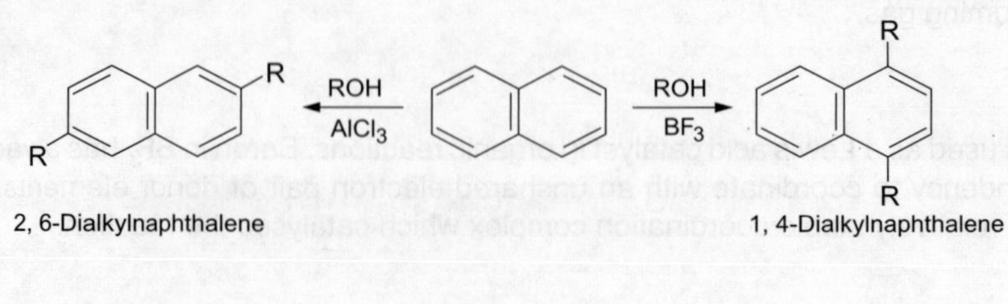

2, 6-Dialkylnaphthalene 1, 4-Dialkylnaphthalene

(ii) Acylation—Ketones react with acid anhydride in the presence of BF_3 to give 1, 3-diketones.

$$CH_3COCH_3 + (CH_3CO)_2O \xrightarrow{BF_3} \underset{\text{Acetyl acetone}}{CH_3COCH_2COCH_3} + CH_3COOH$$

$$\underset{\text{Acetophenone}}{C_6H_5COCH_3} + (CH_3CO)_2O \xrightarrow{BF_3} \underset{\text{Benzoyl acetone}}{C_6H_5COCH_2COCH_3} + CH_3COOH$$

Alcohols and phenols are acetylated with $CH_3CONH_2BF_3$ which is a good acetylating agent.

$$CH_3CONH_2 + BF_3 \longrightarrow CH_3CO\overset{\oplus}{N}H_2\overset{\ominus}{B}F_3$$

$$ROH + CH_3CO\overset{\oplus}{N}H_2\overset{\ominus}{B}F_3 \longrightarrow \underset{\text{Ester}}{RO-\overset{O}{\overset{\|}{C}}-CH_3} + \overset{\oplus}{N}H_3\overset{\ominus}{B}F_3$$

(b) Formation of esters Boron trifluoride catalyses the formation of esters from alcohols, acids, olefins, ethers, etc.

$$RCOOH + R'OH \xrightarrow{BF_3} RCOOR' + H_2O \rightarrow BF_3$$

$$RCOOH + CH_2{=}CH_2 \xrightarrow{BF_3} RCOOC_2H_5$$

$$ROR + R'COCl \xrightarrow{BF_3} RCOOR' + RCl$$

$$ROR + CO + BF_3 \xrightarrow[500\text{ atm}]{125\text{–}180\,^\circ C} RCOOR$$

Alkynyl ethers react with carbonyl compounds in the presence of BF_3 to form α,β-unsaturated esters.

$$R-\overset{O}{\overset{\|}{C}}-R + R'C{\equiv}C-OR'' \xrightarrow{BF_3} R-\overset{R}{\overset{|}{C}}{=}\overset{R'}{\overset{|}{C}}-\overset{O}{\overset{\|}{C}}-OR''$$

(c) Formation of acids

$$ROH + CO + BF_3 \xrightarrow[500\text{ atm}]{125\text{–}180\,^\circ C} RCOOH$$

(d) Nitration and sulphonation Boron trifluoride is an effective catalyst for nitration. Yields are better and the products are pure. It is specially useful for nitrating aromatic rings with negative groups.

$$C_6H_5NO_2 + HNO_3 \xrightarrow{BF_3} \underset{o\text{-Dinitrobenzene}}{C_6H_4(NO_2)_2}$$

Nitronium tetrafluoride is a useful nitrating agent.

$$ArH + \overset{\oplus}{N}O_2\overset{\ominus}{B}F_4 \longrightarrow ArNO_2 + HF + BF_3$$

Boron trifluoride effectively catalyses sulphonation as well.

$$C_6H_6 + H_2SO_4 \xrightarrow{BF_3} C_6H_5SO_3H + H_2O \rightarrow BF_3$$

(e) Reduction of esters Boron trifluoride etherate catalyses the reduction of esters to ethers by $LiAlH_4$.

$$RCOOR' \xrightarrow[Et_2O \rightarrow BF_3]{LiAlH_4} RCH_2OR'$$

(f) Rearrangement Boron trifluoride brings about the Beckmann transformation, Benzidine rearrangement and Fries rearrangement.

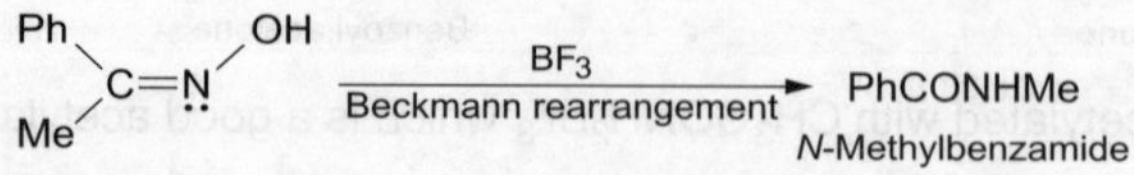

$$Ph-NH-NH-Ph \xrightarrow[\text{Benzidine rearrangement}]{BF_3} H_2N-Ph-Ph-NH_2$$

Benzidine
(4, 4′-Diaminodiphenyl)

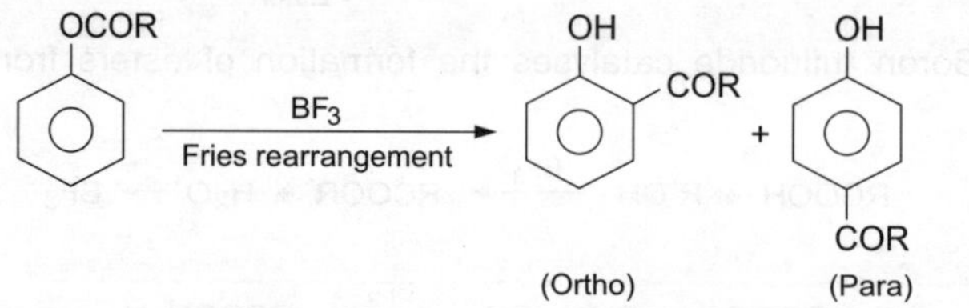

Hydroxy ketones

(g) Formation of amides Nitriles are hydrolysed to acids through the formation of amides. The reaction can be stopped at the amide stage by using BF_3.

$$RCOOH \xleftarrow{H_2O} RCONH_2 \xleftarrow{H_2O} R-C\equiv N \xrightarrow[BF_3]{H_2O} RCONH_2$$

(h) Methylation of alcohols Methylation of alcohols with diazomethane is catalysed by boron trifluoride which increases the acidity of alcohol for the reaction to occur.

$$R-OH + BF_3 \longrightarrow R-\overset{\oplus}{\underset{H}{O}}-\overset{\ominus}{B}F_3 \xrightarrow{CH_2N_2} ROCH_3 + N_2 + BF_3$$

$$\underset{n\text{-Octyl alcohol}}{CH_3-(CH_2)_6-CH_2OH} + CH_2N_2 \xrightarrow{HF-BF_3} \underset{\text{Methyl-}n\text{-octyl ether}}{CH_3-(CH_2)_6-CH_2-O-CH_3} + N_2$$

(i) Polymerization Isobutylene on treatment with BF_3 at –100 °C gives a high molecular weight polymer (about 400–8000 C_4H_8 units) which is sold under the trade name Vistanex.

$$n(CH_3)_2C{=}CH_2 \xrightleftharpoons{BF_3,\ -100\,^\circ C} \underset{\text{Vistanex}}{\left[C(CH_3)_2-CH_2 \right]_n}$$

(j) Analysis of potassium Sodium tetraphenylboride is used for the detection and estimation of potassium in the presence of sodium. The sodium salt is soluble in water but its potassium salt is insoluble in water and is quantitatively precipitated.

The reagent is prepared by reacting phenylmagnesium chloride with boron trifluoride and subsequent treatment with sodium chloride.

$$4C_6H_5MgCl + BF_3 \longrightarrow (C_6H_5)_4\overset{\ominus}{B}\overset{\oplus}{Mg}Cl + 3MgClF$$

$$(C_6H_5)_4\overset{\ominus}{B}\overset{\oplus}{Mg}Cl \xrightarrow[NaCl]{CO_2} (C_6H_5)_4\overset{\ominus}{B}\overset{\oplus}{Na} + MgCO_3$$

Sodium tetraphenyl boride (water soluble)

Boron trifluoride has been used in the Fischer indole synthesis, polymerization of oils, gasoline, etc.

N-BROMOSUCCINIMIDE (NBS)

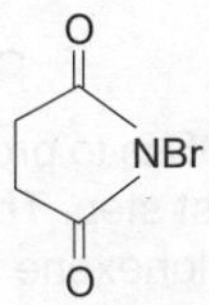

Preparation

The reagent is prepared by gradually adding bromine to an ice-cold solution of succinimide in alkali. *N*-Bromosuccinimide precipitates out immediately.

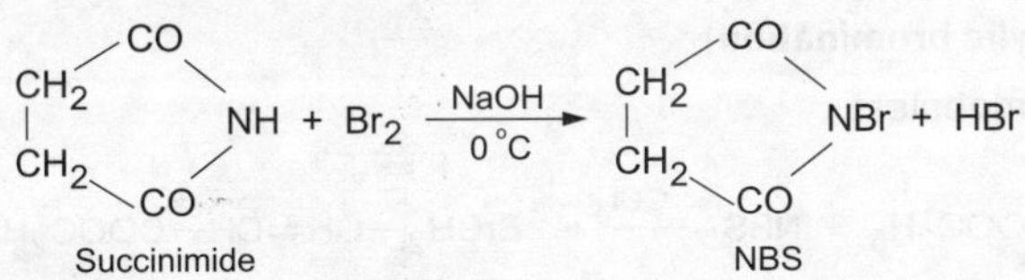

Bromination with NBS is generally carried out in carbon tetrachloride as solvent in which the liberated succinimide is insoluble and easily separated.

N-Bromosuccinimide is a valuable reagent for brominating specifically allylic and benzylic positions. Such reactions are called Wohl–Ziegler bromination. The reagent is also used for brominating positions α- to the carbonyl group and triple bond. When both double and triple bonds are present in a compound, the preferred position for bromination is α- to the triple bond. The reagent can be used to oxidize primary alcohols, secondary alcohols and primary amines.

Specificity of allylic and benzylic position

Allylic and benzylic hydrogens have low bond dissociation energy, it is only 77 kcal, while for vinylic and methane hydrogens it is 104–122 kcal and 102 kcal respectively. Also the allylic or benzylic radical (or ion) formed on dissociation is stabilized by delocalization.

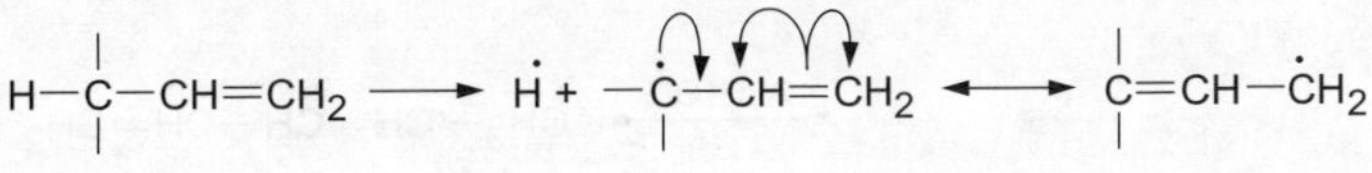

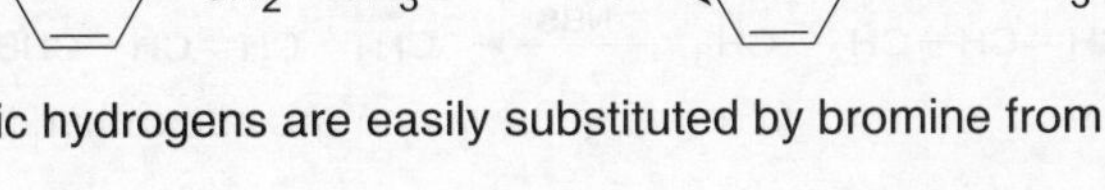

Hence, the allylic and benzilic hydrogens are easily substituted by bromine from NBS.

Mechanism

The reaction proceeds only in the presence of free radical initiators, i.e., peroxide or UV light. Hence the reaction is a free radical reaction. It is suggested that the reaction is initiated by a small amount of bromine atom, $\dot{Br}$. Thus,

$$\dot{Br} + -CH_2-CH{=}CH_2 \longrightarrow -\dot{C}H-CH{=}CH_2 + HBr$$

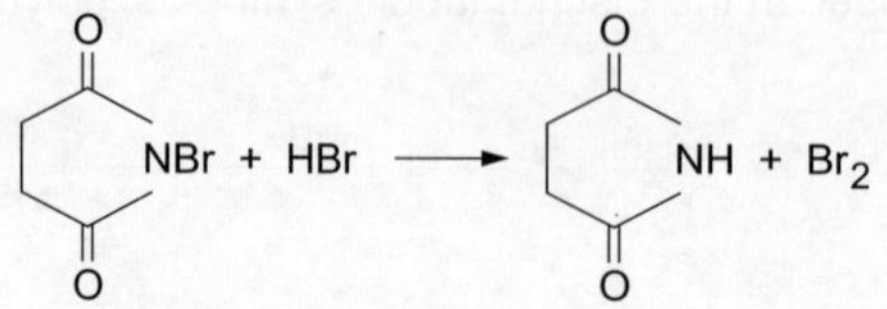

$$-\dot{C}H-CH{=}CH_2 + Br_2 \longrightarrow -CHBr-CH{=}CH_2 + \dot{Br}$$

Function of NBS is to provide a slow constant supply of a low concentration of bromine by reacting with HBr formed in the first step. This is substantiated by the observation that on passing bromine vapours slowly into a solution of cyclohexene in carbon tetrachloride, 3-bromocyclohexene has been obtained.

Uses

1. As brominating agent (allylic bromination)

(a) Preparation of bromoesters

$$CH_3-CH{=}CH-COOC_2H_5 + NBS \xrightarrow{CCl_4} BrCH_2-CH{=}CH-COOC_2H_5 + \begin{array}{l}CH_2CO\\ |\\ CH_2CO\end{array}\!\!>NH$$

Ethyl-γ-bromocrotonate

This compound is used in the synthesis of vitamin A by Reformatsky reaction.

(b) Conversion of monoenes to dienes and trienes

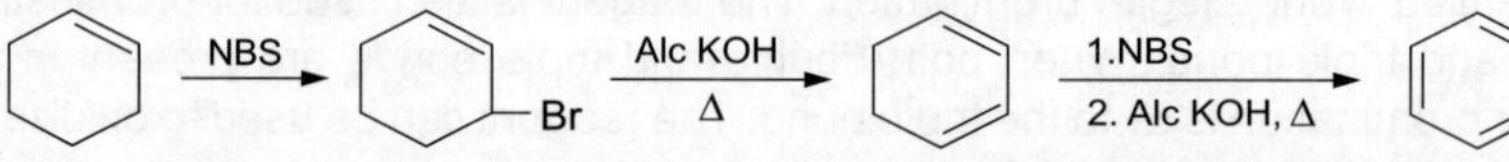

Such allylic bromination followed by dehydrohalogenation has been used in the commerical production of cortisone.

(c) Degradation of olefinic compounds—The reagent can be employed to split off carbons from suitable olefinic compounds, which may be obtained from alcohols.

$$\underset{n\text{-Pentanol}}{CH_3CH_2CH_2CH_2CH_2OH} \xrightarrow[360\,^{\circ}C]{Al_2O_3} CH_3-CH_2-CH_2-CH{=}CH_2 \xrightarrow{NBS} CH_3-CH_2-CHBr-CH{=}CH_2$$

$$\xrightarrow[-\,HBr]{Alc\ KOH} CH_3-CH{=}CH-CH{=}CH_2 \xrightarrow[2H_2O,\ Zn]{1.\ O_3} CH_3CHO$$

Such degradations help in determining the structure of compounds. It may be noted that when an olefine has two different α-positions the preferred position of attack is the secondary carbon for reasons of stability of 2° radical.

$$CH_3-CH{=}CH-CH_2-CH_3 \xrightarrow{NBS} CH_3-CH{=}CH-CHBr-CH_3$$

(d) Conversion of vitamin A_1 to vitamin A_2

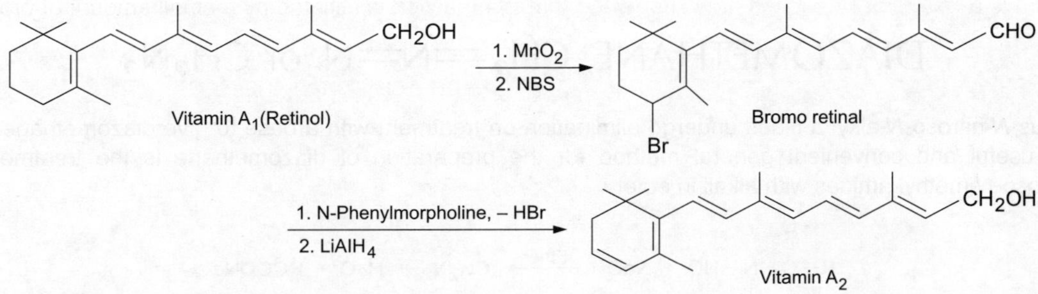

(e) Addition reaction—NBS also exhibits addition reaction but the yield is very poor. However, the addition reaction may be catalysed by tetraalkylammonium salts.

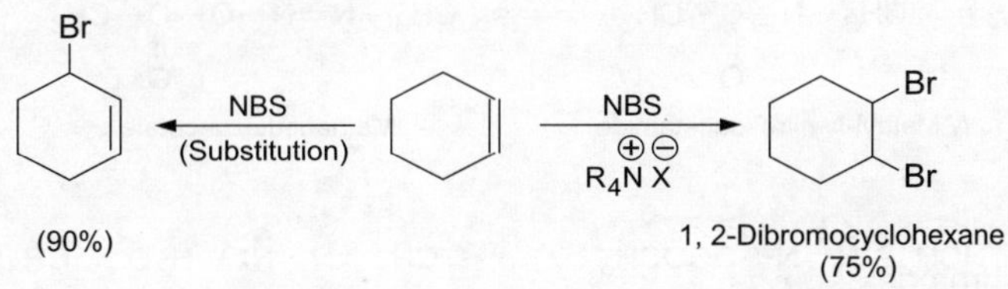

2. As oxidizing agent NBS oxidizes primary alcohols and primary amines to aldehydes and secondary alcohols to ketones. The reaction proceeds readily in the absence of light. Hence the reaction is not radical type. It probably involves attack by positive bromine. The mechanism is not known.

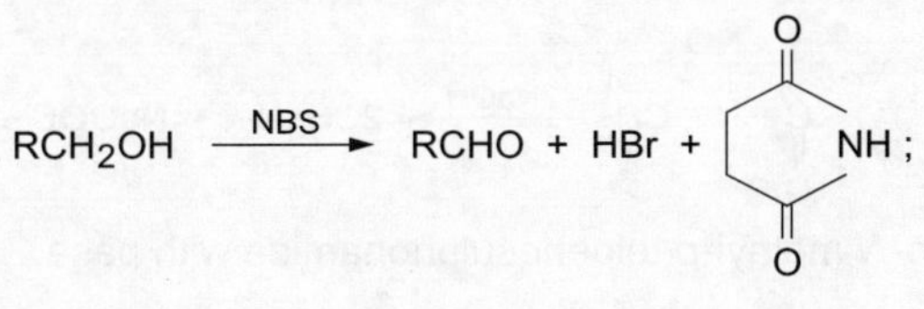

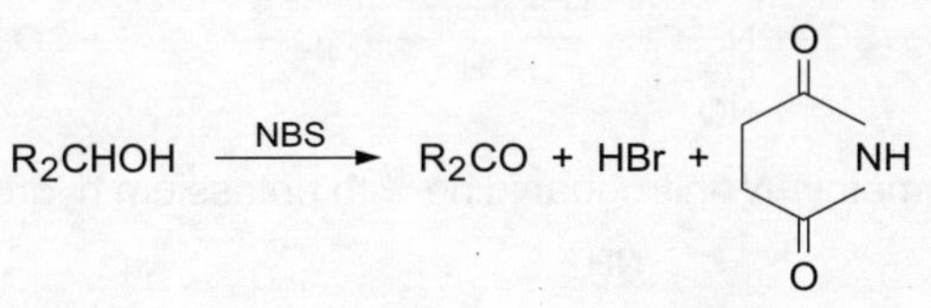

3. Degradation of amino acids α-Amino acids, peptides and proteins are decarboxylated with NBS in aqueous medium.

$$\underset{\alpha\text{-Alanine}}{CH_3CH(NH_2)COOH} \xrightarrow{NBS} CH_3CHO + NH_3 + CO_2$$

NBS has also been employed for allylic bromination in the synthesis of some important natural products.

DIAZOMETHANE, $CH_2{=}\overset{+}{N}{=}\overset{-}{N}$ or CH_2N_2

Various *N*-nitroso-*N*-alkyl amides undergo elimination on treatment with a base to give diazomethane. The most useful and convenient general method for the preparation of diazomethane is the treatment of *N*-nitroso-*N*-methyl amides with alkali in ether.

$$R{-}\overset{\overset{\displaystyle O}{\|}}{C}{-}\underset{\underset{\displaystyle CH_3}{|}}{N}{-}NO + NaOH \xrightarrow{\text{Ether}} CH_2N_2 + H_2O + RCOONa$$

The elimination occurs probably through the tautomer, diazoester of the *N*-nitrosamide

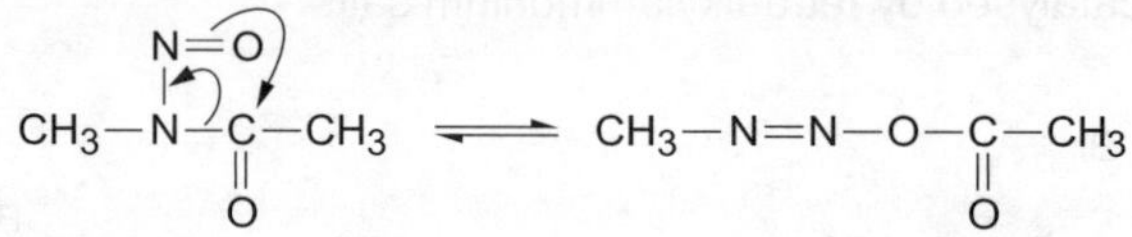

N-Methyl-*N*-nitrosoacetamide Methanediazoacetate

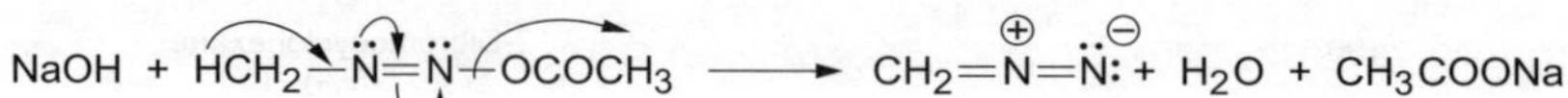

Diazomethane

Preparation

Several *N*-nitroso-*N*-methyl compounds have been used to prepare diazomethane.

1. Alkaline hydrolysis of *bis*-(*N*-nitroso-*N*-methyl) terephthalimide.

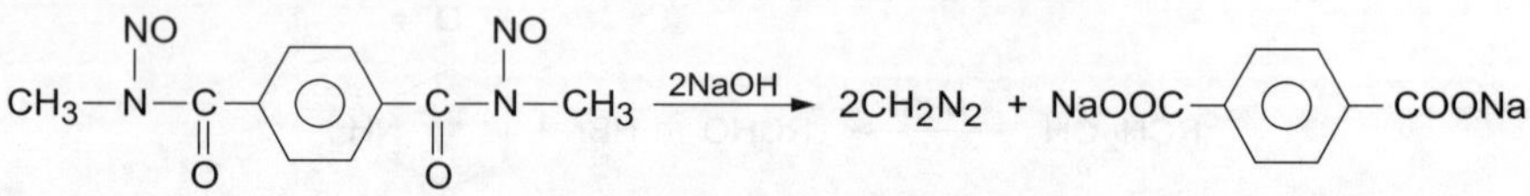

2. Distillation of *N*-nitroso-*N*-methyl-*p*-toluenesulphonamide with base.

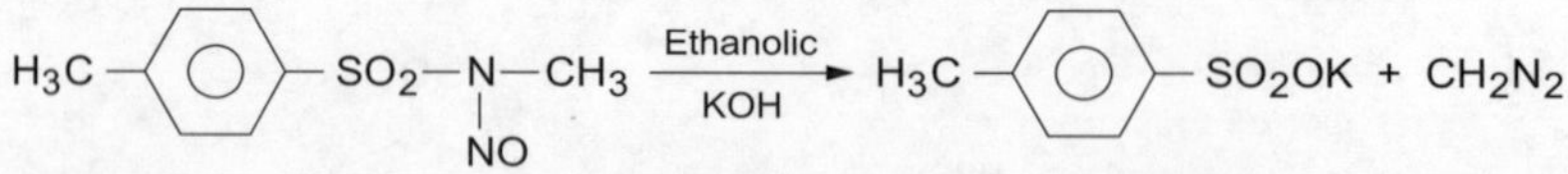

3. Warming *N*-nitroso-*N*-methyl-*N*′-nitroguanidine with potassium hydroxide.

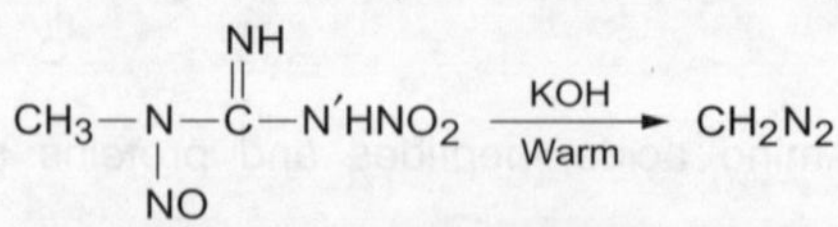

Diazomethane is a yellow gas (b.p. –23 °C). It is highly toxic and explosive. It sometimes explodes even in gaseous state. It decomposes readily. Its ethereal solution may be stored at 0 °C for about 24 h without appreciable decomposition. Diazomethane is a resonance hybrid of the following canonical structures:

$$CH_2{=}\overset{\oplus}{N}{=}\overset{\ominus}{N} \longleftrightarrow \overset{\ominus}{C}H_2{-}\overset{\oplus}{N}{\equiv}N \longleftrightarrow \overset{\oplus}{C}H_2{-}N{=}\overset{\ominus}{N}$$

It is mainly used as a methylating agent for reasonably acidic compounds. The reagent provides methods (Arndt–Estert reaction) for the conversion of acids into their higher homologues. It reacts rapidly even without a catalyst and the yield is high. The reaction is clean since the other product is nitrogen. Completion of the reaction is indicated by the stoppage of the evolution of nitrogen. Hence, inspite of its toxic and explosive nature it is one of the most useful and versatile reagents for preparative purposes.

The reaction is carried out, at about 0 °C by adding ethereal solution of diazomethane to the solution of the substrate in ether till evolution of nitrogen ceases and a yellow colour persists. Sometimes diazomethane is generated 'in situ' by adding potassium carbonate to the alcoholic solution of *N*-nitrosomethyl urea. Some of its important uses are given.

Uses

1. Methylation It is used as methylating agent for acidic compounds such as carboxylic and mineral acids. It also methylates reasonably acidic substance like phenols, enols, etc. Alcohols and amines are methylated only in the presence of catalysts.

(a) Acidic substances—

$$RCOOH \xrightarrow[-N_2]{CH_2N_2} RCOOCH_3\ ; \qquad RSO_3H \xrightarrow[-N_2]{CH_2N_2} RSO_3CH_3\ ;$$

$$C_6H_5OH \xrightarrow[-N_2]{CH_2N_2} C_6H_5OCH_3\ ; \qquad HCl \xrightarrow[-N_2]{CH_2N_2} CH_3Cl$$

Ethyl acetoacetate is O-alkylated.

$$CH_3-\overset{O}{\overset{\|}{C}}-CH_2-COOC_2H_5 \xrightarrow{CH_2N_2} CH_3-\overset{OCH_3}{\overset{|}{C}}=CH-COOC_2H_5 + N_2$$

It is very useful for the preparation of methyl esters of rare and acid-sensitive carboxylic acids.

$$C_6H_5-CH=CH-COOH \xrightarrow{CH_2N_2} C_6H_5-CH=CH-COOCH_3$$

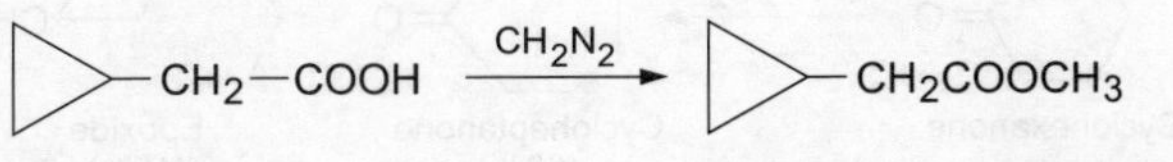

Cyclopropylacetic acid — Methylcyclopropyl acetate

The reagent has been employed for the qualitative and quantitative estimations of carboxyl and enolic groups in various natural products.

(b) Alcohols—Alcohols have weak acidic hydrogens and hence catalyst is required to increase the acidity.

$$R-OH + BF_3 \longrightarrow R-\underset{H}{\underset{|}{\overset{\oplus}{O}}}-\overset{\ominus}{B}F_3 \xrightarrow{CH_2N_2} R-O-CH_3 + BF_3 + N_2$$

$$\underset{n\text{-Octyl alcohol}}{CH_3(CH_2)_6CH_2OH} + CH_2N_2 \xrightarrow{HBF_4} \underset{\text{Methyl-}n\text{-octyl ether}}{CH_3(CH_2)_6CH_2OCH_3} + N_2$$

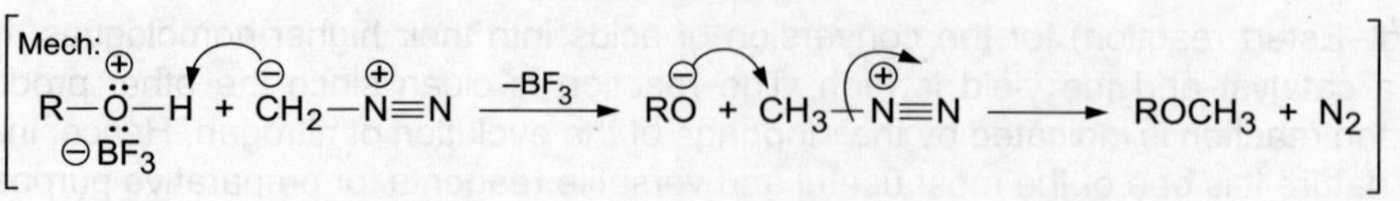

The same mechanism operates for the reaction of diazomethane with acids and amines.

(c) Carbonyl compounds—Aldehydes and ketones react with diazomethane to yield higher ketones and epoxides as side reaction.

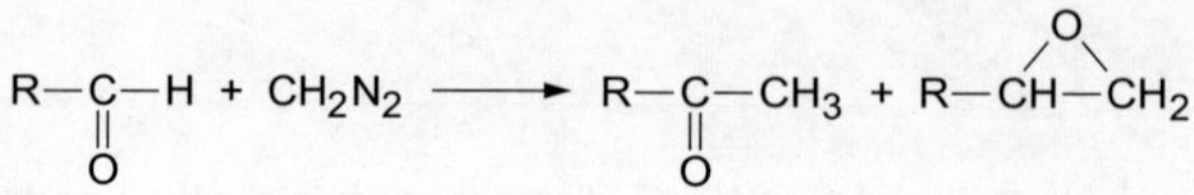

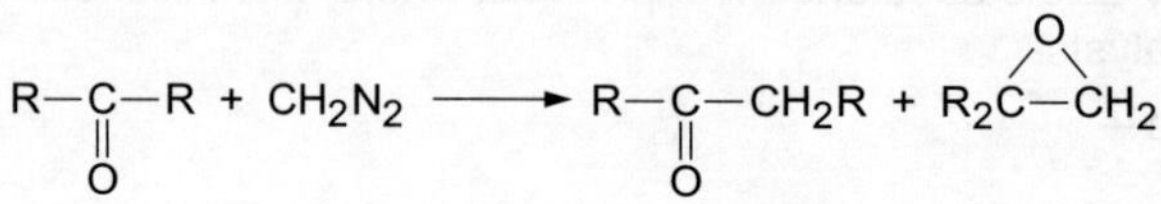

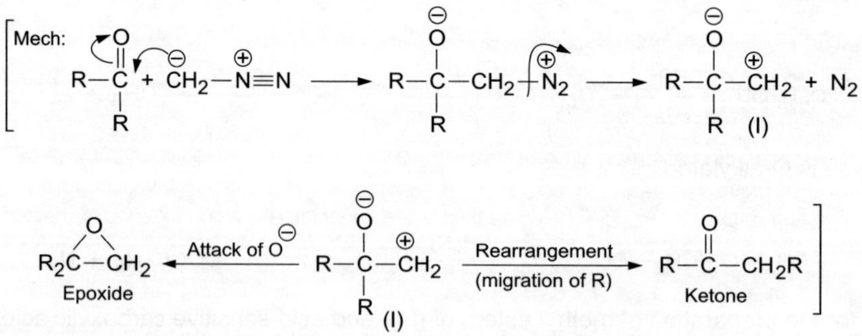

Some cyclic ketones undergo ring expansion.

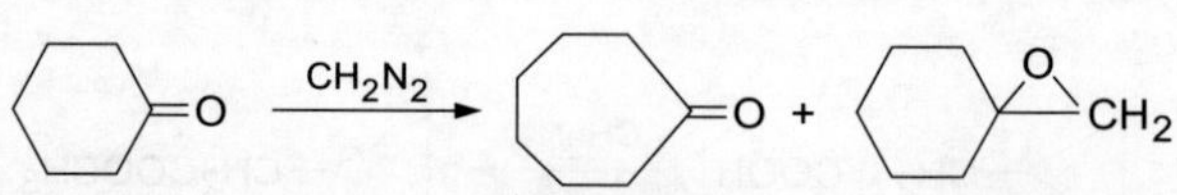

Cyclohexanone   Cycloheptanone (63%)   Epoxide (15%)

(d) Amines—Amines are methylated in the presence of Lewis acid since amines are not acidic enough to react. Hence BF_3 is used as catalyst.

$$R_2NH + CH_2N_2 \xrightarrow{BF_3} R_2NCH_3 + N_2$$

Primary amines give a mixture of secondary and tertiary amines.

2. Arndt–Eistert reaction Acid chlorides prepared from acids are converted to diazoketone with excess of diazomethane.

$$RCOOH \xrightarrow{SOCl_2} RCOCl$$

$$RCOCl + CH_2N_2 \longrightarrow \underset{\text{Diazoketone}}{RCOCHN_2} + HCl$$

$$CH_2N_2 + HCl \longrightarrow CH_3Cl + N_2$$

If excess of diazomethane is not present to react with HCl then chloromethyl ketone is formed.

$$RCOCHN_2 + HCl \longrightarrow RCOCH_2Cl + N_2$$

Diazoketone undergoes Wolff rearrangement in different mediums in the presence of catalyst, Ag_2O (or Ag, Pt, Cu) to yield acids, esters, amides, etc., all with one carbon more (homologization) than the starting acid.

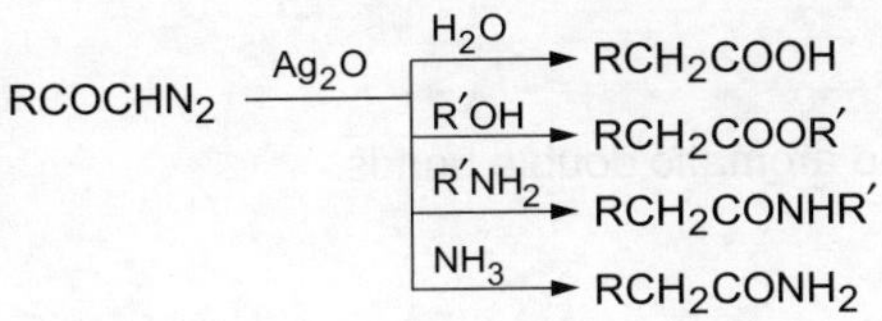

It forms hydroxymethyl ketone with water and formic acid.

$$RCOCHN_2 + H_2O \xrightarrow{HCOOH} RCOCH_2OH + N_2$$

Arndt–Eistert reaction has several important synthetic applications.

3. Synthesis of heterocyclic compounds Diazomethane condenses with ethylenic and acetylenic bonds to give heterocyclic compounds.

(i) 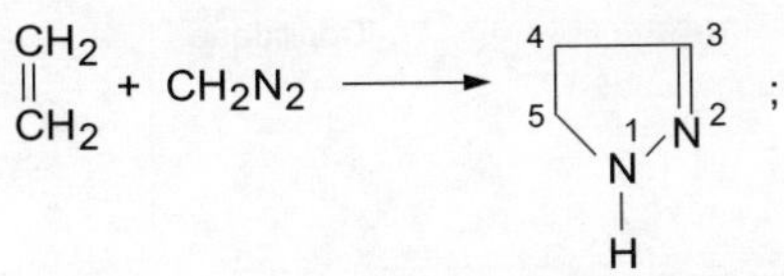

Pyrazoline

(ii) 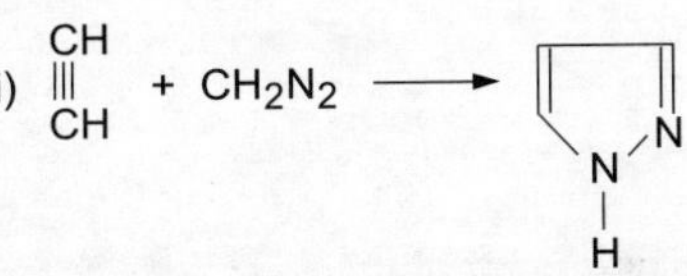

Pyrazole

(iii) 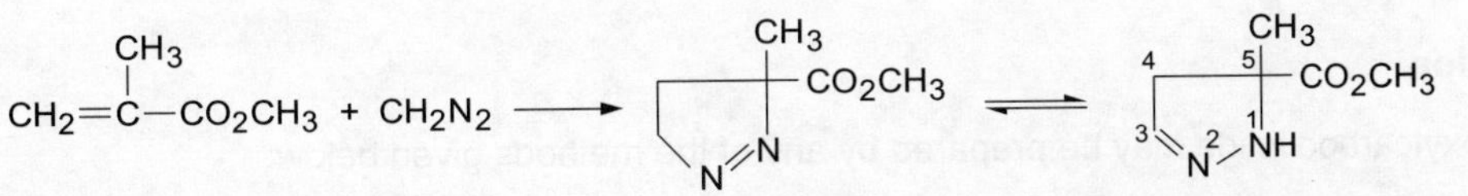

5-Methyl-5-carbmethoxy pyrazoline

Pyrazolines are important intermediates for the preparation of cyclopropane rings. On heating with KOH on platinized asbestos, pyrazolines are decomposed to cyclopropane and nitrogen.

4. Formation of carbene (methylene) Photolysis of diazomethane yields carbene which is extremely reactive species with a very short life period.

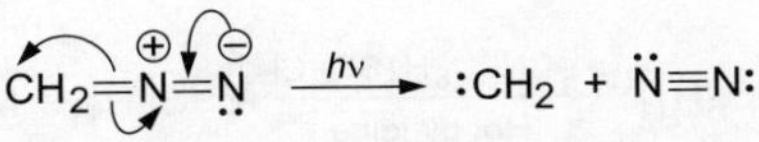

Carbene reacts with hydrocarbons by insertion into carbon–hydrogen bond. The reaction is nonselective and hence useless for synthesis.

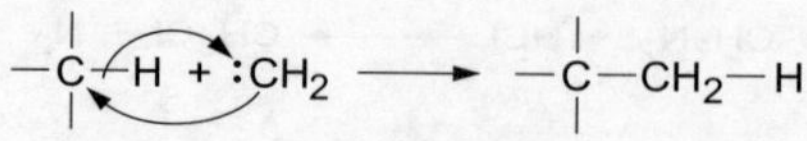

$$CH_3-CH_2-CH_2-CH_2-CH_3 \xrightarrow[UV]{CH_2N_2} CH_3-CH_2-CH_2-CH_2-CH_2-CH_3 + CH_3-\underset{}{\overset{CH_3}{\overset{|}{C}H}}-CH_2-CH_2-CH_3$$

n-Pentane ... *n*-Hexane ... 2-Methylpentane

$$+\ CH_3-CH_2-\underset{\underset{CH_3}{|}}{CH}-CH_2-CH_3$$

3-Methylpentane

Carbene also adds to aliphatic and aromatic double bonds.

(i) 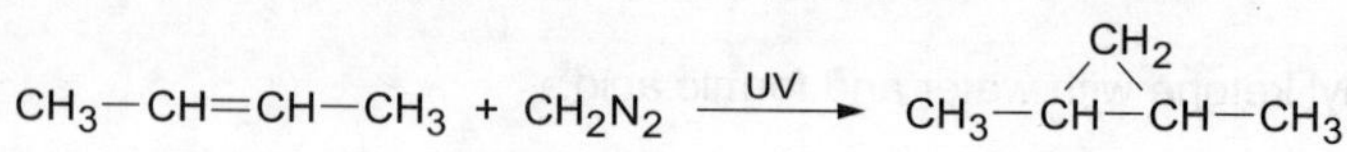

1, 2-Dimethyl cyclopropane

(ii) 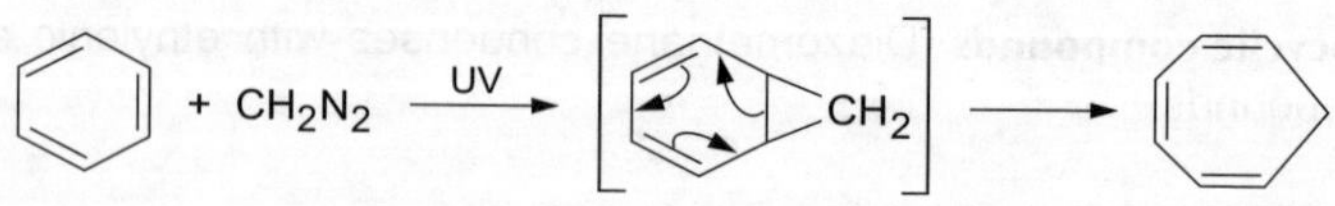

Tropilidene

DICYCLOHEXYLCARBODIIMIDE

Preparation

Dicyclohexylcarbodiimide may be prepared by any of the methods given below:

(i) By the oxidation of *N, N*′-dicyclohexylthiourea with mercuric oxide

$$C_6H_{11}-NH-\overset{\overset{S}{\|}}{C}-NH-C_6H_{11} \xrightarrow{Hg_2O} C_6H_{11}-N=C=N-C_6H_{11} + Hg_2S + H_2O$$

N,N′-Dicyclohexylthiourea ... Dicyclohexylcarbodiimide

(ii) By the dehydration of dicyclohexylurea with *p*-toluenesulphonyl chloride in hot pyridine

$$C_6H_{11}-NH-CO-NH-C_6H_{11} \xrightarrow[\text{Hot pyridine}]{p\text{-}CH_3C_6H_4SO_2Cl} C_6H_{11}-N=C=N-C_6H_{11} + H_2O$$

Dicyclohexylurea ... DCC

The reagent will be represented by the abbreviation, DCC.

Uses

Dicyclohexylcarbodiimide finds application as a dehydrating agent usually under mild conditions. Thus, the reagent has been employed as dehydrating agent in the synthesis of various compounds such as, esters, ethers, anhydrides, amides, lactones, lactams, peptides, etc.

1. Esters Esterification of acids with primary or secondary alcohols is promoted by the reagent.

$$\underset{}{RCOOH} + R'OH + \underset{\text{DCC}}{C_6H_{11}{-}N{=}C{=}N{-}C_6H_{11}} \longrightarrow RCOOR' + \underset{\text{DCC, } H_2O}{C_6H_{11}{-}NH{-}CO{-}NH{-}C_6H_{11}}$$

Mechanism—The reaction is catalysed by acid. The acid reacts with the reagent to form the compound (I) with a good leaving group. Subsequent reaction of the compound (I) with alcohol gives the ester with the expulsion of dicyclohexylurea. The sequential steps of the reaction are given.

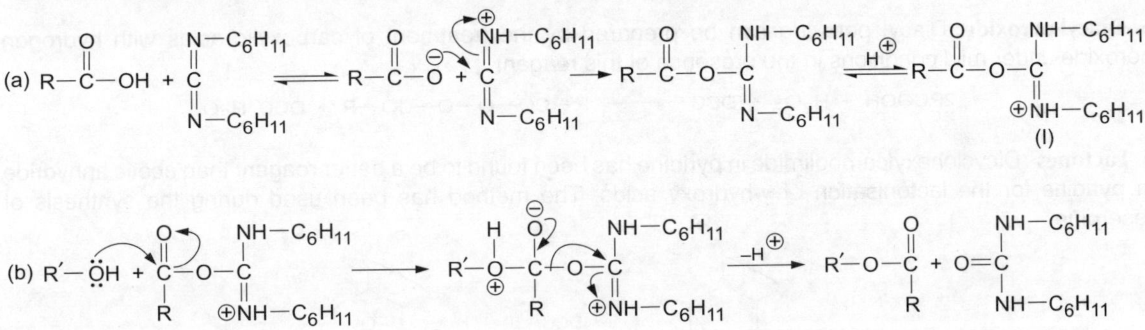

The driving force of the reaction is the formation of a very stable compound, dicyclohexylurea.

2. Amides Amides are not directly obtainable by the treatment of acids with amines. In the presence of this dehydrating reagent however, amides in good yield are obtained at about the room temperature.

$$2RCOOH + R'NH_2 + C_6H_{11}{-}N{=}C{=}N{-}C_6H_{11} \longrightarrow RCONHR' + RCOOH + C_6H_{11}NH{-}CO{-}NHC_6H_{11}$$

Mechanism—It is suggested that the reagent first converts the acid to its anhydride which with amine gives the amide.

The acid first reacts with the reagent, as in the case of esterification to form (I) which reacts with another molecule of the acid to form the anhydride. The anhydride then reacts with the amine to form amide.

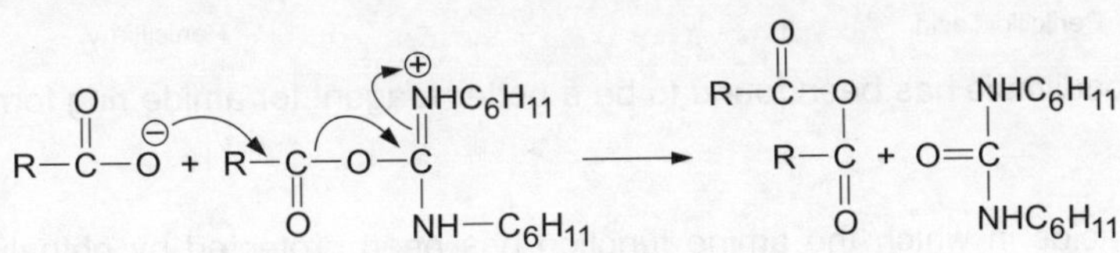

$$(RCO)_2O + R'NH_2 \longrightarrow RCONHR' + RCOOH$$

The reaction has been employed to prepare lactams (cyclic amides).

3. Ethers A mixture of phenol, alcohol and the reagent on prolonged heating under pressure gives aryl alkyl ether.

$$C_6H_5OH + C_2H_5OH + C_6H_{11}N{=}C{=}NC_6H_{11} \xrightarrow[\text{Press.}]{\text{Heat}} \underset{\text{Ethyl phenyl ether}}{C_6H_5OC_2H_5} + \underset{N,\,N'\text{-Dicyclohexylurea}}{C_6H_{11}{-}NH{-}\overset{O}{\overset{\|}{C}}{-}NH{-}C_6H_{11}}$$

4. Acid anhydrides The reagent gives an excellent yield of acid anhydrides from carboxylic acids.

$$2RCOOH + C_6H_{11}N{=}C{=}NC_6H_{11} \longrightarrow (RCO)_2O + C_6H_{11}NH{-}CO{-}NHC_6H_{11}$$

The reaction has been employed to produce symmetrical anhydrides from *N*-substituted amino acids.

$$\underset{\substack{C_6H_5CH_2OCONH \\ \text{N-Carbobenzoxy-}\beta\text{-phenylalanine}}}{C_6H_5{-}CH_2{-}CH{-}COOH} \xrightarrow{DCC} \underset{\substack{C_6H_5CH_2OCONH \\ \text{Anhydride}}}{(C_6H_5{-}CH_2{-}CH{-}CO)_2O} + C_6H_{11}{-}NH{-}CO{-}NH{-}C_6H_{11}$$

The amino group of the amino acid is substituted by carbobenzoxy group to prevent the amino group from reacting with the carboxyl group. The carbobenzoxy group may be easily removed by hydragenolysis after the reaction.

5. Diacyl peroxide Diacyl peroxide can be prepared by the treatment of carboxylic acids with hydrogen peroxide under mild conditions in the presence of this reagent.

$$2RCOOH + H_2O_2 + DCC \longrightarrow R{-}CO{-}O{-}O{-}CO{-}R + DCC, H_2O$$

6. Lactones Dicyclohexylcarbodiimide in pyridine has been found to be a better reagent than acetic anhydride in pyridine for the lactonisation of γ-hydroxy acids. The method has been used during the synthesis of reserpine.

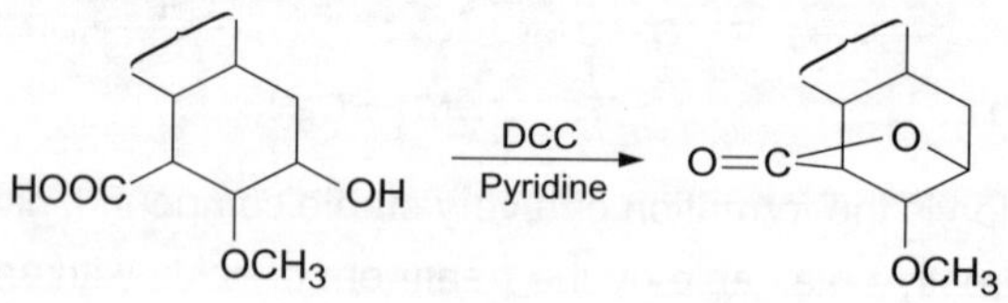

7. β-Lactams Lactams are cyclic amides. β-Lactams are highly strained rings, sensitive to acids while most reagents for amide linkage involve strongly acid reagents. This caused serious problems in the synthesis of penicillin. However, the difficulty was overcome by using dicyclohexylcarbodiimide for the amide ring.

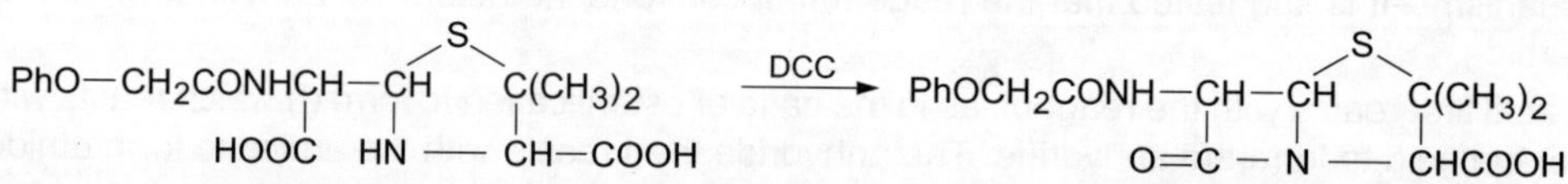

Penicilloic acid

Penicillin V

Diisopropylcarbodiimide has been found to be a better reagent for amide ring formation as it is a very mild reagent.

8. Peptides Amino acids in which the amino function has been protected by phthalyl $\left(C_6H_4\begin{matrix}CO{-}\\CO{-}\end{matrix}\right)$ or carbobenzoxy $(C_6H_5CH_2O{-}CO{-})$ group condense with amino acid esters in the presence of *N, N′*-dicyclohexylcarbodiimide at room temperature to give peptides.

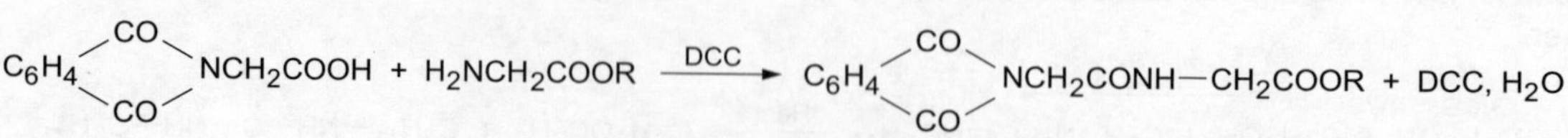

After hydrolysis of the product, the protecting group is removed by treating with hydrazine. (See Gabriel synthesis.)

Phthalyl and carbobenzoxy groups are used as protecting groups since they can be easily substituted and easily removed. Carbobenzoxy group may be removed by hydragenolysis (H_2 + Pt).

9. Barbituric acid Barbituric acid derivatives may be prepared by the treatment of malonic acid with the reagent.

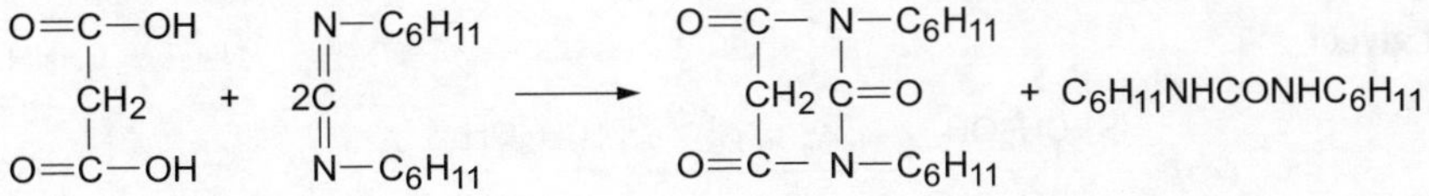

FENTON'S REAGENT ($H_2O_2 + Fe^{2+}$)

Inorganic ions which can change their valence state by losing or gaining one electron (oxidation–reduction) have been used to produce radicals. Thus, ferrous ions (Fe^{2+}) generate from hydrogen peroxide, hydroxyl radicals which can oxidize organic compounds.

A mixture of ferrous sulphate or acetate and hydrogen peroxide known as Fentón's reagent has been used to oxidize organic compounds. The mixture consists of ferric ions, hydroxyl ions and hydroxyl radicals.

$$\overset{2\oplus}{Fe} + H-O-O-H \longrightarrow \overset{3\oplus}{Fe} + H\dot{O} + H\overset{\ominus}{O}$$

In Fenton's reagent the ferrous ion catalyses the oxidation of hydrogen peroxide generating hydroxyl radicals which oxidize organic substances. The oxidation is carried out by adding slowly a solution of hydrogen peroxide into an ice-cold aqueous or alcoholic solution of the organic substance and ferrous acetate or sulphate.

Uses

1. Oxidation of hydrocarbons (a) Hydroxylation—Aromatic hydrocarbons are hydroxylated with Fenton's reagent. The generated hydroxyl radical abstracts a hydrogen from the site of attack and oxidizes the substrate. The yield is, however, poor.

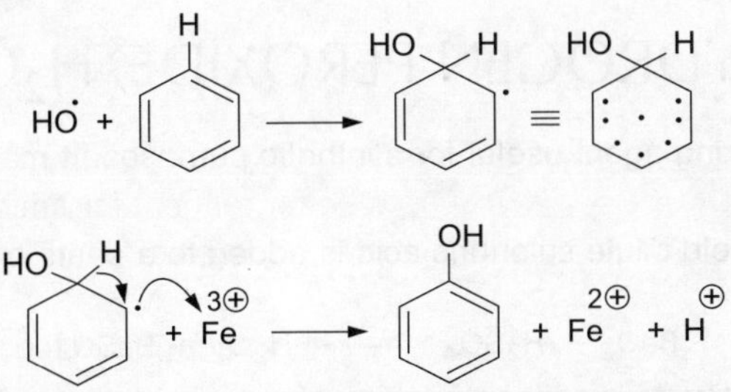

(b) Coupling—The hydroxyl radical may abstract a hydrogen from the susceptible position of the substrate producing radicals which couple. The susceptible reactive positions are supposed to be the α-positions to the phenyl, ether, cyano, carboxyl, ester groups, etc.

Thus,

$$\underset{\text{Anisole}}{2C_6H_5-O-CH_3} \xrightarrow{H_2O_2 + \overset{2\oplus}{Fe}} 2[C_6H_5-O-\dot{C}H_2] \longrightarrow C_6H_5-O-CH_2-CH_2-O-C_6H_5$$

The reaction is, however, not a general one.

2. Oxidation of α-hydroxy acids α-Hydroxy acids are oxidized with Fenton's reagent to α-keto acids.

$$\underset{\text{Lactic acid}}{CH_3{-}CH(OH){-}COOH} \xrightarrow{H_2O_2 \;+\; Fe^{2\oplus}} \underset{\text{Pyruvic acid}}{CH_3COCOOH}$$

3. Oxidation of glycol

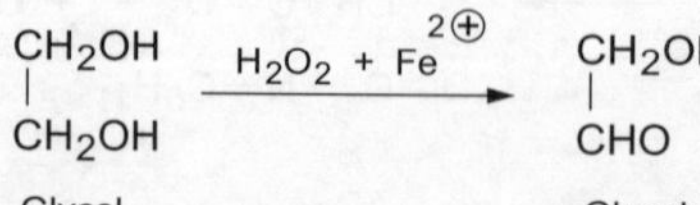

Glycol Glycolaldehyde

4. Oxidation of sugars Aldoses may be degraded to the next lower member with Fenton's reagent (Ruff's method). Aldoses are oxidized to aldonic acid, the calcium salt of which on treatment with Fenton's reagent gives the next lower member.

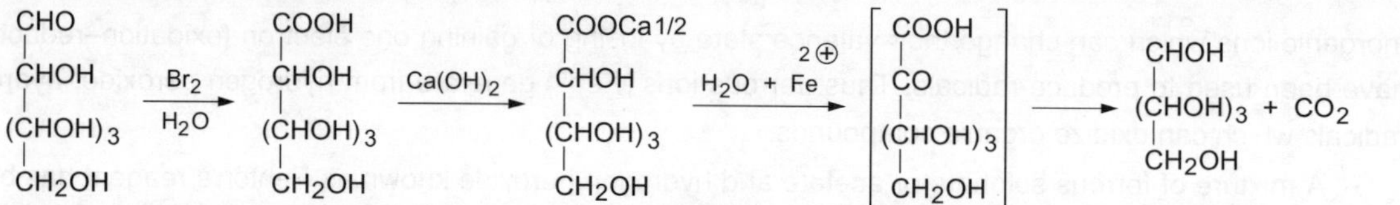

Glucose Arabinose

5. Oxidation of tartaric acid Tartaric acid is oxidized to dihydroxyfumaric acid.

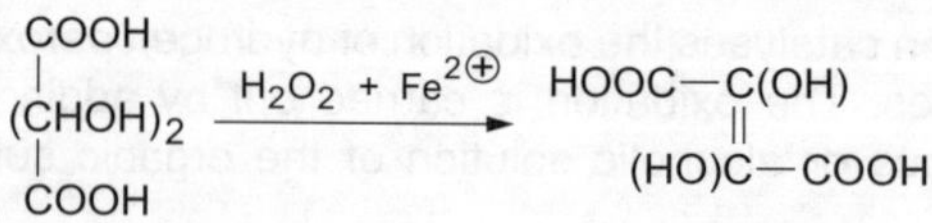

Tartaric acid Dihydroxyfumaric acid

Dihydroxyfumaric acid forms a complex with the ferric ions. The complex has a violet colour in alkaline medium. This is used as a test for tartaric acid.

HYDROGEN PEROXIDE, H_2O_2

Hydrogen peroxide is an oxidizing agent useful for synthetic purposes. It may be prepared by the following methods.

1. From barium peroxide Ice cold dilute sulphuric acid is added to a paste of barium peroxide in water until just acid.

$$BaO_2 + H_2SO_4 \longrightarrow H_2O_2 + BaSO_4$$

The solution is filtered and the filtrate is concentrated by slow evaporation at 70 °C.

2. Electrolytic process Electrolysis of 50% sulphuric acid gives 30% hydrogen peroxide solution.

$$2H_2SO_4 \rightleftharpoons 2\overset{\oplus}{H} + 2\overset{\ominus}{O}SO_3H \;;\quad 2\overset{\oplus}{H} + 2e \longrightarrow H_2$$

$$2\overset{\ominus}{O}SO_3H \longrightarrow \underset{\text{Perdisulphuric acid}}{H_2S_2O_8} + 2e \;;\quad H_2S_2O_8 + H_2O \longrightarrow \underset{\text{Caro's acid}}{H_2SO_5} + H_2SO_4$$

$$H_2SO_5 + H_2O \longrightarrow H_2O_2 + H_2SO_4$$

3. Nonelectrolytic process 2-Ethylanthraquinone is reduced with nickel and hydrogen to 2-ethyl-9-anthrol which is oxidised with oxygen of air to the starting material, 2-ethylanthraquinone and hydrogen peroxide. The reaction is performed in organic solvent and hydrogen peroxide is extracted with water. The method is not suitable for the production of a high concentration of hydrogen peroxide which undergoes explosive decomposition with organic impurities.

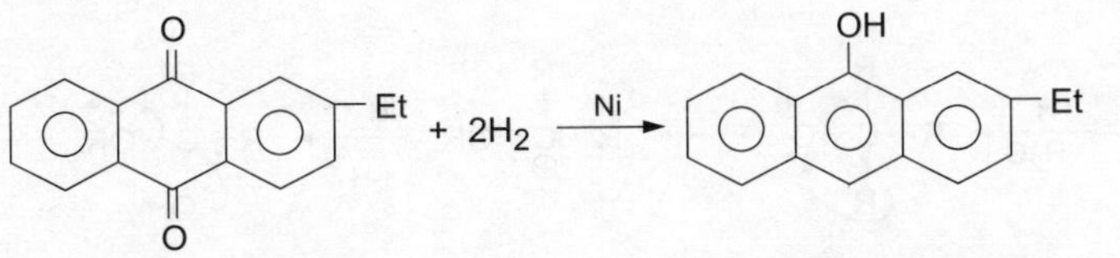

2-Ethylanthraquinone 2-Ethyl-9-anthrol

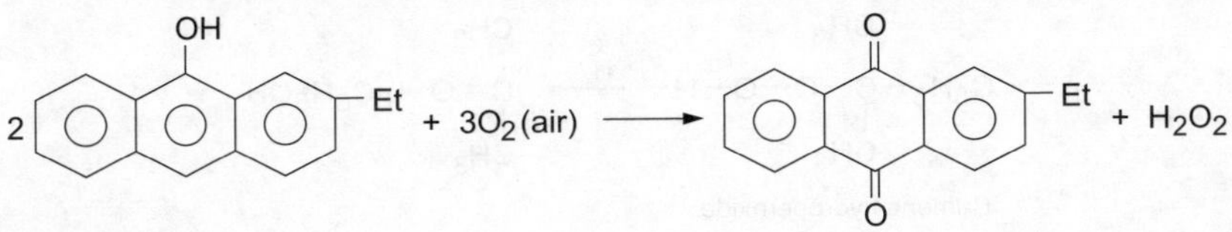

Its structure is suggested to be

$$H{-}O{-}O{-}H \rightleftharpoons H{-}\overset{\overset{\large H}{|}}{\underset{\oplus}{O}}{-}\overset{\ominus}{O}$$

Uses

It is a good oxidizing agent and also catalyses many reactions.

In alkaline medium hydrogen peroxide supplies oxygen nucleophiles as the attacking species for the oxidation.

$$H{-}O{-}O{-}H + H\overset{\ominus}{O} \longrightarrow H{-}O{-}\overset{\ominus}{O} + H_2O\ ; \quad H{-}O{-}O{-}H + 2\overset{\ominus}{O}H \longrightarrow \overset{\ominus}{O}{-}\overset{\ominus}{O} + 2H_2O$$

In acidic medium it probably forms the conjugate acid of H_2O_2 which can transfer $\overset{\oplus}{O}H$ moiety of protonated H_2O_2 to the unshared pair of electrons of the element of the substrate, e.g., alkyl sulphides, amines, etc.

$$H{-}O{-}O{-}H \underset{}{\overset{\overset{\oplus}{H}}{\rightleftharpoons}} H{-}O{-}\underset{\underset{\large H}{|}}{\overset{\oplus}{O}}{-}H \longrightarrow H\overset{\oplus}{O} + H_2O$$

Applications and uses

It is a good oxidizing reagent and catalyses many reactions.

1. Preparation of alkyl hydroperoxides and alkyl peroxides (a) Alkyl hydroperoxides are prepared by reacting alkyl halides or sulphates with alkaline hydrogen peroxide.

$$RX + H_2O_2 \xrightarrow{NaOH} ROOH + NaX + H_2O$$

They may also be prepared from alkenes by sulphuric acid-induced addition of H_2O_2.

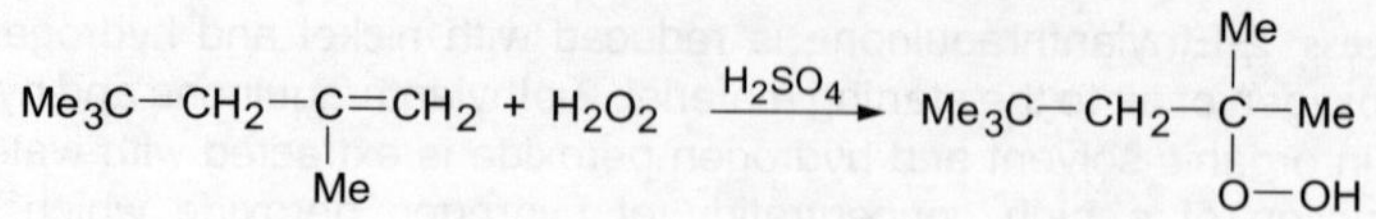

Secondary and tertiary hydroperoxides undergo acid-catalysed rearrangement and cleavage to ketones and alcohols or phenols.

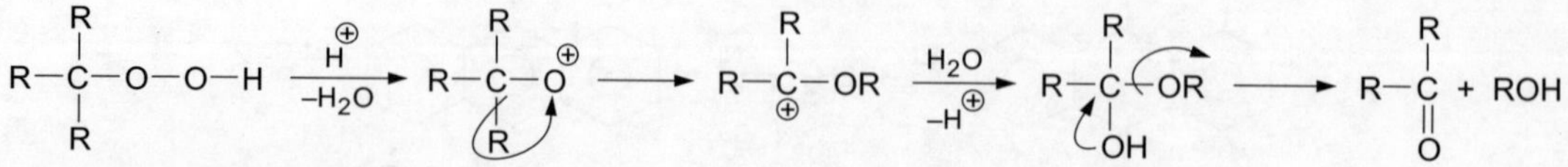

Aryl group migrates in preference to alkyl group. The method has been employed for the industrial production of ketones and alcohols or phenols. Thus,

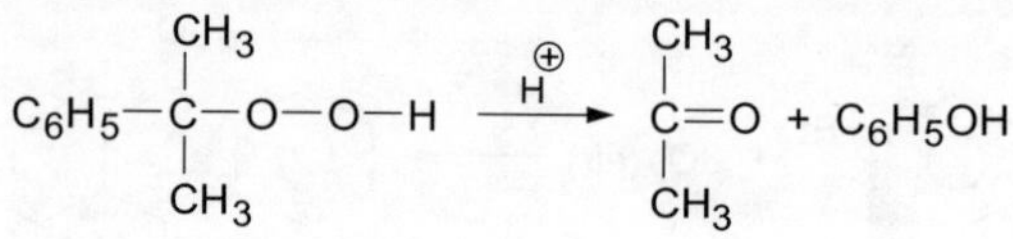

Cumene hydroperoxide

(b) Alkyl peroxides are prepared by reacting alkyl halides with Na_2O_2.

$$2RX + Na_2O_2 \longrightarrow R{-}O{-}O{-}R + 2NaX$$

2. Preparation of acyl hydroperoxides and acyl peroxides (a) Acyl hydroperoxides are prepared by treating carboxylic acids with 90% H_2O_2 in the presence of acid.

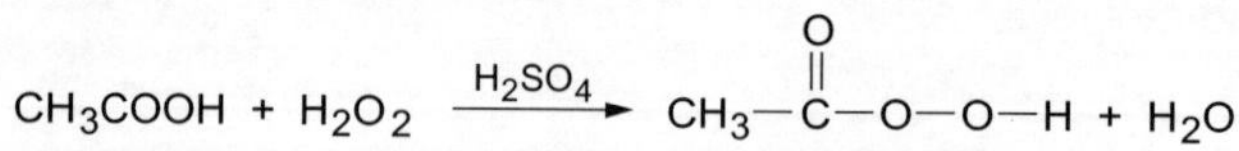

Acyl hydroperoxide
(peracetic acid)

Peracids are important oxidants.

(b) Acyl peroxides are prepared by treating excess of acetic anhydride or acid chloride with alkaline H_2O_2.

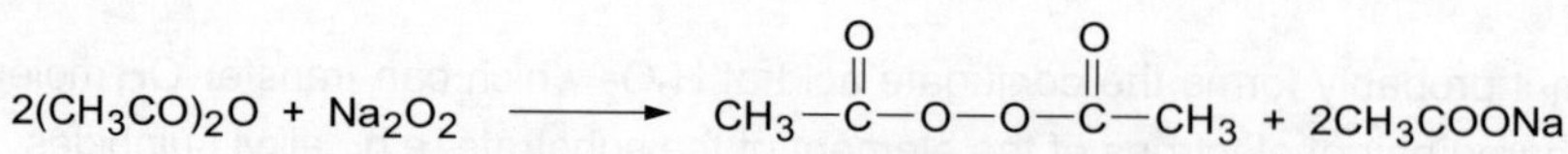

Acetyl peroxide

$$2C_6H_5COCl + Na_2O_2 \longrightarrow C_6H_5{-}CO{-}O{-}O{-}CO{-}C_6H_5 + 2NaCl$$

Benzoyl peroxide

Peracids may be prepared from acylperoxides also.

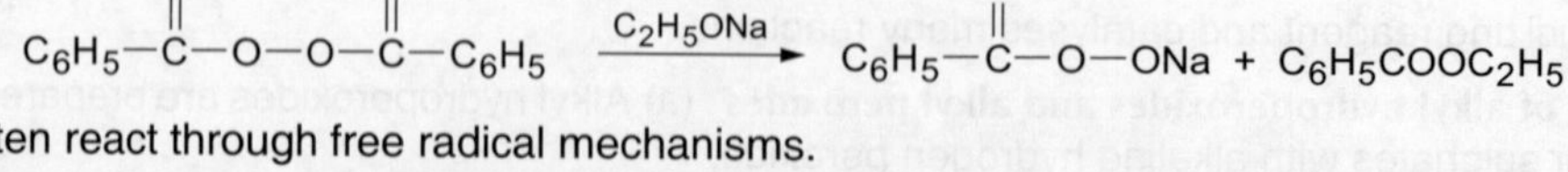

Peroxides often react through free radical mechanisms.

3. Hydroxylation of alkenes With hydrogen peroxide and formic acid, alkenes undergo trans hydroxylation. In contrast, alkaline $KMnO_4$ or OsO_4 gives cis product. Formic acid is first converted by H_2O_2 to performic acid which epoxidates the alkene. Protonation of the oxygen, S_N2 attack by formate anion, and subsequent hydrolysis yields trans diol.

$$H_2O_2 + HCOOH \longrightarrow H{-}\overset{O}{\overset{\|}{C}}{-}O{-}OH + H_2O$$

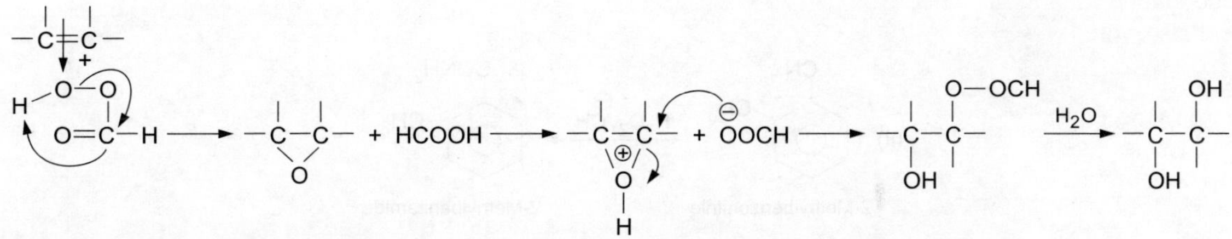

4. Hydroxylation of aromatic hydrocarbons Hydrogen peroxide and ferrous sulphate (Fenton's reagent) react wtih aromatic hydrocarbons to yield phenols.

$$\overset{2\oplus}{Fe} + HO{-}OH \longrightarrow \overset{3\oplus}{Fe} + H\overset{\ominus}{O} + H\dot{O}$$

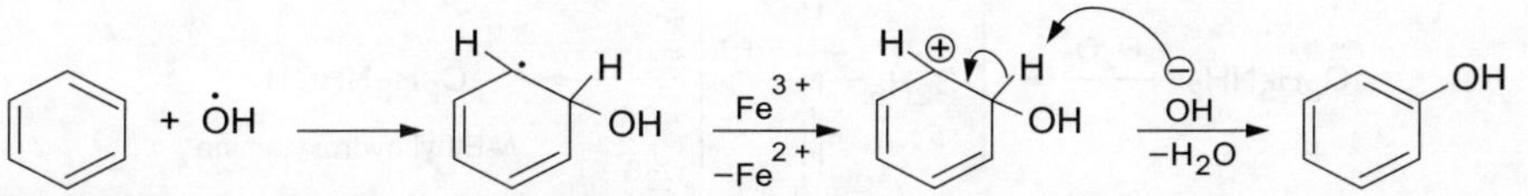

5. Substitution of aldehyde group by hydroxyl group (Dakin reaction) Aldehydic group ortho or para to NH_2 or OH group is converted to hydroxyl group.

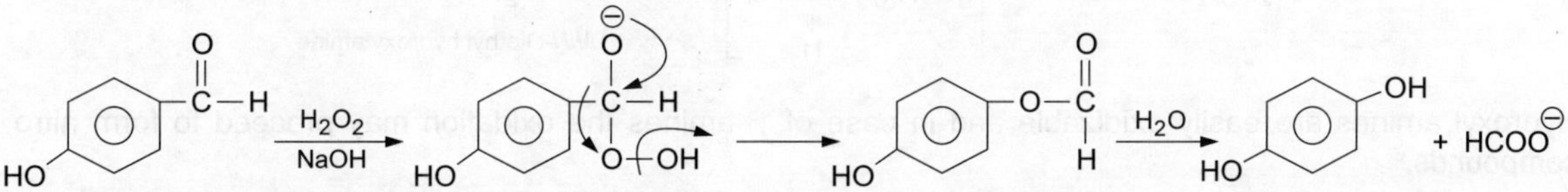

6. Oxidation of trialkyl boranes Trialkyl boranes are oxidized by alkaline hydrogen peroxide to alkyl borates which may be hydrolysed to alcohols.

$$R_3B \xrightarrow[\overset{\ominus}{O}H]{H_2O_2} (RO)_3B \xrightarrow{H_2O} 3ROH + B(OH)_3$$

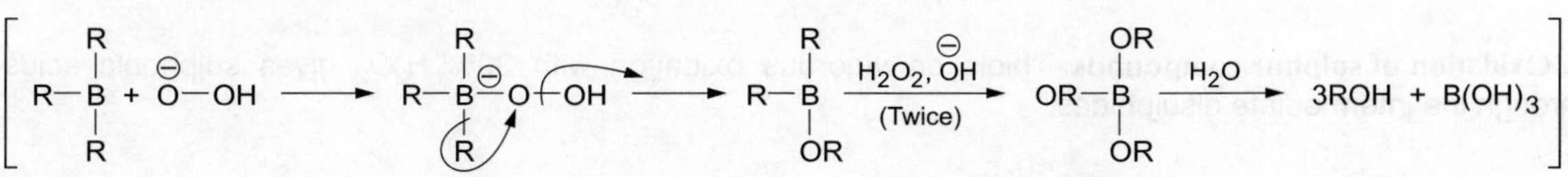

The reaction has been utilized in the preparation of alcohol by hydroboration of alkenes.

$$6CH_3{-}CH{=}CH_2 + B_2H_6 \longrightarrow 2(CH_3CH_2CH_2)_3B$$

$$(CH_3CH_2CH_2)_3B \xrightarrow[25\text{–}30\,^\circ C]{H_2O_2,\ \overset{\ominus}{O}H} (CH_3CH_2CH_2O)_3B \xrightarrow{H_2O} 3CH_3CH_2CH_2OH + B(OH)_3$$

7. Oxidation of nitriles Nitriles are oxidized to unsubstituted amides.

$$\text{(i)}\quad R{-}C{\equiv}N \xrightarrow[\ominus OH]{H_2O_2} RCONH_2$$

(ii)
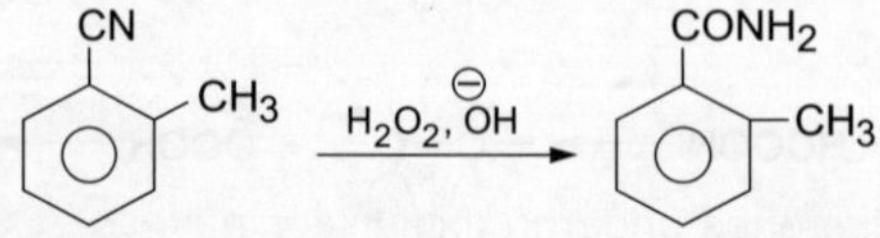

2-Methylbenzonitrile 2-Methylbenzamide

8. Oxidation of amines Tertiary amines are oxidized by H_2O_2 to *N*-oxide.

$$R_3N{:} \xrightarrow{H_2O_2} R_3\overset{\oplus}{N}{-}\overset{\ominus}{O}$$

Primary and secondary amines are oxidized to *N*-alkyl-substituted hydroxyl amines.

$$C_2H_5NH_2 \xrightarrow{H_2O_2} \left[C_2H_5{-}\overset{\oplus}{N}H_2{-}\overset{\ominus}{O}\right] \longrightarrow \underset{N\text{-Ethyl hydroxylamine}}{C_2H_5NHOH}$$

$$(C_2H_5)_2NH \xrightarrow{H_2O_2} \left[(C_2H_5)_2{-}\overset{\oplus}{N}H{-}\overset{\ominus}{O}\right] \longrightarrow \underset{N,N\text{-Diethyl hydroxylamine}}{(C_2H_5)_2NOH}$$

Hydroxyl amines are easily oxidizable and in case of 1° amines the oxidation may proceed to form nitro compounds.

$$CH_3{-}(CH_2)_5{-}NH_2 \xrightarrow{H_2O_2} CH_3{-}(CH_2)_5{-}NO_2$$

Aromatic amines are oxidized to nitro compounds through the intermediate formation of *N*-phenyl hydroxyl amine and nitroso compounds.

$$C_6H_5NH_2 \xrightarrow{H_2O_2} C_6H_5NO_2$$

9. Oxidation of sulphur compounds Thiols on vigorous oxidation with 30% H_2O_2 gives sulphonic acids through the intermediate disulphides.

$$2RSH \xrightarrow{H_2O_2} [R{-}S{-}S{-}R] \longrightarrow 2RSO_3H$$

Sulphides are oxidized to sulphoxides and sulphones depending on the concentration of the oxidant.

(i)
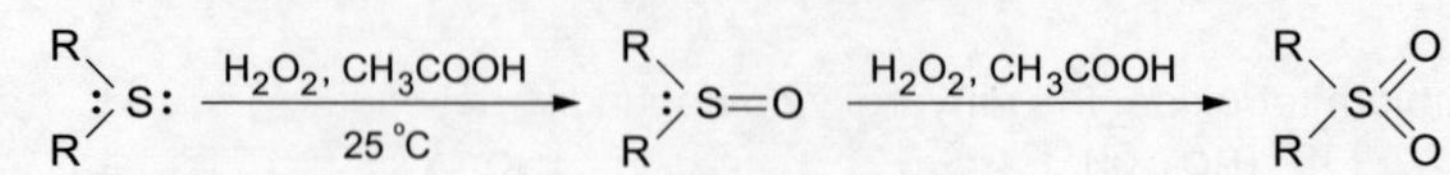

Alkyl sulphide Dialkyl sulphoxide Dialkyl sulphone

(ii) 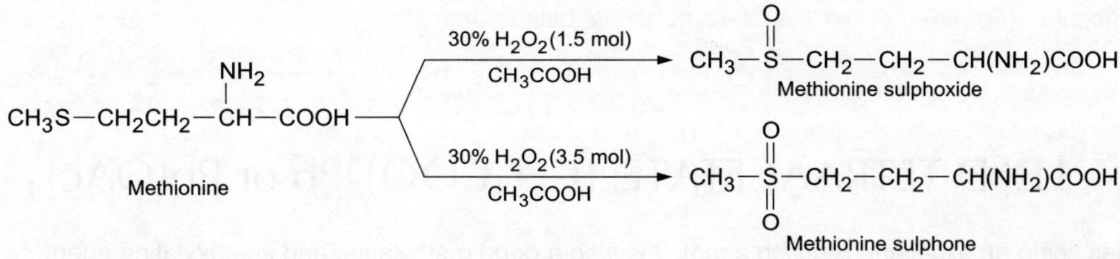

10. Cleavage of α-diketones α-Diketones undergo oxidative cleavage by alkaline H_2O_2 to two molecules of acids.

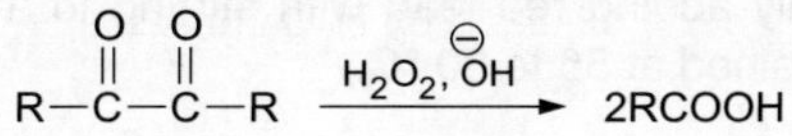

Similarly, α-hydroxy and α-keto acids are cleaved (cf. lead tetraacetate).

(i) 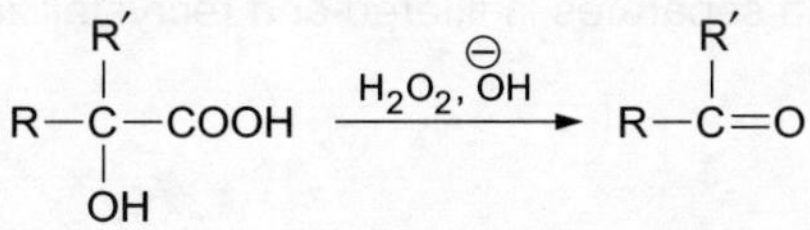

(ii) 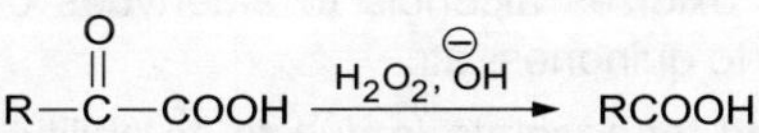

11. Degradation of sugars Aldoses are first oxidized to aldonic acids. Subsequent oxidation of the calcium salt with Fenton's reagent ($H_2O_2 + Fe^{2+}$) converts the aldose to the next lower member.

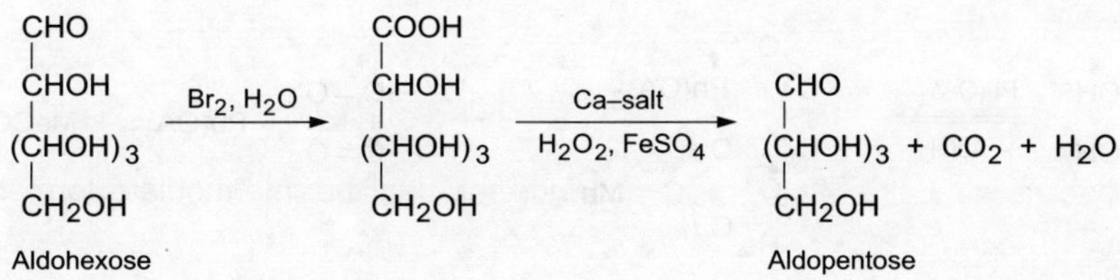

12. Epoxidation of α, β-unsaturated ketones

$$\text{HO—OH} + \overset{\ominus}{\text{OH}} \longrightarrow \text{HO—}\overset{\ominus}{\text{O}} + H_2O$$

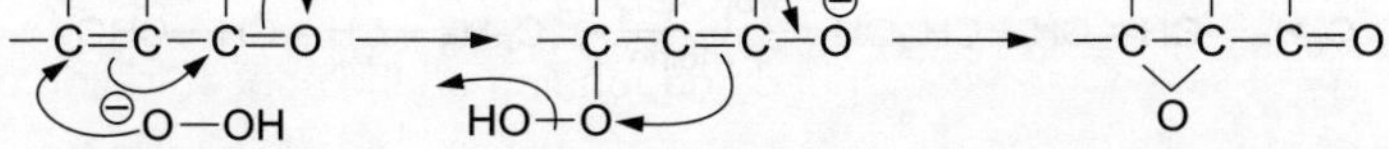

In the presence of osmium tetroxide, the dihydroxy compound is obtained.

$$R_2C{=}CHCOR \xrightarrow[OsO_4]{H_2O_2} R_2C(OH){-}CH(OH){-}COR$$

LEAD TETRAACETATE, $(CH_3COO)_4Pb$ or $Pb(OAc)_4$

Besides being an excellent oxidizing agent, it is also a good methylating and acetoxylating agent.

Preparation

The reagent is prepared by gradually adding red lead with stirring to a mixture of acetic acid and acetic anhydride. The temperature is maintained at 55 to 80 °C.

$$Pb_3O_4 + 8CH_3COOH \xrightarrow[55-80\,^{\circ}C]{Ac_2O} (CH_3COO)_4Pb + 2(CH_3COO)_2Pb + 4H_2O$$

On cooling, lead tetraacetate which separates is filtered and recrystallized from acetic acid.

Uses

The reagent is generally employed as an oxidizing, methylating and acetoxylating agent.

1. As oxidizing agent The reagent oxidizes alcohols to aldehydes or ketones, 1, 2-glycols to aldehydes, ketones or both, hydroxy quinones to quinones, etc.

The oxidizing property of lead tetraacetate is due to its ability to dehydrogenate the substrate while undergoing reduction to lead acetate and two molecules of acetic acid.

The mechanism of the oxidative cleavage of 1, 2-diols is given for illustration. The mechanism was suggested by Criegee.

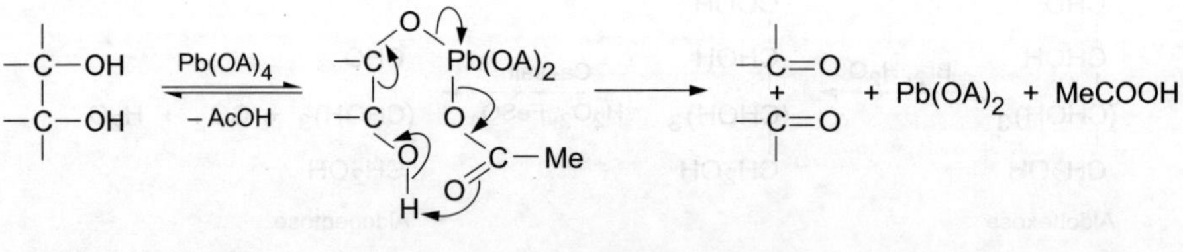

(a) Oxidation of alcohols—Lead tetraacetate with pyridine oxidizes alcohols to aldehydes or ketones at room temperature in good yield. The reagent in pyridine is mild enough not to oxidize aldehyde further.

$$CH_3-(CH_2)_3-CH_2OH \xrightarrow[\text{Pyridine}]{Pb(OAc)_4} CH_3-(CH_2)_3-CHO$$

$$C_6H_5-CH=CH-CH_2OH \xrightarrow[\text{Pyridine}]{Pb(OAc)_4} C_6H_5-CH=CH-CHO$$

$$CH_3-CHOH-CH_2-CHOH-CH_3 \xrightarrow[\text{Pyridine}]{Pb(OAc)_4} CH_3-CO-CH_2-CO-CH_3$$

Alcohols having hydrogen at δ-carbon may be cyclised. Tetrahydrofuran is formed in high yield from *n*-butanol.

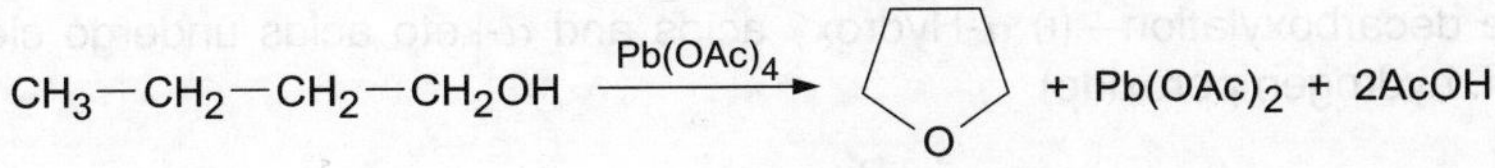

Tetrahydro furan (THF)

(b) Oxidation of 1, 2-glycols—Vic diols are oxidized by lead tetraacetate at room temperature with cleavage of bond to aldehydes, ketones or both depending upon the structure of the glycols.

(i) 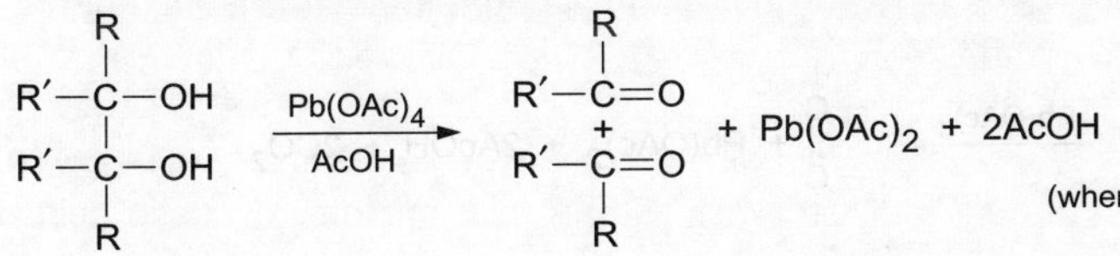

(where R′ = H or alkyl)

(ii) $$CH_3-(CH_2)_7-\overset{OH}{CH}-\overset{OH}{CH}-(CH_2)_7-COOH \xrightarrow[AcOH]{Pb(OAc)_4} CH_3-(CH_2)_7-CHO + OHC-(CH_2)_7-COOH$$

9,10-Dihydroxystearic acid — *n*-Nonaldehyde — Half aldehyde of azelaic acid

The reaction is useful for the determination of the positions of the hydroxyl groups and for that matter the position of the double bond in the olefine from which the glycols are prepared.

Similar oxidative cleavage is observed in compounds having oxygen and nitrogen on adjacent carbons.

(iii) 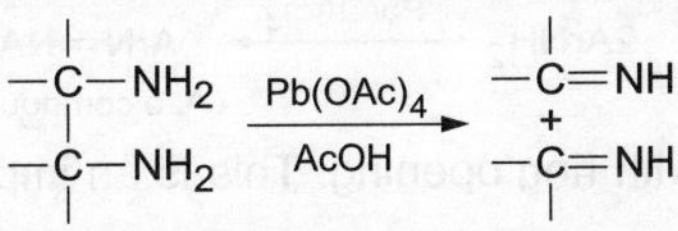

(iv) 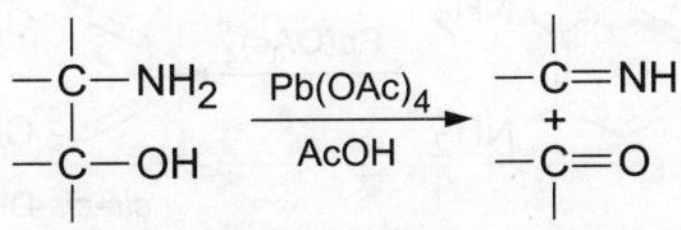

(c) Oxidation of hydroquinones—It is an excellent reagent for oxidizing hydroquinones to quinones. The oxidation is useful for elucidating structures of organic compounds.

(i) 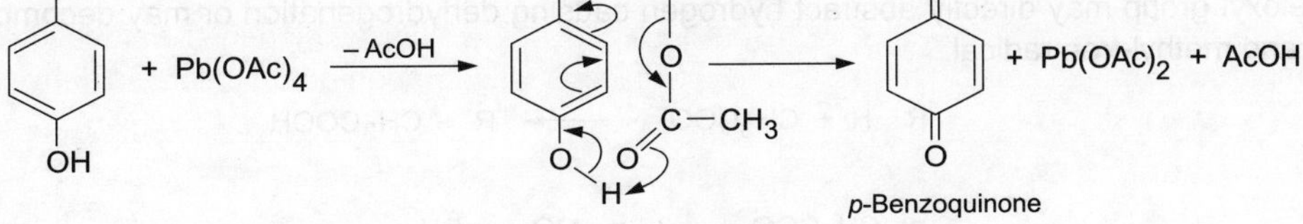

p-Benzoquinone

(ii) 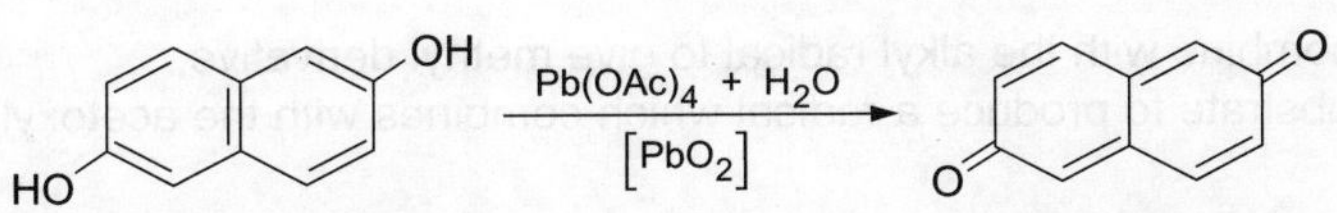

2,6-Dihydroxy naphthalene — *amphi*-Naphthaquinone (2,6-Naphthaquinone)

Lead oxide, PbO_2 is actually the oxidant which is obtained by decomposing lead tetraacetate with water.

(d) Oxidative decarboxylation—(i) α-Hydroxy acids and α-keto acids undergo cleavage with loss of carboxyl groups (cf. hydrogen peroxide).

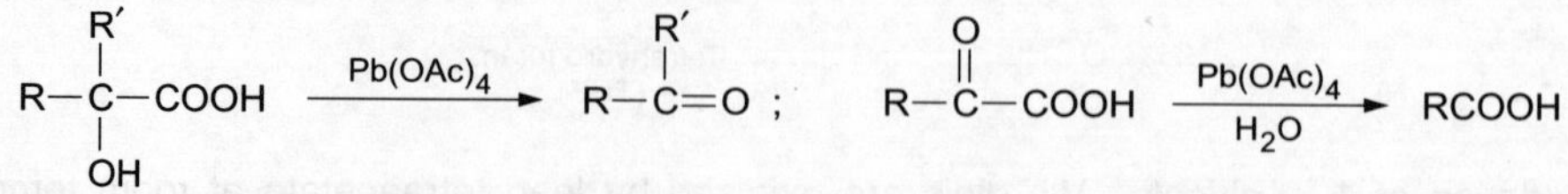

(ii) Compounds having carboxyl groups on adjacent carbons (succinic acid derivatives) undergo bisdecarboxylation.

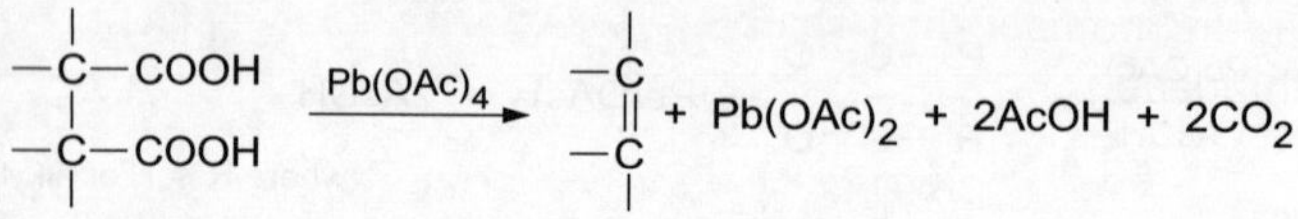

Similarly, malonic acid derivatives undergo bisdecarboxylation with lead tetraacetate.

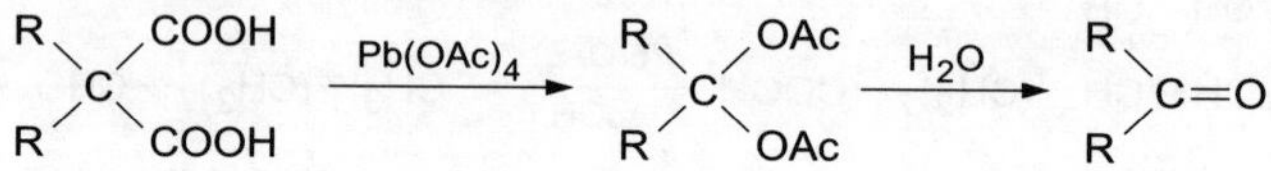

Monobasic carboxylic acids give esters which may be hydrolysed to alcohol but there are many side products.

$$R{-}COOH \xrightarrow{Pb(OAc)_4} R{-}O{-}Ac \xrightarrow{H_2O} R{-}OH$$

(e) Oxidation of amines—Oxidation of aromatic primary amines gives azo compounds.

$$2ArNH_2 \xrightarrow{Pb(OAc)_4} \underset{\text{Azo compound}}{ArN{=}NAr}$$

Ortho-diamines are oxidized with ring opening. This is an important industrial method for cleavage of aromatic rings.

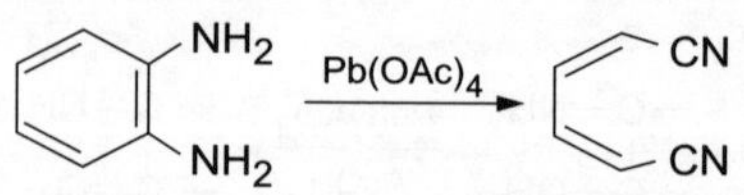

cis-cis-Dinitrile

2. As acetoxylating and methylating agent When boiled with glacial acetic acid, lead tetraacetate breaks up into lead acetate and two acetoxyl radicals.

$$(CH_3COO)_4Pb \xrightarrow[\Delta]{CH_3COOH} (CH_3COO)_2Pb + 2CH_3CO\dot{O}$$

The acetoxyl group may directly abstract hydrogen causing dehydrogenation or may decompose to carbon dioxide and methyl-free radical.

$$R{-}H + CH_3CO\dot{O} \longrightarrow \dot{R} + CH_3COOH$$

$$\text{or } CH_3CO\dot{O} \longrightarrow CO_2 + \dot{C}H_3$$

The methyl radical may combine with the alkyl radical to give methyl derivative, or it may dehydrogenate the substrate to produce a radical which combines with the acetoxyl radical to give acetoxyl derivative.

$$\dot{R} + \dot{C}H_3 \longrightarrow R{-}CH_3$$

$$C_6H_5CH_3 + \dot{C}H_3 \longrightarrow C_6H_5\dot{C}H_2 + CH_4\ ;\ C_6H_5\dot{C}H_2 + CH_3CO\dot{O} \longrightarrow C_6H_5CH_2OCOCH_3$$

(a) Acetoxylation—(i) Carbonyl compounds—The reagent acetoxylates the reactive methyl groups and the active methylene groups.

$$CH_3COCH_3 \xrightarrow{Pb(OAc)_4} \underset{\alpha,\ \alpha'\text{-Diacetoxy acetone}}{AcOCH_2COCH_2OAc}$$

$$CH_3COCH_2COOR \xrightarrow{Pb(OAc)_4} CH_3-CO-\overset{OAc}{\overset{|}{OH}}-COOR$$

(ii) Hydrocarbons—In aromatic hydrocarbons the susceptible positions of attack are benzilic and 9 or 10-positions of anthracene.

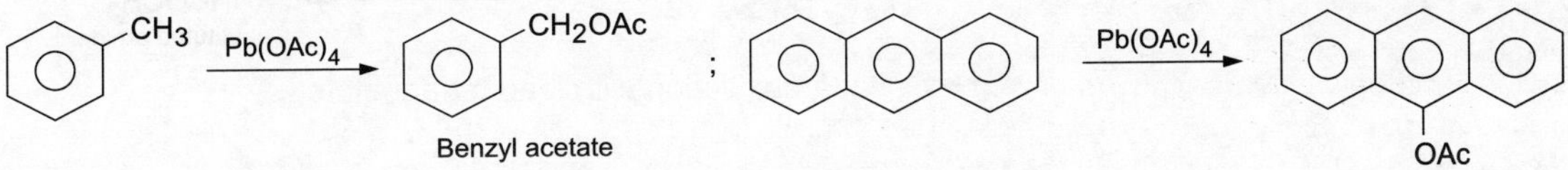

Benzyl acetate ; 9-Acetoxy anthracene

In cyclo alkenes both the double bond and the allylic position are attacked.

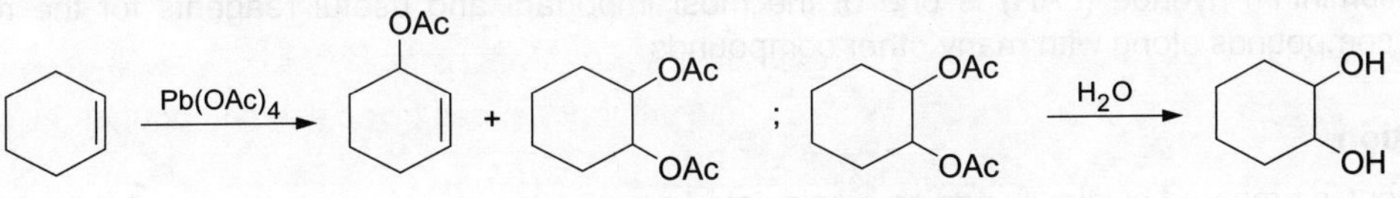

cis- and *trans*- 1, 2-Diacetates ; *cis*- and *trans*- 1, 2-Diacetates ; Diol

It is in fact a process of hydroxylation.

(b) Methylation—Direct methylation can be carried out by boiling the compound with lead tetraacetate and glacial acetic acid.

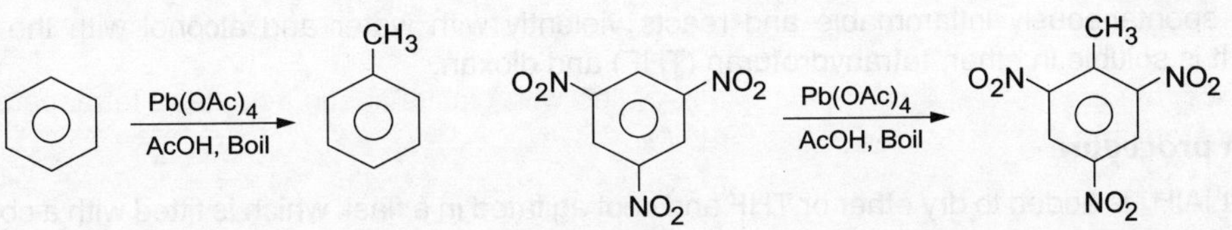

TNB ; TNT

A substitute of vitamin K (antihemorrhagic factor) is 2, 3-dimethyl-α-naphthaquinone which can be prepared by direct methylation.

$$Pb(OAc)_4 \xrightarrow[\text{Boil}]{AcOH} 2Pb(OAc)_2 + 2CH_3CO\dot{O}$$

$$2CH_3CO\dot{O} \longrightarrow 2\dot{C}H_3 + 2CO_2$$

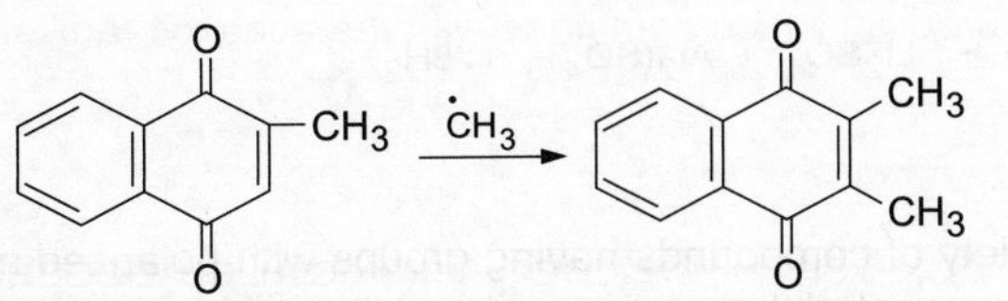

$$+ \dot{H} \quad ; \quad CH_3CO\dot{O} + \dot{H} \longrightarrow CH_3COOH$$

Other reactions

Hunsdieckler reaction (decarboxylative bromination) may be conveniently effected by treating the acid with lead tetraacetate in the presence of halide ion.

$$RCOOH + \overset{\ominus}{Br} \xrightarrow{Pb(OAc)_4} RBr$$

A reaction similar to Hofmann rearrangement may be performed by treating the amide with lead tetraacetate. The initially formed isocyanate and the amine may react to form substituted ureas or the amine may react with the liberated acetic acid from the reagent to yield amide.

$$RCONH_2 \xrightarrow{Pb(OAc)_4} R{-}N{=}C{=}O \xrightarrow{H_2O} RNH_2$$

$$RNH_2 \xrightarrow{R-N=C=O} \underset{\text{Substituted urea}}{RNHCONHR}$$

$$RNH_2 \xrightarrow{CH_3COOH} \underset{\text{Substituted amide}}{RNHCOCH_3}$$

LITHIUM ALUMINIUM HYDRIDE

Lithium aluminium hydride (LAH) is one of the most important and useful reagents for the reduction of carbonyl compounds along with many other compounds.

Preparation

The reagent is prepared by slowly adding a calculated amount of anhydrous aluminium chloride to a paste of lithium hydride in dry ether or THF.

$$4LiH + AlCl_3 \xrightarrow[\text{or THF}]{\text{Dry ether}} \overset{\oplus\ominus}{LiAlH_4} + 3LiCl$$

Precipitated lithium chloride and the unreacted lithium hydride are removed by filtration. The filtrate is evaporated in the absence of air and carbon dioxide when lithium aluminium hydride is obtained as a grey solid. It is spontaneously inflammable and reacts violently with water and alcohol with the evolution of hydrogen. It is soluble in ether, tetrahydrofuran (THF) and dioxan.

Reduction procedure

Powdered $LiAlH_4$ is added to dry ether or THF and kept agitated in a flask which is fitted with a condenser and a dropping funnel. Solution of the substance in ether is then gradually run into the flask so as to maintain a gentle boiling of the mixture. The reduction product is decomposed with water and acid.

$$4R{-}\underset{R'}{C}{=}O + LiAlH_4 \xrightarrow{\text{Ether}} \left[R{-}\overset{H}{\underset{R'}{C}}{-}O \right]_4 \overset{\ominus\oplus}{AlLi} \xrightarrow[H_2O]{H_2SO_4} 4R{-}\overset{H}{\underset{R'}{C}}{-}OH + Al_2(SO_4)_3 + Li_2SO_4$$

(where R′ = alkyl, OH, Cl, etc.)

Excess of $LiAlH_4$ is also decomposed by water and acid.

$$2LiAlH_4 + 4H_2SO_4 \longrightarrow Li_2SO_4 + Al_2(SO_4)_3 + 8H_2$$

Mechanism

The reagent can supply hydride ions to a large variety of compounds having groups with polarized multiple bonds such as, C = O, C ≡ N, C = N, N = O, etc. It is suggested that as the nucleophilic hydride ion attacks the positively charged carbonyl carbon, aluminium complexes with the oxygen, i.e., the reaction is concentrated. The intermediate (I) formed in the first step has three more hydrogens which are similarly transferred to three other molecules of the substrate to yield the complex (II). The latter on hydrolysis with water and acid gives the reduced product.

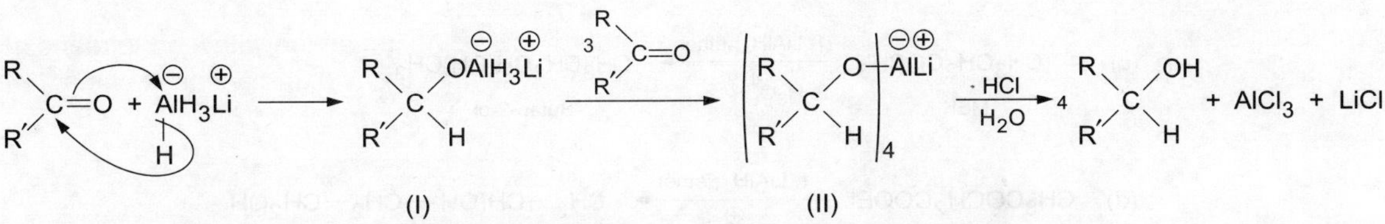

The first step is fast but the subsequent steps are slow because the electron-withdrawing effect of the alkoxyl group inhibits the hydride ion transfer. It is seen that in reducing the cabonyl compound, half the hydrogen is supplied by the reagent and the other half is supplied by the solvent, i.e., water.

It reacts readily with acidic hydrogens. One fourth of the valuable reagent is lost in the formation of hydrogen on reacting with the hydrogens of acids.

$$R-COOH + LiAlH_4 \longrightarrow R-COO\overset{\ominus}{Al}H_3\overset{\oplus}{Li} + H_2$$

Hence acids are better converted to their esters before reduction with lithium aluminium hydride.

Uses

The reagent may be used to reduce aldehydes, ketones, acids and their derivatives, epoxides, etc., to alcohols. The reagent can also reduce nitriles, aliphatic nitro compounds, anilides, azides and isocyanates to amines. The substrates and their reduction products with $LiAlH_4$ are listed below.

Substrates	Reduction products	Substrates	Reduction products
RCHO	RCH_2OH	$(RCO)_2O$	$2RCH_2OH$
RCOR	RCHOHR	$R-C\equiv N$	RCHO or RNH_2
RCOOH	RCH_2OH	$R-NO_2$	RNH_2
RCOOR′	RCH_2OH + R′OH	$Ar-NO_2$	ArNH=NHAr
RCOCl	RCH_2OH	$ArNHCOCH_3$	$ArNHCH_2CH_3$
		R—N=C=O	$RNHCH_3$
$R-\overbrace{CH-CH_2}^{O}$	$RCHOHCH_3 + RCH_2CH_2OH$	RN_3	RNH_2

The list is by no means exhaustive.

1. Reduction of carbonyl compounds The carbonyl compounds are smoothly reduced without affecting double or triple bonds.

(a) $$\underset{\text{Hexanal}}{CH_3(CH_2)_4CHO} \xrightarrow[2.\ H_3O^{\oplus}]{1.\ LiAlH_4,\ \text{ether}} \underset{\text{Hexanol}}{CH_3-(CH_2)_4-CH_2OH}$$

(b) $$\underset{\text{Crotonaldehyde}}{CH_3-CH=CH-CHO} \xrightarrow[2.\ H_3O^{\oplus}]{1.\ LiAlH_4,\ \text{ether}} \underset{\text{Crotyl alcohol}}{CH_3-CH=CH-CH_2OH}$$

Sometimes the double bond is also reduced when a phenyl group is attached to the β-carbon.

$$\underset{\text{Cinnamaldehyde}}{C_6H_5-CH=CH-CHO} \xrightarrow[\text{2. } H_3O^{\oplus}]{\text{1. LiAlH}_4\text{, ether}} \underset{\text{3-Phenylpropanol-1}}{C_6H_5-CH_2\cdot CH_2-CH_2OH}$$

(c) $$\underset{\text{MEK}}{CH_3CH_2COCH_3} \xrightarrow[\text{2. } H_3O^{\oplus}]{\text{1. LiAlH}_4\text{, ether}} \underset{\text{Butan-2-ol}}{CH_3CH_2CH(OH)CH_3}$$

(d) $$\underset{\text{Ethyl acetoacetate}}{CH_3COCH_2COOEt} \xrightarrow[\text{2. } H_3O^{\oplus}]{\text{1. LiAlH}_4\text{, ether}} \underset{\text{Butan-1, 3-diol}}{CH_3-CH(OH)-CH_2-CH_2OH}$$

The reagent is of considerable utility for the reduction of sensitive and expensive carbonyl compounds.

(e) 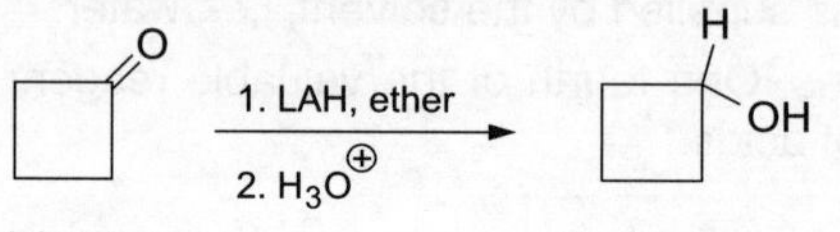

Cyclobutanone Cyclobutanol

2. Reduction of acids and their derivatives Acids are resistant to reduction by all other reagents.

Acids

$$\underset{\text{Palmitic acid}}{CH_3-(CH_2)_{14}-COOH} \xrightarrow[\text{2. } H_3O^{\oplus}]{\text{1. LAH, ether}} \underset{\text{Hexadecanol-1 (cetyl alcohol)}}{CH_3-(CH_2)_{14}-CH_2OH}$$

$$\underset{\text{Crotonic acid}}{CH_3-CH=CH-COOH} \xrightarrow[\text{2. } H_3O^{\oplus}]{\text{1. LAH, ether}} \underset{\text{Crotyl alcohol}}{CH_3-CH=CH-CH_2OH}$$

$$\underset{\beta\text{-Alanine}}{CH_2(NH_2)CH_2COOH} \xrightarrow[\text{2. } H_3O^{\oplus}]{\text{1. LAH, ether}} \underset{\text{3-Aminopropanol-1}}{CH_2(NH_2)CH_2CH_2OH}$$

Acid chlorides

$$CH_3COCl \xrightarrow[\text{2. } H_3O^{\oplus}]{\text{1. LAH, ether}} CH_3CH_2OH$$

Acid anhydrides

$$(CH_3CO)_2O \xrightarrow[\text{2. } H_3O^{\oplus}]{\text{1. LAH, ether}} 2CH_3CH_2OH$$

Esters

$$CH_3-CH=CH-COOC_2H_5 \xrightarrow[\text{2. } H_3O^{\oplus}]{\text{1. LAH, ether}} \underset{\text{But-2-ene-1-ol}}{CH_3-CH=CH-CH_2OH}$$

Amides—Unsubstituted amides give 1° amines while substituted amides give 2° or 3° amines.

$$\left.\begin{array}{l}\text{(i) } RCONH_2 \\ \text{(ii) } RCONHR' \\ \text{(iii) } RCONR'_2\end{array}\right\} \xrightarrow[\text{2. } H_3O^{\oplus}]{\text{1. LAH, ether}} \begin{array}{l}\text{(i) } RCH_2NH_2 \\ \text{(ii) } RCH_2NHR' \\ \text{(iii) } RCH_2NR'_2\end{array}$$

Anilides are similarly reduced to 2° or 3° amines.

$$\left.\begin{array}{l}\text{(i) } C_6H_5{-}NH{-}CO{-}CH_3 \\ \quad\text{Acetanilide} \\ \text{(ii) } C_6H_5{-}N(CH_3){-}CO{-}CH_3 \\ \quad N\text{-Methylacetanilide}\end{array}\right\} \xrightarrow[\text{2. } H_3O^{\oplus}]{\text{1. LAH, ether}} \begin{array}{l}\text{(i) } C_6H_5{-}NH{-}CH_2{-}CH_3 \\ \quad N\text{-Ethylaniline (2° amine)} \\ \text{(ii) } C_6H_5{-}N(CH_3){-}CH_2{-}CH_3 \\ \quad N\text{-Methyl-}N\text{-ethyl aniline (3° amine)}\end{array}$$

3. Reduction of nitro compounds, azides, oximes, nitriles, etc., to primary amines

Nitro compounds

$$CH_3{-}CH_2{-}CH(NO_2){-}CH_3 \xrightarrow[\text{Ether}]{\text{LAH}} CH_3{-}CH_2{\cdot}CH(NH_2){-}CH_3$$

Nitrobenzene, however, gives azobenzene via azoxybenzene.

$$2C_6H_5NO_2 \xrightarrow[\text{Ether}]{\text{LAH}} C_6H_5{-}\overset{\overset{O}{\uparrow}}{N}{=}N{-}C_6H_5 \longrightarrow \underset{\text{Azobenzene}}{C_6H_5{-}N{=}N{-}C_6H_5}$$

Azides

$$\underset{\text{Azide}}{RN_3} \xrightarrow[\text{Ether}]{\text{LAH}} \underset{\text{1° amine}}{RNH_2}$$

$$\underset{\text{Allyl carbinyl azide}}{CH_2{=}CH{-}CH_2CH_2N_3} \xrightarrow[\text{Ether}]{\text{LAH}} \underset{\text{Allylcarbinyl amine}}{CH_2{=}CH{-}CH_2{-}CH_2{-}NH_2}$$

Oximes

$$\underset{\text{Benzophenone oxime}}{(C_6H_5)_2C{=}N{-}OH} \xrightarrow[\text{Ether}]{\text{LAH}} \underset{\text{Diphenylmethyl amine}}{(C_6H_5)_2CH{-}NH_2}$$

Nitriles—Reduction of nitriles with $LiAlH_4$ may give amine or aldehyde depending on the conditions of the reaction.

(a) Aldehydes are given when a solution of $LiAlH_4$ is added to the solution of a nitrile in dry ether or THF at low temperature.

Nitriles

$$R{-}C{\equiv}N \xrightarrow[-\,50\ °C]{\text{LAH, Ether}} \underset{\text{Imine}}{R{-}CH{=}NH} \xrightarrow{H_3\overset{\oplus}{O}} R{-}CHO$$

(b) Amines are obtained when a solution of nitrile is added to the solution of lithium aluminium hydride in ether or THF.

$$R-C\equiv N \xrightarrow[\text{Ether}]{\text{LAH}} \underset{\text{Imine salt}}{R-CH=NLi} \xrightarrow[\text{2. } H_3\overset{\oplus}{O}]{\text{1. LAH, ether}} RCH_2NH_2$$

4. Reduction of halides

$$4(CH_3)_2CH-CH_2Br + LiAlH_4 \xrightarrow{\text{Ether}} 4(CH_3)_3CH + LiAlBr_4$$

5. Reduction of epoxides to alcohols

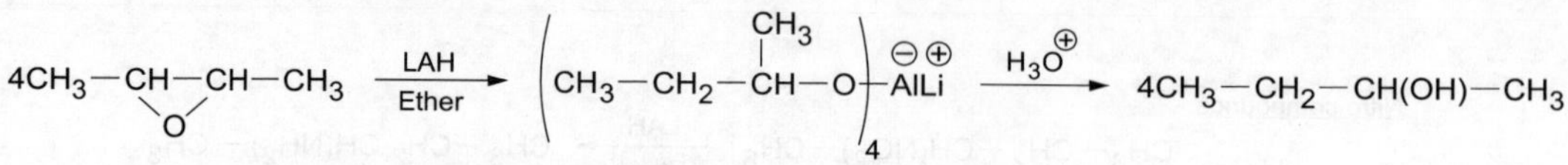

6. Reaction with compounds containing active hydrogens The reagent reacts with alcohols and amines to evolve hydrogen. The method can be used to estimate active hydrogen.

$$4ROH + LiAlH_4 \longrightarrow (RO)_4\overset{\ominus}{Al}\overset{\oplus}{Li} + 4H_2$$

$$4RNH_2 + LiAlH_4 \longrightarrow (RNH)_4\overset{\ominus}{Al}\overset{\oplus}{Li} + 4H_2$$

7. Introduction of deuterium in organic molecules Lithium aluminium deuteride has been used for introducing deuterium in organic compounds.

(i) $$LiAlD_4 + 4C_6H_5-\underset{\underset{Br}{|}}{CH}-CH_3 \longrightarrow 4C_6H_5-\underset{\underset{D}{|}}{CH}-CH_3 + LiAlBr_4$$

(ii)

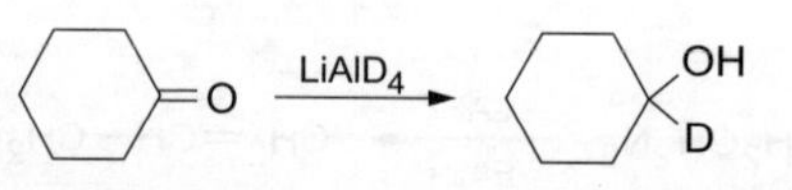

Cyclohexanone Cyclohexanol-1-d

OSMIUM TETROXIDE, OsO_4

Osmium tetroxide is a reagent for *cis*-hydroxylation of carbon–carbon double bond.

Preparation

It is prepared by the oxidation of osmium metal or its compounds by strong heat in the presence of air. More commonly it is prepared by heating osmium metal to red heat in air.

$$Os + 2O_2(\text{air}) \xrightarrow{\text{Red heat}} OsO_4$$

Osmium tetroxide is toxic and volatile. Its vapours are specially dangerous for eyes. Since it is an expensive and toxic substance it is used only for the synthesis of fine chemicals (pharmaceuticals) and for degradative purposes in the elucidation of structures.

For the oxidation purpose, a solution of OsO_4 in ether or *t*-butyl alcohol is added to the solution of the olefine in the presence of a base, e.g., pyridine which catalyses the reaction by coordinating with the resulting osmic ester. The osmic ester is then hydrolysed by refluxing with an aqueous-alcoholic solution of a reducing agent, e.g., sodium sulphite which prevents further oxidation of the product.

Osmium tetroxide, like permanganate, undergoes initial *cis*-cycloaddition with the olefine from the less hindered side to yield *cis*-1, 2-diol as the final product.

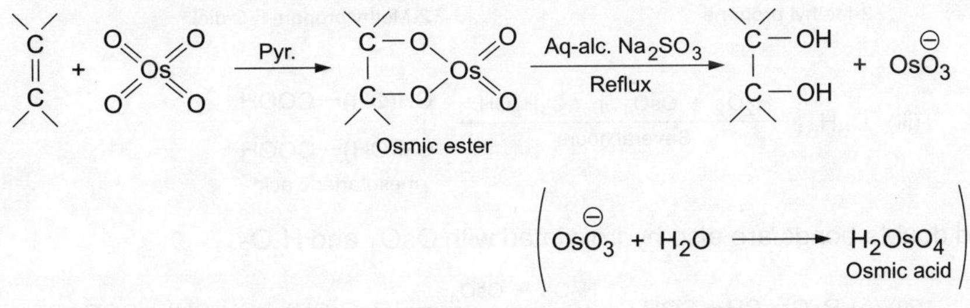

The addition of OsO_4 is slow but almost quantitative. The cyclic osmic ester is insoluble. The reaction generally occurs at room temperature.

Uses

1. Preparation of *cis*-1, 2-diols

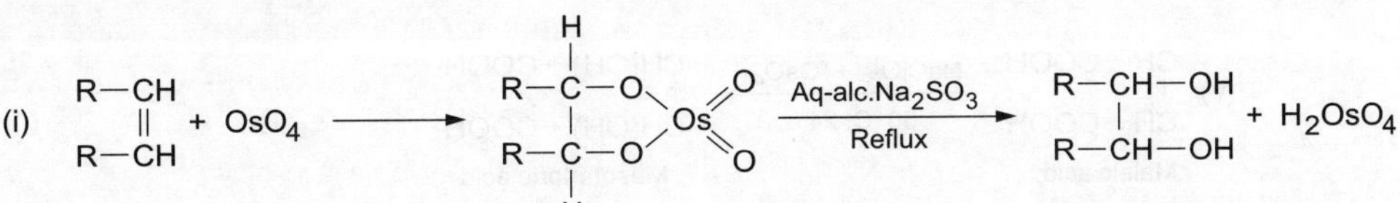

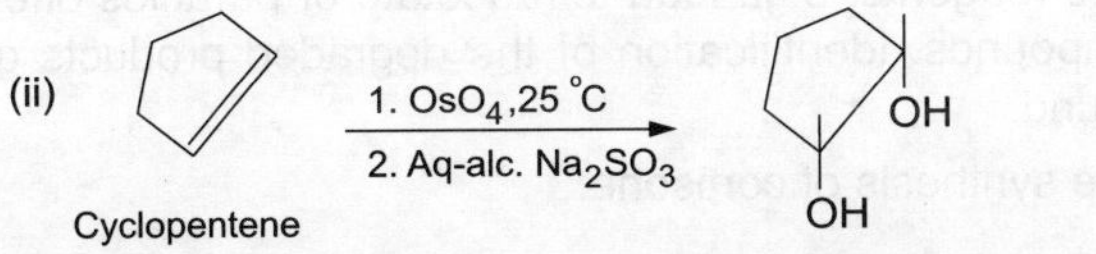

cis-Cyclopentan-1, 2-diol

2. Elucidation of the structures of polynuclear hydrocarbons Anthracene is oxidized by OsO_4 to tetrol (I) which on further oxidation with potassium ferricyanide gives naphthalene-2, 3-dicarboxylic acid (II). The carboxyl groups at positions-2 and -3 indicate ortho fusion of the third ring in anthracene and also linear fusion of the three rings.

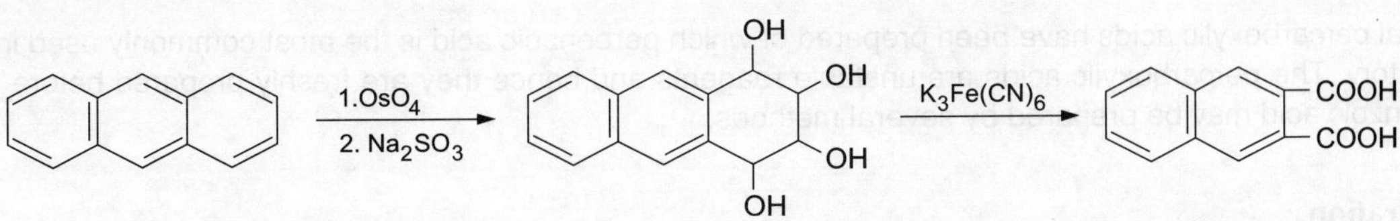

(I) (II)

Similar treatment indicates ortho fusion of the two rings in naphthalene.

3. As a catalyst Since it is an expensive and toxic reagent, it is sometimes used in small catalytic amounts with other oxidizing agents, e.g., H_2O_2 which reoxidize osmium in its lower valence states to OsO_4 to continue the oxidation of the substrate.

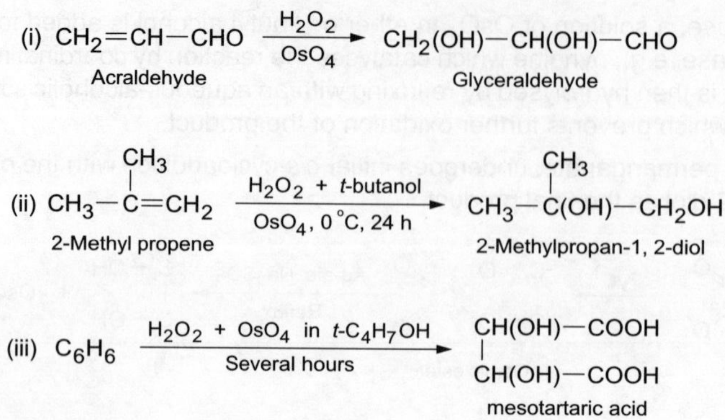

Conjugated double bonds are also hydroxylated with OsO_4 and H_2O_2.

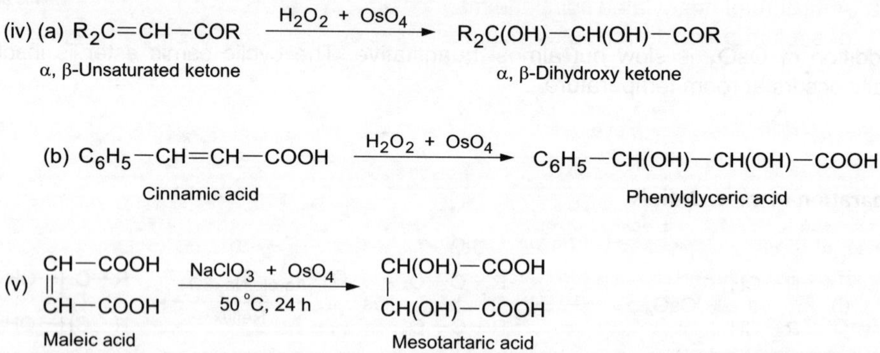

4. Elucidation of the structures of unsaturated compounds Hydroxylation of carbon–carbon double bonds by osmium tetroxide and their cleavage with specific reagents, e.g., lead tetraacetate or peracids offer a good method for the degradation of unsaturated compounds. Identification of the degraded products gives the presumptive structure of the unsaturated compound.

The reagent has also been employed in the synthesis of cortisone.

PERBENZOIC ACID (Peroxybenzoic acid), $C_6H_5CO_3H$

Several percarboxylic acids have been prepared of which perbenzoic acid is the most commonly used in the laboratory. The percarboxylic acids are unstable reagents and hence they are freshly prepared before use. Perbenzoic acid may be prepared by several methods.

Preparation

1. A cold solution of benzoyl peroxide in chloroform is added to a cold (0–5 °C) solution of sodium methoxide in methanol. The product, sodium perbenzoate is extracted with ice-cold water which is acidified with cold normal sulphuric acid and extracted with chloroform. Chloroform is removed by distillation under reduced pressure when perbenzoic acid is obtained as a solid, m.p. 41 °C. The yield is about 82%.

$$C_6H_5-\overset{O}{\overset{\|}{C}}-O-O-\overset{O}{\overset{\|}{C}}-C_6H_5 + CH_3ONa \longrightarrow C_6H_5-\overset{O}{\overset{\|}{C}}-O-ONa + C_6H_5-\overset{O}{\overset{\|}{C}}-OCH_3$$

$$C_6H_5CO_3Na \xrightarrow[CHCl_3]{H_2SO_4} C_6H_5COOOH$$

2. To a solution of benzoic acid in methane sulphonic acid, 70% hydrogen peroxide is added dropwise with constant stirring. The temperature is maintained at 25–30 °C. The stirring is continued for two hours. The mixture is extracted with benzene, washed with ammonium sulphate solution and filtered when perbenzoic acid is obtained. The yield is 80–90%.

$$C_6H_5COOH + H_2O_2 \longrightarrow C_6H_5-\overset{O}{\overset{\|}{C}}-O-OH + H_2O$$

3. A mixture of methylated spirit and magnesium sulphate is added with stirring to an aqueous solution of sodium peroxide (or better hydrogen peroxide and sodium carbonate) at about 20 °C. Benzoyl chloride is then added slowly with stirring to the resulting mixture. The solution is then filtered, acidified with sulphuric acid and extracted with benzene. Perbenzoic acid is obtained on distilling off benzene.

$$C_6H_5COCl + Na_2O_2 \longrightarrow C_6H_5CO_3Na + NaCl$$

$$2C_6H_5CO_3Na + H_2SO_4 \longrightarrow 2C_6H_5CO_3H + Na_2SO_4$$

Procedure

Ethereal or chloroform solution of perbenzoic acid is added to the substrate. The mixture is kept from one to several days (according to the substrate) at room temperature. The mixture is washed with dilute alkali, dried and the solvent distilled off.

Use

Perbenzoic acid is a good oxidant and reacts with olefinic bonds to yield epoxides (oxiranes). Some of its important uses are—

(a) Epoxidation Perbenzoic acid reacts quantitatively with non-conjugated double bonds to form epoxides.

$$R-CH{=}CH-R + C_6H_5CO_3H \longrightarrow R-\underset{\diagdown O \diagup}{CH-CH}-R + C_6H_5COOH$$

Except amino group, other groups such as hydroxyl, ester, aryl, etc., do not interfere. The reaction conditions are mild and the yield is high. Electron-donating groups increase the reaction rate. Thus, 1, 2-dimethyl 1, 4-cyclohexadiene forms epoxide with the alkyl substituted double bond.

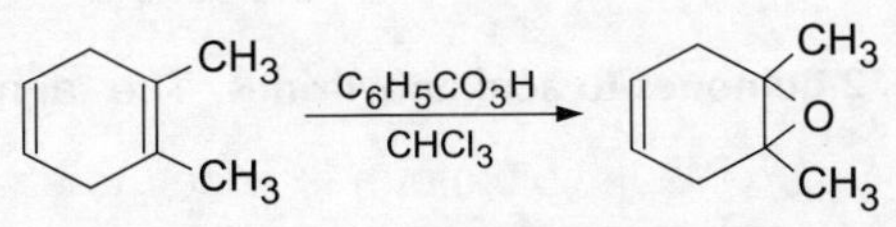

Unsaturated groups adjacent to the olefinic bond decrease the reaction rate by electron withdrawal, e.g., the reaction is very poor with α, β-unsaturated acids or esters. With α, β-unsaturated aldehydes or ketones, Baeyer–Villiger oxidation may compete with epoxidation.

Mechanism of epoxidation—A widely accepted mechanism involves the formation of a cyclic intermediate state which transforms into products.

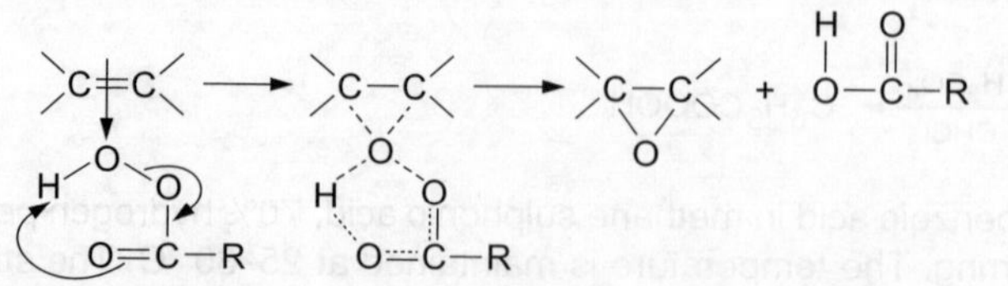

Evidence in favour of this mechanism are—

(I) the reaction is second order (II) reaction occurs readily in nonpolar solvents, i.e., without ion formation and (III) the addition of oxygen is stereospecific, e.g., *cis*-olefin gives *cis*-epoxide.

Epoxides may be transformed into alcohols, diols, carbonyl compounds, etc. Thus,

Alcohol—Epoxides on reduction with $LiAlH_4$ gives alcohols. Cleavage occurs so that a 3° alcohol is formed and if that is not possible then a 2° alcohol is formed.

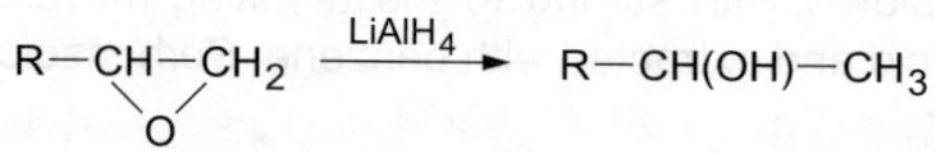

Vic diols—Epoxides are hydrolysed to *trans* 1, 2-diols. the reaction is acid- or base-catalysed.

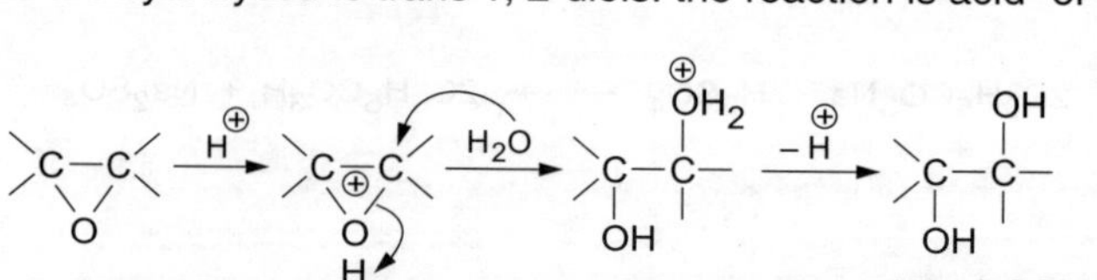

trans 1, 2-Diol

Depending upon reaction conditions the diols may undergo pinacol–pinacolone rearrangement to aldehydes or ketones.

(b) Oxidation of ketones to esters (Baeyer–Villiger rearrangement) Ketones are converted to esters and cyclic ketones to lactones on treatment with perbenzoic acid (or better with CF_3CO_3H). Lactones are formed with ring expansion.

$$C_6H_5COCH_3 \xrightarrow{C_6H_5CO_3H} \underset{\text{Phenyl acetate}}{CH_3-\overset{\overset{\displaystyle O}{\|}}{C}-OC_6H_5} + C_6H_5COOH$$

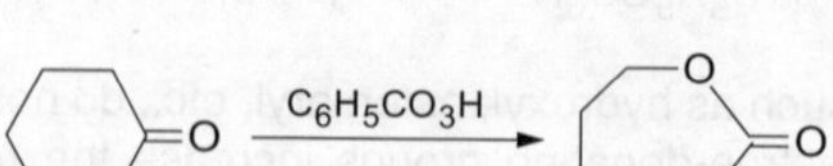

Caprolactone

(c) Oxidation of α-diketones and 1, 2-quinones to acid anhydrides The anhydrides obtained by oxidation may be hydrolysed to acids.

$$CH_3-\overset{\overset{\displaystyle O}{\|}}{C}-\overset{\overset{\displaystyle O}{\|}}{C}-CH_3 \xrightarrow[CHCl_3]{C_6H_5CO_3H} CH_3-\overset{\overset{\displaystyle O}{\|}}{C}-O-\overset{\overset{\displaystyle O}{\|}}{C}-CH_3 \xrightarrow{H_2O} 2CH_3COOH$$

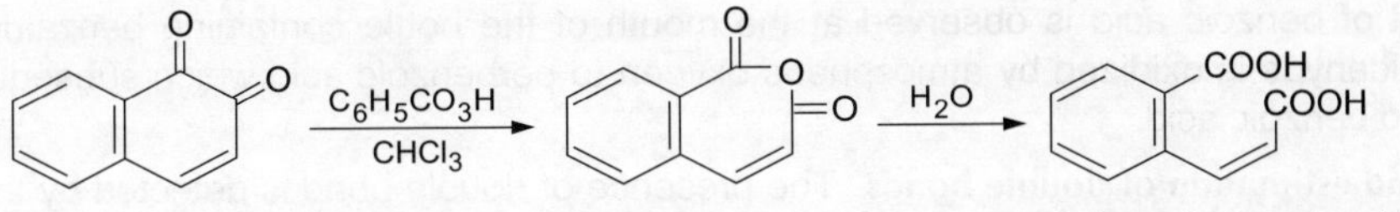

o-Carboxyallocinnamic acid

(d) Oxidation of amines Aliphatic 1° and 2° amines are oxidized to alkyl and dialkyl hydroxylamines respectively.

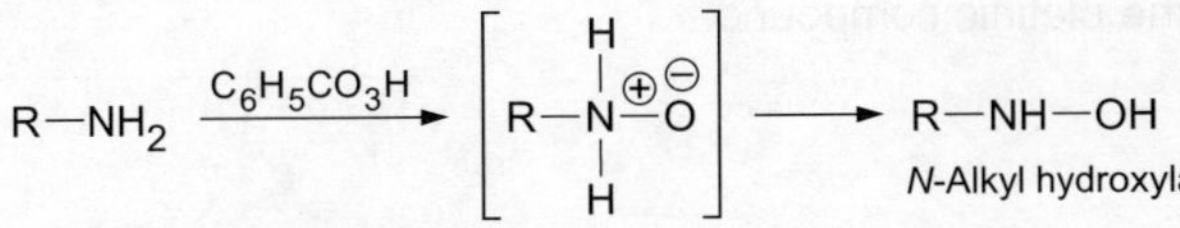

N-Alkyl hydroxylamine

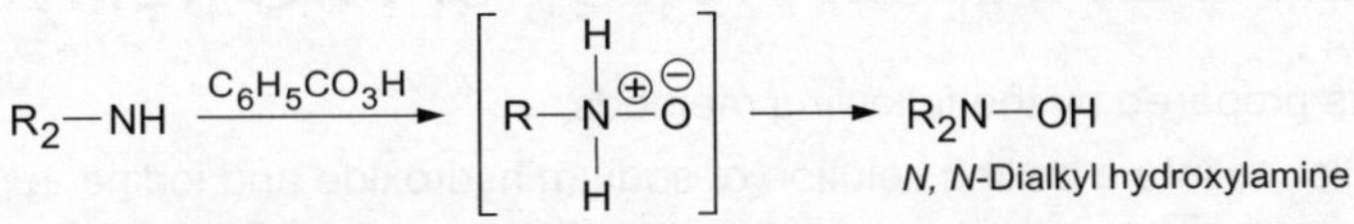

N, N-Dialkyl hydroxylamine

Hydroxylamines are easily oxidized and 1° amine may be oxidized to nitro compound.

$$CH_3-(CH_2)_5-NH_2 \xrightarrow{C_6H_5CO_3H} CH_3-(CH_2)_5-NO_2$$

Aliphatic 3° amines are oxidized to amine oxides and aromatic amines are oxidized to nitro compounds.

$$R_3\ddot{N} \xrightarrow{C_6H_5CO_3H} R_3\overset{\oplus}{N}-\overset{\ominus}{O}\ ; \quad C_6H_5NH_2 \xrightarrow{C_6H_5CO_3H} C_6H_5NO_2$$

Pyridine is oxidized to pyridine-*N*-oxide.

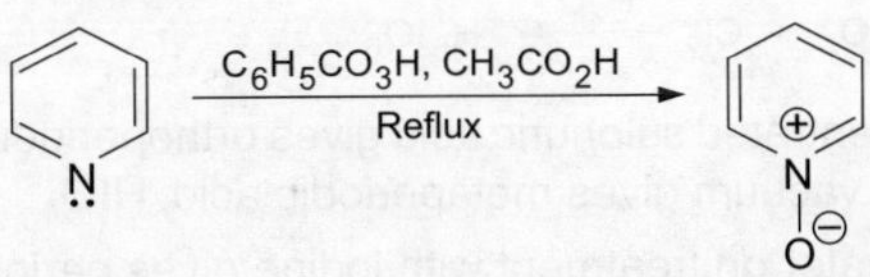

Pyridine-*N*-oxide

(e) Oxidation of azobenzene Perbenzoic acid oxidizes azobenzene to azoxybenzene.

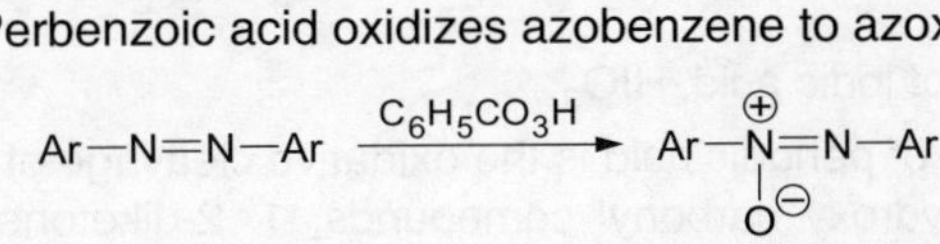

Azoxy benzene

(f) Oxidation of thioethers Thioethers are first oxidized to sulphoxides and on further oxidation to sulphones.

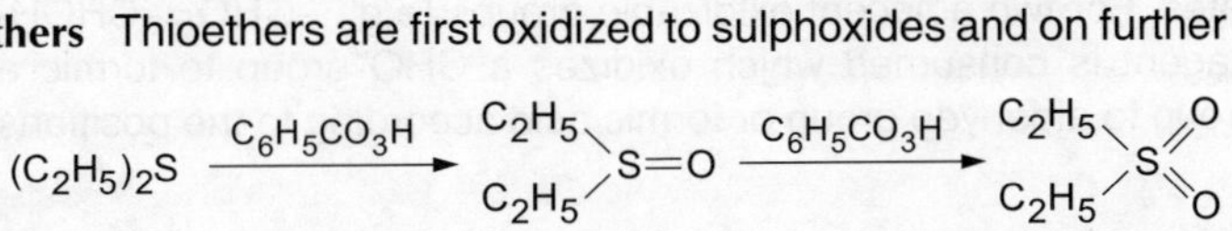

Diethyl sulphoxide Diethyl sulphone

(g) Oxidation of benzaldehyde Benzaldehyde is oxidized to benzoic acid.

$$C_6H_5CO_3H + C_6H_5CHO \longrightarrow 2C_6H_5COOH$$

A white deposit of benzoic acid is observed at the mouth of the bottle containing benzaldehyde. This is because benzaldehyde is oxidized by atmospheric oxygen to perbenzoic acid which subsequently oxidizes benzaldehyde to benzoic acid.

(h) Detection and estimation of double bonds The presence of double bond is detected by the formation of epoxide which may be separated.

For the estimation of double bonds, a known quantity of the olefinic compound is allowed to react with an excess of perbenzoic acid in chloroform for several hours. The unconsumed peracid is determined by iodometry. The number of double bonds in the compound is then calculated from the amount of peracid consumed and the weight of the olefinic compound.

PERIODIC ACID, H_5IO_6 or $HIO_4.2H_2O$

This valuable reagent is prepared by the following methods.

1. On passing chlorine into a boiling solution of sodium hydroxide and iodine, a precipitate of disodium orthoperiodate is obtained. The latter on treatment with aqueous silver nitrate solution gives silver orthoperiodate which on treatment with chlorine in the presence of water gives orthoperiodic acid. It is then filtered.

$$6NaOH + 3I_2 \xrightarrow{\Delta} NaIO_3 + 5NaI + 3H_2O$$

$$NaIO_3 + 3NaOH + Cl_2 \longrightarrow Na_2H_3IO_6 + 2NaCl$$

$$Na_2H_3IO_6 + 5AgNO_3 \longrightarrow Ag_5IO_6 + 2NaNO_3 + 3HNO_3$$

$$Ag_5IO_6 + Cl_2 \xrightarrow{H_2O} H_5IO_6$$

The filtrate on evaporation over concentrated sulphuric acid gives orthoperiodic acid crystals, H_5IO_6 or $HIO_4 \cdot 2H_2O$ which on heating to 100 °C in vacuum gives metaperiodic acid, HIO_4.

2. Perchloric acid solution in water on treatment with iodine gives periodic acid.

$$2HClO_4 + I_2 \longrightarrow 2HIO_4 + Cl_2$$

3. By the anodic oxidation of iodic acid, HIO_3.

The characteristic property of periodic acid is the oxidative cleavage of bonds with adjacent oxidizable groups such as, 1, 2-diols, α-hydroxy carbonyl compounds, 1, 2-diketones, α-amino alcohols, etc. The reagent does not react with 1, 3- or 1, 4-diols or carbonyl compounds. Also, the reagent has no effect on the oxide ring of carbohydrates. For two adjacent oxidizable groups (e.g., –CHOH–CHOH–, –CHOH–CO–, etc.) one molecule of the reagent is consumed which oxidizes a CHO group to formic acid, CH_2OH group to formaldehyde, CHOH group to aldehyde group or formic acid according to the positions of the groups. This is illustrated below.

$$R-CHOH \vdots CH_2OH + HIO_4 \xrightarrow{-HIO_3} R-CHO + HCHO$$

$$R-CHOH \vdots CHOH-R' + HIO_4 \xrightarrow{-HIO_3} R-CHO + R'\,CHO$$

$$R_2C(OH)\vdots CHOH-R' + HIO_4 \xrightarrow{-HIO_3} R_2CO + R'CHO$$

$$R-CHOH\vdots CHOH\vdots CHOH-R' + 2HIO_4 \xrightarrow{-2HIO_3} RCHO + HCOOH + R'CHO$$

$$R'-CO\vdots CHOH-R + HIO_4 \xrightarrow{-HIO_3} R'-COOH + R-CHO$$

$$CH_2OH\vdots CO-CH_2OH + HIO_4 \xrightarrow{-HIO_3} HCHO + HOOC-CH_2OH$$

$$R-CO\vdots CO-R' + HIO_4 \xrightarrow{-HIO_3} R-COOH + R'-COOH$$

$$RCHNH_2\vdots CHOH-R' + HIO_4 \xrightarrow{-HIO_3} RCHO + R'CHO + NH_3$$

$$R-CHOH-CH_2-CHOH-R \xrightarrow{HIO_4} \text{No reaction}$$

Each dotted line represents one mole of periodic acid and the position of the cleavage of bond. The reactions are practically quantitative. The oxidation is carried out at room temperature with the aqueous solution of the oxidant.

Mechanism

The reaction probably proceeds via a cyclic intermediate (II) or (III) resulting from the reaction between the substrate and the ion (I) of the reagent.

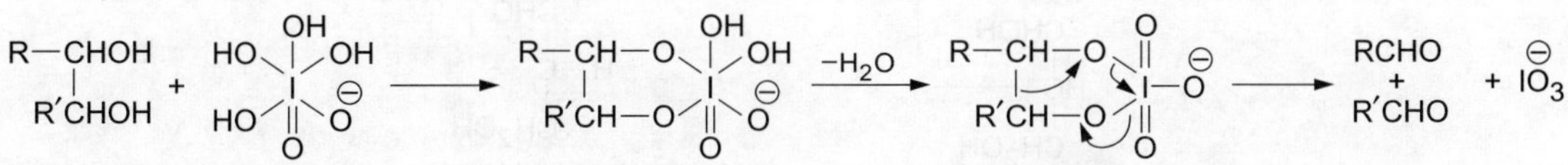

(I) Hydrated ion (II) Dehydrated ion (III)

Uses

Periodic acid has important synthetic and analytical applications. The reagent is very useful in the determination of the structures of carbohydrates and in general of 1, 2-glycols. Different substrates consume different amounts of the oxidant to give different amounts of formaldehyde and formic acid. This is indicative of the structures of the substrates.

Periodic acid can be estimated iodometrically. Similarly, formaldehyde and formic acid produced in the reaction can be estimated. Since the oxidation reactions are practically quantitative, the knowledge of the number of moles of periodic acid consumed and the number of moles of formic acid and formaldehyde liberated can afford valuable informations about the structure and size of the ring of carbohydrates. Identification of the fragments of periodic acid oxidation of glycols provides evidence for the structures of glycols. Qualitatively, the oxidation with H_5IO_6 is indicated by the formation of a white precipitate of $AgIO_3$ with $AgNO_3$ solution.

1. Identification of aldoses Predictable amount of periodic acid consumption per mole of different aldoses is, four moles for aldopentose, five moles for aldohexose, six moles for aldoheptose, etc. Thus, the number of carbons in the aldose can be known from the amount of the oxidant consumed.

$$\underset{\text{Aldopentose}}{CH_2OH \vdots CHOH \vdots CHOH \vdots CHOH \vdots CHO} + 4HIO_4 \longrightarrow 4HCOOH + HCHO + 4HIO_3$$

$$\underset{\text{Aldohexose}}{CH_2OH \vdots CHOH \vdots CHOH \vdots CHOH \vdots CHOH \vdots CHO} + 5HIO_3 \longrightarrow 5HCOOH + HCHO + 5HIO_3$$

2. Distinction of aldohexose and ketohexose Glucose and fructose consume different amounts of periodic acid and give different amounts of formic acid.

$$\underset{\text{Aldohexose (glucose)}}{CH_2OH \vdots CHOH \vdots CHOH \vdots CHOH \vdots CHOH \vdots CHO} \xrightarrow{5HIO_4} 5HCOOH + HCHO + 5HIO_3$$

$$\underset{\text{Ketohexose (fructose)}}{CH_2OH \vdots CHOH \vdots CHOH \vdots CHOH \vdots CO{-}CH_2OH} \xrightarrow{4HIO_4} HCHO + 3HCOOH + HOOC{-}CH_2OH + 4HIO_3$$

From the amount of periodic acid consumed and the amount of formic acid liberated, the two monosaccharides can be identified.

3. Determination of the size of the oxide rings of sugars When glucose is treated with methyl alcohol and hydrochloric acid it gives two isomers of methyl glucosides. The one (I) prepared under hot condition consumes two molecules of periodic acid and gives one molecule of formic acid and no formaldehyde. This fits in with the 1 : 5-oxide ring structure (pyranoside).

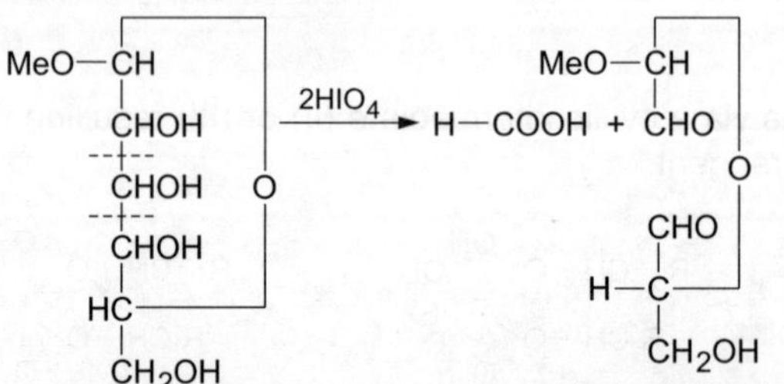

Methyl glucoside (I) Acetaldialdehyde

The other isomer (II) prepared under cold condition consumes two molecules of periodic acid and gives one molecule of formaldehyde but no formic acid. This observation fits in with the 1 : 4-oxide ring structure (furanoside).

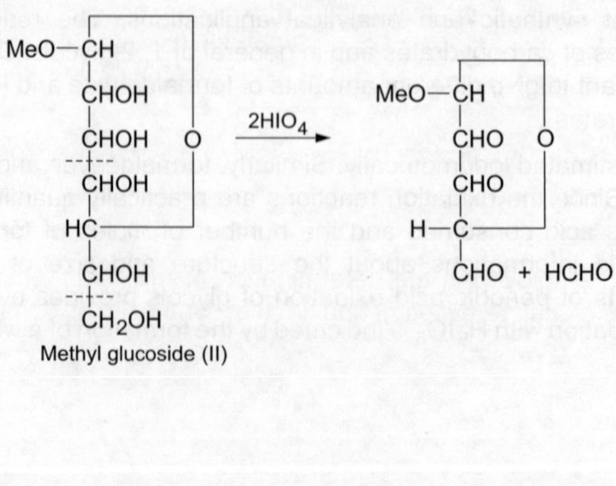

Methyl glucoside (II)

4. Structure of sucrose Each molecule of sucrose consumes three molecules of periodic acid and gives a tetraaldehyde and one molecule of formic acid. Subsequent oxidation of the product followed by hydrolysis gave glyoxalic acid, glyceric acid and hydroxy pyruvic acid. From the degradation products and the number of molecules of periodic acid consumed the C–C linkage of the two moieties in sucrose was established.

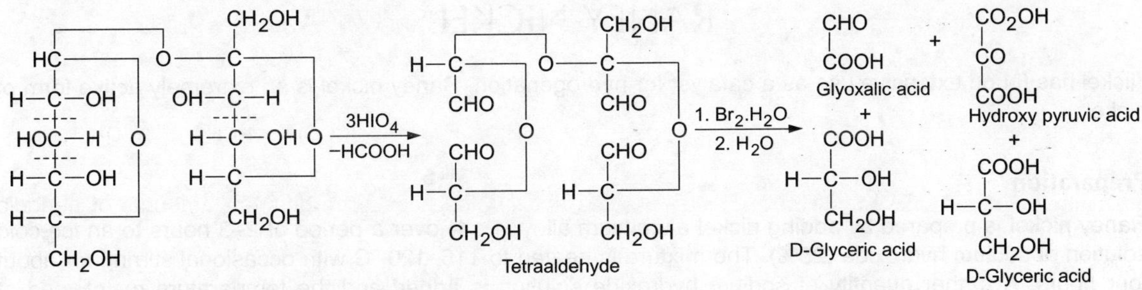

5. Ring size of the sugar residue of nucleosides The sugar residue of nucleosides is a five-membered furanose ring, since it consumes one molecule of periodic acid producing only a dialdehyde.

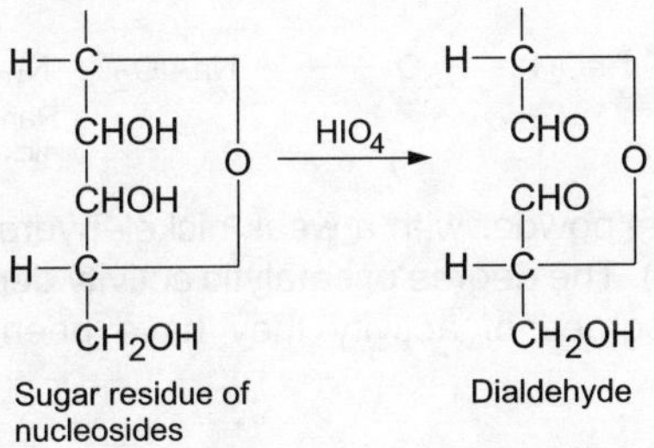

6. Oxidation of alkenes Periodic acid has no reaction on olefins. However, olefins can be hydroxylated to 1, 2-glycols and then oxidized with periodate to carbonyl compounds. Exocyclic olefinic bonds can be oxidized by this method.

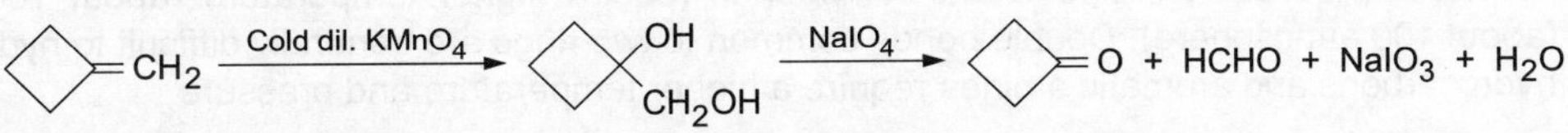

A mixture of dilute aqueous solution of permanganate or hydrogen peroxide and sodium periodate (Lemieux reagent) may be used to oxidize olefins in one step.

$$\underset{\text{Oleic acid}}{CH_3-(CH_2)_7-CH=CH-(CH_2)_7-COOH} \xrightarrow[NaIO_4]{KMnO_4} \underset{n\text{-Nonaldehyde}}{CH_3-(CH_2)_7-CHO} + \underset{\text{Half aldehyde of azelaic acid}}{OHC-(CH_2)_7-COOH}$$

7. Estimation of amino acids Amino acids having hydroxyl group adjacent to the amino group consume one molecule of periodic acid and liberate one molecule of ammonia on oxidation with periodic acid. Evolved ammonia and the oxidant consumed may be estimated and from this the percentage purity of the amino acid can be determined.

$$\underset{\text{Threonine}}{CH_3-\underset{OH}{CH}-\underset{NH_2}{CH}-COOH} \xrightarrow{HIO_4} CH_3CHO + OHC-COOH + NH_3 + HIO_3$$

The reagent has been employed in the determination of the chain length of polysaccharides, in the elucidation of the structure of chloromycetin, and in the synthesis of some natural products such as, cholesterol, reserpine, etc.

RANEY NICKEL

Nickel has found extensive use as a catalyst for hydrogenation. Raney nickel is an extremely active form of nickel.

Preparation

Raney nickel is prepared by adding nickel-aluminium alloy (1 : 1) over a period of 2–3 hours to an ice-cold solution of sodium hydroxide (25%). The mixture is heated to 115–120 °C with occasional stirring for about four hours. A further quantity of sodium hydroxide solution is added and the temperature maintained at 115–120 °C till the evolution of hydrogen ceases. The alkali layer is decanted off and the residue (nickel catalyst) is washed several times with water and then with alcohol. It is stored under absolute alcohol, ether or dioxan in a stoppered bottle.

$$\text{Ni–Al} + \text{NaOH} + H_2O \longrightarrow \text{NaAlO}_2 + \underset{\text{Raney nickel}}{\text{Ni–H}} + H_2$$

Raney nickel is a black spongy metal powder with a weak nickel–hydrogen bond. Hydrogen is bound to the surface of the catalyst (50–100 mL/g). The degree of catalytic activity depends upon the reaction conditions of preparation. Based on different degrees of activity they have been designated as W-1 to W-7 (W = Wisconsin).

Uses

Raney nickel is a widely used powerful reducing agent. Most olefins are reduced at room temperature at about atmospheric pressure while resistant compounds require higher temperature (about 100 °C) and pressure (about 100 atmosphere). Double bonds common to two rings are generally difficult to hydrogenate. Aromatic hydrocarbons and aromatic amines require a higher temperature and pressure.

1. Reduction of carbon–carbon multiple bonds Raney nickel reduces multiple bonds present in aliphatic, alicyclic and aromatic compounds.

(i) $CH_2{=}CH_2 \xrightarrow[\text{Room temp.}]{\text{Ni–H}} CH_3{-}CH_3$ (ii) $HC{\equiv}CH \xrightarrow[\text{Room temp.}]{\text{Ni–H}} CH_3{-}CH_3$

(iii) 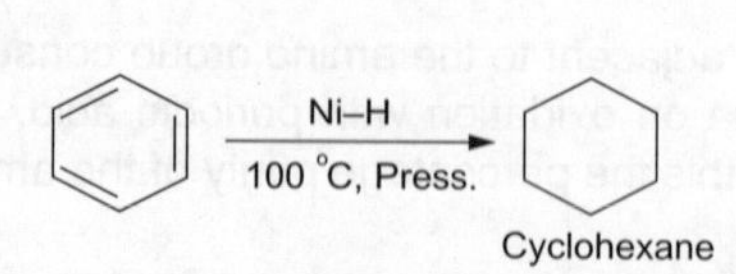

Cyclohexane

(iv) 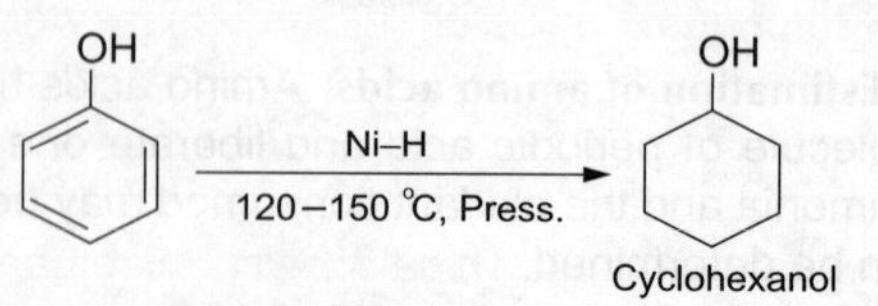

Cyclohexanol

(v) 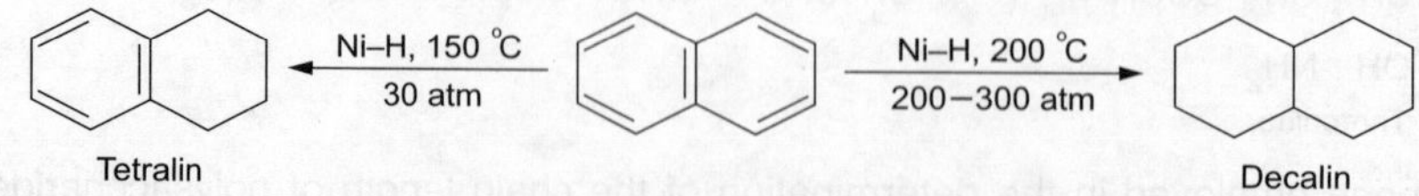

Tetralin Decalin

2. Reduction of aromatic ethers Aromatic ethers are reductively cleaved on heating with Raney nickel. Hydrogen comes from that normally contained in Raney nickel and from the solvent.

$$\text{ArOR} \xrightarrow[\Delta]{\text{Ni–H}} \text{ArH} + \text{RH}$$

When R is aromatic it may be reduced to cyclohexane unless degassed Raney nickel is used.

Mechanism— $$\text{ArOR} \xrightarrow{\text{Ni–H}} \overset{\ominus}{\text{Ar}} + \text{ROH}$$

Ar takes up proton from the solvent and ROH is reduced by hydrogenolysis*.

3. Reduction of nitro group to amino group

$$\underset{\text{Methyl-4-methyl-4-nitropentanoate}}{(CH_3)_2\underset{\displaystyle NO_2}{\underset{|}{C}}{-}CH_2{-}CH_2{-}COOCH_3} \xrightarrow[60\,^\circ C]{\text{Ni–H}} \underset{\text{Methyl-4-methyl-4-aminopentanoate}}{(CH_3)_2\underset{\displaystyle NH_2}{\underset{|}{C}}{-}CH_2{-}CH_2{-}COOCH_3}$$

The product on heating is cyclised to pyrrolidone derivative.

4. Reduction of nitriles Depending upon the conditions of reaction, nitriles are reduced to aldehydes or primary amines.

(a) Nitriles in aqueous acetic acid–pyridine medium are reduced to aldehydes with Raney nickel and sodium hypophosphite.

$$C_6H_5CN \xrightarrow[\text{Pyr–AcOH}]{\text{Ni–H, NaH}_2\text{PO}_2} C_6H_5CHO$$

(b) When nitriles are treated with Raney nickel under pressure, primary amines are formed.

$$R{-}CN \xrightarrow[\text{Press.}]{\text{Ni–H}} R{-}CH{=}NH \xrightarrow{\text{Ni–H}} R{-}CH_2NH_2$$

The primary amine may react with the aldimine to form secondary amine. This may be prevented by carrying out the reaction in the presence of acetic anhydride which converts the primary amine to its acetyl derivative.

5. Reduction of halides Dehalogenation is accomplished by several reagents. The advantage of using Raney nickel is that it removes all the halogens including fluorine. Similarly, phenyl tosylates can be reduced.

$$\text{ArX} \xrightarrow[\text{NaOH}]{\text{Ni–H}} \text{ArH (where X = Cl, Br, I and F)} \;;$$ 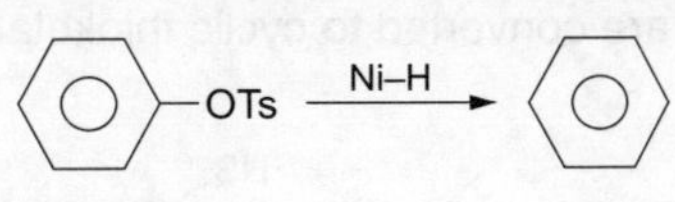

6. Desulphonation Sulphonic groups may be easily replaced by hydrogen.

$$ArSO_3H \xrightarrow[\Delta]{\text{Ni–H, NaOH}} ArH + H_2SO_4$$

7. Desulphurization Thioalcohols, thioethers, disulphides, thioamides, sulphoxides and sulphones are desulphurized by hydrogenolysis with Raney nickel. Hydrogen is not required externally as Raney nickel contains sufficient adsorbed hydrogen for the reaction.

$$\underset{\text{Thioether}}{R{-}S{-}R'} \xrightarrow{\text{Ni–H}} RH + R'H \;;\; \underset{\text{Thioamide}}{RCSNHR'} \xrightarrow{\text{Ni–H}} \underset{2^\circ\text{ Amine}}{RCH_2NHR'}$$

* Hydrogenolysis means the cleavage of carbon-hetero atom bond by catalytic hydrogenation.

Thiophene derivatives which may be considered as cyclic thioethers are desulphurized with accompanying reduction of the double bonds.

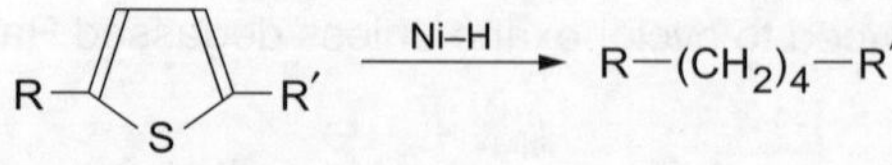

2, 5-Dialkylthiophene

The reaction is very important for the elucidation of the structure of thiophene derivatives e.g., biotin.

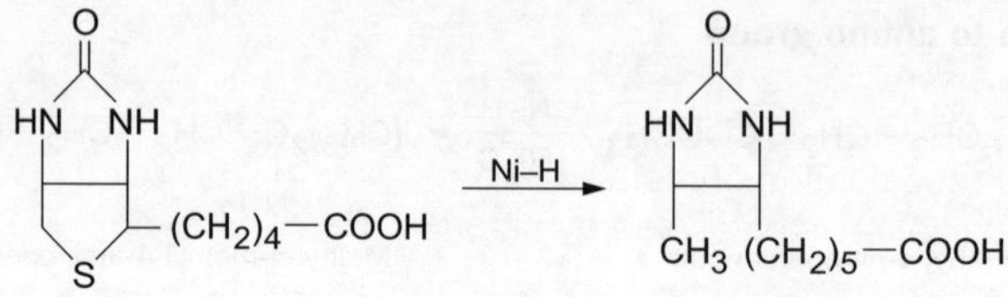

Biotin Dethiobiotin

Desulphurization may also be employed to prepare higher acids and compounds which are otherwise difficult to synthesize.

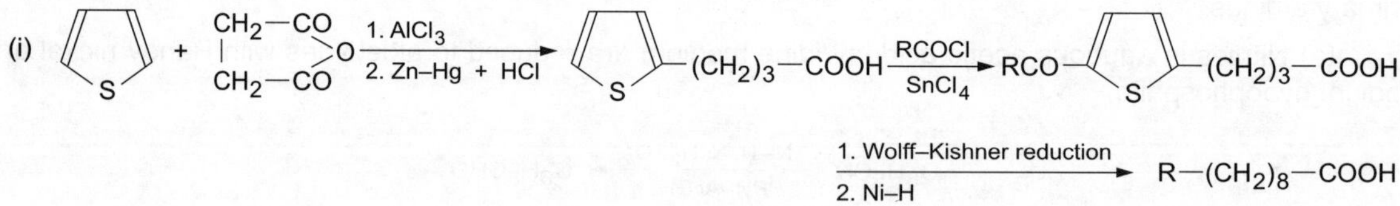

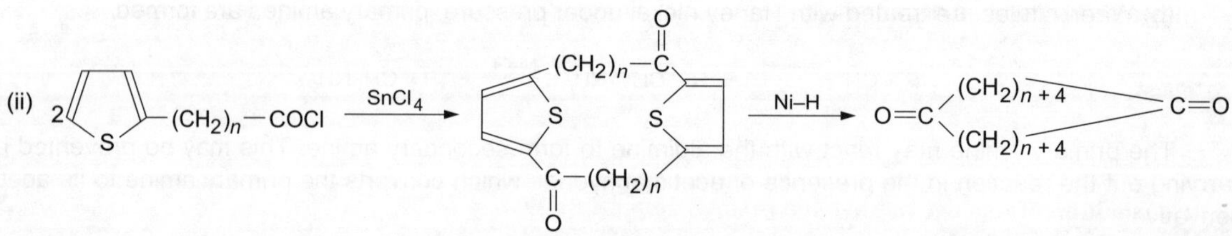

Desulphurization has been utilized for the conversion of a ketonic group to methylene group. When the carbonyl compound to be reduced is sensitive and cannot be reduced by Clemmensen or Wolff–Kishner methods, they are converted to cyclic thioketals with 1, 3-propanedithiol and then desulphurized with Raney nickel.

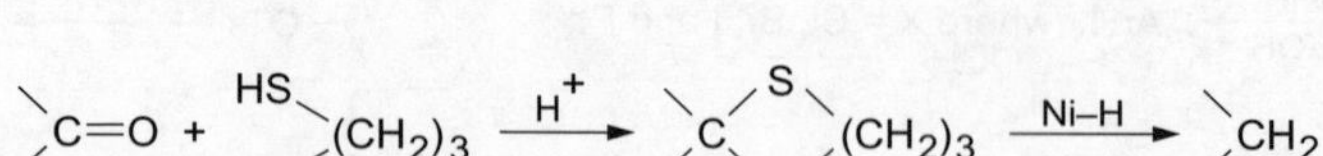

Raney nickel is not poisoned by sulphur compounds.

8. Hardening of oils Raney nickel is employed in the industrial production of hydrogenated oils (vegetable ghee).

Oils are glycerides of unsaturated fatty acids. The unsaturated hydrocarbon part of the fatty acid is partially hydrogenated with Raney nickel at 150–200 °C under pressure to yield the hydrogenated oil.

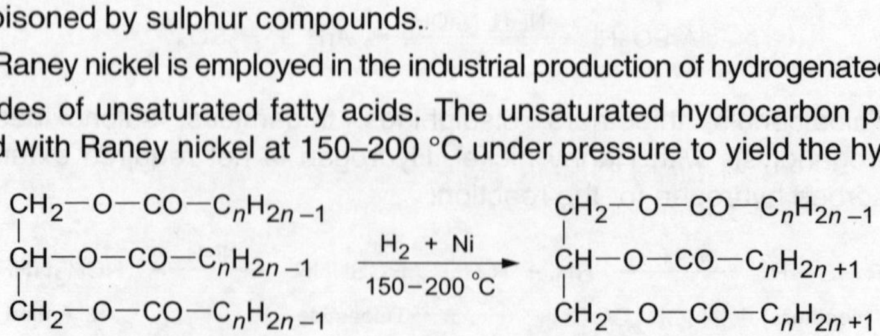

Glyceride of unsaturated fatty acids (oils) Partially hydrogenated oil (vegetable ghee)

SELENIUM DIOXIDE, SeO_2

Selenium dioxide is an important oxidizing agent, specific for the oxidation of reactive methylene and methyl groups.

Preparation

It is prepared by the direct oxidation of metallic selenium. Selenium burns with a blue flame in air producing selenium dioxide. The oxidation is catalysed by nitrogen peroxide.

$$Se + O_2(\text{air}) \longrightarrow SeO_2$$

It is a white crystalline solid, dissolves in water forming selenious acid (H_2SeO_3) and is highly toxic. The reagent, in general, oxidizes active methylene and methyl groups to ketonic and aldehydic groups respectively.

$$-CH_2-\overset{\overset{\large O}{\|}}{C}- \xrightarrow{SeO_2} -\overset{\overset{\large O}{\|}}{C}-\overset{\overset{\large O}{\|}}{C}- \; ; \quad -\overset{\overset{\large O}{\|}}{C}-CH_3 \xrightarrow{SeO_2} -\overset{\overset{\large O}{\|}}{C}-CHO$$

Double bonds, triple bonds and aromatic rings may also activate the methylene group. The reaction is usually carried out in acetic acid or acetic anhydride at a temperature between 100–140 °C. Alcohol or dioxan may also be used as diluents.

Uses

Besides oxidation of the active methylene and methyl groups, the reagent has been employed for allylic hydroxylation, allylic oxidation, dehydrogenation and as a catalyst in some reactions.

1. Oxidation of reactive methyl and methylene groups

(a) $CH_3CHO \xrightarrow{SeO_2} \underset{\text{Glyoxal}}{CHO.CHO}$

(b) $CH_3COCH_3 \xrightarrow{SeO_2} \underset{\text{Methylglyoxal}}{CH_3COCHO}$

(c) $\underset{\text{Acetophenone}}{C_6H_5COCH_3} \xrightarrow{SeO_2} \underset{\text{Phenylglyoxal}}{C_6H_5COCHO}$

(d) $\underset{\text{Diethyl malonate}}{H_2C(COOC_2H_5)_2} \xrightarrow{SeO_2} \underset{\text{Diethyl mesooxalate}}{O{=}C(COOC_2H_5)_2}$

(e) $\underset{\text{Butanone}}{CH_3CH_2COCH_3} \xrightarrow{SeO_2} \underset{\text{Ethylglyoxal (major)}}{CH_3CH_2COCHO} + \underset{\text{Diacetyl (minor)}}{CH_3COCOCH_3}$

(f) 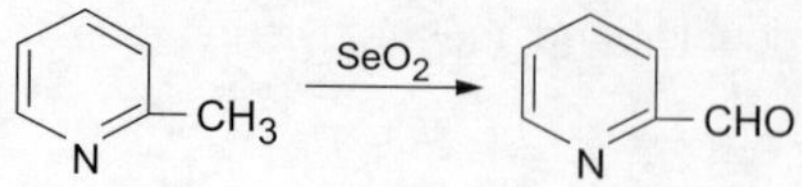

α-Picoline α-Picolinic aldehyde

(g) $$C_6H_5CH_2C_6H_5 \xrightarrow{SeO_2} C_6H_5COC_6H_5$$

Diphenylmethane Benzophenone

Activated ring methylene groups are also oxidized to carbonyl groups.

(h) 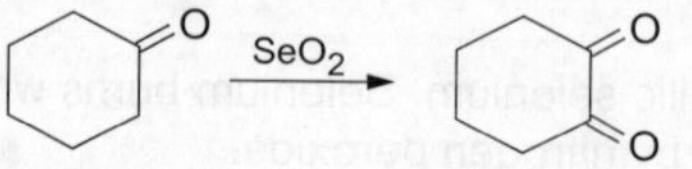

Cyclohexanone Cyclohexan-1, 2-dione

Mechanism

The oxidation is carried out in aqueous acetic acid medium and hence the actual reagent is selenious acid, H_2SeO_3. The mechanism is still not clearly known. It is suggested that the reaction proceeds by the attack of selenious acid on the enol form of the substrate to yield selenate ester which eliminates water and selenium to give the product.

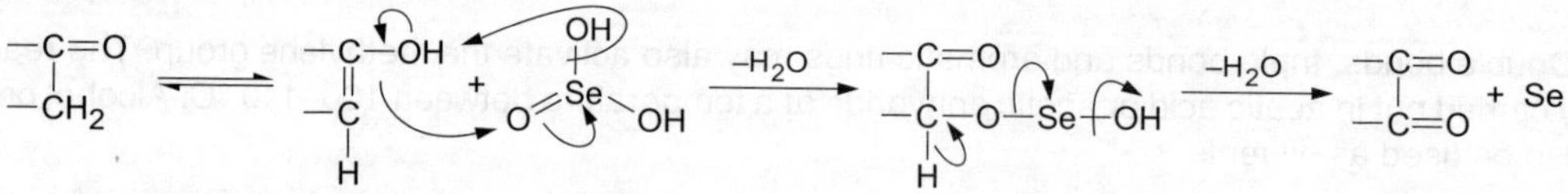

Selenate ester

2. Allylic hydroxylation and oxidation The methylene or methyl group α to the most highly substituted end of the double bond is hydroxylated according to the order of preference of oxidation $CH_2 > CH_3 > CH$ groups.

(i) $$CH_3-CH=C(CH_3)-CH_3 \xrightarrow{SeO_2} CH_3-CH=C(CH_3)-CH_2OH$$

2-Methyl-2-butene 2-Methyl-2-butenol-1

(ii) $$CH_3-CH=C(CH_3)-CH_2CH_3 \xrightarrow{SeO_2} CH_3-CH=C(CH_3)-CH(OH)-CH_3$$

3-Methyl-2-pentene 3-Methyl-3-pentenol-2

(iii) $$CH_3-C(CH_3)=CH-CH_2-CH_3 \xrightarrow{SeO_2} CH_3-C(CH_2OH)=CH-CH_2-CH_3$$

2-Methyl-2-pentene 2-Methyl-2-pentenol-1

In cycloalkenes, the ring methylene group at α-position to the double bond is oxidized to ketonic group.

(iv) 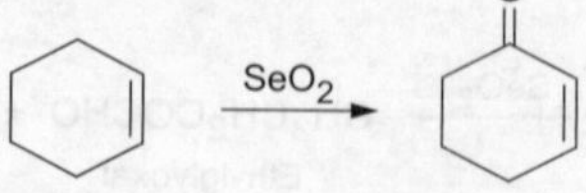

Cyclohexene 2-Cyclohexene-1-one

When the cycloalkene is substituted on the double bond, the methylene group at α-position to the substituted end of the double bond is oxidized.

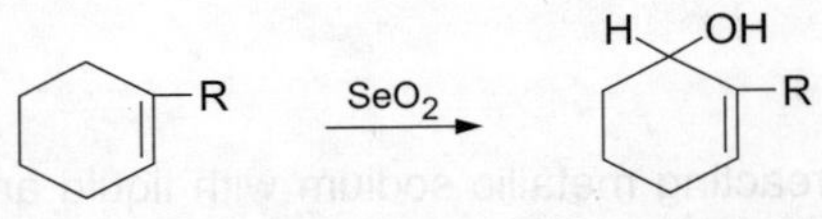

Alkylcyclohexene $\qquad$ α-Hydroxy alkylcyclohexene

Terminal double bonds are oxidized to primary alcoholic groups along with allylic migration of the double bond.

$$\text{(v)}\quad \underset{\text{Pentene-1}}{CH_3-CH_2-CH_2-CH=CH_2} \xrightarrow{SeO_2} \underset{\text{2-Pentenol-1}}{CH_3-CH_2-CH=CH-CH_2OH}$$

3. Dehydrogenation Selenium dioxide has been used for dehydrogenation at elevated temperature.

$$\text{(i)}\quad C_6H_5-CH_2OH \xrightarrow[\Delta]{SeO_2} C_6H_5-CHO$$

$$\text{(ii)}\quad 2CH_3COOH \xrightarrow[\Delta]{SeO_2} \underset{\text{Succinic acid}}{\begin{array}{l} CH_2-COOH \\ | \\ CH_2-COOH \end{array}}$$

$$\text{(iii)}\quad \underset{\text{Hexan-2, 5-dione}}{CH_3-CO-CH_2-CH_2-CO-CH_3} \xrightarrow[\Delta]{SeO_2} \underset{\text{3-Hexene-2, 5-dione}}{CH_3-CO-CH=CH-CO-CH_3}$$

$$\text{(iv)}\quad \underset{\text{Ethyl succinate}}{\begin{array}{l} H_2C-COOEt \\ | \\ H_2C-COOEt \end{array}} \xrightarrow[\Delta]{SeO_2} \underset{\text{Ethyl fumarate}}{\begin{array}{r} EtOOC-CH \\ \| \\ HC-COOEt \end{array}}$$

4. As a catalyst It catalyses the *trans*-hydroxylation of some unsaturated compounds by hydrogen peroxide.

$$\text{(i)}\quad \underset{\text{Maleic acid}}{\begin{array}{l} HC-COOH \\ \| \\ HC-COOH \end{array}} \xrightarrow[SeO_2]{H_2O_2} \underset{\text{DL-Tartaric acid}}{\begin{array}{c} OH \\ | \\ H-C-COOH \\ | \\ H-C-COOH \\ | \\ OH \end{array}}$$

$$\text{(ii)}\quad \underset{\text{Oleic acid}}{CH_3-(CH_2)_7-CH=CH-(CH_2)_7-COOH} \xrightarrow[SeO_2]{H_2O_2} \underset{\text{9,10-Dihydroxystearic acid}}{CH_3-(CH_2)_7-CH(OH)-CH(OH)-(CH_2)_7-COOH}$$

SODIUM AMIDE (SODAMIDE), $NaNH_2$

Preparation

This useful reagent is prepared by reacting metallic sodium with liquid ammonia in the presence of ferric nitrate.

$$Na + NH_3 \xrightarrow{Fe(NO_3)_3.6H_2O} NaNH_2 + \frac{1}{2}H_2$$

Uses

It finds use in various reactions in which the reacting species is the amide anion. Some of its important reactions are given below.

1. Dehydrohalogenation of alkyl halides Sodamide is the most commonly used base for the formation of triple bonds from suitable alkyl halides, e.g.,

$$\underset{\text{gem-Dihalide}}{R-CH_2-CBr_2-R'} \text{ or } \underset{\text{vic-Dihalide}}{RCHBr{=}CHBrR'} \xrightarrow{2NaNH_2} R-C{\equiv}C-R' + 2NaBr + 2NH_3$$

$$R-CH{=}CBrR' \xrightarrow{NaNH_2} R-C{\equiv}C-R' + NaBr + NH_3$$

Thus,

$$\text{(i)}\ \underset{\beta\text{-Bromostyrene}}{C_6H_5-CH{=}CHBr} \xrightarrow{NaNH_2} [C_6H_5C{\equiv}CH] \xrightarrow{NaNH_2} C_6H_5-C{\equiv}CNa \xrightarrow{H_2O} \underset{\text{Phenyl acetylene}}{C_6H_5C{\equiv}CH}$$

$$\text{(ii)}\ \underset{\text{Oleic acid}}{CH_3-(CH_2)_7-CH{=}CH-(CH_2)_7-COOH} \xrightarrow[2.\ NaNH_2\ \ 3.\ H_2O]{1.\ Br_2,\ ether} \underset{\text{Stearolic acid}}{CH_3-(CH_2)_7-C{\equiv}C-(CH_2)_7-COOH}$$

2. Reaction with terminal acetylenic compounds Terminal acetylenic compounds having acidic hydrogens react with sodamide to form sodium acetylenes which may be converted to acids and higher acetylenes.

$$CH_3-C{\equiv}CH \xrightarrow{NaNH_2} CH_3-C{\equiv}\overset{\ominus\oplus}{C\,Na}$$

$$\underset{\text{2-Pentyne}}{CH_3-C{\equiv}C-CH_2-CH_3} \xleftarrow{C_2H_5Br} CH_3-C{\equiv}\overset{\ominus\oplus}{C\,Na} \xrightarrow[2.\ H_3O^{\oplus}]{1.\ CO_2} \underset{\text{Tetrolic acid}}{CH_3-C{\equiv}C-COOH}$$

Internal acetylenes on heating with sodamide in an inert solvent yield terminal acetylenes.

$$\underset{\text{2-Butyne}}{CH_3-C\equiv C-CH_3} \xrightarrow[\text{Paraffin, }\Delta]{NaNH_2} CH_3-CH_2-C\equiv \overset{\ominus\oplus}{CNa} \xrightarrow{H_3O^{\oplus}} \underset{\text{1-Butyne}}{CH_3-CH_2-C\equiv CH}$$

3. Formation of nucleophiles Sodamide reacts with compounds having reactive methyl or active methylene groups (activated by even a single electron-withdrawing group) to yield anions which act as nucleophiles in various reactions.

(a) Alkylation of acids and ketones

(i) $$CH_3-COOK \xrightarrow{NaNH_2} \overset{\ominus}{C}H_2COOK \xrightarrow{CH_2=CH_2} \overset{\ominus}{C}H_2-CH_2-CH_2-COOK \xrightarrow{H_3O^{\oplus}} CH_3-CH_2-CH_2-COOH$$

(ii) $$CH_3COCH_3 \xrightarrow{NaNH_2} CH_3-CO-\overset{\ominus}{C}H_2 \xrightarrow{C_6H_5CH_2Cl} \underset{\text{4-Phenyl butanone-2}}{CH_3-CO-CH_2-CH_2-C_6H_5}$$

(b) Acylation of ketones and nitriles with esters

(i) $$CH_3-CO-CH_3 \xrightarrow{NaNH_2} CH_3-CO-\overset{\ominus}{C}H_2 \xrightarrow{CH_3COOR} \underset{\text{Acetyl acetone}}{CH_3-CO-CH_2-CO-CH_3}$$

(ii) $$R-CH_2-CN \xrightarrow{NaNH_2} R-\overset{\ominus}{C}H-CN \xrightarrow{CH_3COOR'} \underset{\beta\text{-Ketonitrile}}{CH_3-CO-\underset{R}{\underset{|}{C}}H-CN}$$

(c) Formation of β-ketoester

$$CH_3COOC_2H_5 \xrightarrow{NaNH_2} \overset{\ominus}{C}H_2COOC_2H_5 \xrightarrow{CH_3COOC_2H_5} \underset{\text{Ethylacetoacetate}}{CH_3COCH_2COOC_2H_5}$$

(d) Formation of α-cyanoester

$$R-CH_2-CN + \underset{\text{Ethyl carbonate}}{CO(OC_2H_5)_2} \xrightarrow{NaNH_2} \underset{\alpha\text{-Cyanoester}}{R-CH(CN)-COOC_2H_5}$$

4. Cleavage of nonenolisable ketones (Haller–Bauer reaction) Ketones of the type $ArCOCR_3$ are cleaved to give amides, $R_3C\cdot CONH_2$ which are not easily obtainable by other methods. The amides on treatment with nitrous acid give tertiary carboxylic acids.

$$C_6H_5-CO-CR_3 \xrightarrow{NaNH_2} R_3C-CO-NH_2 \xrightarrow{HNO_2} R_3C-COOH$$

The starting compound may be prepared by the repeated treatment of acetophenone with $NaNH_2$ and RI [reaction 3a(ii) above].

5. Cleavage of ethers Ethers on treatment with sodamide undergo cleavage with the formation of olefins.

(i) 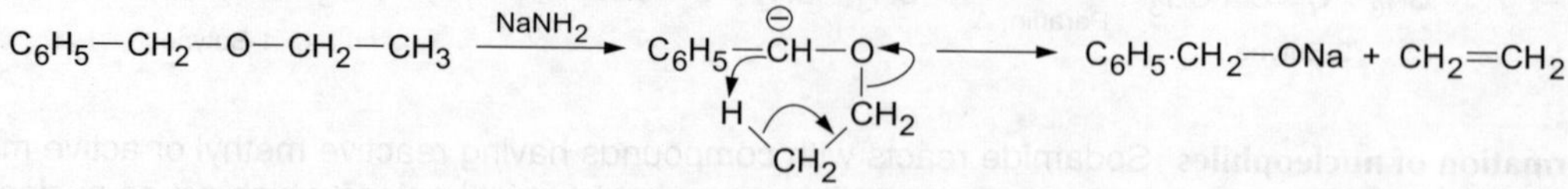

Suitable haloethers undergo dehydrohalogenation accompanied by cleavage so that acetylene derivatives are formed.

$$\text{(ii)}\quad \underset{\text{Diethylchloroacetal}}{ClCH_2{-}CH(OC_2H_5)_2} \xrightarrow[NH_3]{NaNH_2} \underset{\text{Ethoxy acetylene}}{HC{\equiv}C{-}O{-}C_2H_5}$$

Ethoxyacetylene is an useful synthetic intermediate.

(iii) 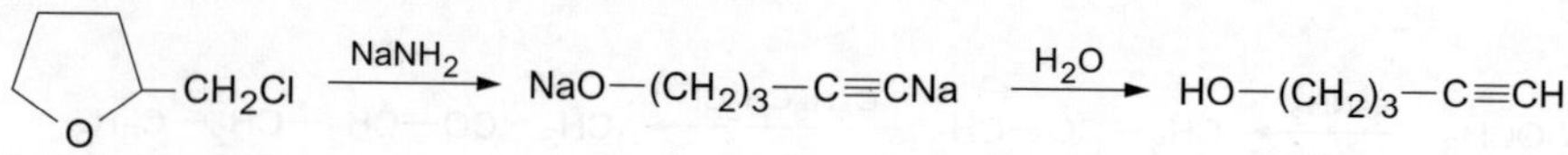

Tetrahydrofurfuryl chloride 4-Pentynol-1

6. Rearrangement of quaternary salts (Stevens rearrangement) Quaternary salts containing an electron-withdrawing group (e.g., –COR, –COOR, $-C_6H_5$, etc.) on the carbon attached to the nitrogen atom undergo rearrangement to tertiary amines on treatment with a strong base such as sodamide.

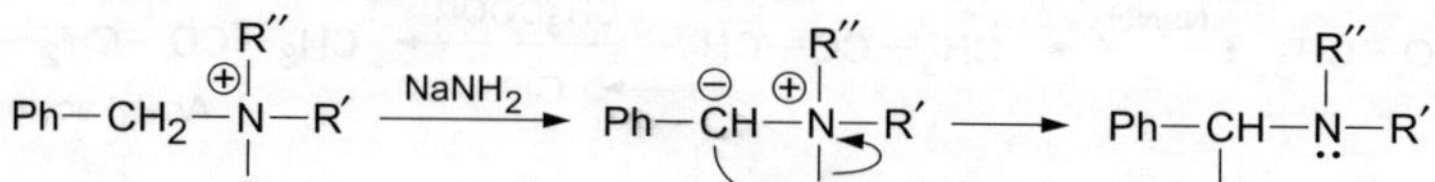

7. Amines from nonactivated aryl halides The halogens of aryl halides are substituted by amino groups on treatment with sodamide.

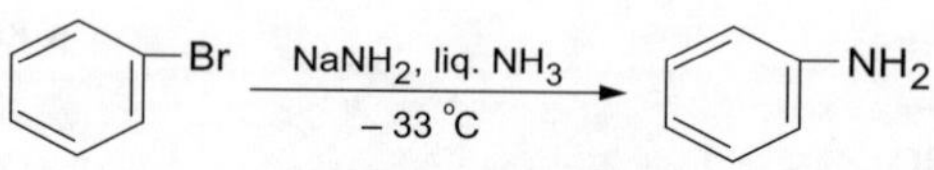

The reaction is believed to proceed through benzyne intermediate.

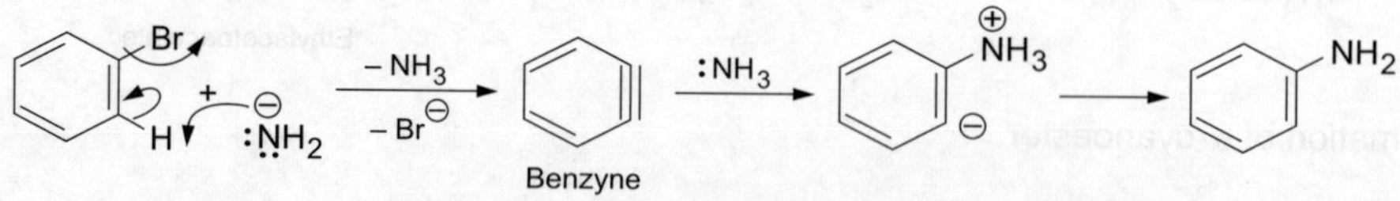

8. Amination of nitrogen heterocyclics (Chichibabin reaction) Pyridine in toluene on treatment with sodamide at 100–200 °C gives 2-aminopyridine. This is a nucleophilic substitution reaction. The attack of the amide ion takes place at the electron-deficient sites, i.e., at 2-, 4- and 6- positions.

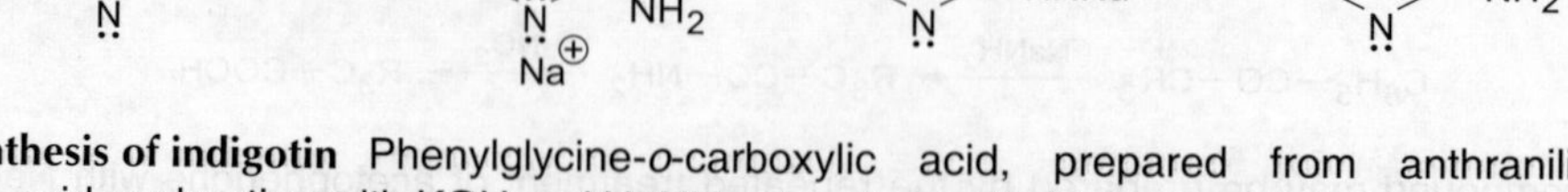

9. In the synthesis of indigotin Phenylglycine-*o*-carboxylic acid, prepared from anthranilic acid and chloroacetic acid, on heating with KOH and $NaNH_2$ gives indoxyl which on oxidation gives indigotin.

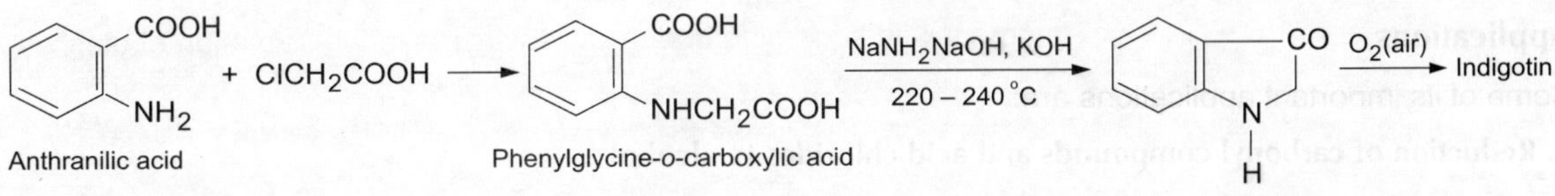

Anthranilic acid Phenylglycine-*o*-carboxylic acid Indoxyl

10. Preparation of organo sodium compound Triphenylmethane reacts with sodamide in liquid ammonia solution to yield triphenylmethyl sodium which is an effective condensing agent.

$$(C_6H_5)_3CH + NaNH_2 \xrightarrow{\text{Liq. } NH_3} (C_6H_5)_3\overset{\ominus\oplus}{CNa} + NH_3$$

SODIUM BOROHYDRIDE, $NaBH_4$

Sodium borohydride is a reducing agent. It reduces by transfer of hydride ions to substrates as in the case of lithium aluminium hydride.

Preparation

It is prepared by heating sodium hydride with trimethoxyborane to 250 °C.

$$4NaH + B(OCH_3)_3 \xrightarrow{250\ ^\circ C} NaBH_4 + 3CH_3ONa$$

The reagent is insoluble in ether but soluble in water or alcohol. Hence, it can be used in hydrolytic solvents, e.g., water or alcohol. The reaction is carried out in ethanol or isopropanol.

It is a milder reducing agent than $LiAlH_4$. Reduction with $NaBH_4$ is more selective. It reduces carbonyl groups of aldehydes, ketones and acid chlorides in the presence of many reducible groups such as nitro, ester, carboxyl, epoxide, nitrile, double bond, etc., which remain unaffected. Double bonds either isolated or conjugated are not affected. The reagent is slowly hydrolysed with water. Hence, reductions which are resonably rapid can be carried out in water without considerable hydrolysis of the reagent. Thus, water soluble sugars can be reduced in aqueous medium.

Mechanism

The mechanism of reduction is similar to that of $LiAlH_4$. The reaction proceeds by complexing the oxygen atom of the carbonyl group with boron and simultaneous transfer of the hydride ion to the carbonyl carbon. All the four hydrogens of the reagent are transferred to the four molecules of the substrate. Subsequent hydrolysis gives alcohol.

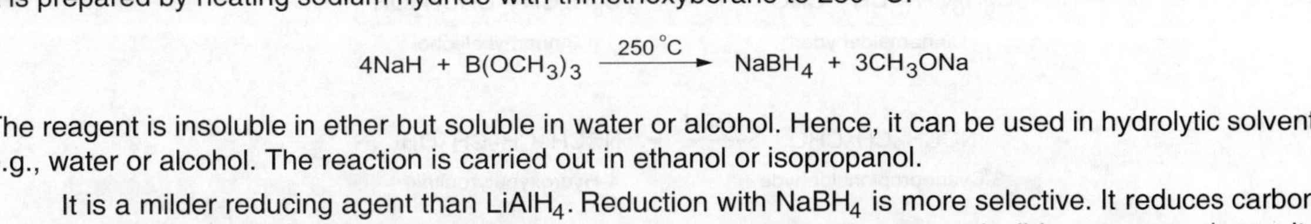

$$NaOH + B(OH)_3 \longrightarrow NaH_2BO_3 + H_2O$$

Applications

Some of its important applications are:

1. Reduction of carbonyl compounds and acid chlorides to alcohol

$$\underset{\text{Ethyl-}\gamma\text{-ketopentanoate}}{CH_3COCH_2CH_2COOC_2H_5} \xrightarrow{NaBH_4} \underset{\text{Ethyl-4-hydroxypentanoate}}{CH_3CH(OH)CH_2CH_2COOC_2H_5}$$

$$\underset{\beta\text{-Benzoyl propanoic acid}}{C_6H_5COCH_2CH_2COOH} \xrightarrow{NaBH_4} \underset{\gamma\text{-Hydroxy-4-phenylbutanoic acid}}{C_6H_5CH(OH)CH_2CH_2COOH}$$

$$\underset{\text{Hexan-2, 5-dione}}{CH_3COCH_2CH_2COCH_3} \xrightarrow{NaBH_4} \underset{\text{Hexan-2, 5-diol}}{CH_3CH(OH)CH_2CH_2CH(OH)CH_3}$$

$$\underset{\text{Glucose}}{CH_2OH(CHOH)_4CHO} \xrightarrow{NaBH_4} \underset{\text{Sorbitol}}{CH_2OH(CHOH)_4CH_2OH}$$

$$\underset{\text{Cinnamaldehyde}}{C_6H_5CH{=}CH{-}CHO} \xrightarrow{NaBH_4} \underset{\text{Cinnamyl alcohol}}{C_6H_5CH{=}CHCH_2OH}$$

$$\underset{\text{3-Cyanopropionaldehyde}}{NCCH_2CH_2CHO} \xrightarrow{NaBH_4} \underset{\text{4-Hydroxybutyronitrile}}{NCCH_2CH_2CH_2OH}$$

$$\underset{\text{Acid chloride}}{RCOCl} \xrightarrow{NaBH_4} \underset{\text{Alcohol}}{RCH_2OH}$$

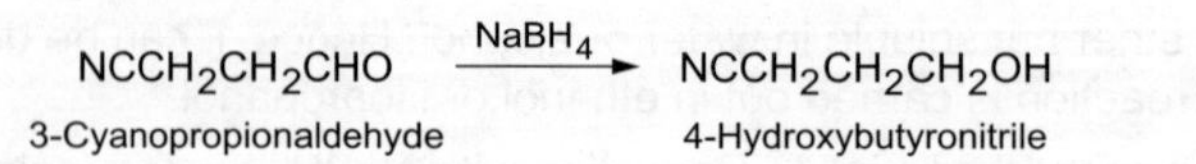

p-Nitrobenzaldehyde *p*-Nitrobenzyl alcohol

In the above compounds it will be seen that only the carbonyl group is reduced and the other functional groups remain unaffected. This high selectivity of $NaBH_4$ makes it the preferred reagent for the reduction of carbonyl groups in sensitive polyfunctional molecules.

2. Reduction of carbonyl group to methylene group *p*-Toluenesulphonyl hydrazine condenses with carbonyl compounds to give tosylhydrazones which on reduction with $NaBH_4$ give hydrocarbons.

$$R_2C{=}O + H_2N{-}NHTs \longrightarrow \underset{\text{Tosylhydrazone}}{R_2C{=}N{-}NHTs} \xrightarrow{NaBH_4} R_2CH_2$$

The method is useful in the synthesis, e.g., ketosteriods.

3. Reduction of ozonides Sodium borohydride reduces ozonides to two molecules of alcohol and ozonides of cycloolefins to diols.

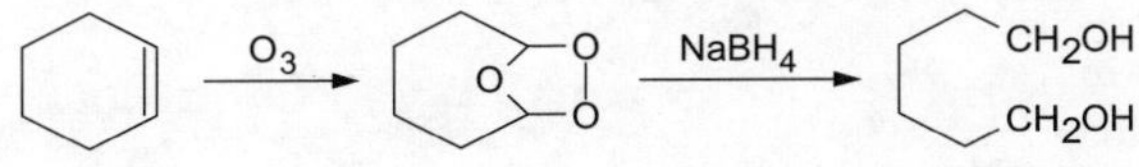

Hexan-1, 6-diol

4. Reductive alkylation of amines When aldehyde or ketone is treated with amines (1° or 2°) in the presence of $NaBH_4$ reductive alkylation occurs.

$$R-\underset{\underset{O}{\|}}{C}-R + R'NH_2 \xrightarrow{NaBH_4} R-\overset{NHR'}{\underset{OH}{C}}-R \xrightarrow[\text{reaction}]{\text{Hydrogenolysis}} R-\overset{NHR'}{\underset{H}{C}}-R$$

5. Reduction of carbon–nitrogen double bond Although sodium borohydride does not reduce nitriles, it reduces carbon–nitrogen double bond.

$$-\overset{|}{C}=\overset{|}{N} \xrightarrow{NaBH_4} -\overset{|}{C}H-\overset{|}{N}H$$

6. Reduction of ester groups Ordinarily ester groups are unaffected by $NaBH_4$ but in the presence of LiCl or $AlCl_3$ in diglyme (diethylene glycol dimethyl ether) they are reduced to alcohols.

$$RCOOR' \xrightarrow[\text{LiCl in diglyme}]{NaBH_4} RCH_2OH + R'OH$$

7. Hydration of olefins Olefins are hydrated under mild condition without rearrangement in high yield on treatment with mercuric acetate followed by $NaBH_4$ 'in situ'.

$$\underset{\text{2-Methyl-1-butene}}{CH_3-CH_2-\overset{CH_3}{\overset{|}{C}}=CH_2} \xrightarrow[2.\ NaBH_4]{1.\ Hg(OAc)_2} \underset{\text{2-Methyl-2-butanol (90\%)}}{CH_3-CH_2-\overset{CH_3}{\underset{OH}{C}}-CH_3}$$

8. Preparation of diborane Diborane which is used for the hydroboration of alkenes is prepared by reacting boron trifluoride with sodium borohydride.

$$\underset{\text{Boron trifluoride}}{4BF_3} + 3NaBH_4 \longrightarrow \underset{\text{Diborane}}{2B_2H_6} + \underset{\text{Sodium borofluoride}}{3NaBF_4}$$

Hydroboration is done 'in situ' either in THF or in diglyme.

$$4BF_3 + 3NaBH_4 + 12R-CH=CH_2 \xrightarrow[\text{Diglyme}]{\text{THF}} 4(RCH_2CH_2)_3B + 3NaBF_4$$

9. Reduction of diazonium borofluoride Diazonium borofluoride can be reduced with $NaBH_4$ in dimethylformamide or alcohol.

$$C_6H_5N_2Cl \xrightarrow{HBF_4} C_6H_5\overset{\oplus}{N_2}\overset{\ominus}{BF_4} \xrightarrow[CH_3OH]{NaBH_4} C_6H_6$$

10. Reduction of azides Azides containing sulphur are not reduced to amines by the usual methods. However, sodium borohydride reduces azides to amines.

WILKINSON'S CATALYST

Wilkinson's catalyst is widely used for homogeneous hydrogenation. The catalyst is a complex of the transition metal rhodium. The name of the complex is tris(triphenylphosphine)chlororhodium (I) and its molecular formula is $RhCl(PPh_3)_3$. The three triphenylphosphine (PPh_3) ligands are bound to rhodium through the unshared pair of electrons on phosphorus.

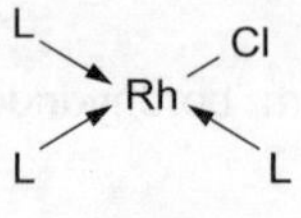

where L = $P(C_6H_5)_3$ or PPh_3

Wilkinson's catalyst
Tris (triphenylphosphine) chlororhodium (I)

The ligands do not directly participate in the reaction but their presence is absolutely essential—they influence the course of the reaction. The function of the metal is to form bonds with the substrate and the reagent and thus bringing them near each other for the reaction to follow.

Mechanism

The catalytic activity is due to the vacant coordination sites in the metal. The active hydrogenation catalyst is formed by the addition of a hydrogen molecule to the complex and loss of one ligand (PPh_3).

It is believed that the reaction proceeds in the following steps:

The complex first exchanges one ligand with a solvent molecule to form $RhCl(PPh_3)_2$(solvent) which then reacts with one molecule of hydrogen to form the dihydrido complex.

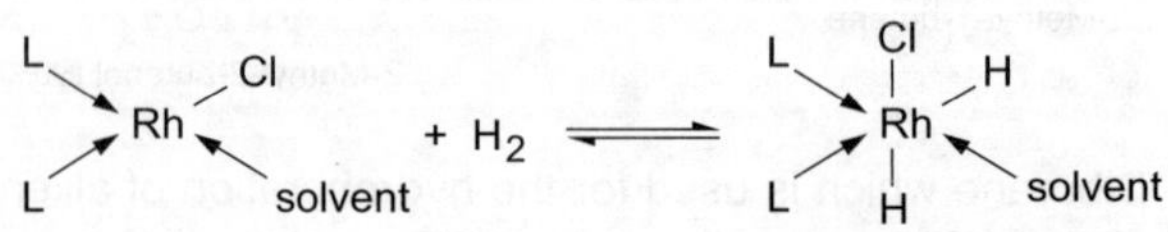

Dihydrido complex

For this the metal uses one of its electron pairs and is itself oxidized from +1 to +3 oxidation state (oxidative addition). The energy liberated in the formation of two metal-hydrogen bonds more than compensate the energy required to break the H–H sigma bond.

The active hydrogenation catalyst is now formed. The alkene then forms a π-complex with the metal probably by replacing the solvent molecule.

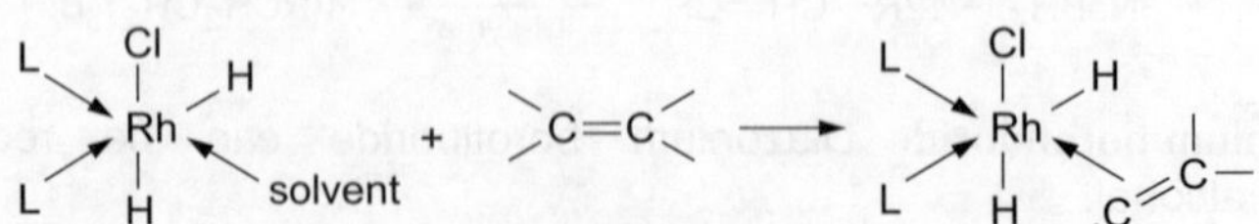

Dihydrido complex
(Active hydrogenation catalyst)

π-Complex

Now that both the reactants are bonded to the metal, the two hydrogens are consecutively transferred to the alkene carbons. One hydrogen migrates from the metal to one of the alkene carbons and the other carbon is bonded to the metal by a σ-bond.

The second hydrogen then migrates to the metal-bonded carbon. The addition being complete, the saturated product leaves the sphere of reaction. The catalyst is regenerated and rhodium returns to +1 state again and the reaction continues.

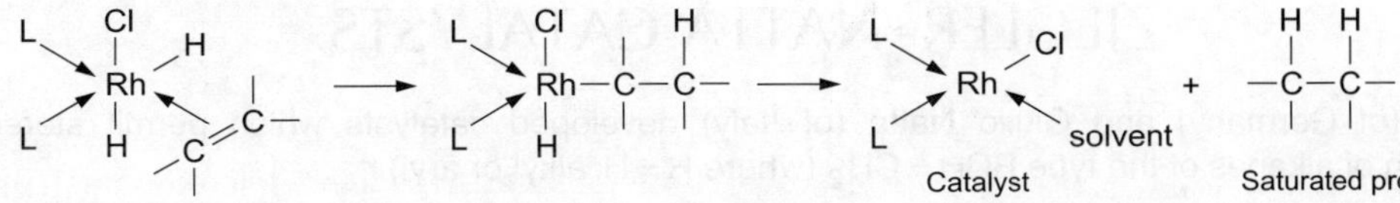

The mechanism is supported by the detection and isolation (in some cases) of intermediates, kinetics studies, NMR spectroscopy, etc.

Stereochemical aspect

It was observed that maleic acid on hydrogenation with Wilkinson's catalyst, using deuterium (D_2) in place of hydrogen gave meso-(2, 3-D_2)butanedioic acid while fumaric acid under the conditions gave racemic butanedioic acid. From this it is concluded that addition of deuterium occurs from the same face of the double bond, i.e., *syn*-addition occurs. The reaction is, therefore, both stereoselective and stereospecific.

This is explained in the following way: Due to the close proximity of the metal (Rh) and hydrogen in the complex, the unsaturated carbons are held from one (or the other) face of the double bond by the metal and hydrogen in the transition state (I). After the migration of hydrogen to one of the doubly bonded carbons, the other carbon is still held from the same face of the double bond by the metal. The second hydrogen is now near the front side of this carbon (II) to which it migrates through the transition state (III) to give the *syn*-addition product and regenerated catalyst (IV).

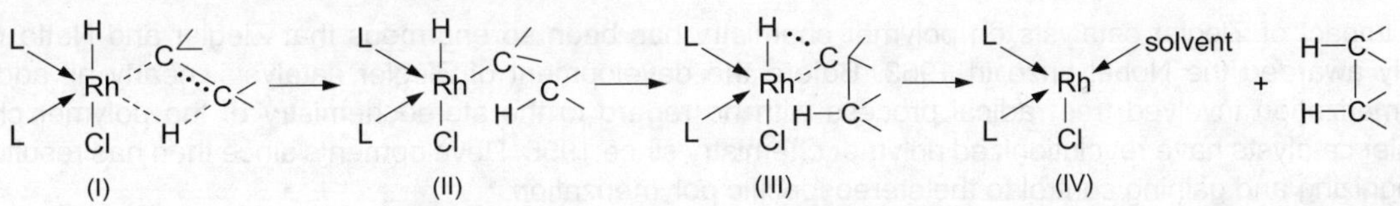

Uses

Geometric isomers on hydrogenation with Wilkinson's catalyst having optically inactive ligands give either meso or a mixture of enantiomers. However, by the use of Wilkinson's catalyst with proper choice of optically active ligands, one or the other enantiomer may be preferentially formed (enantioselectivity).

This method has been employed to prepare L-amino acids which are required for the synthesis of proteins. L-Dopa, an amino acid for the treatment of Parkinson's disease, is being prepared on an industrial scale by this method.

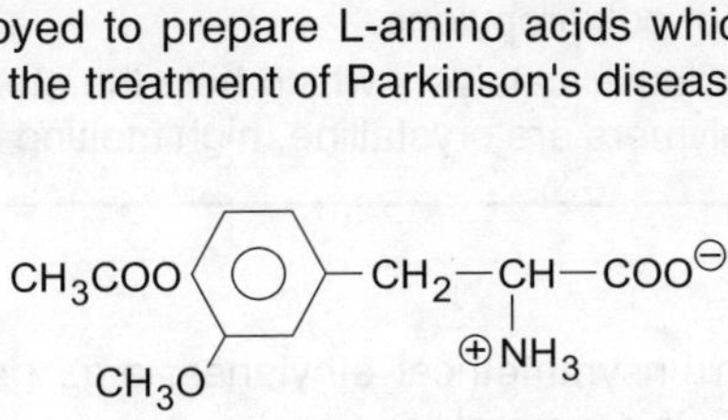

3-Methoxy-4-acetoxyphenylalanine
(L-Dopa)

A number of optically active ligands have been developed to prepare rhodium complexes (Wilkinson's catalyst) to catalyse many types of reactions and useful results are forthcoming. Thus, Wilkinson's catalyst has vast potential. The complex $RhH(CO)(PPh_3)_3$, a Wilkinson's type of catalyst, has been found to be more efficient than the cobalt complex, $Co_2(CO)_8$ for oxo process.

ZIEGLER–NATTA CATALYSTS

Kurl Ziegler (of Germany) and Giulio Natta (of Italy) developed catalysts which permit stereoregular polymerization of alkenes of the type $RCH = CH_2$ (where R = H, alkyl or aryl).

Ziegler catalysts are a combination of organometallics which consists of a complex of triethylaluminium, Et_3Al and a transition metal chloride, $TiCl_4$. When these are mixed in a hydrocarbon solvent a heterogeneous precipitate develops which catalyses polymerization of alkenes at low temperature and pressure.

The method consists in passing the monomer, say propylene under 10 atmospheric pressure into an inert hydrocarbon solvent containing the catalysts at about 100 °C.

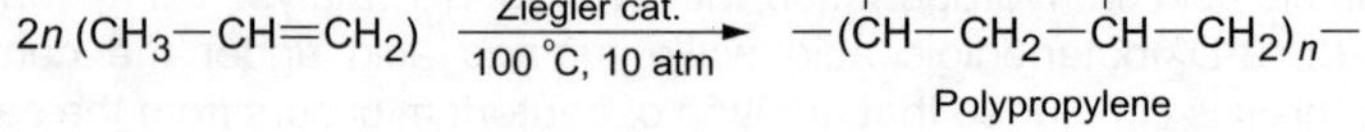

Polypropylene

Ethylene is polymerized to polyethylene in good yield at atmospheric pressure and room temperature by the use of Ziegler process. Isoprene was polymerized by Ziegler catalysts to a substance identical with natural rubber.

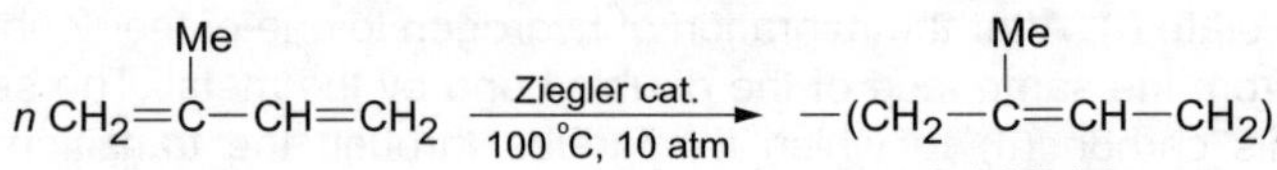

Isoprene

cis-1,4-Polyisoprene (Rubber)

The impact of Ziegler catalysts on polymer chemistry has been so enormous that Ziegler and Natta were jointly awarded the Nobel prize in 1963. Before the development of Ziegler catalysts, nearly all addition polymerization involved free radical process with no regard to the stereochemistry of the polymer chain. Ziegler catalysts have revolutionized polymer chemistry since 1955. Developments since then has resulted in recognizing and gaining control to the stereospecific polymerization.

Polymer chains with branches or irregularly oriented bulky side groups are unable to lie alongside each other for steric reasons. Consequently, they have low crystallinity, are amorphous, low melting and mechanically weak.

Polymerization by radical process under high temperature and pressure gives highly branched polyethylene and irregularly oriented side groups *(atactic)* in polypropylene or polystyrene. In contrast, polymerization by the use of Ziegler catalysts under mild conditions produces unbranched polyethylene and stereoregular (*isotactic*) polystyrene or polypropylene.

Here in lies the usefulness of Zieglar catalysts which help the stereoregularity in the growing chain of the polymer. These stereoregular polymers are crystalline, high melting and mechanically strong.

Stereochemical aspect

In polymers prepared from unsymmetrical ethylenes, e.g., propylene or styrene, every alternate carbon in the chain is asymmetric.

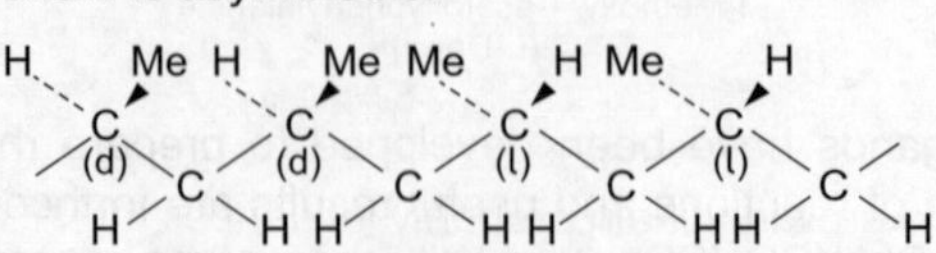

Polypropylene

For stereochemical purposes the carbon chain may be represented as – d – d – l – l – .
The stereochemical sequence of the asymmetric carbons in a polymer chain is described by the term `tacticity' which means the placement of the asymmetric carbon atoms in the chain.
If the stereo arrangement of the asymmetric carbons is (i) always the same, i.e., – d – d – d – d – or – l – l – l – l – it is called *isotactic*, (ii) alternating, i.e., – d – l – d – l – d – l – it is called *syndiotactic* and (iii) random, i.e., – d – l – d – d – l – l – l – it is called *atactic.*
The placement of the asymmetric carbons in the chain, i.e., 'tacticity' has an important bearing on the physical properties of the polymers. Thus, atactic polymers have low crystallinity, low melting points and are mechanically weak. In contrast, isotactic polymers are crystalline, high melting and mechanically strong. The requirement for crystallinity can be satisfied by the stereochemical regularity (*isotactic* or *syndiotactic*) in the chain.

Mechanism

Not much is known about the mechanism of polymerization by this catalyst. Several mechanisms have been suggested but none are so well substantiated. Polymerization by Ziegler catalysts is neither free radical nor ionic types. It is probably a coordination polymerization. As to how each monomer unit adds to the growing chain is not clearly understood.

Ziegler catalysts are a combination of aluminium alkyls (e.g., Et_3Al) and a transition metal halide (e.g., $TiCl_4$). Probably, triethylaluminium reduces the transition metal to a lower valence state producing titanium trichloride, diethyl aluminium chloride and an ethyl-free radical which combine to form the complex, the active catalysts. The active catalysts (hetereogeneous precipitate) is suggested to be an octahedral complex of titanium with a vacant coordination site and an ethyl group bonded to Ti.

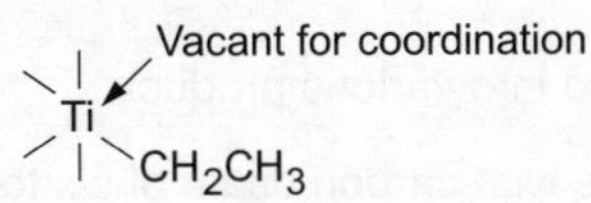

In the generally accepted mechanism, it is suggested that the monomer coordinates at the vacant site of the metal with its pi-clouds to form a pi-bond. Now that both the monomer and the ethyl group are held very close to each other by Ti, the monomer inserts itself between the metal and the ethyl group to form a four-carbon chain. The coordination site is now vacant for the coordination of another monomer unit and the process is repeated.

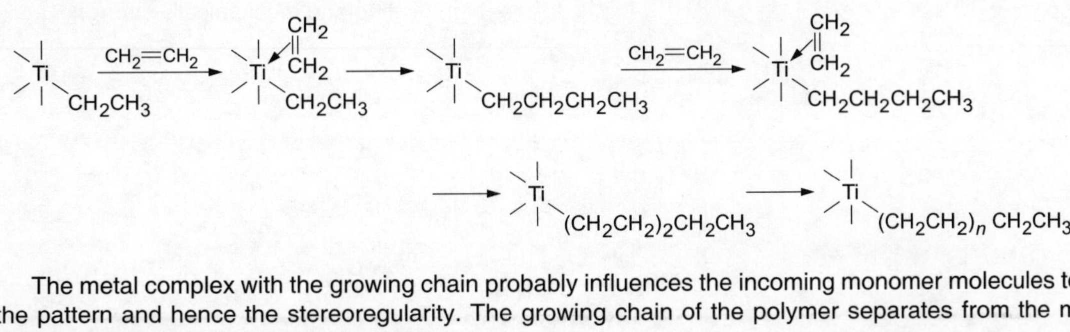

The metal complex with the growing chain probably influences the incoming monomer molecules to fall in the pattern and hence the stereoregularity. The growing chain of the polymer separates from the metal probably through the insertion of a hydrogen.

Applications

Polymers obtained by the use of Ziegler catalysts are superior to those obtained by the free radical process.

(1) It produces linear polymers without branching and gives stereoregular (*isotactic* and *syndiotactic*) polymers which are more dense, crystalline, high melting and mechanically strong. Polypropylene obtained by the use of Ziegler catalysts is extensively used for the preparation of sheets, pipes, synthetic fibres, domestic articles for everyday use, etc.

(2) The copolymer of ethylene and propylene prepared by the use of Ziegler catalysts is an excellent elastomer.

(3) The catalysts permit stereochemical control about the carbon–carbon double bond. Isoprene has been polymerized to all *cis*-1, 4-polyisoprene, a substance practically identical to natural rubber.

(4) Metal alkyls, obtained in the process, on heating in the presence of ethylene and nickel catalyst give straight chain 1-alkenes of even number of carbons.

$$M-(CH_2-CH_2)_n-CH_2CH_3 \xrightarrow[\text{Heat}]{CH_2=CH_2,\ Ni} CH_2=CH-(CH_2-CH_2)_{n-1}-CH_2CH_3$$

These alkenes are used for the manufacture of detergents on a commercial scale.

(5) The metal alkyls on heating in the presence of air give oxides which on hydrolysis give primary alcohols of straight and long chain.

$$M-(CH_2-CH_2)_n-CH_2CH_3 \xrightarrow[30-100\,^\circ C]{\text{Air}} M-O-(CH_2-CH_2)_n-CH_2CH_3 \xrightarrow[\text{Room temp.}]{H_2SO_4,\ H_2O} H-O-(CH_2-CH_2)_n-CH_2CH_3$$

The alcohol may be transformed into various products.

With Ziegler catalysts, polymers with carbon chain of six to twenty carbons are obtained.

Appendix A

Some More Reactions and Rearrangements

CHICHIBABIN REACTION

Amination of pyridine and other nitrogen heterocyclics by alkali-metal amides e.g., sodamide is called chichibabin (Tschitschibabin) reaction.

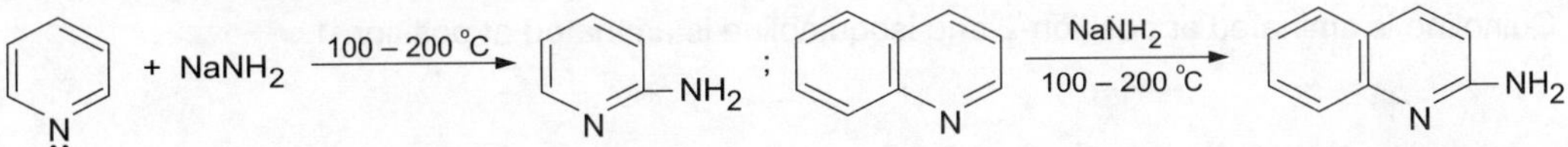

2-Aminopyridine 2-Aminoqunoline

The amino group is substituted at position-2 (and -6) and when these positoins are occupied the amino group is substituted at position-4.

In practice, pyridine dissolved in toluene is heated (100–200 °C) with sodamide when hydrogen is evolved and the sodium salt of 2-aminopyridine is obtained. The latter on hydrolysis with water gives 2-aminopyridine. Excess of sodamide produces 2, 6-diaminopyridine.

Mechanism

Due to heavier nuclear charge on the nitrogen atom compared to carbon atoms, the loose π-electrons of the ring are polarized towards the nitrogen atom. Hence the ring carbons are electron deficient. The electron deficiency is more marked at positions-2, -4 and -6.

This will be evident from its resonance structures.

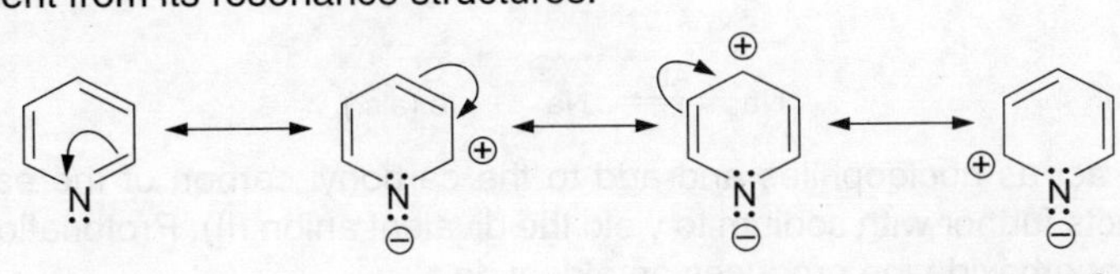

Hence, pyridine undergoes nucleophilic attack by powerful nucleophiles e.g., $\overset{\ominus}{N}H_2$ at these positions.

The reaction occurs by an addition-elimination mechanism. The leaving group is the hydride ion which combines with a proton from the initially formed aminopyridine to evolve hydrogen. The sodium salt of 2-aminopyridine on hydrolysis with water gives 2-aminopyridine and NaOH.

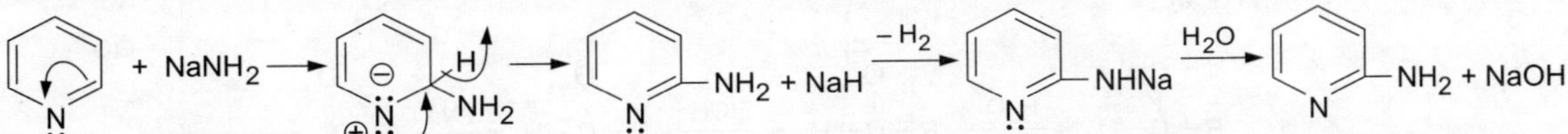

2-Aminopyridine

Formation of the intermediate ion such as (i) for quinoline has been substantiated by NMR spectra.

The nitrogen in the ring of pyridine serves the same general purpose in substitution as do the oxygen of the nitro group in nitrobenzene.

An analogous reaction is Ziegler alkylation which involves alkylation of nitrogen heterocyclic compounds with alkyl lithium.

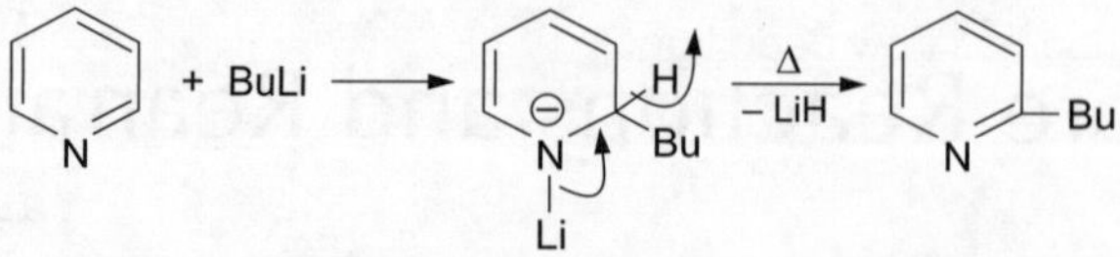

Aminoheterocyclic nitrogen compounds are important synthetic intermediates e.g., 2-aminopyridine is used in the preparation of the drug, sulfapyridine,

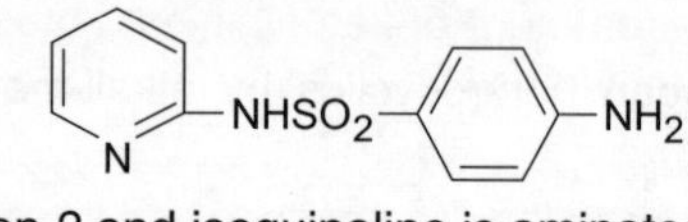

Quinoline is aminated at position-2 and isoquinoline is aminated at position-1.

BOUVEAULT-BLANC REDUCTION

Aldehydes, ketones or esters are reduced to alcohols on treatment with excess of sodium and alcohol. This is known as Bouveault-Blanc reduction.

$$RCHO \xrightarrow[Na]{EtOH} RCH_2OH\ ;\ R'CO_2R'' \xrightarrow[Na]{EtOH} R'CH_2OH + R''OH\ ;\ R''CO \xrightarrow[Na]{EtOH} R''CHOH$$

Mechanism

It was thought earlier that this reduction occured through nascent hydrogen produced from sodium and alcohol. It is now believed that the reaction occurs in several steps involving the transfer of electrons from the metal to the substrate one at a time.

In protonic solvents e.g., alcohol, atoms of strongly electropositive metals (Na, K, etc.) produce solvated electrons.

$$\dot{Na} \underset{}{\overset{Alc}{\rightleftharpoons}} \overset{\oplus}{Na} + \overset{\ominus}{e}\ (alc.)$$

These electrons act as nucleophiles and add to the carbonyl carbon of the ester to produce radical anion (I). The latter reacts further with sodium to yield the divalent anion (II). Protonation of (II) by alcohol and subsequent expulsion of ethoxide ion produces an aldehyde.

Repetition of the above sequence of reactions give alcohol.

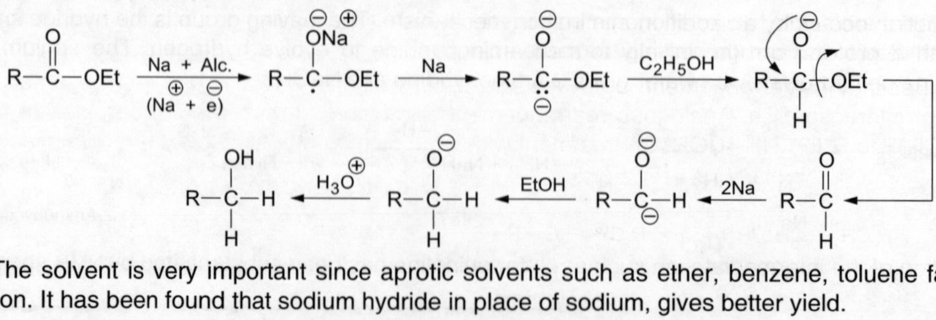

The solvent is very important since aprotic solvents such as ether, benzene, toluene favour acyloin formation. It has been found that sodium hydride in place of sodium, gives better yield.

In the commercial reduction of esters, methyl-isobutyle alcohol is used.

Applications

The method has useful applications in synthesis. It has been applied to reduce esters to alcohols and during the synthesis of many natural products e.g., cadalene, eudalene, abietinol etc. The double bonds in the substrate remain unaffected.

Bouveault-Blanc method has now been largely reduced by $LiAlH_4$ but this method is still in use where selectivity is required.

NEBER REARRANGEMENT

Preparation of α-aminoketones by the treatment of ketoxime tosylates with a base such as alkoxide ion or pyridine and subsequent hydrolysis is known as Neber rearrangement.

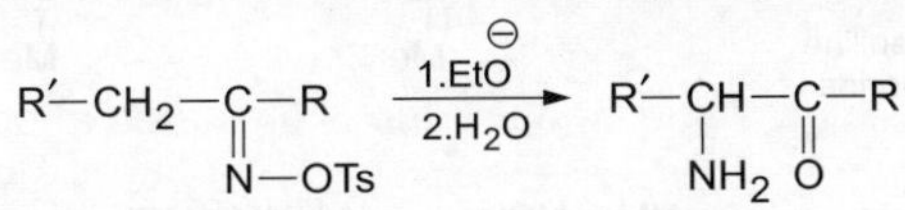

The group R′ is generally aryl but it may be alkyl or hydrogen and group R may be alkyl or aryl only.

Mechanism

The reaction is a base-catalysed intramolecular elimination of tosyl group with the formation of azirine (azacyclopropene) intermediate which has been isolated. Subsequent hydrolysis of azirine affords α-aminoketone.

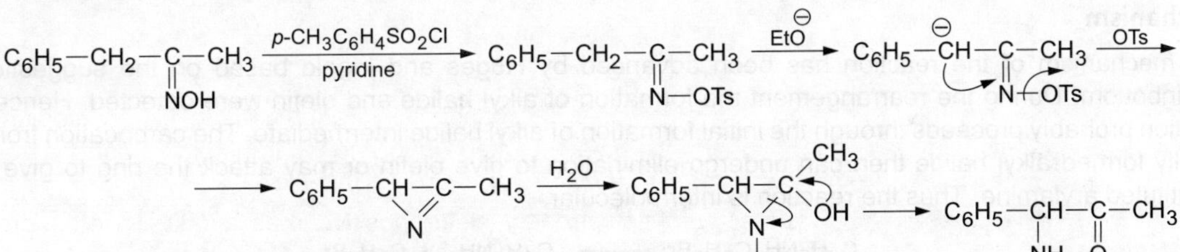

Azirine intermediate
(2-Methyl-3-phenyl-1-azacyclo propene)

Isolation of azirine substantiates the mechanism. Nucleophilic elimination of tosyl group and formation of azirine may be concerted or stepwise i.e., formation of azirine via the formation of nitrine.

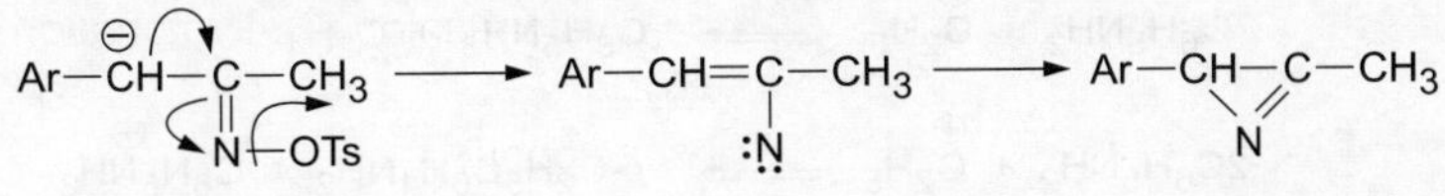

When there are acidic hydrogen atoms on both the α-carbons as in unsymmetrical ketones, the amino group is substituted to the carbon bearing the more acidic hydrogen.

Unlike Beckmann rearrangement, both *syn* and *anti* ketoximes undergo this rearrangemet i.e., the reaction is non-stereospecific. Analogous rearrangement is observed in N, N-dichloroamines of the type $R'CH_2CH(NCl_2)R$ to $R'CH(NH_2)COR$. On treatment with base the compound first forms chloroimine with the loss of HCl.

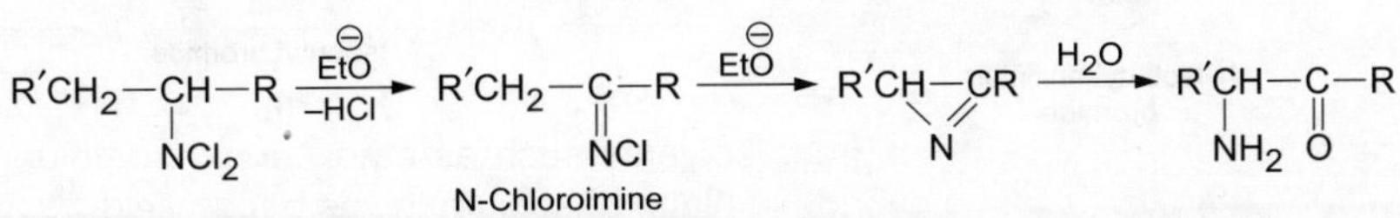

N-Chloroimine

α-Amino ketones have important synthetic applications.

HOFMANN–MARTIUS REARRANGEMENT

Mono and dialkyl aniline hydrochlorides or bromides as also quaternery salts of aniline on strong heating (200–300 °C) undergo rearrangement which involves the migration of the alkyl groups from the nitrogen to the para position and if the para position is occupied, then to the ortho position of the aromatic ring. This is known as Hofmann–Martius rearrangement.

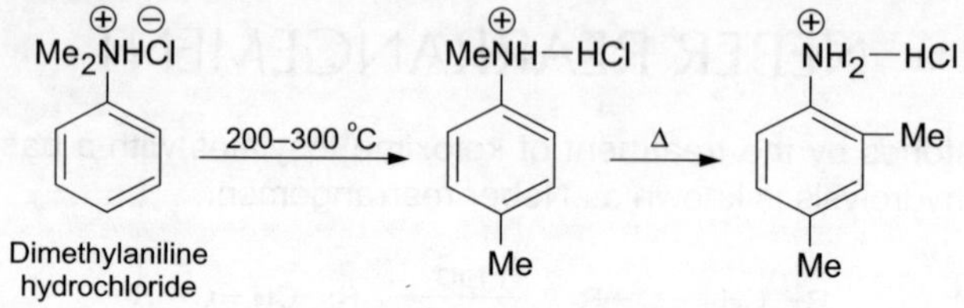

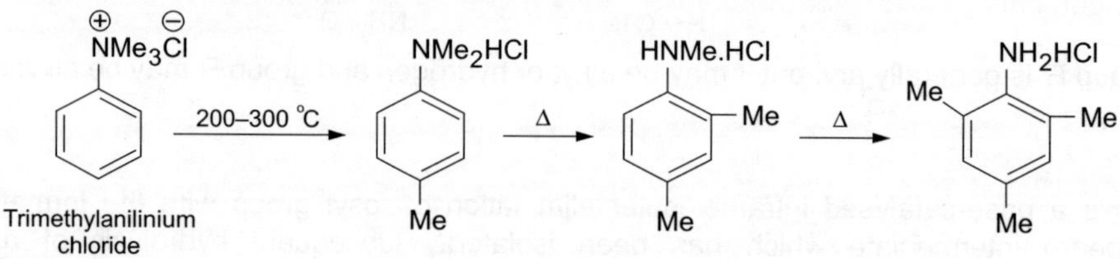

Mechanism

The mechanism of the reaction has been advanced by Huges and Ingold based on the suggestion of Hickinbottom. During the rearrangement the formation of alkyl halide and olefin were detected. Hence, the reaction probably proceeds through the initial formation of alkyl halide intermediate. The carbocation from the initially formed alkyl halide then can undergo elimination to give olefin or may attack the ring to give alkyl substituted arylamine. Thus the reaction is intermolecular.

$$C_6H_5\overset{+}{N}H_2C_2H_5\overset{-}{Br} \rightleftharpoons C_6H_5NH_2 + C_2H_5Br$$

$$C_2H_5Br \rightleftharpoons \overset{\oplus}{C}_2H_5 + \overset{\ominus}{Br}$$

$$C_6H_5NH_2 + \overset{\oplus}{C}_2H_5 \rightleftharpoons C_6H_5\overset{\oplus}{N}H_3 + C_2H_4$$

$$2C_6H_5NH_2 + \overset{\oplus}{C}_2H_5 \rightleftharpoons p\text{-}C_2H_5C_6H_4NH_2 + C_6N_5\overset{\oplus}{N}H_3$$

The mechanism is supported by the observation that if the alkyl group is primary it undergoes isomerisation before attacking the ring.

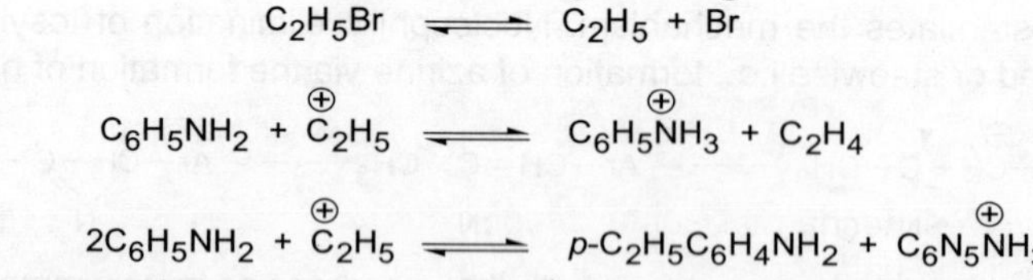

$$Me_2CHCH_2Br \rightleftharpoons Me_2CH\overset{\oplus}{C}H_2 + \overset{\ominus}{Br}$$

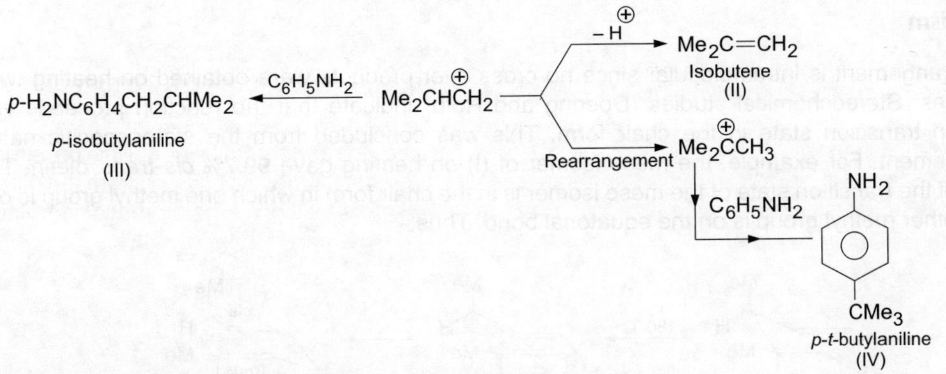

Thus formation of (II), (III) and (IV) can only be explained due to the formation of the intermediate (I) derived from N-Isobutyl anilinium bromide.

Rearrangements of this kind, groups from the N-atom migrating to the ring, have been observed in aniline derivatives. Thus, Orton rearrangement involves migration of chlorine to the ring carbon, e.g., N-chloroacetanilide to *p*-chloroacetanilide. Fischer-Hepp rearrangement involves migration of NO (nitroso) group.

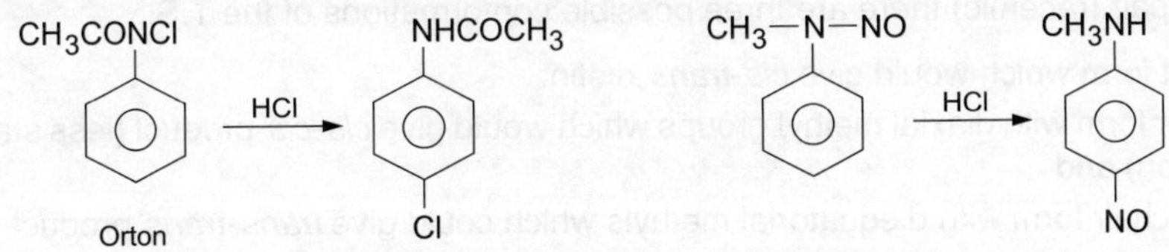

Quaternary salts of pyridine also undergo analogous rearrangement. Pyridine methoiodide on strong heating gives 2- and 4-methylpyridine hydrochloride

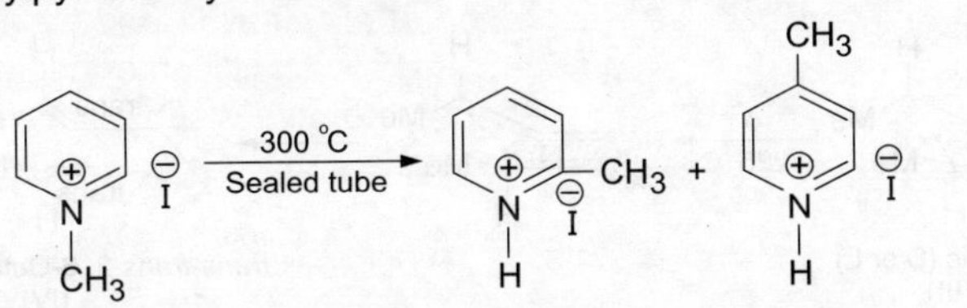

COPE REARRANGEMENT

Cope rearrangement involves the thermal isomerization of 1, 5-dienes with shift of double bonds and breaking of 3,4-σ-bond. Any 1, 5-diene undergoes this rearrangement.

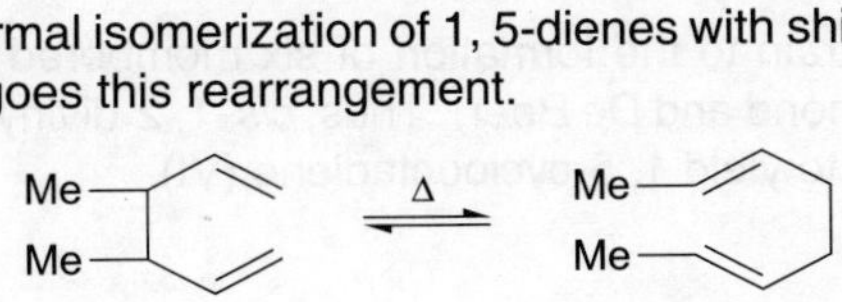

3, 4-Dimethyl-1, 5-hexadiene (I) ⇌ 2, 6-Octadiene (II)

The reaction is reversible and produces an equillibrium mixture of the dienes. That isomer, however, predominates which is thermodynamically more stable. The reaction is facile (occuring at lower temperature) when there is a phenyl or carbethoxy group at 3- or 4-positions. This is due to conjugation of the groups with the double bonds in the product with consequent stablizatoin. When catalysed by transition metal compounds, Cope rearrangement of simple 1, 5-dienes can occur at room temperature.

Mechanism

The rearrangement is intramolecular since no cross over products were obtained on heating two different 1, 5-dienes. Stereochemical studies (Doering and Roth) indicate that the reaction proceeds via a cyclic six-carbon transition state in the chair form. This was concluded from the stereospecific nature of the rearrantgement. For example, the meso isomer of (I) on heating gave 99.7% *cis-trans* olefin. This is only possible if the transition state of the meso isomer is in the chair form in which one methyl group is on the axial and the other methyl group is on the equatorial bond. Thus,

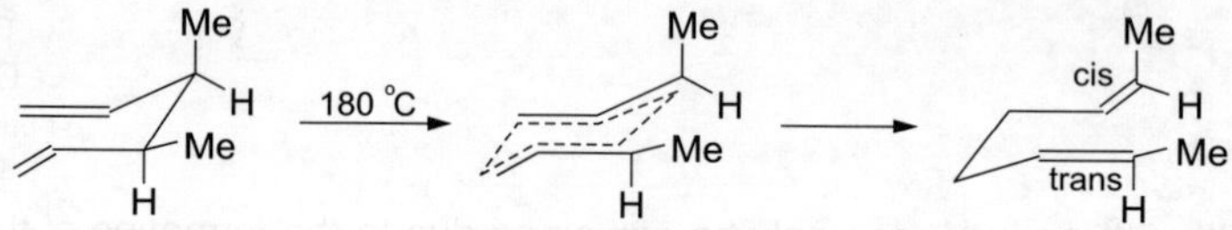

Meso T.S. *cis-trans*-2, 6-Octadiene (99.7%)

If the cyclic T.S. had been in the boat form, the product would be either *cis-cis* or *trans-trans*, since there are two boat forms for the meso-isomer.

For the DL pair (racemic) there are three possible conformations of the T.S.:

(i) one boat form which would give *cis-trans* olefin,

(ii) one chair form with diaxial methyl groups which would give *cis-cis* product (less stable due to diaxial interaction) and

(iii) another chair form with diequatorial methyls which could give *trans-trans* product

In practice the product from DL-isomer (III) is mainly *trans-trans* olefin (IV).

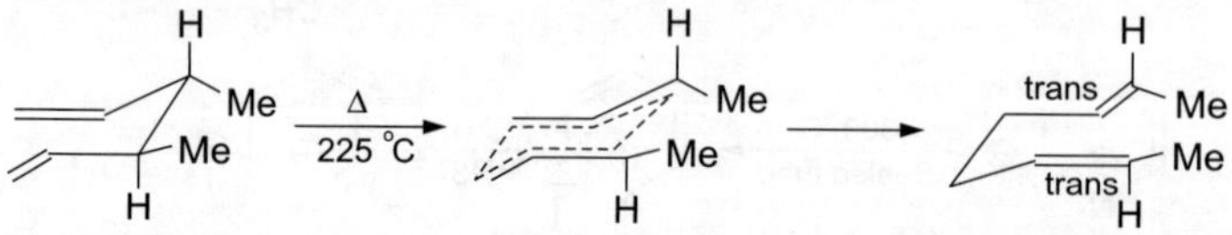

Racemic (D or L) (III) T.S. *trans-trans*-2, 6-Octadiene (90%) (IV)

It is therefore suggested that the isomerization proceeds via a cyclic six-carbon T.S in the energetically preferred chair conformation. The mechanism of Cope rearrangement is similar to Claisen rearrangement which involves six-centered rearrangement of five carbons and one oxygen.

When there is steric restrain to the formation of six membered cyclic T.S. the reaction may proceed through radical pathway (Hammond and De Boer). Thus, *cis*-1, 2-divinylcyclobutane (V) rearranges through a boat-like six-carbon cyclic T.S. to yield 1, 5-cyclooctadiene (VI).

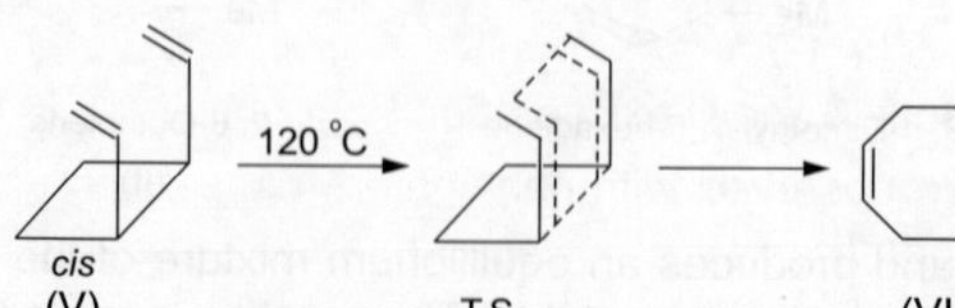

cis (V) T.S. (VI)

However, the trans-isomer (VII) unable to attain the cyclic T.S. due to strain, rearranges via a radical pathway to give a mixture of (VI) and 4-vinylcyclohexene (VIII), the latter being the major product.

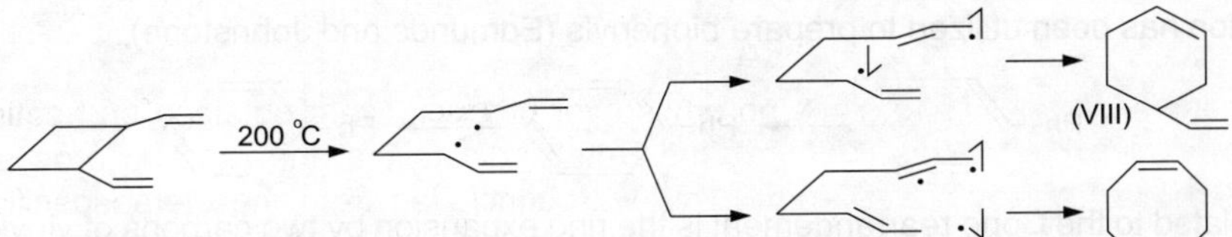

trans (VII) (VIII) (VI)

Divinylcyclopropane similarly undergoes the rearrangement with ring expansion by four carbons. (Vogel et. al.)

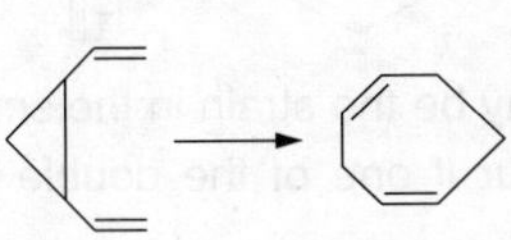

Thus, Cope rearrangement may involve either concerted or biradical mechanism the latter preferred by some substrates. The biradical two steps mechanism may be formulated as below for 1, 5-diene.

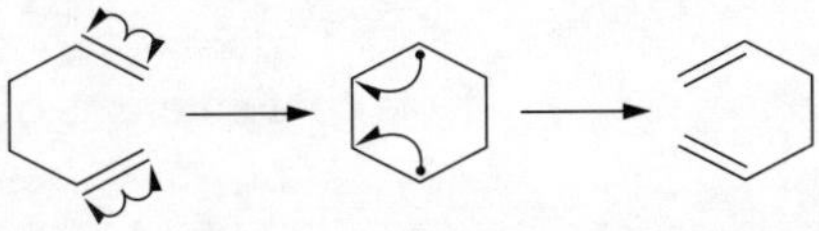

It is seen that 1, 6-bond is formed before the breaking of 3, 4-bond. There is yet another suggestion involving diionic mechanism (Gompper and Ulrich).

Cope rearrangement is not reversible when there is a hydroxy substituent at 3- or 4-position in 1, 5-dienes since the product tautomerizes to stable aldehyde or ketone.

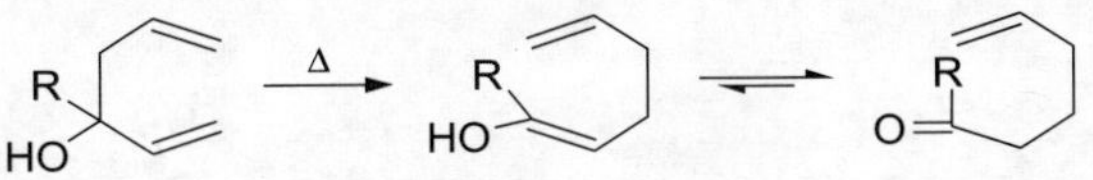

R = H or Alkyl.

This is known as oxyCope rearrangement (Berson and Jones). The reaction has great synthetic importance.

It is seen that Cope rearrangement of symmetrical 1, 5-dienes gives the product which is indistinguishable from the starting material. This is known as degenerate Cope rearrangement.

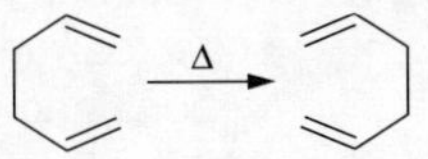

Similarly, degenerate carbocation rearrangement is also known

$$\underset{\text{A}}{CH_3-CH_2-\overset{\oplus}{C}H-CH_3} \xrightleftharpoons{\text{Migration of H}} \underset{\text{B}}{CH_3-\overset{\oplus}{C}H-CH_2-CH_3}$$

Spectral analysis indicate both A and B exist as equillibrium pair.

Cope rearrangement is also observed with conjugated trienes with the difference that the 3, 4-bond changes from double to a single bond.

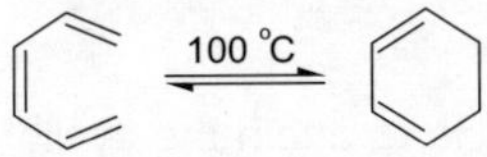

The reaction has been utilized to prepare biphenyls (Edmunds and Johnstone)

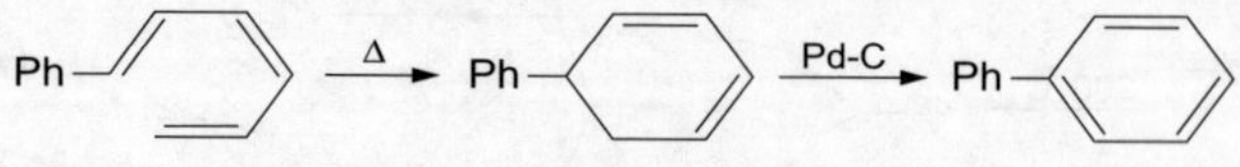

Closely related to the Cope rearrangement is the ring expansion by two carbons of vinylcycloalkanes of small rings via a four-centered T.S. (Overberger & Borchert)

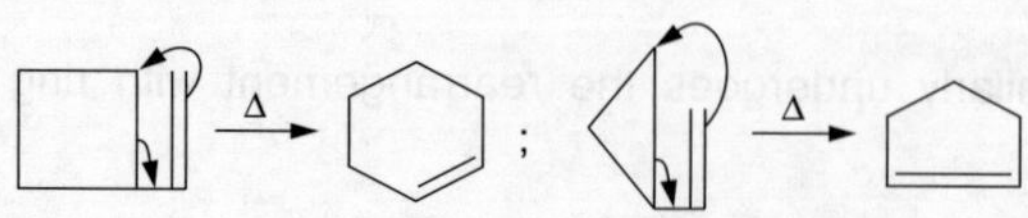

The driving force of the rearrangement may be the strain in the small rings.

Cope rearrangement does not occur if one of the double bonds is a part of an aromatic ring e.g., 4-phenyl-1-butene.

EXERCISES (CHAPTER 1)

1. Which canonical form in each of the following sets is the major contributor to the respective hybrid?

(i) 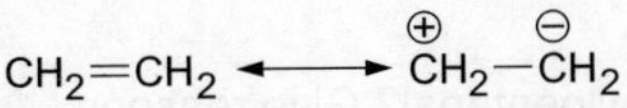

(ii) 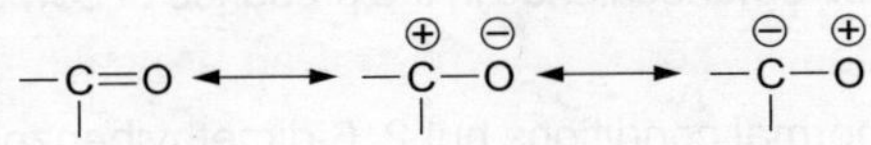

(iii) 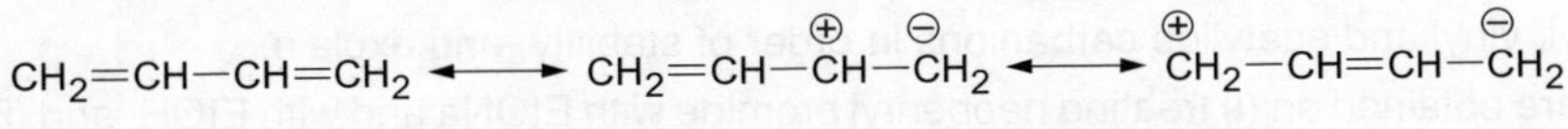

(iv) 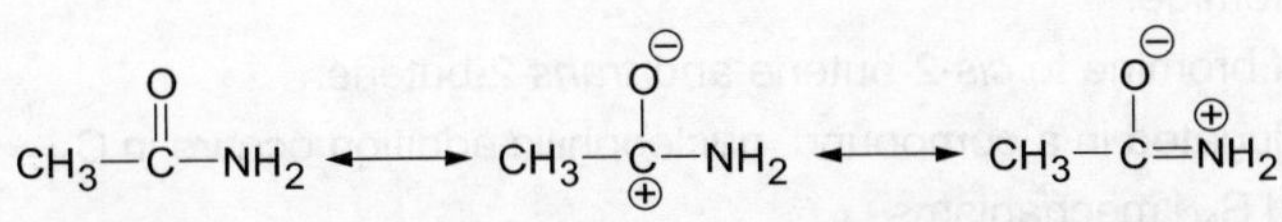

2. Give proper signs between the two sets in each of the following and describe the phenomena.

(i) 

(ii) 

3. In which of the two sets is resonance stability greater and what is the consequence?

(i) 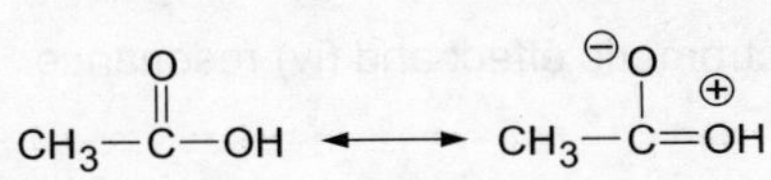

(ii) 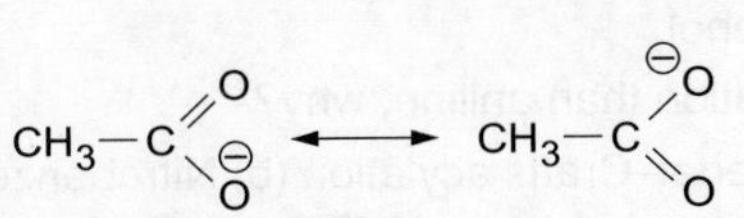

4. Classify the following reactions and give the mechanisms of the reactions.

$$C_6H_6 + HNO_3 \xrightarrow{H_2SO_4} C_6H_5NO_2\ ; \quad C_6H_5Cl + NaNH_2 \xrightarrow{\text{Liq. } NH_3} C_6H_5NH_2$$

$$Me_3CBr + NaOH \longrightarrow Me_3C(OH)\ ; \quad CH_3CHO + NH_2OH \longrightarrow CH_3CH{=}NOH$$

5. Explain:
   (a) Aniline is a weaker base than cyclohexylamine.
   (b) In water 2° amine is a stronger base than 3° amine.
   (c) Formic acid is stronger than acetic acid.
   (d) Propenoic acid is stronger than propanoic acid.
   (e) The order of –I effect of hybrid orbitals is $sp > sp^2 > sp^3$.
   (f) Phenol is acidic but ethyl alcohol is neutral.
   (g) Phenol is a weaker acid than acetic acid.
6. (a) What is the major product of dehydration of 3-hydroxy-4-methylpentanal? Give reasons.
   (b) What product is obtained on treating benzene with iodinemonochloride in the presence of Lewis acid?
   (c) Explain the addition of HBr in 1, 3-butadiene.
7. (a) 2, 6-Dimethylphenyl acetic acid is esterified under normal conditions but 2, 6-dimethylbenzoic acid is esterified under drastic conditions, why?
   (b) Arrange alkyl, vinyl and acetylide carbanions in order of stability, and explain.
8. What products are obtained on (i) treating neopentyl bromide with EtONa and with EtOH, and (ii) addition of HBr to propylene and to vinyl bromide.
9. Give the mechanism of addition of bromine to *cis*-2-butene and *trans*-2-butene.
10. When C = C and C = O are conjugated in a compound, nucleophilic addition occurs in C = C, why?
11. Write short notes on S_N1, S_N2 and S_Ni mechanisms.
12. Discuss Hofmann rule. How has it been used in the structure determination of heterocyclic compounds?
13. Discuss the stereochemistry of S_N2 reaction.
14. What predominant products (i.e., *o*-/*p*- or *m*-) are obtained on nitration of chlorobenzene and chlorination of nitrobenzene?
15. Give the energy diagrams of (i) S_N1 vs S_N2 for the hydrolysis of 1° halides and 3° halides, and (ii) electrophilic substitution in benzene with (a) activating and (b) deactivating groups.
16. Explain: (a) The nucleophilicity order of halides is $\overset{\ominus}{I} > \overset{\ominus}{Br} > \overset{\ominus}{Cl}$ in protic solvents but the order is reversed in aprotic solvents.
    (b) Pure racemic modification is not obtained in S_N1 reaction.
17. Write notes on (i) hybridization, (ii) inductive effect, (iii) electromeric effect and (iv) resonance.
18. Give the mechanism of nitration of phenol.
19. (a) Arrange the following compounds in order of increasing reactivity towards electrophilic substitution: benzene, nitrobenzene, chlorobenzene, toluene and phenol.
    (b) Acetanilide is less reactive towards electrophilic substitution than aniline, why?
20. Explain: (a) More than one equivalent of $AlCl_3$ is used in Friedel–Crafts acylation (b) Nitrobenzene is the favoured solvent in Friedel–Crafts reaction (c) Polyacylation is not observed in Friedel–Crafts acylation.
21. Give the mechanisms of addition–elimination and elimination–addition of nucleophilic aromatic substitution.
22. Place the groups —OH, —Cl, —NH_2, —NO_2, —CHO, —COOH and –OR in the following three catagories:
    (i) *o*-/*p*-directing with activation
    (ii) *o*-/*p*-directing with deactivation
    (iii) *m*-directing with deactivation
23. Write brief notes on Saytzev elimination and Hofmann elimination.

24. What products are obtained on treatment of neopentyl bromide with (i) alcohol, and with (ii) sodium ethoxide? Explain the reactions.
25. Elimination of HCl from the β-isomer of hexachlorocyclohexane is very much slower than from its other isomers, why?
26. (a) Discuss briefly the stereochemistry of carbocation rearrangements. (b) Give all the products obtained on deamination of (i) cyclobutylamine and (ii) cyclobutylmethylamine, with HNO_2.
27. Explain:
    (a) Aldehydes are more reactive than ketones.
    (b) The enolate form of EAA is less soluble in water but more soluble in cyclohexane.
    (c) *o*-Hydroxybenzoic acid is stronger acid than its other isomers.
    (d) Elimination of HCl from chlorofumaric acid is faster than from chloromaleic acid.
28. Write short notes on E1, E2 and E1cB mechanisms.
29. Explain:
    (a) The stereochemistry of nucleophilic addition to carbonyl group.
    (b) The reaction of *p*-chlorotoluene with strong NaOH at elevated temperature.

EXERCISES (CHAPTER 2)

1. Discuss the mechanism and applications of the following rearrangements:
   (a) Allylic, (b) Beckmann and (c) Hofmann.
2. Discuss the acid-catalysed rearrangement of 1, 2-diols to ketones. Describe its synthetic applications.
3. Define and discuss the mechanism of Cannizzaro reaction and give an account of its applications. Explain why *p*-dimethylaminobenzaldehyde does not undergo Cannizzaro reaction.
4. Describe the mechanism and some important applications of any three of the following rearrangements:
   (a) Hofmann (b) Wagner–Meerwein (c) Curtius (d) Claisen (e) Pinacol–Pinacolone
5. Explain allylic rearrangement. Discuss S_N1', S_N2' and S_Ni' reactions involved in allylic rearrangement.
6. Name any three reactions which involve rearrangement of electron-deficient carbon. Discuss the mechanism and applications of any two of them.
7. Define and discuss Aldol condensation. Give the mechanism of the reaction and its important applications.
8. (a) Discuss acyloin condensation between esters of monobasic acids and between esters of dibasic acids. Give the mechanism.
   (b) Mention the products obtained when diethyl sebacate is treated with (i) sodium and alcohol and (ii) sodium in the presence of tolune and then with acetic acid.
9. How will you establish the intermediate formation of a cyclopropanone ring in Favorskii rearrangement? How does such an intermediate, cyclopropanone ring open when the ring is unsymmetrically substituted?
10. Compare Friedel–Crafts alkylation and acylation. With the help of Friedel–Crafts reaction how will you synthesize naphthalene and phenanthrene?
11. (i) Give the mechanism of the reactions when benzene is treated with (a) *t*-butyl chloride in the presence of aluminium trichloride and (b) 2-methyl propylene in the presence of sulphuric acid.
    (ii) What products are formed when *t*-butyl benzene is treated with bromine in the presence of aluminium trichloride? Suggest the mechanism.
12. (a) 'In Friedel–Crafts acylation the product, ketone, complexes with aluminium trichloride'. This is a boon rather than a nuisance, why?

(b) More than one molar proportion of aluminium trichloride is required in Friedel–Crafts acylation, why?

(c) Give the synthetic applications of Friedel–Crafts acylation.

13. Discuss Mannich reaction indicating the components and the mechanism of the reaction. Mention some important synthetic applications.
14. Discuss the mechanism of Wolff rearrangement. How has the reaction been utilized in Arndt–Eistert homologation of acids.
15. Write explanatory notes on
(a) Clemmensen reduction, (b) Wolff–Kishner reduction and (c) Meerwein–Ponndorf reduction. Compare their merits.
16. How will you establish that in Beckmann rearrangement, the group *trans* (syn) to the hydroxyl group migrates? Mention the important applications of Beckmann rearrangement.
17. Describe Claisen condensation. Give the mechanism of the reaction. Esters having only one α-hydrogen undergo Claisen condensation only in the presence of a very strong base (e.g., sodium triphenylmethyl), why? What is the essential difference between Aldol and Claisen condensations?
18. Write the important resonance structures of diazomethane. Give the mechanism and applications of Arndt–Eistert synthesis and show how diazomethane is used in preparing the intermediates di-zoketone in this synthesis.
19. Define and discuss the mechanism of Cannizzaro reaction mentioning crossed and intramolecular Cannizzaro reaction. How has it been established that a direct transfer of hydride ion takes place from one aldehyde to the other? Give some of its applications.
20. Discuss the mechanism of Claisen condensation. How will you synthesize a β-ketoester without α-hydrogen? Give examples of crossed Claisen condensation between an ester having α-hydrogen and an ester having no α-hydrogen.
21. Discuss the mechanism of the following:
(a) Perkin reaction, (b) Benzoin condensation and (c) Mannich reaction.
22. Name the reaction and give the mechanism which involves the conversion of a ketone to an ester with peracids. How has it been proved that the oxygen of the ketone is present as the carbonyl oxygen of the ester? Why is trifluoroacetic acid more effective for the transformation than other peracids? Give some of the applications of this reaction.
23. Discuss the mechanism and applications of any two of the following reactions:
(a) Perkin (b) Michael (c) Wittig (d) Mannich (e) Reimer–Tiemann
24. How is Wittig's reagent prepared? How does it react with aldehydes and ketones? Give the mechanism and applications of the reaction.
25. Describe Favorskii rearrangement of open chain and cyclic α-haloketones.
Give all the steps for the transformation of 1, 3-dibromo-3-methyl-2-butanone to β-methyl crotonic acid under Favorskii conditions.
26. Define, giving the mechanisms of the reactions involved and some important uses of the following:
(a) Claisen condensation, (b) Claisen rearrangement and (c) Claisen–Schmidt reaction.
27. What products are obtained when hydrazoic acid in the presence of sulphuric acid is allowed to react with (i) carboxylic acids, (ii) aldehydes and (iii) ketones. Name the reaction and give the mechanism in each case.
28. Mention briefly the types of the two components which may be used in a 4 + 2 cycloaddition reaction to obtain varied types of six-membered rings. Give the mechanism involved and the scope of the reaction.
29. Discuss any two of the following reactions giving the mechanism and some of their important synthetic applications:
(a) Mannich reaction (b) Reformatsky reaction (c) Sommelet reaction.

30. Discuss Diels–Alder reaction. Give the mechanism of the reaction and its synthetic applications.
31. Describe any three of the following giving the mechanism and important applications:
(a) Fries rearrangement (b) Oppenauer oxidation (c) Ullmann reaction (d) Benzilic acid rearrangement.
32. Name three important rearrangements involving electron-deficient nitrogen. Discuss their mechanism and synthetic applications.

EXERCISES (CHAPTER 3)

1. Discuss the preparations and important uses of any three of the following reagents:
(a) Diazomethane (b) Peracetic acid (c) *N*-Bromosuccinimide (d) Lead tetraacetate (e) Lithium aluminium hydride
2. Discuss the important synthetic applications of the following organic reagents:
(a) Selenium dioxide (b) Raney nickel (c) Hydrogen peroxide (d) Osmium tetroxide
3. Give the preparations, important uses and the mechanism of the reactions brought about by any three of the following reagents:
(a) Periodic acid (b) Lead tetraacetate (c) Lithium aluminium hydride (d) Sodium borohydride
4. How is diazomethane prepared and stored? Write the important resonance structures of diazomethane. Give the mechanism of methylation of phenols, alcohols, amines and acids with diazomethane.
5. Discuss the important uses of the following:
(a) NBS (b) Fenton's reagent (c) Dicyclohexylcarbodiimide (d) Anhydrous aluminium trichloride (e) Sodamide
6. Give the preparation of periodic acid. Illustrate with examples its use in oxidative cleavage of adjacent oxidizable groups and the mechanism involved. How has it been used in the determination of the size of oxide ring of glucose?
7. Write short notes on:
(a) Aluminium isopropoxide (b) Sodium borohydride (c) Osmium tetroxide (d) Raney nickel (e) Anhydrous aluminium trichloride
8. Describe the preparations and important applications of the following organic reagents:
(a) Sodamide (b) Raney nickel (c) Lead tetracetate (d) Dicyclohexylcarbodiimide
9. Discuss the uses of any four of the following:
(a) Hydrogen peroxide (b) Sodamide (c) Sodium borohydride (d) Fenton's reagent (e) Periodic acid (f) Selenium dioxide
10. Illustrate with examples the specific uses of the following:
(a) Selenium dioxide in the oxidation of the active methylene groups, allylic hydroxylation and dehydrogenation
(b) Raney nickel for the synthesis of higher fatty acids through desulphurization
(c) Periodic acid in the determination of the size of the oxide ring of carbohydrates and in the structure determination of chloromycetin
(d) Diazomethane in methylation of carbonyl compounds, synthesis of pyrazoline and in the estimation of amino acids
(e) Lead tetraacetate as acetoxylating, methylating and oxidizing reagent
11. (a) Discuss the use of periodic acid in the (i) determination of the size of the oxide ring of sugars (ii) oxidation of exocyclic double bond and (iii) estimation of amino acids.
(b) How will you detect potassium in the presence of sodium by the use of boron trifluoride?

12. How will you bring about the following transformations by the use of suitable organic reagents?
    (a) Cyclohexene to benzene
    (b) Ketones to higher ketones and epoxides
    (c) Benzene to tropilidene
    (d) Maleic acid to *meso*-tartaric acid
    (e) *o*-Diamine to dinitrile
    (f) Cyclohexene to hexan-1, 6-diol
13. Write short notes on:
    (i) Ziegler–Natta catalysts (ii) Wilkinson's catalyst
14. What is meant by the term `tacticity'? Describe briefly the preparation, mechanism of reaction and some important uses of Ziegler–Natta catalysts.
15. Describe the preparation of Wilkinson's catalyst and the mechanism of hydrogenation of alkenes by this catalyst. Give some of its important uses.

Simple Problems and Their Solutions

[Students are advised not to look up the solutions before trying. In case of difficulty they should look up the appropriate section in the text, think and then try to solve the problem. Only after this they should look up the solution.]

1. How will you distinguish between
   (a) methyl alcohol and ethyl alcohol
   (b) 1-propanol and 2-propanol
   (c) diethyl ether and *n*-butyl alcohol
   (d) ethane, ethylene and acetylene
   (e) 1-butyne and 2-butyne
2. Ethyl alcohol has a higher boiling point than diethyl ether. Why?
3. Compare the basicity of aliphatic and aromatic 1° amines.
4. An alkane of mol. wt. 84 gives one monochloro derivative. What is the structure of the alkane?
5. Amongst a group of isomeric amines, tertiary amine has the lowest boiling point. Why?
6. How will you obtain 1, 4-pentadiene and trimethyl amine from pyridine?
7. Mention the products formed on treating cyclobutylamine with nitrous acid.
8. The hydrogen atom of the carboxyl group is more easily replaced than the hydrogen of the alcoholic group.
9. 1, 2-dimethyl propanol(I) on dehydration with sulphuric acid gives 2-methyl butene-2(II) as the major product. Why?
10. How is methylene cyclohexane obtained from cyclohexanone?
11. The base strengths of 3° amines are less than that of 2° amines. Explain.
12. Amides are practically neutral. Why?
13. *o*-hydroxy benzoic acid is a stronger acid than its isomers. Why?
14. Which of the two carbocations is more stable. State reason.

$$CH_3-\overset{\oplus}{C}H-CH_3 \qquad CH_2=CH-\overset{\oplus}{C}H_2$$

(1) (2)

15. Explain with an example what is meant by β-elimination.
16. Give the mechanisms of acid-catalysed and base-catalysed dehydration of an alcohol.
17. Phenol is acidic but ethyl alcohol is neutral. Explain.
18. Arrange the following in order of increasing rates of addition:

$$\underset{1}{CH_2=CH_2},\ \underset{2}{MeCH=CHMe},\ \underset{3}{Me_2C=CMe_2},\ \underset{4}{CH_2=CH-COOH},\ \underset{5}{EtCH=CH_2}$$

19. Mention the products and the rule governing the formation of the products.

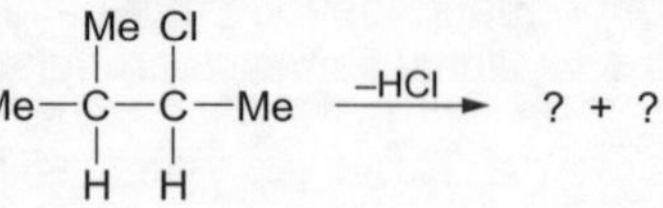

20. *N*, *N*-dimethylaniline undergoes ready coupling but its 2, 6-dimethyl derivative does not. Why?

21. Complete the following reactions:

(i) $R_2C(OH)—CHOH—R' + HIO_4 \xrightarrow{-HIO_3} ? + ?$

(ii) $R—CO—CO—R' + HIO_4 \xrightarrow{-HIO_3} ? + ?$

(iii) $R—CHOH—CH_2—CHOH—R \xrightarrow{HIO_4} ?$

22. How is exocyclic olefinic bond oxidized?

23. How will you bring about the following conversions?
   (i) Cyclohexene to cyclohexene-I-one
   (ii) Acetic acid to succinic acid
   (iii) Maleic acid to DL-Tartaric acid
   (iv) Pyridine to 2-Amino Pyridine
   (v) 3, 4-Dimethyl- 1, 5-hexadiene to 2, 6-Octadiene

24. Acetyl chloride has lower boiling point than acetic acid.

Solutions

1. (a) Ethyl alcohol gives a yellow crystalline precipitate of iodoform with alkaline iodine solution while methyl alcohol does not.

   (b) 1-propanol is a 1° alcohol and reacts with Lucas reagent ($ZnCl_2$ / HCl) to form an alkyl halide only on heating. 2-propanol is a 2° alcohol and reacts with Lucas reagent after some time (5 minutes) to form an alkyl halide which being immiscible in 2-propanol forms a cloudy liquid. 3° alcohol reacts immediately to give an alkyl halide at room temperature.

   (c) *n*-butyl alcohol reacts with sodium to give bubbles of hydrogen gas due to its OH group. Diethyl ether does not react with sodium as it has no OH group.

   (d) Ethylene and acetylene being unsaturated, add bromine but ethane is a saturated hydrocarbon and so does not add bromine. Acetylene gives silver acetylides with $AgNO_3$ / NH_3 solution but ethylene does not.

   (e) A 1-butyne ($C_2H_5C \equiv CH$) like acetylene gives a red precipitate with ammoniacal cuprous chloride solution and a white precipitate with ammoniacal silver chloride solution. 2-butyne ($CH_3C \equiv CCH_3$) having no acidic hydrogen does not react with these reagents.

2. In an alcohol a hydrogen atom is covalently linked to a strong electronegative O-atom. The σ-bond is thus distorted towards the O-atom resulting in a polar bond. This polarity in the $\overset{\delta-}{O}—\overset{\delta+}{H}$ bond causes association of alcohol molecules. The unusual high boiling point of an alcohol is due to the energy required to break the H-bond and vaporize the alcohol molecules. Diethyl ether has no polar bond for association and hence has a relatively low boiling point.

3. The lone pair of N-atom of aromatic amines is involved in resonance with the ring and hence is not easily available for protonation. On the other hand the lone pair of the nitrogen atom of aliphatic amines are freely available for protonation. Hence aliphatic amines are relatively more basic than aromatic amines.

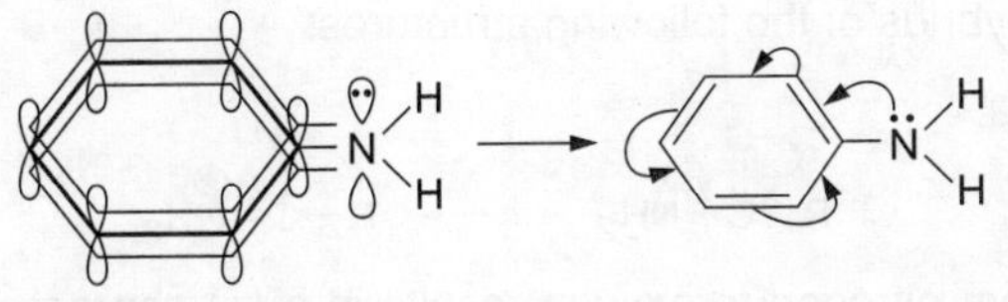

Aromatic amine

4. The general formula of an open-chain alkane is C_nH_{2n+2} and that of a closed-chain alkane is C_nH_{2n}.

When the alkane is an open chain

$C_nH_{2n+2} = 84$

or $12n + 2n + 2 = 84$

or $14n = 82.$

$\therefore$ $n = \frac{82}{14}$ (not a whole number).

Hence, the compound is not an open-chain alkane.

When the alkane is a closed chain

$C_nH_{2n} = 84$

or $12n + 2n = 84$

or $14n = 84.$

or $n = 6.$

Hence the compound is a closed chain of 6 carbons.

Therefore, the compound is cyclohexane which can give only one monochloro derivative as all the twelve hydrogen atoms are equivalent.

5. Primary and secondary amines having polar bonds $\left(\overset{\delta-}{N} - \overset{\delta+}{H}\right)$ form intermolecular hydrogen bonding, while tertiary amines having no hydrogen atom on the N-atom cannot form an H-bond. Thus 1° and 2° amines are associated and need higher energy to break the H-bond and vaporize the liquid. Hence 1° and 2° amines have higher b.p.'s with respect to 3° amines in a group of isomeric amines.

6. See page 65; Hofmann elimination

7. See page 70.

8. The hydrogen atom of the carboxyl group is easily replaced since the carboxylate ion is resonance stabilized on the departure of hydrogen.

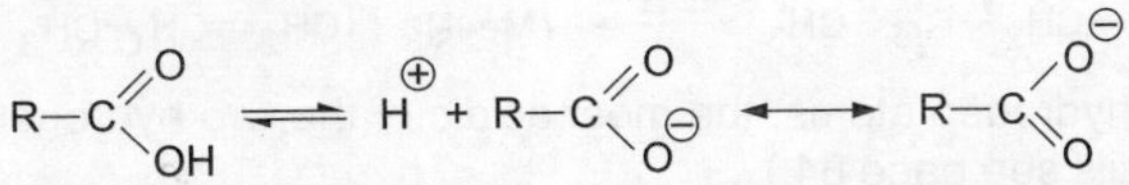

Hydrogen atom of the alcoholic group is however not easily replaced since the charge on the alkoxide ion is localized and has no factor for stability.

9. See page 18.

10. See page 185; Wittig reaction

11. The base strength of amines in water is due not only to the electron availability on the nitrogen atom, but also to the extent of solvation by hydrogen bonding of the cation formed by the uptake of a proton. The solvation then depends upon the number of hydrogen atoms attached to the nitrogen atom. It is seen that the cations of 2° and 3° amines have each two and one hydrogen atom respectively. Therefore, the basicity order is 2° amine > 3° amine.

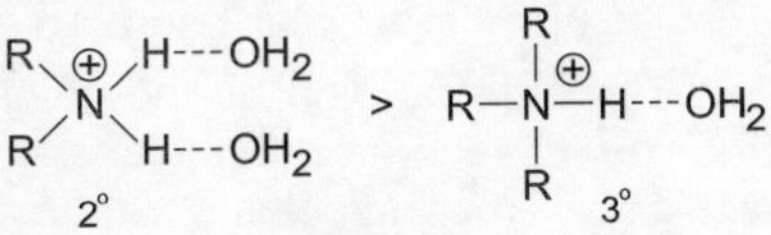

Protonated amines

This is, however, true only in protic solvents. In aprotic solvents (e.g., chlorobenzene) the basicity order is 1° < 2° < 3° amines.

12. The basicity of nitrogeneous compounds depends on the availability of the lone pair of the N-atom. Amides are resonance hybrids of the following structures:

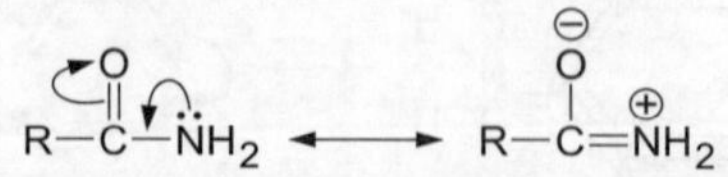

The shift of electrons from nitrogen to oxygen results in a (+) charge on the N-atom. The lone pair of electrons of the N-atom is therefore less available for protonation, i.e.,amides are practically neutral.

13. The ionization of *o*-hydroxy benzoic acid is promoted due to stabilization of its anion by intramolecular hydrogen bonding.

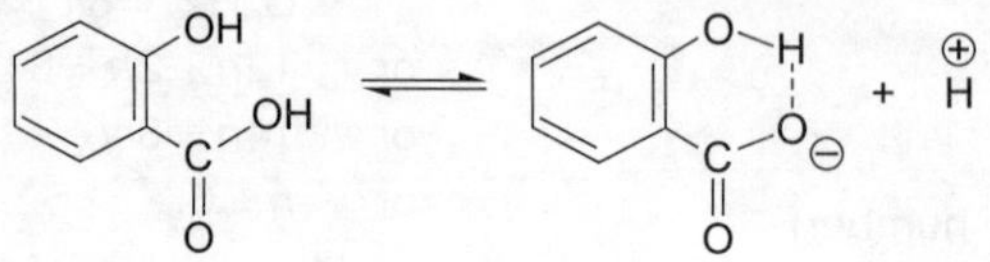

The intramolecular H-bonding is not possible in its other isomers in which the OH and COOH groups are far apart for H-bonding.

Hence it is the *strongest acid* of the three isomers.

14. The stabilities of ions depend upon charge delocalization through inductive effect, no bond resonance (hyperconjugation) and resonance. In (1) two +I effects are operating for stabilization as also six feeble hyperconjugative effects. On the other hand cation (2) is stabilized by strong resonance energy of two equal energy structures.

$$CH_2{=}CH{-}\overset{\oplus}{C}H_2 \longleftrightarrow \overset{\oplus}{C}H_2{-}CH{=}CH_2$$

Hence, carbocation (2) is more stable than the carbocation (1).

15. Hofmann elimination is known as β-elimination. The reaction involves abstraction of a proton from the β-carbon with the simultaneous expulsion of the leaving group.

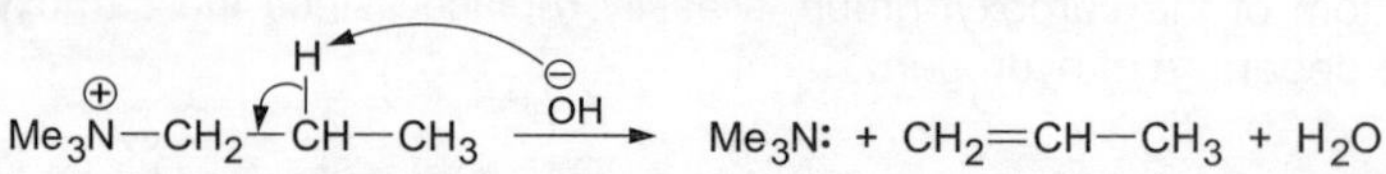

In case of alternate β-hydrogen atoms, the most acidic of the two hydrogen atoms is abstracted by the base. (For further details see page 64.)

16. See page 82.
17. See page 17 also.

Both phenol and phenoxide ions are resonance hybrids. Charge separation in the resonance structures of phenol makes it less stable than the phenoxide ion where charge delocalization is observed. Hence phenol prefers ionization, i.e., it is acidic.

The ionization of alcohol gives alkoxide ion which has no stability because the charge cannot delocalize.

$$R{-}OH \rightleftharpoons R\overset{\ominus}{O} + \overset{\oplus}{H}$$

Hence, alcohol is neutral.

18. See page 35.
19. See page 60.
20. See page 20.
21. See page 234.

22. Periodic acid has no reaction on olefins. Hence olefins are first hydroxylated to 1, 2-glycols and then oxidized with periodic acid to carbonyl compound.

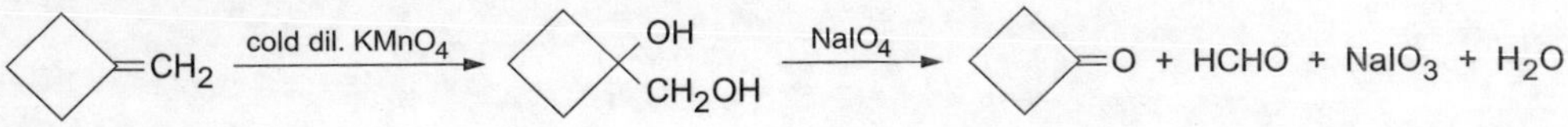

23. See page 241, 242, 242, 254 and 258.
24. Since acetyl chloride has no hydroxyl group, intermolecular hydrogen bonding is absent and hence the association of molecules is also absent. Therefore they are low boiling. On the other hand intermolecular hydrogen bonding in acid molecules through the hydroxyl hydrogen and carbonyl oxygen makes the acids higher boiling.